KU-763-420

OXFORD MEDICAL PUBLICATIONS

Oxford Specialist Handbooks in Psychiatry

Forensic Psychiatry

Oxford Specialist Handbooks published and forthcoming

Oxford Specialist Handbooks in Psychiatry
Forensic Psychiatry

Nigel Eastman

Professor of Law and Ethics in Psychiatry
Honorary Consultant Forensic Psychiatrist,
St George's, University of London, UK

Gwen Adshead

Consultant Forensic Psychotherapist
Broadmoor Hospital, UK

Simone Fox

Consultant Clinical and Forensic Psychologist
South-West London & St George's Mental Health NHS Trust
Lecturer, Royal Holloway, University of London, UK

Richard Latham

Consultant Forensic Psychiatrist
East London NHS Foundation Trust, UK

Seán Whyte

Consultant Forensic Psychiatrist, Community Forensic Team
South-West London & St George's Mental
Health NHS Trust, London, UK

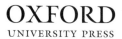

OXFORD
UNIVERSITY PRESS

OXFORD
UNIVERSITY PRESS

Great Clarendon Street, Oxford OX2 6DP

Oxford University Press is a department of the University of Oxford.
It furthers the University's objective of excellence in research, scholarship,
and education by publishing worldwide in

Oxford New York

Auckland Cape Town Dar es Salaam Hong Kong Karachi
Kuala Lumpur Madrid Melbourne Mexico City Nairobi
New Delhi Shanghai Taipei Toronto

With offices in

Argentina Austria Brazil Chile Czech Republic France Greece
Guatemala Hungary Italy Japan Poland Portugal Singapore
South Korea Switzerland Thailand Turkey Ukraine Vietnam

Oxford is a registered trade mark of Oxford University Press
in the UK and in certain other countries

Published in the United States
by Oxford University Press Inc., New York

© Oxford University Press, 2012

British Library Cataloguing in Publication Data
Data available

Library of Congress Cataloguing in Publication Data
Data available

Typeset by Cenveo, Bangalore, India
Printed in China
on acid-free paper through
Asia Pacific Offset

ISBN 978–0–19–956282–4

10 9 8 7 6 5 4 3 2 1

Dedication

In memory of Dr James MacKeith, a compassionate forensic psychiatrist who dedicated his wisdom and integrity to both caring for his patients and informing legal process.

Preface

When the first author of this handbook entered forensic psychiatry there were two views of the specialty, identified with either side of the Atlantic. To the British forensic psychiatrist, his or her role was to practise clinical psychiatry with mentally disordered offenders and, where necessary, to know a little of the law and of legal process. Clinical involvement with law was pursued simply as necessary in order to treat patients, and with a predominantly paternalistic ethical stance. Law was seen merely as a necessary means to aid clinical practice in pursuit of patient welfare, and sometimes as representing an irritating intrusion into the proper exercise of medical paternalism. The anger amongst many psychiatrists that greeted Larry Gostin's two-volume legal critique of psychiatry and defence of patient's rights, *A Human Condition*, in 1975 offered further evidence of an emerging tension between psychiatry and law. This was then stoked by passage of the Mental Health Act 1983 in England & Wales, which increased the legal regulation of psychiatry, enhanced the powers of Mental Health Review Tribunals and increased checks on clinical decision making via psychiatrists appointed by the Mental Health Act Commission.

The same UK forensic psychiatrists looked critically across the Atlantic at their American counterparts, who embraced a relationship with the legal system through an industry of expert witness work, and who, aside from a few, showed relatively little interest in treating patients. They were viewed as too-close bedfellows of the justice system, and as having abandoned proper clinical practice.

The past three decades have witnessed progressive change in forensic psychiatry in the UK and Ireland. The pioneering generation of forensic psychiatrists has passed, and the attitude of later generations towards the law and legal process is significantly more accommodating. Gradually the relationship has become one of mutual respect and interest. Academically, 'psycho-legal studies' is emerging as an interface discipline in its own right, offering a forum within which to explore and inform the relationship between the theory and practice of psychiatry and of law. It is also now the case, for example, that a significant proportion of trainee forensic psychiatrists not only train in their clinical speciality but also undertake some form of legal training, most commonly an LLM in Mental Health Law. This is a sign of recognition within the specialty, as it has expanded and matured, that clinical forensic psychiatry cannot be practised effectively or ethically without a real understanding of how the two disciplines relate, one to the other.

We suggest in the 'Welcome' page to this handbook that 'forensic psychiatry comprises the psychiatry of mental disorder and offending behaviour, plus law in relation to all psychiatry'. The former is represented in detail in the handbook. However, so is the latter, since it is not possible either effectively or ethically to guide an offender patient through the justice system so as to ensure they receive the treatment they need (for their own benefit and that of society), or properly to assist the justice system in dealing with mentally disordered offenders, without a real understanding of legal process and of the interface between law and psychiatry.

The necessity of understanding 'law and psychiatry' is not limited to those that practise the designated speciality of forensic psychiatry. It applies to all psychiatrists who are regulated by, operate within, or make use of the law. General psychiatrists using mental health legislation, for example, need an understanding of law in order not only to treat their patients but also to pay proper regard to their civil rights. Similarly, it is not possible for lawyers effectively to represent or prosecute someone with a mental disorder without some understanding of that disorder.

This handbook is similar to others in the OUP series in its attempt to offer a 'user friendly quick reference' approach. However, it differs from others in addressing not one discipline but two, and the relationship between them. As such, it is intended not only for trainees in forensic psychiatry but also for experienced other psychiatrists, all of whom effectively practise 'forensic psychiatry' as we have identified it to be. It is also for all lawyers who need to understand psychiatric concepts and thinking and how they relate to law and legal process.

For a psychiatrist to relate closely to the legal system and to understand it is not to be used by it. Rather, knowledge and understanding is likely to encourage a boundaried relationship suffused with mutual respect, and the enjoyment of difference. Doctors and lawyers do not need to become fully acquainted with each other's professions and epistemologies. However, each does need to have enough understanding of the other to operate effectively at the interface of their disciplines. We hope that this handbook will make a contribution to enhanced understanding and enjoyment on both sides.

NE
GA
SF
RL
SW
2011

Acknowledgements

In writing and compiling this handbook, we have benefited from the hard work and good advice of a considerable number of our colleagues and friends, and from the support of our families and employers. We would like to thank in particular the following psychiatrists, psychologists, lawyers, judges, academics and other colleagues, for giving their time so freely to comment on drafts of parts of the handbook and to suggest corrections and improvements:

Dr Karen Brown
Dr Bee Brockman
Dr Colin Campbell
Dr Simon Christopherson
Ms Emma Chrobok
Mr James Cronin
Dr Claire Dimond
Dr Bridget Dolan
Dr Ceri Evans
Mr Chris Giles
Dr Paul Gilluley
Prof Donald Grubin
Mr Robert Halsey
Mr Christopher Hart
Mr Anthony Haycroft
Mr John Horne
Ms Julia Houston
Dr Tina Irani
Mr Ashley Irons
Dr John Kent
Dr Fiona Mason
Prof Andy Macleod
Prof James Maguire
Prof David Ormerod
Dr Catherine Penny
Ms Natasha Pettit
Ms Helen Pote
Dr Keith Rix
Mr Stephen Rose
Ms Sarah Mackenzie Ross
Mrs Lisa Whyte
Dr Zoe Wiseman

We would also like to thank the junior doctors and students who tried out portions of the handbook for us; and Susan Crowhurst, Helen Liepman and especially Charles Haynes at OUP for their advice, support, and patience.

Contents

Symbols and abbreviations

📖	cross-reference
☙	controversial topic
⚠	warning
▶	important
5HT	5-hydroxy tryptamine, also known as serotonin
AA	Alcoholics Anonymous
ABC	Acceptable Behaviour Contract
ABH	actual bodily harm
AC	approved clinician (E&W)
ACCT	assessment, care in custody and teamwork
ACT	assertive community treatment
AD	absolute discharge
ADHD	attention-deficit hyperactivity disorder
AMHP	approved mental health practitioner (E&W)
AMP	approved medical practitioner (Scotland)
AOT	assertive outreach team
APA	American Psychiatric Association
ASBO	antisocial behaviour order
ASD	autistic spectrum disorders
ASPD	antisocial personality disorder
ASSET	assessment tool, used by YOTs
ASW	approved social worker (NI)
AWIA	adults with incapacity (Scotland) Act 2000
BCE	before the common era (equivalent to BC, before Christ)
BME	black and minority ethnic
BPD	borderline personality disorder
BP	blood pressure
CAF	common assessment framework
CAMHS	child & adolescent mental health services
CBT	cognitive-behavioural therapy
CCRC	Criminal Cases Review Commission (UK)
CD	clinical director, conditional discharge, or conduct disorder
CE	of the common era (equivalent to AD, Anno Domini)
CFT	community forensic team
CIN	child in need

CJD	Creutzfeldt–Jakob disease
CJS	criminal justice system
CLIA	Criminal Law (Insanity) Act 2006 (RoI)
CMHT	Community Mental Health Team
CoP	Court of Protection (E&W)
CPA	care programme approach (E&W) or continuing power of attorney (Scotland)
CPN	community psychiatric nurse
CPS	Crown Prosecution Service (E&W)
CPSA	Criminal Procedure (Scotland) Act 1995
CQC	Care Quality Commission (England)
CT	computed tomography
CTO	Community Treatment Order (E&W), or Compulsory Treatment Order (Scotland)
DA	dopamine, or dopaminergic
DBT	dialectical behaviour therapy
DoH	Department of Health (E&W)
DMP	designated medical practitioner (Scotland)
DoLS	deprivation of liberty safeguards (E&W)
DSM-IV	APA *Diagnostic and Statistical Manual*, 4th edition
DSPD	dangerous & severely personality disordered
DTO	detention and training order (E&W)
DVLA	Driver and Vehicle Licensing Agency (UK)
ECHR	European Convention on Human Rights
ECG	electrocardiogram
ECT	electroconvulsive therapy
ECtHR	European Court of Human Rights
EDR	expected date of release
EEG	electroencephalogram
EIT	early intervention (in psychosis) team
EMIS	Egton Medical Information Systems (computerized medical records)
EPA	enduring power of attorney (RoI)
EPP	extended sentence of imprisonment for public protection
EPSE	extra-pyramidal side effects
ERASOR	estimate of risk of adolescent sexual offence recidivism
ETS	enhanced thinking skills
E&W	England & Wales
EU	European Union
EWO	Education Welfare Officer
FBI	Federal Bureau of Investigation (US)

FME	forensic medical examiner (previously known as police surgeon)
fMRI	functional magnetic resonance imaging
FTTMH	first tier tribunal (Mental Health) (E&W)
GAD	generalized anxiety disorder
GBH	grievous bodily harm
GMC	General Medical Council (UK)
GP	general practitioner
HCR20	Historical, Clinical & Risk management 20-item scale
HMP	Her Majesty's Prison
HSE	Health Service Executive (RoI)
ICD10	WHO *International Classification of Diseases*, 10th edition
ICJ	International Court of justice, The Hague
IM	intramuscular
IMCA	Independent Mental Capacity Advocate (E&W)
IMHA	Independent Mental Health Advocate (E&W)
IMR	inmate medical record (in prison)
IPP	indeterminate sentence of imprisonment for public protection
IPT	interpersonal therapy
IQ	intelligence quotient
ISSP	intensive supervision and surveillance programme
IV	intravenous
LA	local authority
LALY	liberty-adjusted life year
LASCH	LA secure children's home
LD	learning disability
LED	licence expiry date
LPA	lasting power of attorney (E&W)
LRA	Lunacy Regulation (Ireland) Act 1871
LREC	Local Research Ethics Committee (UK)
LSU	low secure unit
MACI	millon adolescent clinical inventory
MAO	monoamine oxidase (MAOA, type A; MAOB, type B)
MAPPA	Multi-Agency Public Protection Arrangements (E&W, Scotland)
MAPPP	Multi-Agency Public Protection Panel
MBT	mentalization-based therapy
MC	Medical Council (RoI)
MCA	Mental Capacity Act 2005 (E&W)
MDO	mentally-disordered offender

MDT	multidisciplinary team
MHA	Mental Health Act (E&W 1983; RoI 2001)
MHC	Mental Health Commission (NI, RoI)
MHCTA	Mental Heath (Care and Treatment) (Scotland) Act 2003
MHNIO	Mental Health (Northern Ireland) Order 1986
MHO	Mental Health Officer (Scotland; a social worker)
MHRT	Mental Health Review Tribunal (NI, RoI)
MHT	Mental Health Tribunal (Scotland; also see 📖 footnote p.IV.309)
MHU	Mental Health Unit (of the Ministry of Justice, E&W)
MI	motivational interviewing, or mental illness
MoJ	Ministry of Justice
MREC	Multi-centre Research Ethics Committee (UK)
MRI	(structural) magnetic resonance imaging
MST	multi-systemic therapy
MSU	medium secure unit
MWC	Mental Welfare Commission (Scotland)
NA	Narcotics Anonymous, or noradrenaline
NAPO	National Association of Probation Officers (E&W)
NFA	no fixed abode, or no further action
NHS	National Health Service (UK)
NI	Northern Ireland
NICE	National Institute of Health and Clinical Excellence (UK)
NIMHE	National Institute for Mental Health in England
NOMS	National Offender Management Service (E&W)
NPD	non-parole date
NPS	National Probation Service (E&W)
NPSA	National Patient Safety Agency (UK)
NSF	National Service Framework (E&W)
OASys	offender assessment system
OCD	obsessive–compulsive disorder
ODD	oppositional-defiant disorder
ONS	Office for National Statistics (UK)
ONSET	an assessment tool used by YOTs
PACE	Police and Criminal Evidence Act 1984 (E&W)
PCL-R	Psychopathy Checklist (Revised)
PCL-YV	Psychopathy Checklist (Youth Version)
PD	personality disorder
PDD	pervasive developmental disorders
PED	parole eligibility date
PET	positron emission tomography

PICU	psychiatric intensive care unit
PPANI	Public Protection Arrangements for Northern Ireland (cf MAPPA)
PPG	penile plethysmograph
PRN	pro re nata ('as required')
PSR	pre-sentence report
PTSD	post-traumatic stress disorder
QALY	quality-adjusted life year
QTc	Q-T interval (corrected for heart rate)
RC	responsible clinician (E&W)
RCPsych	Royal College of Psychiatrists (UK)
REC	Research Ethics Committee
RiO	Records in Operation (a computerized medical records system)
RoI	Republic of Ireland
RMO	responsible medical officer (Scotland, NI)
R&R	reasoning & rehabilitation programme
RSA	Road Safety Authority (RoI)
RSU	regional secure unit (may comprise both MSU and LSU)
RSVP	risk of sexual violence protocol
SAVRY	structured assessment of violence risk in youth
SCT	supervised community treatment
SED	sentence expiry date
SM	substance misuse
SMI	severe (and enduring) mental illness
SOAD	second opinion appointed doctor
SOAP	sex offender assessment pack
SOTP	sex offender treatment programme
SPECT	single photon emission computed tomography
STC	secure training centre
TBI	traumatic brain injury
TBS	Terbeschikkingstelling (Dutch system similar to DSPD)
TC	therapeutic community
TD	tardive dyskinesia (persistent oro-facial dyskinesia)
TWOC	taking (a vehicle) without consent
UK	United Kingdom
UN	United Nations
US	United States (of America)
VBP	values-based practice
WEMSS	women's enhanced medium secure service (E&W)
WHO	World Health Organization

WMA	World Medical Association
WPA	Welfare Power of Attorney (Scotland), or World Psychiatric Association
YISP	Youth Inclusion and Support Panel
YJA	Youth Justice Agency (NI)
YJB	Youth Justice Board (E&W)
YJS	Youth Justice System (cf. CJS)
YOI	young offenders institute
YOT	youth offending team
YRO	youth rehabilitation order

Part I

Introduction to the handbook

Introduction

Welcome

We hope you enjoy using this, the first *Oxford Handbook of Forensic Psychiatry*; we have enjoyed writing it. Whether you might be an established psychiatrist brushing up on the *Pritchard* criteria (📖 p.V.474) before entering the witness box, a trainee psychiatrist drafting your first risk assessment (📖 p.II.128), a professional from another discipline or specialty compiling an unanticipated court report (📖 pp.V.556–V.584), or a lawyer looking for guidance on psychiatric expert witnesses (📖 pp.V.532–V.539), we hope you will find it a useful and reassuring pocket or briefcase guide.

Forensic psychiatry comprises the psychiatry of mental disorder and offending behaviour, plus law in relation to all psychiatry. The handbook therefore refers to, but does not cover in detail, large areas of other subjects, such as general psychiatry, forensic and clinical psychology, criminal law, criminology, and other aspects of forensic mental healthcare.

Also, no page covers a topic comprehensively, as this would lead to vast duplication of material with the same points being raised on many different pages to which they are relevant. Instead, we have made extensive use of cross-references from one page to another.

We have used the following conventions throughout the handbook:

- Abbreviations are used in the handbook wherever you would encounter them in clinical or legal practice. You can find a list of abbreviations on 📖 p.xi
- We indicate cross-referenced topics by the Oxford handbook symbol, 📖, and Part and page number immediately following the topic—e.g. functional psychosis (📖 p.II.54)
- Diagnostic terms are those of the DSM-IV (📖 p.App. 1.601) except where otherwise specified.

We have relied heavily on the work of a large number of other authors in the compilation of this handbook; we thank them all, and we acknowledge their copyright in their work. That said, any errors or omissions are our responsibility alone. We welcome corrections and clarifications: please contact us care of Oxford University Press at 🖱 http://www.oup.com/uk/medicine/handbook if you can help us to improve the handbook.

A note on jurisdictions

We have had to take account of the fact that laws and aspects of legal systems relevant to the forensic psychiatrist differ from one country to another. We cannot, in a book of this size, cover multiple jurisdictions equally thoroughly. Our main focus is on the three UK jurisdictions (England & Wales, Scotland, and Northern Ireland), plus the Republic of Ireland. Where we are aware of differences of approach elsewhere in the world that illustrate important points of principle, particularly in the United States (US), the European Union (EU), and in Commonwealth countries that tend otherwise to follow the same principles as English law, we have attempted to explain this, so far as space allows.

Using this handbook

Our philosophy

This book is for everyone who is interested in, or encounters practitioners of, forensic psychiatry and related disciplines. It focuses on the relationship between psychiatry and law, and is intended to be of value to clinicians and lawyers working at the interface between the two disciplines.

We aim to enable readers to find out some of the key facts and issues within a given topic simply, rapidly, and in an easily digestible form. The handbook therefore promotes brevity and ease of reference, at the expense of detail.

To keep the text of the handbook brief and punchy (insofar as that is possible with ethical and legal topics), we have frequently had to omit detailed discussion of issues, and we have had to simplify many others. Here are some examples that illustrate the different ways in which we have omitted and abbreviated:

- The prevalence figures for the mental disorders listed on
  📖 pp.II.54–II.88 are derived from a variety of studies that use different definitions of the disorders in question, occasionally use different prevalence periods (although it is usually 1 year), and cover different populations.
- The definition of murder on 📖 p.IV.345 omits mention of the fact that killing a person with the intention of causing a different person serious harm can also be murder, as well as other technical details of the offence.
- The discussions of the construction and measurement of 'crime' on
  📖 p.II.19, the social context of sexual offending on 📖 p.II.25, and the association of violence and mental disorder on 📖 p.II.31, all do no more than skim the surface of major and wide-ranging controversies in criminology, sociology, philosophy, social psychology, and psychiatry.

Readers seeking detailed coverage of the topics in this handbook should therefore consult a textbook of law, psychiatry, psychology, criminology or ethics, as appropriate. In particular, as regards psychiatry the focus of discussion of individual clinical conditions here is very much forensic, and therefore not comprehensive. Hence, for general information on the diagnosis, aetiology, treatment, or prognosis of conditions, we would direct you to the *Oxford Handbook of Psychiatry*, or a general psychiatric textbook. Likewise, if you are in search of definitive and comprehensive legal information, consult a relevant legal text, or lawyer.

The organization of the handbook

The handbook is divided into four main Parts (II–V), which are intended to be complementary in presenting both clinical forensic psychiatry and legal psychiatry (📖 p.I.7). We have therefore used detailed cross-referencing of topics between the different aspects of forensic psychiatry in the book.

Thus, for example, a clinician dealing with a man exhibiting personality disorder (PD) might:

- begin by looking at various pages within Part II, which deal with the clinical assessment and treatment of PD and its behavioural manifestations from a specific forensic perspective; then

- be cross-referred to pages in Part IV for information about a criminal charge and process faced by his patient; then
- refer to Part V for information about legal representations of PD in law, for example, in terms of criminal responsibility, including in the context of intoxication; then
- within the same Part, he might cross-refer for advice concerning provision of an expert report to the Crown Court in relation to trial; and
- he might then, at a later stage, wish to seek guidance on how he might ethically decide whether to recommend treatment in hospital under mental health law, in the knowledge that his risk assessment (or other data he presents) could be used by the court instead as a basis for the imposition of indeterminate penal sentencing on the grounds of risk to the public, addressed in Part III.

We also offer occasional vignettes to test out your thinking within topics. However, we suggest you also utilize your own case examples similarly.

A lawyer dealing with the same man, to her not a patient but a defendant (ethically very distinct), might:

- look for guidance in understanding the clinical concepts in the psychiatrist's court report, or the risk assessment offered to the court, within Part II; and then
- be referred to pages in Part V, concerning 'the forensic psychiatrist in the legal system', in order to know what are proper methods and standards in psychiatric report writing and therefore how best to support (if she is for the same side) or attack (if she is for the other side) the evidence that will be given orally at trial; she may then
- at the sentencing stage, when puzzled by ethical conundra apparently facing the psychiatrist in relation to providing a risk assessment for 'risk-based' penal sentencing, turn to a relevant page in Part III.

Our approach to the law

Although we have written extensively about many areas of law in the handbook, we have self-consciously not tried to write a legal textbook. The aim of the handbook is to summarize and describe areas of law of relevance to the interface between law and psychiatry (📖 p.IV.293). This necessarily implies that we will not always write in the technically precise manner of legal texts, but by sometimes adopting a different approach we hope that the handbook will be of use both to medical and to legal experts, from their different sides of the divide.

One of the difficulties of writing a handbook of law and psychiatry is that fact and opinion in both fields is changing rapidly, particularly in Britain and Ireland in the early years of the 21st century. We have tried to ensure that we have reflected accurately the position in the four jurisdictions of the UK and Ireland as of early 2011, and have also referred to impending changes where appropriate, such as the NI Mental Capacity (Health, Welfare and Finance) Bill (📖 p.App. 2.624).

Clinical forensic psychiatry and legal psychiatry

Forensic psychiatry comprises clinical forensic psychiatry and legal psychiatry.

Clinical forensic psychiatry is concerned with the assessment and treatment of mental disorder where that disorder appears to be associated (not necessarily causally) with offending behaviour, whether or not the patient has been convicted. Although clinical forensic psychiatry deals with mentally disordered offenders (MDOs),[*] to limit the subject to that would be analogous to a subspecialty of 'self-harm psychiatry', with forensic psychiatry being 'harm to others psychiatry'. Hence, clinical forensic psychiatry is also particularly closely engaged with law, and 'legal psychiatry', so that a clear understanding of law is necessary in order to practise clinically. For example, it is not possible to negotiate your patient out of the criminal justice system and into mental healthcare without knowledge of the relevant law (📖 pp.IV.403–IV.417). Clinical forensic psychiatry can be pursued effectively and ethically only if it is based on substantial knowledge of the law and legal process, and its interface (📖 p.IV.293) with psychiatric practice.

Legal psychiatry comprises all law relating to mental disorder, and to the treatment and care of those suffering from mental disorder. The relationship between psychiatry and the law is bilateral, comprising the giving of psychiatric evidence (📖 pp.V.586–V.597) in a wide variety of civil and criminal legal contexts, and the use of law for clinical purposes and for the regulation of clinical practice. This relationship is at the heart of forensic psychiatry, within which it is particularly strongly represented, by comparison with other branches of psychiatry.

Why all psychiatry is forensic psychiatry

Having emphasized the close association specifically of clinical forensic psychiatry with the law, all psychiatrists must be acquainted with those areas of the law that bear directly on treating and managing their patients. These include mental health law (📖 pp.IV.374–IV.423), mental capacity law (📖 pp.IV.424–IV.439), the law and procedures relating to public protection (📖 pp.V.468, II.203, III.242–III.248) and report-writing (📖 pp.V.556–V.584), for mental health tribunals (📖 p.V.567), and for courts (📖 pp.V.569–V.583). Psychiatrists do not all need to become quasi-lawyers, but they do need to be able to recognize and understand legal questions, to know how to prepare evidence relevant to those questions, and to understand how lawyers and courts reason and make decisions, particularly at the interface with psychiatry.

---

[*] Throughout the handbook we use the term 'mentally disordered offenders' to include people exhibiting offending behaviour: conviction is not a necessary pre-condition for assessment or treatment by forensic psychiatric services.

Tensions between law and psychiatry

The purposes of a discipline and the interests of its practitioners determine the constructs it uses. Hence, constructs in psychiatry are determined essentially by its pursuit of human welfare, including through understanding disorder in order to reverse it or its effects. By contrast, law pursues abstract justice, albeit this may sometimes involve balancing the welfare of different parties against one another, or against societal welfare. Even within a discipline, different branches often give rise to different approaches to determining constructs.

Since criminal law at trial, for example, is concerned with responsibility or culpability (📖 p.IV.296), its definitions of mental disorder (and there are a number) are characteristically tight, and address justice* and not human welfare. By contrast, the constructs utilized in sentencing, sometimes relating to public protection (📖 pp.IV.361, V.549), are often more loosely defined, although again without reference to the welfare of the individual concerned (except where sentencing occurs by way of mental health legislation). Certainly within both, indeed all, criminal domains the constructs derived are wholly different from biological or psychological constructs adopted within medicine, psychiatry, and clinical psychology, which are concerned chiefly with aetiology, and/or with treatment (📖 p.II.145). Examples of different constructs of mental disorder derived for different legal purposes include (within criminal law) fitness to plead (📖 p.V.474), insanity (📖 p.V.489), diminished responsibility (📖 p.V.491), automatism (📖 p.V.483), the reliability of confessions (📖 p.V.479) and extended or indefinite sentences (📖 pp.IV.361–IV.366) for public protection. Within branches of civil law there are, for example, constructs for damages in relation to 'nervous shock' or personal injury (📖 p.V.515), and broader notions such as fitness for childcare (📖 p.V.511).

Ultimately, the purposes of all mental health sciences are focused on the welfare of the patient, who should expect to receive some health benefit from treatment, albeit sometimes with additional gain accruing to others, e.g. potential third-party victims. Law is concerned with justice for all, including concern for the rights of both the defendant and victims. Hence, the manner of striking the balance between pursuit of patient welfare and public protection is bound to be different between mental healthcare professionals and legal agencies. Psychiatry and law address related concerns with potentially different values (📖 pp.III.225–III.289). Negotiating the interface (📖 p.IV.299) between the two is therefore ethically, and legally, both difficult and crucially important.

Reference

Semple D, Smyth R (2009). *Oxford Handbook of Psychiatry*, 2nd edn. Oxford: Oxford University Press.

---

*Justice from the perspective of the individual (i.e. proportionality, 📖 p.IV.297, or 'just deserts'). There are other meanings to justice—see the discussion in 📖 footnote p.IV.294 and elsewhere.

How forensic services are related

As has been described elsewhere (📖 p.I.7), the term 'forensic' refers to legally related work, and within psychiatry also to the clinical services provided for mentally disordered offenders. Some of these services will be psychiatric, or forensic psychiatric, but many others will not be. This page seeks to explain the different forensic services and areas of practice.

Criminal justice and court services

Almost all professional groups can offer forensic testimony: so there are forensic entomologists and forensic accountants as well as the more familiar forensic pathologists. Psychologists and psychiatrists who give expert testimony are acting as 'forensic' professionals, regardless of their usual clinical practice.

Clinical mental health services provided to offenders may be offered by general psychiatrists, rehabilitation psychiatrists, substance misuse services, or those psychiatrists (often forensic psychiatrists) working in secure settings. For some time, the term 'forensic' was only applied to those services that managed offenders and/or 'risky' patients: but it is now expected that many other services will also manage such patients.

Mental health services in prison

Since 2006, in the United Kingdom (UK) the National Health Service (NHS) has provided inreach services to prisons (📖 p.II.217); usually consisting of community psychiatric nurses, and some psychiatric/psychological consultancy, often with a dedicated healthcare centre. These personnel may be general adult practitioners, or sometimes forensic practitioners. Prisons may also ask for opinions from the catchment area psychiatrist. In many areas of the country, forensic psychiatrists will generally only be asked for an opinion if a prisoner is thought to need specialist psychiatric treatment in secure conditions.

In addition to the psychiatric services into prisons, the prison service also retains its own psychology service primarily staffed by forensic psychologists.

Secure psychiatric services

The 'forensic' professionals who work in secure mental health services (📖 p.II.209) include the same range of professionals expected in any mental health service. Thus there will be psychiatrists, psychologists, arts psychotherapists, medical psychotherapists, nurses, healthcare assistants, occupational therapists, social workers, and pharmacists. Confusingly, some secure services will also employ forensic psychologists because of their expertise in offender management programmes. Generally, however, the distinguishing feature of any 'forensic' mental health professional is that they have experience of working with very disordered men and women, usually with long and/or significant histories of violence, and often in long-stay residential care.

Specific staff groups

Forensic psychiatrists are psychiatrists, medically qualified initially, who have further training in the subspecialty of forensic psychiatry. Typically, though not always, they chair or lead multidisciplinary clinical teams. They often hold legal responsibility for the patient as responsible clinician (RC) or responsible medical officer (RMO, 📖 p.IV.379) under mental health law.

Clinical psychologists working in forensic settings have undertaken a general training in clinical psychology to doctorate level. They are almost always members of a multidisciplinary team but will generally be especially responsible for the coordination and delivery of psychological assessment and interventions of a variety of types. Increasingly they are specialists within clinical psychology (as are forensic psychiatrists within psychiatry).

Forensic psychologists are, by training, quite distinct from clinical psychologists, and also typically have a master's degree in their subject. They usually directly address offending behaviour, often not in the context of mental disorder. Hence they often carry out risk assessments and oversee the psycho-educational programme for offenders, typically in prisons. They may or may not have any general mental health experience.

Forensic psychotherapists are trained psychotherapists who have specialized in working with mentally disordered offenders. They may or may not be medically qualified. They may work in specialist services or provide consultation and supervision for forensic multidisciplinary teams. They may deliver individual or group interventions.

Criminologists study crime and criminals, and do not, in the UK, have direct involvement in the care of mentally disordered offenders. The impact of criminological research is, however, widespread and seen throughout this handbook, since many mentally disordered offenders are driven to offend not only in the context of their mental disorder but also by criminogenic factors.

Probation officers may be involved in supervision of mentally disordered offenders in the community, usually in collaboration with mental health professionals. Interventions may include measures aimed at risk reduction and rehabilitation. They also take on particular roles with sex offenders, and commonly coordinate sex offender interventions, sometimes with mental health service involvement. There may be interaction between probation officers and forensic psychiatrists in the production of reports used for sentencing convicted offenders, sometimes resulting in 'joint working' thereafter.

The history of forensic psychiatry

The modern forensic psychiatrist in the West combines up to three historical roles: the physician tending the mentally unwell; the superintendent of the asylum; and the expert witness to the court. All three have their own origins.

Physicians

Physicians—appliers of specialized knowledge in order to treat the sick, distinct from a religious role of ministering to the sick—can be recognized as such in Egypt as long ago as the 27th century BCE. A theme common to early medicine across many cultures, including Europe, India, China, and the Islamic world, is that physicians dealt only with physical health: mental ill-health was not seen as a 'medical' problem at all, but rather as a personal, family one, mostly dealt with informally by extended family networks. Only with the beginning of the industrial era in the West from the 18th century onwards, and the associated dislocation of families and disruption of kinship networks, did mental illness become a social problem requiring the intervention of specialized social actors and social institutions. People who were rich or of high social status were able to afford personal physicians to treat their illnesses.

The Madness of George III

George III probably suffered from porphyria, which can present with psychiatric symptoms such as anxiety, depression, paranoia, and hallucinations. No expense might be spared in treating the King, who naturally had a personal physician. However, even Dr Francis Willis (an enlightened physician for the 1780s, who treated many mentally ill patients with respect and kindness, in his own home) had little to offer the King beyond restraint, blistering, fresh air, and physical labour—in addition to antimony. Ironically, the antimony given to suppress 'ravings' contained arsenic, which is thought to have exacerbated the King's porphyria.

Asylum superintendents

People with mental illness who were poor or of low social status were committed to lunatic asylums, which were originally non-medical institutions. Over time these went from being progressive institutions that aimed to offer a human sanctuary to the distressed, to overcrowded 'bins' whose chief aim was the removal of the obviously mentally ill from the streets. Treatment was rarely available. Each asylum was presided over by a superintendent, who might or might not be medically qualified, but even if so, did not treat inmates personally, but merely oversaw the unqualified 'lunatic attendants'. 19th-century asylums included those developed specifically to deal with the 'criminally insane', first at the Bethlem Hospital and then Broadmoor Hospital, built for the purpose.

Expert witnesses

The role of the expert witness (📖 p.V.534) can be traced back to the Roman Empire, with courts accepting evidence from physicians, amongst others. However, as dealing with mental illness was not yet seen as part of medicine, judges and juries regarded themselves as competent to decide questions of insanity. Only in the 19th century, as asylums spread and those administering them came to be seen as experts, did courts begin to defer to psychiatric expert witnesses.

Psychiatrists

With the dissemination in the early 20th century of new scientific (or sometimes pseudo-scientific) developments, such as Kraepelin's identification and classification of psychotic disorders, Charcot's research on hypnosis and hysteria, and Freud's establishment of psychoanalysis, practitioners of psychiatry, who now had an institutional home in the asylums, were recognized as a single profession with a specialized body of knowledge. Psychiatrists, now so called, edged out office-based neurologists from the treatment of mental illness.

Psychiatry consolidated its professional position during the 20th century, with armies turning to it after World War I and II to treat their 'shell-shocked' soldiers (which led to the development of group therapy, 📖 p.II.171), and with the discovery of antipsychotics (📖 p.II.159)—which presaged the ascendancy of biological psychiatry and the sidelining of psychoanalysis. During the latter half of the century, psychiatric subspecialties developed alongside the biological/psychoanalytic division, such as child psychiatry, liaison psychiatry (providing advice and psychiatric care to patients of other specialties), and community psychiatry.

Forensic psychiatrists

The forensic subspecialty was a relatively late arrival, separating from mainstream general psychiatry largely because of two developments, one institutional and one ethical. In the UK, although there had been an isolated body of (with hindsight) recognizably 'forensic' practitioners in prisons and the special hospitals (📖 p.III.209), the development of the regional secure units (📖 p.II.210) from the 1980s onwards led to the establishment of a group of psychiatrists with a distinctively different job—i.e. caring for patients detained in a secure hospital environment, or in prison, who were numerous enough to develop their own sub-professional identity and their own faculty of the Royal College of Psychiatrists. In a very different vein, and partly to sidestep any perceived compromise of their ethical position as doctors (📖 p.III.245), many psychiatrists in the US who had traditionally concentrated on assessment of defendants or litigants for the courts, rather than treating patients, redesignated themselves as 'forensicists' and sought separate recognition in the American Academy of Psychiatry and Law. Thus, somewhat divergent ethical and clinical traditions of forensic psychiatry were established in the US and Europe, according to whether the doctor's primary duty was seen as being to the patient, or (through public protecion) to the State.

Part II

Clinical forensic psychiatry

Clinical and social aspects of crime

Crime to the forensic psychiatrist

Forensic psychiatry and crime

Forensic psychiatrists are only involved with a subgroup of criminal offenders. Reasons for referral to forensic psychiatry include:

Concerns that the (alleged) offender is mentally disordered

- Where the offender has a history of mental illness
- Before trial (📖 p.V.448), where mental disorder may be a ground for diversion (📖 p.II.216) on bail or while on remand
- At the sentencing stage (📖 pp.IV.361–IV.372), where hospital treatment (📖 p.IV.405) may be an alternative to prison (📖 p.V.456)
- While an offender is serving a sentence, especially in prison
- After an offender has been released and is under licence (📖 p.IV.365) or some other supervision.

Concerns that the offence is unusual and odd

- Crimes involving great or unusual cruelty to the victim
- Crimes odd in being committed by someone unusual, such as a child, woman, or elderly person
- When a defence team hopes that a psychological explanation may appeal to a jury or judge, and affect the likelihood of conviction; or be taken in mitigation (📖 IV.362) of the offence
- When the prosecution think that psychological or psychiatric testimony may properly lead to an extended (📖 pp.IV.362, IV.367) or indeterminate sentence (📖 p.IV.364) on risk grounds.

Concerns that the person needs treatment

- To improve their mental health, or
- To reduce their risk of offending, or both.

Conflicts and confusions

Forensic psychiatrists disagree on their role in the criminal justice system (📖 pp.I.8, III.245):

- Some argue that their predominant role is to *diagnose and treat mental disorders* such as psychotic disorders; with no duty on them to address risk of offending except insofar as it is functionally linked to mental disorder.
- Others argue that their role is to *assist in the psychological explanation* of serious crimes, and if possible to *reduce the risk of reoffending* by whatever means, including non-therapeutic means.

Each position raises its own problems for the profession and for the individual practitioner, because the association between mental disorder and violence (📖 p.II.31) is not straightforward, nor, usually, can the violence be managed (📖 p.II.191) by addressing the mental disorder alone; because British (or at least English) society in particular expects forensic psychiatrists to contribute to public protection (📖 p.V.468); and because there are unavoidable ethical role conflicts (📖 pp.III.244, III.258, III.261) between being a doctor and working with the criminal justice system. Each strand of opinion resolves these conflicts in its own way.

Violence, crime, and mental disorder

Crime statistics (📖 p.II.18) provide a picture of criminal rule breaking behaviour. The commonest type of criminal rule breaking is theft and other types of acquisitive offences, including burglary. Only 20% of recorded crime involves physical violence (Fig. 2.1); and only a minority of those offences will cause serious physical harm.

Debate continues as to whether violence is a normal aspect of human behaviour in certain circumstances (given its prevalence in all human societies), or whether it represents an essentially abnormal behaviour indicating at least an unusual mental state (given its comparative rarity as a form of social rule-breaking). Whichever view is correct, mental disorders are properly seen as a risk factor for violence (📖 pp.II.130, II.144), through creating appropriate circumstances for violence, or generating the relevant unusual mental state. This is supported by a large number of published studies.

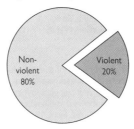

Fig. 2.1 Criminal rule-breaking.

Vignette: a case for forensic psychiatry?

Jason is an 18-year-old man who killed his girlfriend by setting her alight, and locking her in her bedroom. The prosecution claimed that he did this because she rejected him. He is convicted of murder.

Is there a role for forensic psychiatry?

No: Although this is a particularly unpleasant killing, there is no indication for mental health services to be involved unless there is any evidence that Jason was psychotic at the time. Killing someone in an unpleasant way is not *prima facie* evidence of mental illness or distress.

Yes: Killing is an unusual behaviour, and sadistic killing is particularly unusual; especially in young men. To kill in such a way itself suggests an abnormal psychological state which may be associated with a high risk of future violence. Treating Jason might improve his psychological health and reduce his risk.

Prevalence and measurement of crime

There are several difficulties with establishing how rates of crime differ, either between different countries or regions, or in the same place over time. Court records and rates of conviction and imprisonment can be useful, but the most commonly cited and reliable measures of crime are national and international police records of crime (e.g. the European Sourcebook) and household surveys of victimization (such as the BCS and the ICVS).

Sources of comparative crime statistics

- British Crime Survey (BCS)
- US National Crime Survey
- European Sourcebook of Crime & Criminal Justice Statistics
- Home Office Research Development & Statistics (RDS) publications
- UN International Crime Victims Survey (ICVS)
- US Department of Justice World Factbook of Criminal Justice Systems.

These measures give an indication of the prevalence of specific crimes and, if repeated, can be used to estimate trends over time. Rates are expressed in terms of acts per unit population for a given period.

For example, the 2011 BCS shows that the number of assaults (□ p. II.36) per 100,000 population in E&W fell from 1930 to 1488 between 2006–7 and 2010–11. More generally, it shows that total crime in E&W, which had previously risen inexorably throughout the 20th century, fell steadily from 1996 to the present.

Comparative prevalence figures for different countries can be found on pages for individual crimes, e.g. homicide (□ p.II.35), stalking (□ p.II.40), and sexual assault (□ p.II.42). Some broad international patterns, all expressed as numbers per 1000 citizens per year, include:

- Relative to population size, Anglo-Saxon countries such as the US, UK, Canada, Australia, and New Zealand have higher rates (all 7.0–7.5) than continental European countries (1.0–5.3)
- However, the US, Russia, and many Eastern European countries have higher rates of murder (0.04–0.05) than Australia, New Zealand, the UK, and other Western European countries (0.01–0.02)
- South Africa has the world's highest assault (12.0) and, after Colombia, murder (0.5) rates
- Property offences, such as burglary, do not show this differential between Anglo-Saxon and other European countries—all have rates in the same range (4–21)
- In general, Middle Eastern and other Islamic countries report lower rates of most crimes than Western or former Eastern-bloc countries
- The US prosecutes more of its adult population (48) than other Anglo-Saxon countries (New Zealand 31, UK 24, Canada 11) and Finland (31); other European countries have even lower prosecution rates (1–11).

The data from which such interpretations are made are not perfect, however. Problems with official figures include:

- Misleading and internationally inconsistent definitions of crimes (e.g. rape (📖 p.II.42) includes consensual sex with a minor in the US, whereas in E&W this is a different crime (see 📖 p.II.44))
- Crimes may not be reported to the police, depending on the local culture and expectations (e.g. a man may not report domestic violence by his wife, fearing ridicule by the police; or if reported, it may not be recognized as 'domestic violence' but categorized differently)
- The statistics are typically collected for local political reasons (e.g. to assess the performance of the police service), not to describe social reality in a neutral fashion
- They are not a complete record of criminal offences known to the authorities. For example, in E&W some include 'Notifiable offences' (those tried in a Crown Court, 📖 p.IV.320) but not 'Summary offences' (those that can be dealt with by lower courts)
- There are changes over time in what is counted for the purposes of inclusion into the official records.

Victimization surveys attempt to overcome these difficulties. They are typically surveys of a randomly selected representative group conducted by a neutral organization. Their limitations include:

- Omission of crimes without identifiable victims (e.g. fare evasion, drug possession) or where victims cannot be surveyed (e.g. young children)
- Recall and response biases determined by surveyed victims (e.g. greater chances of remembering more traumatic crimes; e.g. middle class respondents might classify some acts as crimes that working class ones might regard as non-criminal behaviour).

Both sets of figures, some sociologists argue, cannot ever be reliable because whatever their source they rely on someone interpreting and classifying a series of events, and this process of the construction of meaning is inevitably determined as much by social structures, ideologies, and values as by anything intrinsic to the events themselves.

Vignette: when is a crime not a crime?

A man walks through a city park. He approaches a group of children playing. The children include him in their group and the man joins in their game for a short while. Presently the man and two of the children wander amongst some nearby bushes. The man removes his trousers and brings out his penis in front of the children.

Whether your reaction is that the man is a paedophile in the process of abusing two or more children, or a socially inept and possibly learning disabled young man urinating in a socially inappropriate fashion, depends on your personal ideology and that of your society or culture.

Psychology & philosophy of volition

Philosophy of volition

For millennia, and since at least the time of Aristotle, who advocated this in his *Nicomachean Ethics*, people have usually been held responsible and blamed only for those acts that they chose to do, as opposed to acts that are involuntary (such as when someone pushes you and you cannot avoid stumbling into and therefore assaulting another person). Aristotle also identified a category of less-blameworthy acts that were chosen in circumstances in which the alternatives open to the individual were worse, such as stunning an intruder when that is the only way to stop them sexually assaulting your partner.

The mental faculty of choosing immediate actions is known as *volition*, as distinct from pursuing long-term goals. Much of philosophy and economics assumes that people rationally choose actions so as to maximize the probability of achieving as many of those goals of possible. Evolutionary psychology suggests, however, that although humans have numerous 'reasoning instincts' governing specific situations, there is no general reasoning system capable of overriding other systems, and therefore the assumption of rational choice may not hold in all situations.

Another philosophical view, determinism, states that all actions are caused by what preceded them, with no room for free will. Despite the fact that at the quantum physical level events are non-deterministic (that is, there is a significant component of apparent randomness), it might still be the case that the brain and therefore the mind function as a deterministic system. If this is the case, most determinists ('incompatibilists') hold that people cannot therefore meaningfully be held responsible for their actions.

Neuropsychology of volition

This has mainly been studied in relation to impairment of volition: compulsive behaviours, impulsivity, addictions and other behaviour suggestive of akrasia (weakness of will). The volitional system in the brain involves the dorso-lateral prefrontal cortex (DLPFC) and the supplementary motor area (SMA), with the former being activated in choosing a particular action, but the latter only if the chosen action is to be carried out rather than merely imagined. The experience of making choices is distinct from general intellectual function; and is integrated with conscious awareness, emotional attributions, systems of belief, values, and temporal assessment.

It has been hypothesized by Damasio and others that, whereas long-term goals are selected consciously and through intellectual processes, emotional processing is essential to volition, and that it is this discrepancy that explains the common experience of repeatedly choosing something that conflicts with one's goals (e.g. overeating when trying to lose weight, or smoking cigarettes when trying to quit, or shopping for luxuries despite wishing to pay off a large overdraft).

Disorders affecting volition

Neurological disorders such as Alzheimer's disease and other dementias (📖 p.II.85), or Parkinson's disease and other movement disorders, affect the experience of volition; as can acute intoxication with substances such as cannabis. Chronic schizophrenia (📖 p.II.55) can also cause a state of avolition, typically in conjunction with alogia, anhedonia, and flattened affect.

Legal and moral responsibility

The assignment of criminal responsibility often rests on an assessment of the defendant's volition, i.e. on how (not why) they chose to act.[*] Choices can include the choice to do nothing (which may lead to crimes of omission, 📖 p.IV.332); therefore, being reckless (📖 p.IV.336) or negligent (📖 p.IV.336) can represent choices as much as can an intention (📖 p.IV.334) to commit an offence.

In moral philosophy, knowledge of the wrongness of the action is required for it to be morally blameworthy. The law rarely has such a requirement (see 📖 pp.IV.332–IV.343); in fact, it is a general principle that 'ignorance of the law is no excuse'. Moreover, the law ignores the question of whether the individual even had the capacity to take into account the wrongness of the action, and with the exception of children (📖 p.IV.338) holds individuals responsible even if they lacked a capacity for moral reasoning unless they have other deficits of mental function that render them unfit to plead (📖 p.V.474). This reflects the different, although overlapping, social functions of law and morality (📖 p.IV.294).

Personal beliefs and professional opinion

The different views of professionals about the nature of volition and free will may have an impact on their professional stance and behaviour. Those who take a strict determinist view may not see the mentally ill as having any control over their volitions and by extension their offending behaviour; those who take a more experiential view, or who have strong religious views, may be more inclined to want them held at least partially responsible even when the illness is severe and involves a loss of touch with reality. These views also have significant influence on how risk is assessed and managed. Practitioners should be aware of their own views and how they may influence their professional judgement or the objectivity of their opinion (📖 p.V.551) in certain cases.

Types of violence

Definitions

The term violence is often used interchangeably with aggression, and also criminal violence, but these should be distinguished. There is some disagreement about how broadly each term should be defined, but conventional comparative definitions are:
- *Aggression* refers to intentionally hurting or gaining advantage over another person, without necessarily involving physical injury
- *Violence* involves the use of strong physical force against another person, which may be accompanied by aggression and which causes harm to others

---

[*] Except in offences of strict liability (📖 p.IV.337).

- *Criminal violence* involves directly injurious behaviour which is against the law. This includes murder, manslaughter, assault, and robbery. Sexual offences (📖 p.IV.348) and arson (📖 p.IV.350) are also acts of criminal violence.

Each infers actual or potential consequent harm.

Instrumental violence is violence used as a means to attain a goal; it is usually planned and is not precipitated by increased arousal (e.g. violence used to carry out a robbery). The exception is sadistic violence, where pain and cruelty are used not only to control a victim, but also to generate sexual arousal and excitement.

Expressive (or reactive) violence is accompanied by strong affects, such as hostility, fear, anger, or loss. The primary goal in harming the victim is the expression (or communication) of these affects. The violence occurs in response to, or in conjunction with, feelings of arousal (due to fear, frustration, anger, resentment) in the perpetrator. It is usually impulsive (although may be planned). Examples include a response to being threatened or a confrontation in a pub.

An act of violence may be seen as either instrumental or expressive, although many combine features of both, e.g. violence may be used to carry out a robbery of a victim (instrumental) but also as an angry reaction to the victim first accusing the perpetrator of something (expressive).

Gang violence

Peer groups play an important role in the development of violence and delinquency (📖 p.II.23). Involvement with deviant peers is the most proximate influence on the onset of delinquency, including its escalation to violence. In North America two-thirds of serious violent delinquents are gang members.

Victims of violence

The victims of violence can be men, women, or children, but the contexts in which they each become a victim tend to differ. The common factor is their vulnerability at the time.

- *Violence against strangers* Few victims of serious violence (such as rape or homicide) are strangers to the perpetrator. The majority of violent offences committed by mentally disordered offenders occur within a family setting, and less than 10% of victims are strangers. Males are more likely than females to be the victim of stranger violence. Stranger violence is more likely to occur in public places with alcohol being consumed. Violence against strangers is usually less severe than violence against acquaintances or those well-known to the perpetrator. A very small subgroup of child sex offenders target children who are unknown to them.
- *Intimate partner/domestic violence* One in four women (but very many fewer men) experience domestic violence at some point in their lifetime. Younger populations are more likely to report a higher prevalence of domestic violence than older populations. Both men and women can be the victim of domestic violence, although women's injury rates are higher, and they often also suffer sexual attacks, such as rape or indecent assault. Feminist theories of male domestic violence indicate the role of power and control. Economic dependency in women and

emotional dependency in men independently contribute to the risk of partner abuse and also reduce the likelihood that the victimized person will terminate the relationship. Women are more at risk of assault and murder if they leave their abusive male partner. Rapes may often be carried out by new suitors or ex-partners who have been rejected.

- *Family violence* Evidence suggests that homicide is mainly a domestic affair, with a large proportion of victims being the partner or child of the perpetrator. 80% of the children killed each year are killed by their parents; newborns being most at risk. About two-thirds of assaults perpetrated between parents are witnessed by their children; and violence between parents is often accompanied by violence to children. Physical abuse of children occurs in 10–16% of families, and carries a mortality rate of up to 10%. Sexual abuse of children occurs in 8–10% of households; and is more common where there is domestic violence or physical abuse of children. Severe abuse in childhood and witnessing family violence is predictive of later violence and delinquency, as well as mental health problems.

Social factors in crime and delinquency

The idea that crime can be 'explained' by underlying social factors arises within some models of criminology. It has been politically controversial, especially through some right-wing politicians being unwilling to accept any kind of causative link between social factors and crime for fear that to do so would undermine the presumption that individuals are criminally responsible (p.IV.338) for their own criminal acts. Some criminological models verge on political science.

Whether in any sense causative or not, however, most studies of crime and social factors have found a strong association between the two. (This is reflected in aspects of so called 'actuarial' approaches to risk assessment, p.II.130, and risk assessment tools, p.II.133, relating to violence at an individual level.) Commonly identified factors include:

- Economic and health factors (see also p.II.31):
  - Poverty
  - Unemployment
  - Chronic physical or mental illness
- Familial factors:
  - Parental inadequacy (e.g. poor role model, erratic discipline, inadequate supervision) leading to inadequate child socialization
  - Parental criminality
  - Intra-family violence
  - Large family size
  - Child abuse and neglect
- Peer factors:
  - Antisocial/delinquent peers
  - Gang membership
- School factors:
  - Low educational ability
  - Low academic attainment
  - Lack of parental involvement

- Societal factors:
  - Inequality of social standing and power
  - Poor access to, or low perceived value of, education
  - Poor housing
  - Prejudice, on grounds of race, poverty, geography, etc.
  - Poor family and neighbourhood support
  - Lack of community cohesion and leadership

Delinquency

Delinquency—that is, antisocial and criminal behaviour in children (📖 p.IV.356) and teenagers—is frequently cited as a critical predictor of adult criminality and is itself associated with the factors already listed, particularly those regarding family breakdown and poor parenting. Despite this, parental attitudes and behaviours, while still predictive, are less good predictors of future delinquency than family income or deprivation.

The peak ages for recorded crime across the lifespan are 14–15 years (see 📖 p.II.30); as many as 81% of all adolescents will commit a criminal act bringing them into contact with the police (e.g. shop lifting, possession of illicit substances) but will have no future contact with the police. Such crime is typically a social phenomenon, in that it will be committed with peers, or through interactions with peers. A minority of adolescents (9%) will commit a serious offence. Those who show signs of delinquency earliest commit most acts over the longest period such that in some deprived areas 9% of males are responsible for half of all crimes.

Social factors in crime prevention

Many governments attempt to reduce crime rates by tackling the social and economic problems previously listed, in the hope that this will lead people who might otherwise have committed crime to engage in more pro-social behaviour, such as obtaining a job and paying taxes. (This makes a particular assumption about criminals' motivation for committing crime.)

Such governments have therefore directed resources towards improving public housing, increasing access to education, expanding social services, and improving local health services, amongst other measures. Some studies have found an apparent resultant reduction in crime rates, but the picture is complex: for example, a reduction in one form of crime (e.g. joyriding, 📖 p.IV.356) may occur at the same time as a rise in another form (e.g. robbery, 📖 p.IV.355); moreover, the effect of the public spending directed this way may be impossible to disentangle from simultaneous changes in other socioeconomic factors, such as an economic boom or bust, or increased rates of mobile phone possession amongst school-age children.

A crucial related problem in investigating the association between mental disorder and crime (📖 p.II.31) is that individual, or social, 'criminogenic' factors unrelated to mental disorder make such a major contribution to criminal behaviour by MDOs that it is difficult to tease out what is the 'residual' contribution of mental disorder.

Sexual offending and its social context

To an even greater extent than other offences, sexual offences are overwhelmingly (though not exclusively) committed by men, and overwhelmingly (but not exclusively) against women and to a lesser extent children. They have attracted a great deal of sociological, criminological, and political dispute about why certain men offend in this way.

The individual and social positions

❧ Psychology and psychiatry have traditionally given an account of sexual offending as caused by individual psychopathological problems which can be clustered into diagnoses and disorders. On this account, the impulse to commit sexual offences (📖 p.IV.348) is itself evidence of individual deviance; and treatment or educational programmes need to be offered to correct this.

However, other accounts of sex offending take a more systemic and social view; arguing that there are social and cultural factors that make sexual offending more likely. A key fact supportive of the argument is that there are societies where sexual offending is almost unknown; whilst rates of sex offending are highest in societies where derogatory attitudes to women or children are tolerated or supported; for example, where there is easy access to cheap pornography. In addition, many sex offenders are also prolific criminal offenders or violent offenders, suggesting that the sexual offending is better understood as part of a generally antisocial stance and lifestyle.

The counter argument to this view is that only a small proportion of men (let alone women) are sexual offenders; and they come from across the social spectrum. Supporters of the individual deviance account would argue that sex offenders do appear to present with persistent and recognizable distortions of beliefs and cognitions (📖 p.II.47) about their victims that drive offending behaviour and are not found in non-offenders.

Supporters of the social deviance position would argue that, actually these distortions and beliefs are widespread in the community; and that detected sex offenders represent only those who are excessively antisocial or criminally incompetent. They would argue that the overall rate of sex offending in the community would therefore be reduced if social attitudes towards the vulnerable (including women and children) were changed. Specifically, social theorists argue that contempt for the vulnerable is common in capitalist societies; and that sexual offending is better understood as control and humiliation of the vulnerable, rather than as disorder of individual appetites. Further, social theories of sexual deviance would suggest that mental health professionals prefer to emphasize individual disorders, rather than examine the attitudes they themselves might share: that is, that the explanation of the sexual offending (the narrative) is suggested by their attitudes, rather than the reverse.

Difference between sex offenders

A complexity in the debate is that not all sex offences are the same. There is real difference between:
- The fetishist who collects sex toys (a legal activity)

- The person who looks at illegal internet pornography[*]
- The serial rapist
- The recidivist paedophile, and
- The parent who abuses their stepchild.

It is unlikely that one explanation will account for these heterogeneous behaviours: not all of which will be detected or result in criminal prosecution. What is more likely is that the social deviance account will fit some offenders well; and the individual deviance account will fit others better. For example, individual deviance may provide a better theoretical understanding for a man who starts to abuse his daughter in the context of his wife's illness/absence: but social deviance might explain the same behaviour in a man who is also physically or emotionally abusive to his wife.

Personality disorder and sexual offending

The individual deviance/pathology model may extend to seeing sex offending as only one aspect of pervasive psychopathology, especially as part of personality disorder. This may have implications for both the therapeutic response (📖 p.II.176), if any, and perhaps legal compulsion (📖 p.IV.405).

Multiple perspectives

As with most dichotomies, to focus on one to the exclusion of the other is unwise. When assessing sex offenders (📖 p.II.94), it is useful to consider their social attitudes towards women and children; and their expression of this to the professional. It is also salutary to recognize that there is research that indicates that significant subgroups of normal men share rape-supportive attitudes.

However, it is also important to consider the individual factors that may have facilitated this person's offending behaviour, not least because it is likely to be easier to intervene at the level of the individual.

Training

It is essential that all those working with sex offenders have an understanding of both social and individual deviance accounts of sexual offending. A sole focus on individual disorders or psychiatric diagnosis is likely to mislead both the clinician and the offender patient.

Ethnicity, crime, and psychiatry

Thinking about ethnicity in forensic psychiatry

Defining ethnicity is complicated, because it overlaps with other concepts such as race, skin colour, religion, culture, nationality, and immigration status. In general, people define their own ethnicity.

---

[*] This varies from one jurisdiction to another. At present in the UK, it comprises child pornography, and 'extreme' pornography (realistically depicting scenes that are life threatening or involve serious damage to the anus, breasts, or genitals, or involve animals or corpses).

People who do not describe themselves as 'white British' make up 15% of the population of the UK. However they are over-represented in both the prisoner population and amongst psychiatric service users, especially in secure services (p.II.209). This issue is pronounced in those areas of the UK where there are large minority ethnic populations, such as inner cities, where so-called black and minority ethnic (BME) groups may be in the majority.[*]

Forensic psychiatric patients are drawn from both general psychiatry (p.II.220) and the criminal justice system (p.IV.330), and BME groups are therefore doubly over-represented.

Concerns about racism

There have been repeated concerns that both the criminal justice system and mental health services are influenced by racist attitudes and beliefs. It is argued that the (largely white British) professional groups who operate these systems discriminate against people from BME groups; either by assuming that they are more likely to be criminal or that they are more likely to be mentally ill (or both, in the case of forensic psychiatry). This is not to argue that those professionals hold racist views as such, although a few may do: merely that being aware of patients' racial origins, and making different assumptions about them as a result, is sufficient for discrimination to occur, however unintended.

There is no direct evidence of racism within psychiatric services, but there is evidence that BME patients, and especially those from Afro-Caribbean backgrounds, are more likely than other patients to be:

- Diagnosed with schizophrenia
- Admitted to hospital compulsorily instead of voluntarily
- Secluded and restrained (p.II.156), or forcibly medicated; and
- Given more severe sentences (p.IV.361), e.g. of imprisonment (p.IV.364).

The situation is complicated by the fact that it is not clear how differences of identities and diversity of values can be defined easily, so as still to be personally respectful. For example, a young man who has been born and raised in the UK may still define himself as African by heritage; but another young man with a similar history may define himself as British. A young woman who has recently migrated from India may have little in common with her British-born Asian psychiatrist. There is a danger that in perceiving difference, one may create difference that is more apparent than real. In addition, some differences may be practically significant (such as religious identity and ritual observance), but not morally significant. For example, no citizen is allowed to kill another person, no matter what their religious beliefs.

Taking difference seriously in forensic psychiatry

The over-representation of BME groups (and foreign nationals) in both prisons and mental healthcare systems does at least raise the question of whether these systems may be treating ethnic and national difference in

---

[*] At the 2001 census, BME groups made up more than 50% of the population of the London Boroughs of Brent and Hackney, and approached 50% in other inner city areas.

a discriminatory way. Given that this may be the case, it is important that forensic healthcare professionals pay attention to the identity and experience of these men and women, particularly during the process of assessment (📖 p.II.113). It may be helpful, therefore, to talk to a wide variety of sources from within the same community, not just the family. It is also important to consider that a patient from a BME or other ethnic group may suffer increased distress and alienation from their community if facing criminal charges or incarceration.

It has also been suggested (by the Bennett inquiry, 📖 p.App. 5. 654) that more staff in forensic units be recruited from BME groups and other countries apart from the UK. There is a danger, however, that this kind of response will lead to a focus on differences that should not be relevant (such as skin colour), and to ignorance of differences that are highly relevant (such as who has power and control).

In summary, the concept of 'empowerment' implies treating each patient as an individual; and not making assumptions about their identity and values. No patient should ever be excluded from accessing potential treatments, or subject to more punitive or coercive risk management measures (📖 p.II.190), on the basis of judgements about ethnicity or culture.

Neurobiology of violence and antisocial behaviour

✒ Biological explanations of criminal behaviour in general and violence in particular have been sought for centuries, with the Victorian craze for phrenology[*] representing just one of the better-known examples. A recent flurry of findings in neurobiological research (some of which are summarized here) has led to another increase in interest in the field, in the hope that violence and criminal rule-breaking can be explained biologically. However, it still remains the case that all we have are glimpses of associations, not yet any biological explanation (in terms of brain structure and function, or genetics) for something as complex as human volition (📖 p.II.20).

A key question is whether violent behaviour can be explained directly by biology, or whether biology can only explain psychologically-defined phenotypes (e.g. psychopathology), which in turn explain behaviour. Many studies purport to correlate psychological and biological descriptions.

There is a danger of 'over defining' any relationship found between biology and behaviour, extrapolating from it to ethical or even legal conclusions, such as making inferences about criminal responsibility (📖 p.IV.338) and agency (📖 p.IV.339).

---

[*] The pseudo-science of determining personality traits and behavioural patterns from palpable lumps and depressions on the skull, thought to represent the size of underlying brain regions, which themselves were arbitrarily deemed to have specific psychological functions.

Functional neuroimaging studies

In additional to structural abnormalities, several studies, using different methodologies, have concluded that individuals with significant antisocial personality traits (📖 p.II.60) have dysfunction of the frontal and temporal lobes. PET (positron emission tomography) studies have associated reduced metabolism in the frontal cortex with aggression, violence and murder. SPECT (single photon emission computed tomography) studies have associated reduced frontal lobe perfusion with antisocial behaviour.

Abnormalities in activation of areas of the frontal lobes have been found on fMRI (functional magnetic resonance imaging) scans during the processing of emotional stimuli by antisocial and psychopathic (📖 p.II.66) individuals, and in response inhibition tests in which the subject has to withhold their usual response to a stimulus.

More generally, a number of neuroimaging and other studies have linked damage to the frontal lobes (such as after traumatic brain injury, 📖 p.II.82), especially damage to the prefrontal cortex, to personality change and social disinhibition.

Genetic and related neuroendocrine studies

Meta-analysis of twin and adoption studies suggests that around 40% of the variability in antisocial behaviour between individuals is explained by genetic factors. Whilst there is increasing evidence that genetic and environmental factors interact with respect to antisocial behaviour, some types of antisocial behaviour appear to be more heritable than others (e.g., children with callous-unemotional [CU] traits, 📖 p.II.66). Genetically-mediated deficiencies in MAOA (monoamine oxidase type A) activity have been associated with increased levels of violence and aggression, leading to at least one successful claim that an alleged murderer should be acquitted on the grounds of his low levels of MAOA. Moreover, MAOA activity seems to mediate experiences of childhood abuse and maltreatment, such that children with high MAOA levels are less likely to display antisocial behaviour when older than are similarly abused children with low MAOA levels.

In mice, the targeted disruption of certain genes has been associated with aggressive behaviour; many such genes have a role in brain development and the function of neurotransmitter systems implicated in aggression (e.g. neuronal nitric oxide synthase and the serotonergic system).

The evidence from human studies suggests that testosterone has a role in social dominance but is less clear regarding its role in aggression.

Callous-unemotional traits and psychopathy

Children with significant CU traits and adults with psychopathy are less able to recognize facial emotional expressions, especially fearful expressions; and they have reduced physiological and behavioural responses to such expressions observed in others.

The deficit may be partly attentional: children with CU traits fail to concentrate on the eyes when looking at faces, and telling them to look in the eyes before responding improves their accuracy. It has been hypothesized that a failure from birth to attend specifically to the eyes may impair attachment and bonding with the parent, thereby impairing emotional development.

The amygdala is known to be involved in the processing of emotional stimuli, particularly stimuli indicating fear and submission, and adults with psychopathy show reduced amygdala activation to facial recognition stimuli compared to controls. It is also involved in stimulus-reinforcement learning, and impairment of this function may explain why adults exhibiting psychopathy find it difficult to learn from punishment or other negative outcomes. Structural abnormalities in the main white matter tract connecting the amygdala with the orbitofrontal cortex, the uncinate fasciculus, have also been associated with psychopathy.

People with CU traits also show endocrine abnormalities, including persistently low levels of cortisol (a hormone involved in responding to stress). Low cortisol, and decreased cortisol response to stress, appear to be related to cold, unemotional violence (of the sort committed by people with psychopathy), whereas serotonergic dysfunction appears to be associated with emotional, explosive violence.

Crime and violence from the developmental perspective

Adolescence-limited and lifecourse-persistent violence

There is considerable continuity of aggression and violent behaviour across the lifespan. Childhood aggression is highly predictive of future aggression and violence. Aggressive behaviour in the classroom is a predictor of adolescent delinquency, and aggression in middle childhood predicts conduct problems in adolescence. The predictive relationships have been shown across different cultures.

There appear to be two distinct developmental trajectories in relation to antisocial behaviour, the result of individual combinations of risk and resilience factors. With the adolescence-limited trajectory, violence and antisocial behaviour starts early in adolescence (around age 12), peaks around age 15–16, and disappears almost entirely by age 21. In the lifecourse-persistent trajectory, instead of peaking around age 15, the rate of violence and antisocial behaviour continues to rise steadily until the mid-20s, after which it declines slowly, falling to a low level only in the mid-40s.

Within the lifecourse-persistent group, a subgroup has callous and unemotional traits (🕮 p.II.29) which are linked with the later emergence of psychopathy (🕮 p.II.66); the remainder have higher levels of anxiety and lower IQs, and are likely to develop ASPD (antisocial personality disorder; 🕮 p.II.60).

Offending during adolescence

In the UK, very few children under the age of 12 behave in a way that could result in prosecution (for any offence, not just those involving antisocial behaviour or violence) if they were over the age of criminal responsibility (🕮 p.IV.338). The rate of such behaviour rises to a peak at age 15 for girls and 18 for boys.

During adolescence, more than half of boys and a third of girls commit an offence, though they may well not be prosecuted for it. Much of this offending behaviour consists of status offences (📖 p.IV.356) that can only be committed by people with the status of 'adolescent', such as underage sex (📖 p.IV.349) or truancy* (📖 p.IV.356). However, by age 17 for girls and age 21 for boys, offending behaviour ceases for all bar a small minority.

There is a typical progression of offence type with increasing age. Very loosely, those aged 12–13 tend to commit criminal damage (📖 p.IV.350) and minor assaults (📖 p.IV.346); those aged 15–16, theft (📖 p.IV.354) and similar property offences; and those aged 18–21, drug offences and later also vehicle offences such as theft of or from vehicles, or joyriding.

Risk factors for persistence of violence

Longitudinal studies have found a number of childhood risk factors that are predictive of later violent offending in adolescence and adulthood. These include: individual characteristics (e.g. low intelligence, poor problem solving skills, low empathy, impulsivity, and risk taking); family environment (e.g. parental conflict, harsh and inconsistent discipline, low supervision and monitoring, parental criminality and unemployment, and large family size); peer factors (e.g. antisocial delinquent peers, gang membership); school factors (e.g. low attainment, exclusion, truancy, lack of parental involvement) and community factors (e.g. socioeconomic deprivation, high crime neighbourhood).

Protective factors against persistence of violence include being first born, small family size, being an active and affectionate infant, resilient temperament, high IQ, positive disposition, receiving large amounts of attention from care-givers and social bonding (e.g. pro-social relationships with peers, family and teachers).

The greater the number of risk factors that are present in a child's early life, the greater the likelihood of later violent offending. There are similar risk factors for males and females, although socioeconomic deprivation and child-rearing factors (such as low family income and poor parental supervision) are more important for females, and parental characteristics are more predictive of offending for males.

The earlier the onset of offending behaviour, the more likely it is that the person will commit more offences and have a longer criminal career. In one study, men who started offending at age 10–16 committed three-quarters of all crimes leading to conviction.

Do mental disorders cause violence?

✒ This is a highly contentious and politicized topic. In the 1980s, the then-dominant view within the profession was that patients were no more likely to be violent than any other member of the population, were unfairly stigmatized, and should usually be free within the community once their mental disorder had been treated to the fullest extent possible (which in the case of personality disorder was widely held to be a very limited extent).

---

*Although only the adolescent can 'commit' truancy, it is actually their parent or guardian who commits the offence of failing to secure their regular attendance at school.

From the mid-1990s onwards, it became the dominant view of politicians and the media, and of a significant section of the profession, that some patients were inherently dangerous, substantially more likely to be violent than the rest of the population, and should potentially be detained on grounds of risk to the public even after treatment* (📖 p.II.146) options had been exhausted. This shift in views resulted chiefly from several high profile incidents of violence by patients, and only to a limited extent from new scientific evidence.

The scientific evidence

From the mid-1980s onwards, evidence began to accumulate of a greater than average frequency of violence amongst people with mental disorder. Studies were mainly of two kinds: those looking at the incidence of mental disorder in known criminal populations (e.g. prisons); and those measuring levels of offending in mentally disordered groups and the general population. In chronological order, studies found that:

- Psychosis was much more common in prisoners in E&W remanded (📖 p.IV.330) for a violent offence than in prisoners remanded for a non-violent offence
- Approximately 10% of patients with schizophrenia (📖 p.II.54) in the community reported a violent act in the previous 12 months, compared with 2% of those without mental disorder. The rate of violence was 12 times higher in those with alcohol dependence, and 16 times higher in those with drug dependence. This was found in various cities in the US and also in Sweden
- Rates of arrest and self-reported violence in New York were higher in all patient groups than in the non-patient group
- In the community in the UK, comorbid personality disorder almost doubled the risk of violent behaviour
- Around 70% of people with psychopathy (📖 p.II.66) in Canada reoffended within 5 years of release from prison, three times more than people without psychopathy
- The prevalence of schizophrenia in perpetrators of homicide (📖 p.II.35) in the UK was 5%, as opposed to 1% in the general population
- In the UK, the population attributable risk of violence (i.e. the reduction in the frequency of people committing five or more violent incidents in 5 years that would result if the risk factor in question was removed entirely from the population) was 2% for psychosis, 20% for ASPD, 33% for all personality disorder, 55% for hazardous drinking, and 21% for drug dependence
- In a Swedish population study, 9% of homicide offenders had schizophrenia, 12% another psychotic disorder, and 54% a principal or secondary diagnosis of personality disorder.

---

* This gloss assumes that by 'treatment' we mean interventions that are effective in improving the patient's condition and thereby their risk to others, whereas there is a lively debate about whether essentially palliative and potentially public-protective measures can count as 'treatment'.

The statistical significance of the association of violence (but not crime in general) with schizophrenia is as great as that between cigarette smoking and carcinoma of the lung, and consistent across a variety of different studies. The associations with personality disorder, and alcohol and drug misuse, are also robust, and considerably greater in magnitude.

To put this in perspective, however, it should be remembered that people with mental illness are at much higher risk than the general population of being victimized (📖 p.II.139) and of suicide and self-harm (📖 p.II.137). That is, the rate of violence towards people with mental illness (by others or by the person themselves) is considerably greater than their rate of violence towards others. Moreover, factors unrelated to mental disorder are even more strongly related to violence, most notably being male, being aged 15–30, being socioeconomically deprived, and (especially) having a past history of violence.

Interpreting the evidence with your patient

As with all evidence, some thought is required in applying it to an individual patient. First, you must decide whether the available statistical evidence applies to your patient. If they have an eating disorder as their primary diagnosis, or are aged over 65, for example, the evidence previously discussed on risk of violence does not cover them and is a poor guide to their risk.

Say, though, that your patient has schizophrenia, or personality disorder, or misuses substances: will they be violent? The other crucial point to bear in mind is that the studies discussed in this section relate to the group as a whole, not the individual. 10% of the group of which the patient is a member might commit a violent act in the next year, but that does *not* mean that your patient has a 10% risk of committing a violent act in the next year. Think about your own car insurance, if you drive: your insurance company might correctly allocate you to a group 5% of whom will have an accident this year, based upon your age and profession; but if you routinely drive while drunk your risk will be very much higher than that, whereas if you only ever use the car to drive to church on Sundays, it will be much lower. In the same way, your patient's personal risk depends on their personal circumstances (such as the presence of active delusions, their engagement with your service, their insight, etc.), not only their group membership. This is why an individualized formulation (📖 p.II.110) as part of their risk assessment (📖 p.II.130), perhaps assisted by an HCR20 (📖 p.II.133) if necessary.

Vignette: should I be worried?

The following vignette is a worked example of the principles already set out on interpreting the evidence associating mental disorder and violence with a specific patient.

Mrs B and her son S both suffer from chronic paranoid schizophrenia. Mrs B arrived in the UK from India in the 1970s as a teenage girl; she was diagnosed 5 years later, when her husband took her to A&E because she attacked him with a hammer in his sleep, saying he was a *raksa* (devil) and she had to kill him to save her son. Mr B did not press charges against his wife, even though he was quite seriously injured; instead, she was admitted to hospital under the Mental Health Act, section 2 (📖 p.IV.383). She was discharged a month later on oral trifluoperazine, which he ensures she takes every day. She has suffered no further relapses.

SB was born in the UK in 1988. His family encouraged him to study, and he was academically successful. He suffered his first psychotic episode at university in 2007, after he began using cannabis with a group of university friends. He is now cared for by an Early Intervention in Psychosis team and, although they have not been able to persuade him to stop using cannabis entirely, he has accepted depot *risperidone* and has not yet had a second psychotic episode.

Mrs B has a history of serious violence—an attack on her husband that, had she been prosecuted, could have resulted in conviction for GBH (assault occasioning grievous bodily harm; 📖 p.IV.346). She has schizophrenia, so the studies listed on 📖 p.II.32 would appear to suggest that she is in a group roughly 10% of whom will commit a violent act (possibly another attack on her husband with a weapon) in the next year. However, these studies were conducted on mostly male Americans and Europeans. Although she has lived in the UK for most of her life, it is not at all clear that the research findings are any guide to the risk that she will commit another violent act. Therefore, her risk of violence assessment (📖 p.II.132) must look at her personal risk factors, such as her stable marriage, the care she receives from her husband, her regular daily activities, her lack of current symptoms, her abstinence from alcohol and drugs, and so on. The result of this assessment might well be that her risk of a further act of violence is low—but might highlight the scenario of her husband predeceasing her and her losing that essential care while grieving, in which case she might need additional support to prevent a relapse and possible violence.

Mr SB has no such history of violence. However, he does have schizophrenia, and he is a regular user of cannabis, factors that together place him in a group of whom perhaps 20% or more will commit a violent act in a given year. The relevant research is more applicable to him than to his mother, because he is male and was born and raised in the UK. Despite the lack of a history of violence, this group membership is a good reason to conduct a separate risk assessment for S. When this assessment considers his personal risk factors (possibly, for example, worsened academic and employment prospects because of the effect of the schizophrenia on his cognitive function; a lack of an intimate relationship; low self-esteem; cutting himself off from his family; and so on), it might conclude that he does pose a significant risk of violence, and that he needs support in the community now to improve his self-esteem, help him find employment, and assist him in re-establishing contact with his family, amongst other interventions.

Homicide

Homicide is the killing of one human being by another. When it amounts to murder (📖 p.IV.344), it is conventionally regarded as the most heinous offence (although modern concepts of genocide and crimes against humanity (📖 p.IV.358) are arguably more heinous); and yet at the same time it can be legally sanctioned, such as in wartime or in self-defence (📖 p.IV.340).

Mental disorder and homicide

☀ The precise nature of the association between mental disorder and homicide needs to be considered carefully (see also 📖 p.II.32). Certain mental illnesses, particularly schizophrenia and other psychotic disorders (📖 p.II.54), are associated with an increased risk of serious assault or homicide, but personality disorder (particularly ASPD, 📖 p.II.60 and psychopathy, 📖 p.II.66) and substance misuse (📖 p.II.56) are very much greater risk factors, and a significant proportion of homicides are committed by people with no mental disorder:

- ⚠ People with schizophrenia commit approximately 5% of homicides in E&W, whereas they form about 1% of the population
- Between 1980 and 2004 in E&W the number of homicides committed by people with mental disorder fell from 120 to 20 per year, and also fell significantly as a proportion of all homicides
- In a Swedish population study, 9% of homicide offenders had schizophrenia, 12% another psychotic disorder, and 54% a principal or secondary diagnosis of personality disorder
- Roughly 10% of people convicted of homicide have some form of abnormal mental state at the time of the offence (mania or hypomania, depression, delusions, hallucinations, or other psychotic symptoms), and of these two-thirds have psychosis
- ⚠ Approximately 10% of homicides are committed by people who have had some contact with mental health services in the past year.

Victims

Victims of homicides by people with mental disorder are more likely to be acquaintances than strangers. There is debate as to whether the rate of homicide by people with mental disorder is stable or falling in the UK. Women with mental disorder who commit homicide are most likely to kill family members.

Infanticide and related behaviours

The intentional killing of an infant (a child aged up to 12 months) by its mother is conventionally regarded as separate from other homicides in many cultures, because of the effect childbirth and the stresses of early child-rearing are believed to have on the mother's mind. There is a separate infanticide offence (📖 p.IV.344) in some jurisdictions.

Infanticide is associated with:

- A diagnosis of depression
- Postpartum psychosis
- Maternal childhood sexual abuse.

Neonaticide is the killing of a newborn child. It has been suggested that neonaticide is not typically associated with mental disorder.

Filicide is the killing of a child (of any age) by a parent. One proposition for a categorization of filicide is:

- Altruistic
- Psychotic
- Accidental
- Unwanted child
- Spousal revenge.

Up to 50% of women who kill their children will have some form of mental disorder. Categorization oversimplifies and most cases will be multifactorial.

Murder-suicide

Murder-suicide—that is, the suicide of the perpetrator directly after the homicide—is uncommon but often results in high levels of media attention. Most occur in intimate relationships and are perpetrated by men. Substance misuse and previous criminal history is of less significance than with other homicides. Depression is suggested as being more common in perpetrators of murder-suicide when compared to other homicide (20–60%).

Clinical issues

Many people charged with a homicide offence will have a psychiatric assessment. There are a number of specific clinical (📖 pp.II.90–II.111) and legal and practical (📖 pp.II.112–II.125) issues that must be taken into account when assessing someone alleged to have killed, including the risk of suicide (📖 p.II.136) by the perpetrator.

Murder-suicide rates have been found to be between 0.2–04 per 100,000 citizens per year. See Table 2.1 for simple homicide rates.

Table 2.1 Crimes recorded by the police—rates per 100,000 citizens per year, 2007

Crime	England & Wales	Scotland	Northern Ireland	Republic of Ireland
Homicide	1.4	2.2	1.7	2.0

Rates derived from Eurostat homicide statistics. Intentional killing of a person, including murder, manslaughter, euthanasia, and infanticide. Excluding attempted (uncompleted) homicide. Excluding causing death by dangerous driving, abortion and help with suicide.

Non-fatal assaults

Non-fatal assault in this context is taken to exclude sexual assault. Any attempt to compare statistics is hampered by differing definitions of assault. In E&W approximately one million offences against the person are recorded each year (some of these offences will not result in any injury) but this encompasses the very broad definition of assault; see also Table 2.2. The majority of injuries sustained include bruising, black eyes, and minor cuts:

- Most serious violence (including homicide): 2%
- Less serious wounding: 45%
- Assault without injury: 23%
- Harassment: 25%
- Other: 5%.

Jurisdictions vary (see 📖 p.IV.346 for a discussion of laws on assault) but in English law a person is guilty of *common assault* if he intentionally or recklessly causes another person to apprehend the application of immediate unlawful force. Assaults therefore include being put in fear of violence, and can include psychological assaults. Some types of stalking behaviour fall within this definition. A person is guilty of *battery* if he intentionally or recklessly applies unlawful force to the body of another person. The distinction between assault and battery is often misunderstood, especially by non-lawyers.

Consent

Assault is defined by the presence or threat of unlawful force. Force is defined as 'unlawful' if there is an absence of consent; and if the force is not justified in terms of self-defence, necessity, or the reasonable discipline of a child. In theory, it is possible for people to consent to the use of force against them; although this remains legally contentious where certain types of injury result (such as for the purpose of sexual pleasure).[*]

It is the gaining of consent that protects doctors from charges of battery; although in practice, failure to gain consent results in civil actions not criminal because of the lack of malicious intent involved.

Offenders

The majority of offenders who commit non-fatal assaults are young men aged between 16–30 and this group are also most likely to be victims. The next most likely group of victims are women who are victims of domestic violence.

Clinical issues

The majority of people treated in forensic psychiatric settings have committed non-fatal, non-sexual assaults. There is a strong relationship between mental disorder and committing assault (📖 p.II.31).

Men who are repeatedly violent and who are imprisoned may be offered psycho-education groups in prison during their sentence.

In prison samples, 9% of people convicted of non-fatal violence have been found to have schizophrenia. Other studies have repeatedly found higher rates of mental disorder in people convicted of non-fatal assaults.

---

[*] The legal ruling that consent could, at least sometimes, be no defence to a charge of battery arose from wartime cases in which a soldier would consent to another shooting them (for example) in the foot, to enable them to avoid further active service. It has been extended in E&W to cases in which an individual consented to sexual violence against them (for example, nailing their penis to a board) for the purpose of masochistic pleasure, although such rulings have been partly overturned by the European Court of Human Rights (📖 p.IV.326).

Many perpetrators of non-fatal assaults are under the influence of alcohol at the time; and substance misuse services may meet the needs of service users with histories of non-fatal assaults. Antisocial personality disorder is highly prevalent in populations of people convicted of non-fatal assault but it is unusual for this group of people to be assessed or treated by forensic psychiatrists; unless there is also an established history of mental illness, or some other psychological disorder.

Table 2.2 Crimes recorded by the police—rates per 100,000 citizens per year, 2007

Crime	England & Wales	Scotland	Northern Ireland	Republic of Ireland
Violent crime	2033	524	1850	1453

Rates derived from Eurostat violent crime statistics. Violence against the person (such as physical assault), robbery (stealing by force or by threat of force), and sexual offences (including rape and sexual assault).

Fire-setting behaviours

There are 3500 fires deliberately started per week in the UK. This results in 50 injuries and two deaths on average, and costs around £25 million per week (see also Table 2.3). About one in four fires is intentionally set. Arson (p.IV.350) is the crime of maliciously, voluntarily and wilfully setting fire to a building or other property that is owned by another, or for an improper purpose, such as to collect insurance. Not all fire-setting behaviours result in a charge of arson, and not all fire-setting is pathological. Distinguishing pathological arson related to mental disorder is not always easy.

Pathological fire-setting as defined in ICD10 (p.App. 1.601), is characterized by multiple acts of, or attempts at, setting fire to property or other objects, without apparent motive, and by a persistent preoccupation with subjects related to fire and burning. There may also be an abnormal interest in fire-engines and other fire-fighting equipment, in other things associated with fires, and in calling out the fire service.

Pyromania is defined in DSM-IV as a pattern of deliberate setting of fires for pleasure or satisfaction derived from the relief of tension experienced before the fire-setting. Pyromania can only be diagnosed if there has been purposeful setting of fire on at least two occasions. There is usually arousal before the act and relief or gratification after the act. It is in the category of impulse control disorders.

Juvenile fire setters (e.g. aged 10–18 in E&W) account for at least half of all arrests for fire-setting. The majority of fires are started by children aged 5–10 years, who do not understand the dangers of playing with fire.

Even though the majority of child-set fires are started out of curiosity, not malice, the damage caused, both in human and economic costs, is real and sometimes devastating. Factors determining criminal intent include the fire setter's age, the nature and extent of the individual's fire-setting history, and the intent.

More *female* patients than males in high secure hospitals have an index offence of arson. There are also high prevalence rates of self-harm among this group. Women are more likely to set fire to property which is invested with emotional meaning (communicative act). Motives include revenge, hatred, and jealousy.

Clinical issues

There are various theoretical models of arson including: pyromania/ abnormal fascination with fire/displaced sexual drive; displaced aggression; or a communicative act. There is no definite association between sexual gratification and fire-setting. Fire-setting may be chronic or episodic; some may set fires frequently as a way of relieving tension, others apparently do so only during periods of unusual stress in their lives. Psychiatric disorders may be present in fire-setters. However, there is no direct relationship between particular mental disorders and arson.

- 14–65% of arsonists fulfil criteria for personality disorder
- 8–35% of arsonists fulfil criteria for psychosis
- 8–48% of arsonists fulfil criteria for learning disability
- 35–66% of offenders are intoxicated, and alcohol misuse is likely to be a significant factor.

Assessment of a fire setter needs to include: investigation of early experience of fire; personality assessment; a functional analysis—antecedent events, including general setting conditions, specific psychosocial stimuli and triggering events, and positive consequences that might reinforce future fire-setting (fire-setting is a powerful act that might result in the perpetrator gaining a lot of attention); and the individual's current understanding of fire-setting and risk.

Additional clinical factors that should be specifically considered are:
- Parental violence and alcoholism
- History of attempted suicide
- Psychotic or revenge motive
- Social skills
- Other family dysfunction
- Evidence of sadistic traits or psychopathy (📖 p.II.66).

Treatment in addition to the treatment of any underlying mental disorder, amounts to risk management (📖 p.II.202) and might include fire-safety training, increasing responsibility for dangerousness of arson, social/coping skills, anger and/or aggression management, self-esteem work, and relapse prevention.

Table 2.3 Crimes recorded by the police—rates per 100,000 citizens per year, 2007

Crime	England & Wales	Scotland	Northern Ireland	Republic of Ireland
Criminal damage	1916	2204	1599	945
Arson	73	90	128	47
BCS vandalism	4973			
FB deliberate fires	118			

BCS refers to the British Crime Survey (📖 p.II.18)—that is, figures as reported by victims.
FB refers to figures from the Fire Brigade on the presumed causes of fires.

Stalking behaviours

Definitions

The essence of the various definitions of staking is intruding upon, or attempting to communicate with, the victim in an unwanted fashion. Examples of stalking behaviours are shown in Box 2.1. For research purposes, the behaviours are typically required to occur at least 10 times and to last at least 2 weeks, but victims may perceive themselves as being stalked well before (or sometimes only well after) that threshold has been met.

Box 2.1 Examples of stalking behaviours

- Unwanted telephone calls, emails, letters, faxes, or notes
- Following the victim or loitering near their home or workplace
- Giving unwanted gifts or ordering unwanted services (taxi, pizza, etc.)
- Issuing threats, including death threats
- Intimidating, slandering, libelling, or officially complaining about them
- Damaging property at their home or workplace
- Physical or sexual assault.

Relevant crimes

The more serious behaviours associated with stalking are often crimes in their own right, such as assault (📖 p.IV.346), sexual assault or rape (📖 p.IV.348), making threats to kill (📖 p.IV.357) or criminal damage (📖 p.IV.350). In addition, a few jurisdictions such as Scotland and New York define specific stalking offences,[*] and many others, including E&W, define harassment offences (📖 p.IV.358).

---

[*] Defined in New York extremely broadly, as when a person 'intentionally, and for no legitimate purpose, engages in a course of conduct directed at a specific person, and knows or reasonably should know that such conduct' would cause 'material harm' to their mental or emotional health, or would be likely to 'cause reasonable fear' of material harm to their own health, safety, property or employment, or that of their family, friends or acquaintances.

Epidemiology

A variety of victim studies have shown that 2–15% of Western populations have been stalked, with the lower figures found in large-scale random population samples and higher ones in selected samples (e.g. university counselling services). Mean figures tend to be around 8% of the population, with higher rates for women and lower for men.

⚠ Psychiatrists and other mental health workers appear to be at particular risk; one study of British psychiatrists found that 10.7% met the research definition of having been stalked, and 21.3% experienced themselves as having been stalked.

There is much less evidence on what proportion of the population, or of offenders, or of patients, exhibit stalking behaviours.

Typology

There is no single agreed classification of stalkers. One widely-adopted typology is that of Mullen, which comprises:
- *Intimacy seekers* responding to loneliness by attempting to establish a close relationship
- *Rejected* responding to an unwelcome end to a close relationship by actions intended to lead to reconciliation, or reparation, or both
- *Incompetent* would-be suitors seeking a partner by socially inappropriate methods
- *Resentful* responding to a perceived insult by actions aimed at revenge and vindication
- *Predatory* pursuing desires for control and sexual gratification.

Clinical issues

Two studies found that, amongst stalkers known to have a mental disorder, the commonest conditions were functional psychoses (📖 p.II.54) and personality disorder (📖 p.II.58). Another study of patients in high security suggested that the following factors were associated with stalking:
- A sexual index offence, or a sexual motive for the index offence
- A lack of physical contact with the victim
- Little or no previous acquisitive offending (📖 p.IV.354)
- Amongst those who kill, a finding of diminished responsibility (📖 p.V.491).

Risks

Stalking behaviours often escalate, and often come to include violent behaviours; stalking is therefore a risk factor for violence. Stalking with a sexual motive may be a risk factor for sexual violence.

Prognosis

Stalkers of all types tend, by definition, to persist in their behaviours, and they often find it difficult to desist even with support and/or when facing criminal sanctions. However, change is possible, particularly in those with an underlying mental disorder that can be treated.

Management

Key principles of management include:
- Having the victim avoid confrontation (or indeed, any further contact) with the stalker, as this will only reinforce the behaviour
- If the victim has a professional relationship with the stalker, transferring their care to another professional immediately
- Offering counselling and support to the victim and putting them in touch with professional and legal advice; advising them to inform their employer etc. of the stalking at the earliest opportunity
- If the stalker has a mental disorder, treating the underlying disorder if possible.

Sexual offending against adults

Sexual offending must be distinguished from the much larger category of sexually inappropriate behaviour (see also ⌨ pp.II.94, II.134, II.197). Whereas the former refers to specific legally-defined crimes such as rape, buggery and sexual assault (⌨ p.IV.348), which may differ in the detail of their definition from one jurisdiction to another, the latter is a term often used in clinical scenarios to describe any inappropriate behaviour or action deemed to have a sexual motive. This can range from implicit sexualized suggestions and other incidents that would not amount to an offence, to acts of serious sexual violence.

Sexual offending as an aspect of mental disorder

DSM-IV and ICD10 (⌨ p.II.109) contain a number of paraphilias (⌨ p.II.74, the DSM term; the ICD term is 'disorders of sexual preference'), although many would consider their definitions to be outdated. They are clinical categories defined by behaviour and do not automatically correspond to a criminal offence; they include exhibitionism, fetishism, frotteurism, paedophilia, sadomasochism, fetishistic transvestism, and voyeurism. All are grouped under the general heading.

Epidemiology

Sexual offences account for approximately 1% of the crimes recorded by the police in E&W. These statistics (see Table 2.4) represent an underestimate of offences. Sexual offences are often not reported; allegations are withdrawn because the victim finds the process too unpleasant or wishes to move on; the evidence may be too weak for the prosecution to proceed or the court to convict. Surveys of victimization (⌨ p.II.19) give much higher estimates of sexual offending: for example, the 2000 British Crime Survey found that 18% of rapes (as defined by the victim) were reported; another UK study found that 6% of reported rapes resulted in conviction.

Sexual offences are very often committed by someone known to the victim. For example, only 14% of rapes in one 2007 UK study were committed by a stranger; another study of unreported rapes found that 56% were committed by a current or ex-partner, 16% by other acquaintances, 11% by 'dates', 10% by 'other intimates', and 8% by strangers.

Table 2.4 Crimes recorded by the police—rates per 100,000 citizens per year, 2007

Crime	England & Wales	Scotland	Northern Ireland	Republic of Ireland
Rape	23.4	20.5	23.9	8.3
Sexual assault	42.9	32.4	21.3	18.7
Other	26.7	74.5	24.6	7.9

Rates include rape and sexual assault against men as well as women in most jurisdictions. Scottish figures include attempted rapes. 'Other' varies between jurisdictions and includes offences such as grooming, soliciting for prostitution, incest, lewd behaviour and 'unlawful carnal knowledge'.

Association between sexual offending and mental disorder

Sexual offences are not generally correlated with any specific mental disorder, and the link, if any, between sexual offending and mental disorder is not as thoroughly researched as is the link with violent offending.

▶The great majority of sex offenders do not have a major mental illness (no more than 10%). Even in those that do, there may be no causal or contributory relationship between the disorder and the offending. However, there is good evidence that functional psychotic disorders (📖 p.II.54) can be associated with some sexual offences through:

- Disinhibition, arousal, or irritability secondary to psychosis
- Direct 'psychotic drive' (e.g. command auditory hallucinations)
- Cognitive impairments or distortions secondary to psychosis
- Poor social skills related to negative schizophrenic symptoms.

Overall, the psychosexual profiles of mentally ill and non-mentally ill sex offenders are similar, however, and the presence of mental illness alone can provide only a partial explanation of sexual offending. In particular, research suggests that those with psychotic disorders may be psychotic when assessed but often this appears to be a reaction to the stress of arrest and imprisonment, with no evidence that they were psychotic at the time of the offence; and very few such offenders suggest that such symptoms explain their behaviour.

Other mental disorders may be associated with sexual offending, including personality disorder (📖 p.II.58, found in 30–50% of sex offenders—especially ASPD, 📖 p.II.60, and psychopathy, 📖 p.II.66); substance dependence (📖 p.II.56), learning disability (📖 p.II.80), Asperger's syndrome (📖 p.II.76), and brain damage (📖 p.II.82). Studies of personality in sex offenders show that some (but not, for example, rapists) tend to have more schizoid, avoidant, depressive, dependent, self-defeating and schizotypal personality traits, compared to other offenders.

The importance of conviction

When people with major mental disorders commit sexual offences, there is a strong tendency for them to be diverted (📖 p.II.216) out of the criminal justice system to hospital. While this might enable them to receive initial treatment more rapidly than if they remain in the criminal justice system, it can complicate (or even render ineffective) any future psychological work, as the lack of a conviction allows the patient to deny their commission of, or responsibility for, the offending behaviour.

Sexual offending against children

Sexual offences against children, mostly by adults (referred to in this section as 'child sexual offending') can involve the same act as sexual offences against adults, but they are usually separately classified. Internet-based child sexual offending is increasingly considered as a separate category requiring new assessment tools and treatment interventions.

Child sexual offending as an aspect of mental disorder

The mental disorder most strongly identified with sexual offending against children is paedophilia (📖 p.II.74). DSM-IV describes paedophilia as a paraphilia in which a person has acted on intense sexual urges towards children, or experiences recurrent sexual urges towards and fantasies about children that cause distress or interpersonal difficulty.

Defining paedophilia as a mental disorder carries no implication about criminal responsibility, or the lack of it; nevertheless, the term 'paedophile' has been adopted in popular culture, particularly in the UK, to refer to anyone convicted of a sexual offence against a child, although the broader use of this term does not accurately reflect the heterogeneity of this group of offenders. Many authors prefer the term 'child molester', because it does not presume a pathological basis for the behaviour.

Epidemiology

Recorded rates of offences against children are generally unreliable. A few of the better-established statistics are:

- Up to 40% of people report having experienced some type of sexual abuse as a child although the rates vary markedly in different studies
- Girls are 2–5 times more likely than boys to suffer sexual abuse
- The incidence of sexual crimes perpetrated against children in the UK is 0.5–2 per 1000 children per year
- 70–90% of sexual abusers are someone the child knows; 33–50% of abusers of girls, and 10–20% of abusers of boys, are family members
- Less than 5% of reported offences against children are committed by women
- The actual proportion of abuse perpetrated by women against children may be as high as 20%, based upon victim studies
- Up to 15% of sexual offences are committed by adolescent offenders.

As with sexual offending against adults (📖 p.II.42), sexual offences against children frequently go unreported, and even if reported to the police or social services, rarely result in conviction. One 2004 study estimated that fewer than 2% of such offences result in conviction. Moreover, even convicted offenders are seldom reconvicted for committing such offences again: as few as 20%, according to one estimate.

Association between sexual offending and mental disorder

There is no known causal relationship between mental disorder and child sexual offending. Some recent studies suggest that psychosis, personality disorder and substance abuse are all less common amongst child sexual offenders than rapists (for whom, like other sex offenders against adults, 📖 p.II.43, there is more evidence of association with mental disorder).

There is some evidence to suggest that mood disorders and anxiety disorders are unusually prevalent in child sex offenders and that on personality assessment child sex offenders have more prominent neurotic and affective traits when compared to rapists.

Mental disorder in women convicted of all sexual offences may be more common than in men, although the relatively small numbers involved make it difficult to offer definitive statements. A greater proportion of female perpetrated sexual offences are against children compared to male perpetrated sexual offences.

Internet-based offending

The Internet has made child pornography more affordable, accessible and anonymous than ever before. It has either revealed an enormous previously unrecognized sexual interest in children, or has resulted in an enormous increase in such interest. There are estimated to be a total of over 100,000 hits every day on illegal child pornography websites.

People charged with Internet-based child sex offences often have difficulties with sexual self-regulation and significant numbers of life events prior to arrest. It has been postulated that emotional dysregulation and intimacy deficits are the primary drivers for Internet-based offenders; and that viewing child pornography helps people with depressive and negative mood states find solace.

The majority of Internet-based offenders have no previous convictions. The great majority of solely Internet-based offenders do not reoffend, or escalate to committing contact sexual offences. However, Internet-based offenders with a previous conviction for any other offence are more likely to reoffend or escalate.

The following typology of Internet-based offenders has been proposed:
- *Emotional satisfaction:* people who are emotionally distressed and who seek solace and comfort through the use of Internet pornography
- *Intimacy deficits:* socially isolated people, who may satisfy some of their needs for intimacy by using Internet pornography
- *Hypersexuality:* people with high levels of sexual behaviour who use Internet pornography compulsively.

Other types of sexual offending

Indecent exposure

This is the offence of removing clothes so as to reveal the genitals or (in some jurisdictions) other sexual parts of the body (see 📖 p.IV.348). It may occur as exhibitionism, or a paraphilia (📖 p.II.74) in which such behaviours cause distress and interfere with normal daily life—but there is no general association between indecent exposure and mental disorder. The focus of most research is on contact sexual offences and there is a tendency for indecent exposure sometimes to be regarded as a nuisance rather than a criminal act.

- Up to 4% of men and 2% of women report witnessing at least one exhibitionist act, making indecent exposure one of the commonest sexual offences
- Up to a third of exhibitionists will also commit a contact sexual offence.

There is no established risk assessment tool specifically for indecent exposure, but it is suggested that the same risk factors as for other sexual offences are relevant. In addition, exhibitionism is associated with decreased satisfaction with life, and with higher scores on tests of impulsivity and risk-taking.

Previous attempts to categorize exhibitionists have revolved around motivation. A common distinction drawn, although it has not been empirically validated, is between the inhibited, guilty exhibitionist (who if male, typically has a flaccid penis during the exposure) and the angry, aggressive exhibitionist (who, if male, typically has an erect penis).

Voyeurism

Voyeurism is the behaviour of spying on people undressing or engaging in sexual activity. If done knowingly without the consent of those spied upon, it is an offence in some jurisdictions, including E&W, Scotland, and NI (see 📖 p.IV.349). Up to 11% of men and 4% of women admit to engaging in behaviour of this nature. There is no known association between voyeurism and mental disorder.

Pornography offences

Use of deviant (sometimes illegal) pornography may be associated with coercive sexual behaviour and sexual aggression although the nature of the association is not fully understood. The association is frequently suggested to be mediated via other risk factors. There is no known link with any mental disorder.

Incest

There is no known association between mental disorder and sexual activity with children, siblings or other family members.

Bestiality

The prevalence of bestiality is not known. There is some suggestion of high prevalence of bestial behaviour amongst adolescent offenders (10% in one study) and that this group may have higher rates of mental disorder. There is limited evidence to suggest that bestiality is more common among psychiatric patients when compared to general medical patients.

Necrophilia

Necrophilia (sexual activity with a corpse) is not known to be associated with any psychiatric disorder.

Abuse of position

Certain sexual offending may relate to perpetrators abusing their position and power against vulnerable victims, including children and people with mental impairment. Doctors, teachers, staff at children's homes or learning disability hostels, prison officers and others all have opportunities to abuse their position of trust in this way. There is no association with mental disorder, except insofar as people with mental disorder are at increased risk of victimization (📖 p.II.141).

Motivations for sexual offending

A variety of psychological and criminological theories have been suggested to explain why people (mostly men) sexually offend, and the processes by which this occurs. Key aspects include sexual arousal, justificatory beliefs and traits of antisocial personality disorder (📖 p.II.60).

The main theories are summarized here, except those seen as outdated (e.g. the assertion by some feminist theorists that rape is a normal behaviour for men, albeit one that almost all men manage to suppress).

Factors contributing to sexual offending

- Predispositional and *biological vulnerabilities* such as hormonal abnormalities or an inability to distinguish aggressive and sexual impulses
- *Childhood experiences* of physical or sexual abuse, neglect or family disruption, especially experiences that predispose to anxious, insecure or dismissive attachment styles
- Deviant *sexual preferences* including coercive sexual fantasies and sexual arousal to images of children—though both are reported in non-offender populations as well as amongst offenders
- *Intimacy deficits*: difficulty establishing and maintaining intimate relationships, and strong feelings of loneliness for which others are blamed
- Underlying beliefs and *cognitive distortions*. In the context of sexual offending, the latter are errors of thinking that typically exclude others' perspectives, particularly those of a victim, and allow justification of otherwise unacceptable behaviours. They may result from inability to process information adequately. Examples include:

Child sex offenders
- The child was sexually mature
- The child knew what they were doing
- Children enjoy sexual contact
- It doesn't do any harm
- I'm helping the child's sexual development
- Adults can do what they want with children.

Adult sex offenders
- Women are devious
- Women use sex for their own gain
- She got what she deserved
- Women never say what they mean
- Women like to be dominated
- Men cannot control themselves.

Schema held by sex offenders

These core beliefs about the nature of the world, also known in this context as 'implicit theories', underpin offence-facilitating distorted cognitions. Two have been proposed for all sex offenders:

- *Entitlement:* the offender may believe he is superior to his victims and therefore entitled to demand any sexual activity he desires
- *Dangerous World:* the offender feels the need to gain control over a hostile and abusive world. Women or children may be considered easy targets for control, and children a 'safe haven' from the world.

The following three schema are specific to child sex offenders:

- *Children as Sexual Beings:* the offender believes that children are inherently sexual and capable of choosing to participate in sexual acts
- *Nature of Harm:* the belief that there is no harm in sexual activity with children and it may in fact be beneficial to them. There may be a view that physical harm is the only way of causing harm
- *Uncontrollable World:* a fatalistic belief that events, emotions, and sexual feelings are out of the offender's control.

Further schema for adult sex offenders are:

- *Unknowable Women:* the offender believes women are fundamentally different to men and cannot be understood; from the man's perspective they appear devious and encounters are therefore adversarial
- *Women as Sex Objects:* the belief that women are always sexually receptive, even if they do not realize it, and cannot be hurt by sexual activity as long as there is no physical harm
- *Uncontrollable Male Sex Drive:* the offender believes that men's sexual energy can reach dangerously high levels if women do not provide opportunities for sexual release, and that an aroused man cannot stop until he reaches orgasm.

Widely-accepted schema for adult female sex offenders have not yet been established.

Theories of sexual offending

Sexual offending against children

- *Finkelhor's four conditions model.* Four complementary factors that provide motivation for sexual offending: emotional congruence (children seen as special and as meeting offender's emotional needs); sexual arousal to stimuli involving children; blockage (inability to meet emotional needs through adult relationships); overcoming internal and external inhibitions (e.g. beliefs, opportunity, the child's resistance)
- *Wolf's multifactor model.* Childhood adversity leads to personality traits associated with the development of deviant sexual interests and of low-self esteem. The result is a cycle of fantasy, grooming or offending, cognitive distortion, and further worsened self-image
- *Ward & Siegert's pathways model.* Different routes to offending: deviant (impersonal, purely physical) sexual scripts; intimacy deficits (treating children as 'pseudo-partners'); emotional dysregulation (offending as a way of managing anger, low mood or low self-esteem); antisocial cognitions; and a combination of the four other pathways.

Sexual offending against adults
- *Hall & Hirschmann's quadripartite model.* Four key vulnerabilities contribute to sexual offending: sexual arousal; cognitions justifying sexual aggression; affective dyscontrol; antisocial personality traits. Offending occurs when a 'critical threshold' is passed
- *Malamuth's confluence model.* Childhood experiences lead to individual differences in six key variables related to sexual promiscuity and hostile masculinity, shown to predict 'rape proclivity': sexual arousal to rape; dominance as a motive for sex; hostility towards women; attitudes facilitating aggression towards women; antisocial personality traits; and sexual experience.

Other types of offending

Criminal offences need to be distinguished from behaviours that may indicate psychopathology. If psychiatrists are involved in assessing individuals charged with or convicted of non-violent offences, then their aim should be to ensure that the criminal offence is not a social or behavioural manifestation of psychopathology that could be addressed therapeutically; or could indicate increased risk of future violence.

Property crime

The bulk of non-violent offences recorded by the police in E&W are offences involving theft of property: from homes, cars, or commercial property. These offences make up 48% of police recorded crime; and even this may be an under-representation of actual offences committed. Other types of property offence recorded are vandalism and criminal damage.

Perpetrators of theft are rarely mentally ill or personality disordered; social factors (📖 p.II.23) are more relevant. They are likely to be disadvantaged or poor; and to come from urban economically deprived areas.

Some offenders may steal to finance a drug or alcohol addiction. For some young offenders, repetitive property crime may be the start of an offending trajectory (📖 p.II.30) that will escalate in severity. For other young offenders, property crime will reflect temporary delinquency. Repetitive thefts of single items may reflect an obsessive compulsive disorder or a paraphilia (📖 p.II.74).

In terms of risk assessment, the question is whether the pattern of acquisitive crime is combined with violent offending or other types of crime; which may suggest a more generally antisocial attitude.

Breaching legal sanction

A common form of other recordable offence is breaches of legal sanctions: violations of court orders, failures to pay fines and breaches of probation or parole. As previously described, the pattern of offending is important: repetitive breaches of legal sanctions may be indicative of impulsivity or highly antisocial attitudes. Repetitive breaches of sanctions regarding interpersonal contact with ex-partners or children may suggest an erotomanic attachment or stalking (📖 p.II.40); or paranoid or hostile attachments in the context of domestic violence (📖 p.II.21). Stalking behaviours may first be identified as breaches of legal sanction.

Fraud and crimes of deception

Fraud and other acts of deception covers a wide variety of criminal behaviours. There is no suggestion of a specific relationship between mental disorder and these offences, although repetitive fraud or deception may be associated with psychopathy (p.II.66) or with factitious disorder (p.II.87). If mental disorder is present then the assessment of harm potentially caused by fraud is complex and may invoke a conundrum regarding the location of hospital treatment if required; large scale fraud may not satisfy the risk criteria for secure psychiatric services but the severity of the offence in law may well require this.

Drug offences

A conviction for a drug offence will not ordinarily indicate forensic psychiatric involvement, although drug misuse is common amongst mentally disordered offenders. Serious drug offences committed by people with mental disorder who require treatment may imply difficulties in assessing the risk of harm (supplying illegal drugs may be harmful in a societal sense but not in the direct and individual way that harm is usually addressed), and as with fraud there may be the necessity for secure detention during treatment because of the exigencies of the criminal justice system.

There are many hundreds of other specific offences and offence behaviours which have not been described here, because they are relatively uncommon and/or are of little relevance to forensic psychiatry.

Why divide violent & sexual offending?

The division of violent from sexual offending is in a contemporary sense purely legally determined, but it has wider implications for individual and societal attitudes. The demarcation of some public wrongs as 'sexual' has a long tradition in law. However, the earliest sexual offences were largely confined to rape, sexual abuse of children and anal sex (even if consensual).

Patriarchal dominance

The distinct offences of rape, abduction, or forced marriage reflected the position of women as the property of their fathers or husbands. Whilst it was recognized that there was an offence against the woman herself, the wrong done was also a financial one, since important property arrangements between social subgroups were made through marriage. Rape was therefore not only a criminal offence; it contained elements of a civil wrong or tort (p.V.512).

Religious belief

The criminalization of anal sex (first known as sodomy, then later buggery) has its roots in Judeo-Christian religious proscription. Consent, or injury were both irrelevant, because of its perceived offensive nature; and both parties were subject to punishment.

Incorporation into modern law

Sexual abuse of children was regarded in the 18th century as an offence against the person. Indecent assaults on women and children were also the subject of criminal proceedings in the 18th and 19th centuries.

Consent versus assent

The 20th century saw a much more marked distinction drawn between sexual and other offences, such that they are recorded and thought about separately. The commonest form of sexual offence is sexual assault (📖 p.IV.348), and the next most common is unlawful sexual intercourse, such as intercourse with a child under 16. The basis for the distinction may rest on issues of *consent*. Non-sexual offences against the person involve the use or threat of unlawful force (📖 p.II.36); whereas in indecent assault, or unlawful sexual intercourse, unlawful force (or even the implicit threat of it) is not required, and the 'victim' may have agreed to the act (i.e. assented), even if they have not legally consented*.

Is it a question of force?

In most jurisdictions, violent and non-violent sexual offences are classified together in law, and separated from non-sexual violent offences. This classification obscures the intrinsically violent nature of sexual offences such as sexual assault, perhaps because in cases where the victim assented or passively complied as a result of the fear they experienced, there may be a perception that no force was used. This is despite the fact that the mere threat of force causing fear of violence is sufficient for non-sexual offences such as common assault (📖 p.IV.346) and affray (📖 p.IV.352).

Rape

In rape (📖 p.IV.348) in particular, there is a danger that the offence may continue to be seen as a non-violent offence because of its separate classification in law, and perhaps because of concerns about false allegations. The prevalence of false allegations is unknown, but they are likely to be over-represented because, by definition, they are always reported, whereas true allegations are known to be under-reported.

The separation of rape from violent offences in law is not necessarily justified. Risk factors for rape include previous convictions for violence or other criminality, high levels of psychopathy (📖 p.II.66) and sexual arousal to violent material. Most convicted rapists have previous convictions for violence; and a subgroup graduate from non-contact sexual offences such as indecent exposure to sexual assault and ultimately rape.

What questions are raised?

- To what extent should we base definitions of offences on the victim's perception of violence, as opposed to the intent of the perpetrator?
- Does it make sense to distinguish the use of force against one area of the body from other areas of the body?
- How should we categorize those offences that are genital in nature and content, but do not involve physical force or contact, such as indecent exposure; offences involving pornography; and those

---

* Because, for example, they are too young to have the capacity to consent (see Gillick competence, 📖 p.IV.428).

'offences' committed by consenting adults, such as sadomasochistic practices[*]?

A proposal

The classification of sexual offences and violent offences separately potentially creates a mindset that illegal sexual acts are not violence. Reclassification in the following terms would partially address this issue.

- All violence, sexual, or otherwise classified together
- Offences of breach of social taboos classified separately.

Statistics and measurement of crime would therefore correlate with the legal classification.

[*] Sadomasochistic acts can be prosecuted as assault in E&W despite the consent of the 'victim', and despite the ECtHR ruling that it was possible for the victim to consent to being assaulted in this way, because the ECtHR also ruled that States could nevertheless criminalize such behaviour on the grounds of its social unacceptability.

Mental disorders in forensic psychiatry*

* This chapter provides clinical information in a manner which emphasizes the forensic aspects of the conditions described, focusing mainly on associated risks of harm, and the management of those risks. For comprehensive clinical information concerning each clinical condition we recommend that you consult the *Oxford Handbook of Psychiatry*, or another general psychiatry or specialist text.

Functional psychosis

Much of the forensic psychiatric research on mental disorder and violence has used severe mental illness or psychosis as the focus of study. Psychotic states are states of mind that include:

- Altered perception of external reality
- Distorted cognitions
- Disordered mood (mania, depression, fear)
- Hyperarousal secondary to these.

Prevalence of functional psychosis

- General population: 0.4%
- General psychiatric patients: at least 5%
- Prisoners: 10% male remand; 7% male sentenced; 14% female (both)
- Forensic psychiatric patients: 76%.

Specific psychotic symptoms and violence

Paranoid symptoms involve an abnormal altered interpretation of relationships with others, especially imagining a relationship where none exists (e.g. believing that a news broadcast contains a special coded message for you). Persecutory delusions are paranoid delusions in which the other person is perceived as intending harm.

The risk of acting violently is increased if paranoid symptoms are present, regardless of the specific diagnosis. By definition, patients experiencing paranoia have incorporated other people into their psychotic experiences, and those others may therefore be at risk of harm (from what the patient thinks is necessary self-defence, for instance). This risk is unpredictable in terms of time course, and degree of harm. The violent act may be a result of confusion, panic or fear caused by their symptoms.

Such paranoid psychotic states can occur:

- In schizophrenia and bipolar disorder (📕 p.II.67)
- As a more circumscribed delusional disorder
- Transiently in borderline personality disorder (📕 p.II.61), and
- In conjunction with drug intoxication with (for example) cocaine and amphetamines, or alcohol dependence (📕 p.II.56).

Encapsulated fixed paranoid beliefs may exist in the absence of other types of disordered reality testing (such as hallucinations). Paranoid delusional disorder, which commonly occurs as an exacerbation of paranoid personality disorder (📕 p.II.64), may be particularly resistant to treatment, resulting in persistently high risk to others.

Threat and control override (TCO) symptoms occur most commonly in paranoid schizophrenia. TCO symptoms cause the patient to feel gravely threatened by someone who appears to intend to cause harm and involve the perception of loss of self-control through the operation of external forces (e.g. made actions, severe persecutory delusions or command auditory hallucinations). Unlike other psychotic symptoms, TCO symptoms have been shown in some research studies to be associated with violence[*] but this finding has not been universally replicated. Such symptoms may also be associated with more severe offences.

Schizophrenia and schizoaffective disorder

There is an association between a diagnosis of schizophrenia or schizoaffective disorder and violence, demonstrated in studies employing various epidemiological methods. Violence risk is increased approximately four-fold, but this is a small effect compared to factors such as substance misuse, gender, age, and other risk factors for offending (📖 p.II.23).

The association appears to depend on the presence of acute psychotic symptoms, particularly paranoid and TCO symptoms as discussed earlier.

Delusional disorders

Delusional disorders may be associated with violence in the individual patient. An increased risk of violence may occur in conjunction with the following categories of delusions:

- Persecutory delusions (believing the victim means you harm)
- Misidentification delusions (e.g. believing the victim is in fact another person whom you intend to harm)
- Delusions of jealousy (e.g. believing that the victim is cheating on you)
- Delusions of love (believing that the victim is in love with you, whereupon a sign of rejection that cannot be rationalized away may result in violence)
- Querulous delusions (beliefs that give ground for complaint against the victim).

Morbid jealousy (Othello syndrome) is a syndrome that can occur in conjunction with many psychiatric diagnoses and is not necessarily psychotic. The core feature is an abnormal belief of partner infidelity.[†] This is often accompanied by intensive seeking of evidence to support the belief. It may be difficult to distinguish from paranoid personality disorder, or from extreme but non-pathological jealousy.

Erotomania (De Clerambault's syndrome) is a syndrome that usually affects women. The core feature is that a person of importance is in love with her. The belief is often considered to be psychotic and seen in people diagnosed with schizophrenia or delusional disorder.

---

[*] This research finding refers to an association at the population level: that is, the group of patients with TCO symptoms are more often violent than those without such symptoms. See the discussion on considering population versus individual risks as part of risk assessment (📖 p.II.130). The statements elsewhere in these topics about certain symptoms increasing risk of violence in patients are clinically-observed correlations in individual patients, but not backed up by large-scale research studies.
[†] The diagnosis is independent of whether the partner is, in fact, being unfaithful, since it is based upon failure of reality testing.

Induced delusional disorder is a form of delusional disorder experienced by an individual in prolonged, intimate contact with a person with psychosis. It is also known as 'folie à deux'—arguably wrongly, as the dominant partner is independently delusional. It is a rare condition, but sometimes associated with violent offending by both individuals (for example, see the case of *R v Windle*, 📖 p.App. 3.648).

Who is at risk?
▶ Contrary to the media perception, most victims of violent crime perpetrated by people with psychosis are not strangers but are relatives, partners, or acquaintances. Approximately 60% of victims are family members with no more than 10% being completely unknown to the perpetrator with schizophrenia.

☞ What is the risk?
- ⚠ People diagnosed with a serious mental illness/psychosis are approximately 4–6 times as likely to commit a violent offence
- The link between psychosis and non-violent offending is not well established
- Less than 10% of all violence is attributable to severe mental illness
- In any given year the probability of a person diagnosed with schizophrenia committing homicide is approximately 1 in 3000
- Approximately 5–10% of homicides are committed by people with schizophrenia (higher figures come from Sweden, lower from UK).

The presence of comorbid personality disorder increases the risk of violence in patients with functional psychosis almost twofold; drug or alcohol abuse also increases it very significantly. See 📖 pp.II.31–II.34 for more details.

Alcohol & drug misuse and dependence

Misuse of alcohol or drugs is common in MDOs. ▶Moreover, having a mental disorder doubles the risk of alcohol misuse or dependence, and quadruples the risk of drug misuse or dependence; having comorbid mental illness and personality disorder increases the risk still further. The management of substance misuse is therefore an integral part of the role of the forensic psychiatrist—but its treatment in a forensic setting (📖 p.II.148) is particularly difficult.

Prevalence of substance misuse
- General population: misuse 17%; dependence 4.7% alcohol, 2.2% drugs
- General psychiatric patients: 39%
- Sentenced prisoners: 50–63% of men, 33–39% of women
- Remand prisoners: 58% of men, 36% of women
- Forensic psychiatric patients: 40% alcohol, 51% drugs.

The frequency of substance misuse in prison and secure psychiatric hospitals is an indicator of the failure of even intrusive security procedures to prevent contraband items being smuggled into such institutions (see also 📖 p.II.152). On entering prison, substance misusers tend to stop using drugs such as cocaine and amphetamines, but to continue or even begin using heroin; the same does not hold true in secure psychiatric hospitals, where cannabis is the drug of choice, and more readily available.

Comorbidity with other mental disorders

Substance misuse in combination with mental illness or personality disorder, or both, is extremely common amongst forensic psychiatric patients, as indicated by the high rates of substance misuse in this group already described. For example, one study found that a fifth of male patients with schizophrenia were dependent on alcohol by age 27.

> *Features of misuse/dependence that predispose to violence*
> • Acute intoxication—e.g. through disinhibition and disorganization of behaviour
> • Withdrawal states—e.g. through agitation or paranoia
> • Dependence—e.g. through compulsion to obtain the substance.

Associations with offending behaviour

Alcohol and drug misuse is more strongly linked to offending and violence than any other mental disorder. Recent alcohol use is a major risk factor for violent offending, chiefly through its disinhibiting effect on behaviour; half of those who commit assault are drunk at the time, as are two-thirds of those who kill. Illicit drug use is, by contrast, more a risk factor for acquisitive offending, in order to raise money to buy drugs. Recent drug use can be associated with violence, but in the absence of a co-existing psychotic disorder (📖 p.II.54) only certain drugs are associated with increased rates of violence:

• Positive association: cocaine, crack cocaine, amphetamines, anabolic steroids, alcohol, benzodiazepines, cannabis
• No association: opiates, nicotine.

Other aspects of alcohol and substance misuse that may be relevant to offending include:

• The direct effects of withdrawal
• The neuropsychiatric sequelae of prolonged misuse
• The social context (peer group, socioeconomic deprivation, childhood maltreatment), and
• Personality characteristics (e.g. impulsivity and sensation seeking).

▶The combination of substance misuse and mental disorder greatly increases the likelihood of violent offending: by a factor of 25 for patients with schizophrenia who misuse alcohol, compared with a factor of 3.6 for patients with schizophrenia who do not misuse alcohol. Another study showed that, whereas 18% of patients with a major mental disorder will commit violence during the course of a year, the figure rises to 31% for those with comorbid substance misuse, and 43% for those who also have personality disorder (📖 p.II.58).

Other harms associated with misuse and dependence

- *Self-neglect:* chronically intoxicated or dependent users may fail to care for themselves
- *Self-harm and suicide:* dysphoria is caused by withdrawal, and is much more likely to lead to self-harm in those disinhibited by earlier substance use
- *Being a victim of violence:* one third of assault victims are drunk at the time.

Personality disorder

Personality disorders (PDs) are pervasive disorders of affect, arousal, and self-regulation, which result in personal or interpersonal distress or dysfunction. They are disabling conditions, emerging in middle childhood (or at least by very early adulthood), and manifested in adulthood in a variety of signs and symptoms, usually in the context of social relationships. They are frequently comorbid with mental illness and/or substance misuse. There are three main forms (or clusters) in DSM*: cluster A (odd, eccentric), cluster B (flamboyant), and cluster C (avoidant, obsessional).

Prevalence of PD

- General population: 4–44% (24–30% in primary care settings)
- General psychiatric patients: 50%
- Prisoners: 78% male remand, 64% male sentenced, 50% female
- Forensic psychiatric patients: 60–70%.

Whereas all PDs may be found in primary care and general psychiatry, forensic services deal primarily with Cluster B PDs, particularly antisocial (ASPD; 📖 p.II.60), borderline (BPD; 📖 p.II.61), and narcissistic PD (NPD; 📖 p.II.63). These are also associated with rule-breaking and offending, and are more commonly found in forensic populations.

Comorbidity with other mental disorders

It is rare to find an individual with just one PD in forensic clinical populations. Most patients are diagnosed with at least two PDs, and comorbidity with other conditions is extremely common. In BPD, comorbidity with depression is the most common, whereas in ASPD, substance misuse is the most common comorbid condition. In secure forensic services, ASPD and BPD are often comorbid with chronic psychotic illnesses such as schizophrenia.

Symptoms increasing risk of violence in PD

- Altered perception of external reality—brief psychosis or dissociation
- Paranoid cognitions and lowered threat perception threshold
- Dysregulated mood states: especially anger
- Hyperarousal secondary to the three causes above
- Lack of empathy or contempt for distress in others
- Impulsivity and lack of capacity to reflect on actions.

---

* This is the case in DSM-IV (📖 p.II.69). However, at the time of writing the proposed revisions in DSM-5, due for publication in 2013, would sweep away the PD cluster classification and replace it with a new diagnostic model. See 📖 p.App. 1.616 for more information.

How do symptoms impact on risk of offending or violence?

▶ Although risks of self-harm, suicide, and early mortality from any cause are greatly increased in some PDs, the majority of patients with PDs present no increased risk of violence to others. However, there are specific symptoms that do increase the risk of violence in patients with PD.

These symptoms occur most frequently in cluster B disorders, especially BPD and ASPD. Cluster A patients have symptoms related to poor reality testing and paranoid cognitions, but do not have the dysregulated mood or the impulsivity of those in cluster B. Similarly, cluster C individuals may have dysregulated mood states, but not the paranoia which occurs in cluster A. It is often the combination of the symptoms that increases the risk of violence in people with BPD and ASPD. The risk is further increased with other comorbid conditions that are themselves associated with violence, e.g. schizophrenia and substance abuse.

PDs may be manifested as behavioural signs, usually in the context of interpersonal dysfunction. The behavioural signs of ASPD are antisocial and illegal behaviour, whereas the behavioural signs of BPD are repetitive interpersonal dysfunction, which may involve violence.

Assessing risk associated with symptoms and signs in PDs

Most patients with PDs mainly present a risk to themselves, although there is also a strong association with violence (🕮 pp.II.31–II.34). Beyond general approaches to violence risk assessment (🕮 p.II.132), when assessing risk of violence in a patient with PD it is important to consider the following:

- Is there a history of physical violence to self or others; especially in the form of convictions for violence?
- Is there a history of antisocial and unempathic attitudes to the vulnerable, or to carers?
- Is there any insight or curiosity about their capacity for violence, or do they blame others?
- Is there comorbid Axis I or substance misuse disorders? These may increase impulsivity, impair reality testing or act as disinhibitors.

Who is at risk from violent offenders with PD?

▶ As for mental illness, most victims of violent crime perpetrated by people with PDs are family members, partners, or otherwise known to the offender. ⚠ Healthcare professionals may also be at increased risk from offender patients with PD. Children may be at particular risk from women with PDs.

PD and psychiatric injury

PD can also be relevant to claims for compensation after injury (🕮 p.V.514), because it may increase the plaintiff's vulnerability to injury (the so-called eggshell skull rule, 📖 p.V.515), in that damage caused by the defendant may be exacerbated by the presence of the victim's PD (claims for histrionic PD in particular have been upheld).

Antisocial personality disorder

Antisocial personality disorder (ASPD) is commonly associated with offending and rule-breaking behaviour. This is to some extent is a function of the diagnostic criteria, which include persistent criminality and irresponsible behaviour. However, ASPD also includes symptoms such as persistent antisocial attitudes including lack of empathy and impulsivity, which make offending more likely. Individuals with ASPD frequently have a history of conduct disorder* (📖 p.II.79) and ADHD (📖 p.II.77); for the diagnosis of ASPD using the DSM-IV (📖 p.II.109), conduct disorder with onset before 15 years in a required diagnostic criterion. However, although a substantial proportion of young people are delinquent and show brief periods of antisocial behaviour, only a subgroup show antisocial behaviour and attitudes that persist into adulthood (📖 p.II.30), and form the basis for an ASPD diagnosis.

ASPD is distinct from psychopathy (📖 p.II.66). Almost all patients with psychopathy also meet the diagnostic criteria for ASPD, but few patients with ASPD display signs of psychopathy.

Prevalence and comorbidity of ASPD

- General population: 6% (10% male, 2% female)
- General psychiatric patients: 40–50%
- Prisoners: 63% male remand, 49% male sentenced, 21–31% female
- Forensic psychiatric patients: 40–70%.

Individuals with ASPD are rarely seen in primary care, as they are usually not help-seekers. ASPD is common in users of substance misuse services. In forensic populations and the prison population, the prevalence is 40–70%: partly because ASPD individuals by definition are likely to carry out behaviours that will lead to them being selected for these populations. ASPD is more commonly diagnosed in males. However, as for BPD, in more severe manifestations of the condition, the gender gap is reduced. In forensic psychiatric services, ASPD is commonly comorbid with BPD.

How do symptoms impact on risk of offending or violence?

The majority of patients with ASPD are criminal rule breakers, whose main focus is on property crime and deception; especially in the context of comorbid drug use. However, a minority are violent to others. Specific symptoms that increase the risk of violence in ASPD are:
- Drug-induced disturbances of perceived reality
- Paranoid attitudes and cognitions; especially likely if drugs that increase paranoia are abused, such as alcohol, cocaine or amphetamines

---

*Indeed, in DSM-IV conduct disorder is a diagnostic criterion.

- Hyperarousal for any reason
- Persistent lack of empathy from childhood, especially if there is evidence of contempt for distress in others
- Impulsivity and lack of capacity to reflect on actions
- Grandiosity contributes to contempt for others: is especially common in those who also have narcissistic traits.

Assessing risk associated with symptoms and signs in ASPD

▶ An ASPD diagnosis increases the risk of violence (📖 pp.II.31–II.34) by a factor of 10. Beyond general approaches to risk assessment (📖 p.II.130), when assessing risk in a patient with ASPD a persistent history of violence, especially one which is escalating in its physical severity, may be an indicator of increased risk; particularly if the patient denies responsibility and locates the blame in others. Comorbid BPD may increase the risk in the context of hostile attachments to others, and dissociation (📖 p.II.73). Paranoid states of mind make individuals with ASPD more likely to misperceive threat in its absence or to overestimate a genuine threat, and to carry weapons; and impulsivity implies that they are more likely to use them. As with other diagnoses, the risk of violence is increased if there are comorbid conditions that can be also associated with violence, such as severe mental illness and substance abuse.

Who is at risk from violent offenders with ASPD?

In principle, any person is at risk from an individual in their environment with ASPD. However, those who form attachments to them (e.g. girlfriends or partners) and others who spend most time with them are at greatest risk.

Borderline personality disorder

Borderline personality disorder (BPD) is characterized by pervasive negative affect and affect dysregulation, resulting in hyperarousal and sometimes transient psychotic states. Symptoms include intense anger or distress, dissociative phenomena such as depersonalization and derealization, and very intense repetitive intrusive thoughts of harming self or others, which may be experienced as pseudo-hallucinatory 'voices'.

Signs of BPD include the formation of acute and intense attachments to others who are in some form of caring relationship with the patient: commonly children, partners, or professional carers. These attachments tend to oscillate, so that intense positive regard may be followed with intense hatred, especially if the relationship is threatened in any way. Other signs of BPD include physical attacks on the body in the form of self-harming behaviours and impulsive suicidal behaviour, which varies in intensity and lethality.

Early neurobiological findings suggest that BPD is associated with impaired functioning of the anterior insula, and that this region may be involved in trust and cooperative behaviour. The development of BPD has also been associated with hyper-responsivity of the hypothalamic–pituitary–adrenal axis.

Prevalence and comorbidity of BPD

- General population: 6% (10% male, 4% female)
- General psychiatric patients: 30–50%
- Prisoners: 23% male remand, 14% male sentenced, 20% female
- Forensic psychiatric patients: 24–60%.

BPD is prevalent in specialist services, such as psychotherapy, eating disorders, substance misuse and forensic services. BPD is more commonly diagnosed in women, although the gender gap is less obvious in more severe conditions where individuals suffer from several personality disorders, and may have comorbid mental illness.

BPD patients are typically less able than others to contain their distress, soothe themselves, or negotiate solutions with others, and therefore often act out their feelings rather than acknowledging and managing them. Acting out feelings such as anger and hatred, for example, can involve self-harm, or harm to others—or splitting a group of staff, with many aligning themselves with the split in the patient's mind. Recognizing that such splitting is occurring is often a first step to recognizing the presence of BPD; addressing it is central to successful treatment.

How do symptoms impact on risk of offending or violence?

The majority of patients with BPD chiefly present a risk to themselves, in terms of self-harm or suicidal behaviours. However, there are specific symptoms of BPD that increase the risk of violence:

- Altered perception of external reality (during brief psychotic states or dissociative states)
- Paranoid cognitions and lowered threat perception threshold
- Dysregulated mood states, especially involving anger
- Hyperarousal secondary to the previously listed symptoms
- Presence of additional antisocial features, such as lack of empathy or contempt for distress in others
- Impulsivity and lack of capacity to reflect on actions
- Severe and repetitive self-harm may be an indicator of increased risk.

As in other conditions, the risk of violence is increased if there are other comorbid conditions that can be also associated with violence, such as severe mental illness and substance abuse.

Assessing risk associated with symptoms and signs in BPD

Perceived abandonment is likely to increase arousal and perceived threat, and may therefore result in increased risk of violence (see also 📖 pp.II.31–II.34) as well as increased risk of self-harm. Special care should therefore be taken if there are abrupt changes in routine or physical/psychological security; such as bereavements, new accommodation or change of professional carer. (See also 📖 p.II.61.)

Those with BPD tend to become dependent upon care, and may perceive attempts are made to withdraw elements of a care package or to discharge them as rejection and abandonment, resulting in acting out through self-harm or violence. Thus there is a particular risk with BPD that patients remain inappropriately detained in secure conditions.

Who is at risk from violent offenders with BPD?

BPD is prevalent in perpetrators of family violence of either sex, and in physical abusers of children. Those individuals who are the subject of an intense attachment by a patient with BPD (the strength of which they may not realize) may be particularly at risk; especially if they seek to end the relationship. Healthcare professionals may easily be misperceived as uncaring or abandoning, which may provoke violent behaviour in BPD patients.

Narcissistic personality disorder

The history of narcissism predates the description of narcissistic personality disorder. Narcissus was a figure of ancient Greek mythology who fell in love with his own reflection. The term 'narcissistic personality structure' was introduced by Kernberg in 1967, and 'narcissistic personality disorder' (NPD) was first proposed by Kohut the following year.

Signs of NPD include a pervasive pattern of grandiosity (in fantasy or behaviour), a need for admiration, and a lack of empathy; patients may have a grandiose sense of self-importance, be preoccupied with fantasies of success, power, brilliance, beauty or ideal love, believe that they are special and unique, have a strong sense of entitlement, exploit others to meet their own needs, and be arrogant, haughty and envious.

The causes of NPD are unknown; there are no established neurobiological associations as there are with ASPD (📖 p.II.60) and BPD (📖 p.II.61). The

Prevalence and comorbidity of NPD

- General population: 1%
- General psychiatric patients: 2–16%
- Prisoners: 8% male remand, 7% male sentenced, 6% female
- Forensic psychiatric patients: 26%.

following developmental hypotheses have been proposed:
- An oversensitive temperament at birth
- Excessive and unbalanced admiration, indulgence, praise, or criticism
- Severe emotional abuse in childhood
- Unpredictable or unreliable care giving from parents
- Being valued by parents as a means to regulate their own self-esteem.

How do symptoms impact on risk of offending or violence?

People with NPD commonly feel rejected, humiliated and threatened when criticized. To protect themselves, they often react with disdain, rage, and/or defiance to any slight criticism, real or imagined; this can include a violent reaction.

Although individuals with NPD are often ambitious and capable, the inability to tolerate setbacks, disagreements, or criticism, along with lack of empathy, make it difficult for such individuals to work cooperatively with others or to maintain long-term professional achievements; also, the individual's self-perceived fantastic grandiosity is typically not commensurate with his or her real accomplishments. This may lead to a desire to seek notoriety through alternative routes, including high-profile offending.

At the same time, their exploitativeness, sense of entitlement, lack of empathy, disregard for others, and constant need for attention adversely affect their interpersonal relationships. This can lead to domestic violence, sexual violence, and other offending behaviour.

Narcissistic traits are evident in a small group of high-risk paedophile sex offenders who believe themselves to be attractive to pubescent boys.

As in other conditions, the risk of violence is increased if there are comorbid conditions that can be also associated with violence (such as severe mental illness, psychopathy, and substance abuse).

Assessing risk associated with symptoms and signs in NPD

People who are diagnosed with NPD use splitting as a defence mechanism. They do this to preserve their self-esteem, by seeing the self as purely good and the others as purely bad. The use of splitting also implies the use of other defence mechanisms, including devaluation, idealization, and denial. A psychological assessment may indicate the degree to which these defence mechanisms are being employed, which may relate to the risk of violence.

Who is at risk from those with NPD?

Any individual who challenges the defences of the individual with NPD may be at risk. Similarly, any individual in a position where they may be exploited may be at risk of becoming the victim of offending.

Paranoid personality disorder

Paranoid personality disorder (PPD) is characterized principally by a pervasive pattern of suspiciousness and distrust of others, coupled with a pronounced misperception of others' intentions as hostile when objectively they are neutral or even positive.

Signs of PPD include unfounded suspicions that others are deceiving, harming, or exploiting them, or that partners are unfaithful to them; preoccupation with unjustified doubts of others' trustworthiness or loyalty; reluctance to confide in others because of fear this will be used against them; bearing persistent grudges; and perceiving slights and threats that are not obvious to others. For the diagnosis to be made, it must be clear that these symptoms occur in the absence of paranoid psychosis (📖 p.II.54).

Prevalence and comorbidity of PPD

- General population: 0.5–7% (12% male, 3% female)
- General psychiatric patients: 7–10%
- Prisoners: 29% male remand, 20% male sentenced, 16% female
- Forensic psychiatric patients: 18%.

There is no clear evidence as to the cause of PPD, nor any established neurobiological association. There is some evidence of increased rates of PPD amongst close relatives of those with schizophrenia or delusional disorder, hinting at a genetic or shared environmental association. One psychological theory is that children exposed to extreme anger and rage from adults over a prolonged period, with no way to predict or to avoid these outbursts, learn that this kind of behaviour in others is to be expected at any time, and go on to develop the thinking patterns of PPD.

How do symptoms impact on risk of offending or violence?

The extreme distrust of others experienced by people with PPD generates a very strong desire to be autonomous and self-sufficient, plus a need to feel in control of those around them. Patients are often highly critical of others, rigid in their patterns of thinking and behaving; they have a strong tendency to isolate themselves. It is hard for them to accept criticism or to collaborate productively with others, and this impairs both employment prospects and the chances of establishing meaningful friendships or intimate relationships.

An inability to secure employment may lead to acquisitive offending as an alternative, and an inability to secure a sexual relationship might predispose to sexual offending. More directly, pervasive misperceptions of others as hostile or as seeking to cause harm can lead to violence, often sudden, unpredictable and unprovoked violence from the perspective of the victim and witnesses. Violence in PPD is often reactive, but may also be premeditated, when the individual acts to pre-empt a perceived threat.

Assessing risk associated with symptoms and signs in PPD

The reluctance of people with PPD to reveal their mental state or inner thoughts makes acute risk assessment more difficult; at least until a working relationship has been established (which may well be impossible to achieve), people with severe PPD must be presumed to be capable of significant violence at any moment.

Certain environmental factors may be associated with periods of increased risk: for example, being forced to live in the presence of others, such as in a secure ward or shared prison cell; or being required to collaborate in some way with others, especially if they are likely to evaluate or challenge their behaviour, such as in group therapy (📖 p.II.171).

Who is at risk from those with PPD?

Almost anyone who comes into contact with a person with severe PPD is potentially at risk of violence, if a chance comment or action (such as when driving) is misperceived as sufficiently threatening.

Psychopathy

Psychopathy is a particular form of personality disorder, characterized by extremely antisocial attitudes towards other people (though it is not present as a diagnosis in ICD10 or DSM-IV, 📖 p.II.109). It is distinct from ASPD (📖 p.II.60),[*] although there are overlapping features, and some consider psychopathy to be approximately a severe subset of ASPD.

Current research suggests that there is a primary form, which manifests itself early in childhood as callous and unemotional traits, and a secondary form, which emerges later in life. Psychopathy is the result of a complex interaction of genetic vulnerability, limbic system abnormality and early childhood adversity.

Prevalence and comorbidity of psychopathy

- General population: 3.6%
- General psychiatric patients: no data
- Prisoners: 15–30%
- Forensic psychiatric patients: 15–30%.

Psychopathy has not been widely studied outside criminal populations. In high secure prisons and psychiatric hospitals, the prevalence is 15–30% of detainees. People with psychopathic traits rarely seek help, and are not commonly seen in general psychiatric services. It has been suggested that non-criminal high-functioning psychopaths may be found in any social group, and even that such traits may be adaptive in some occupations or environments.

The most reliable and widely used measure of psychopathy is Hare's Psychopathy Checklist (PCL-R, 📖 p.II.102). Scores above 25–30 are associated with clinical psychopathy. Individuals with any disorder may score for psychopathy, although medium or high scores will rarely be found outside forensic settings. Individuals who score in the clinical range for psychopathy will usually also have ASPD and a substance misuse problem.

PCL-R psychopathy[†] is said to comprise two factors:

- Factor 1 (Callous-unemotional): arrogant interpersonal style, grandiose, glib, deceitful; lacks empathy, lacks remorse, shallow and labile emotions, deficient affective experience
- Factor 2 (Antisocial): impulsive behavioural style, sensation-seeking, lack of planning; irresponsible, parasitic lifestyle.

How do symptoms impact on risk of offending or violence?

Psychopathy is a disorder which increases the risk of violence (📖 pp. II.31–II.34) substantially, especially in those who are antisocial rule breakers generally. Studies of released prisoners indicate that high PCL-R scores are associated with recidivism. PCL-R scores are therefore routinely used as part of violence risk assessment (📖 p.II.132) for serious offenders.

---

[*] The current concept of psychopathy is derived from Pritchard's concept of 'moral insanity' and Cleckley's work *The Mask of Sanity*, whereas the broader concept of ASPD has separate roots in Henderson's 1939 classification, *Psychopathic States*.

[†] There is a lively debate in the literature about whether there is a 'true' construct of psychopathy, derived from Cleckley's original work and excluding most of the PCL-R's factor 2 and whether psychopathy has become over-identified with the PCL-R construct itself.

Specific features of psychopathy that increase the risk of harm to others are:

- Predatory attitudes towards others; seeing them as deserving of being conned or exploited
- Grandiosity and paranoia
- Contempt for others' distress
- Intelligence and planning capacity
- Remorselessness
- Impulsivity and lack of capacity to reflect on actions.

Psychopathy may manifest itself as repeated offending behaviour, including crimes of deception, theft, and violence, and as interpersonal dysfunction, which may or may not involve interpersonal violence.

Risks associated with symptoms and signs in psychopathy

The risks of psychopathy are self-evident. It is unlikely that clinicians will see many individuals with psychopathy who do not already have established risk histories. When assessing risk in this group, it is important to consider the following:

- Is the level of violence escalating?
- Are there any other risk factors present, such as an Axis 1 disorder or substance misuse?
- Is there an identifiable victim?
- Is there a lack of anxiety or remorse for past offences?

Who is at risk from violent offenders with psychopathy?

Any vulnerable person is potentially at risk from individuals with high levels of psychopathy. Some individuals with psychopathy harm strangers, usually in the context of robbery or exploitation of some other kind. Some predatory psychopaths specifically target women or children for harm, and may spend some time in grooming their victims beforehand. Men with mild to moderate degrees of psychopathy may be perpetrators of domestic violence and cruelty to children within the home.

Note on terminology
Psychopathy should never be confused with the legal term 'psychopathic disorder', which is usually taken to mean 'personality disorder' and was until 2008 a category of disorder in the E&W Mental Health Act (📖 p.IV.373). Very few of those detained under this category had any degree of psychopathy. Clinicians should refrain from the use of the word 'psychopath', particularly to describe any criminal person. Not all criminals are psychopaths, and not all psychopaths are criminals.

Bipolar disorder

The main disorder that gives rise to mania (or hypomania) is bipolar disorder, but it can also arise in unipolar mania, puerperal psychosis and cyclothymia, and in a variety of organic (📖 pp.II.82–II.86) and drug-induced (📖 p.II.56) states. Bipolar disorder is often commonly known as manic depression. For risks associated with bipolar depression, see 📖 p.II.69.

Prevalence of bipolar disorder
- General population: 0.7%
- General psychiatric patients: 4%
- Prisoners: 1% whether male or female, sentenced or remand
- Forensic psychiatric patients: approximately 5%.

Comorbidity with other mental disorders

Between 65% and 90% of all people with bipolar disorder have one or more comorbid mental disorder, typically anxiety-related disorders (📖 pp.II.70, II.72) or impulse-control disorders (e.g. ADHD, 📖 p.II.77); these are commonly under-diagnosed. In offenders, 50% have alcohol or drug dependence (📖 p.II.56) or psychopathy (📖 p.II.66), and recidivism is more common if these problems are not addressed. If present, alcohol and substance misuse generally increases during the manic phase, and also to a lesser extent during depressive phases.

Manic features that may predispose to violence & offending

- Elation
- Hyperarousal
- Psychosis (see also 📖 p.II.54), especially intrusive hallucinations or grandiose or persecutory delusions
- Impaired judgement
- Impulsivity
- Irritability
- Intolerance of frustration
- Hypersexuality.

Associations with offending behaviour

It is uncertain whether bipolar disorder is associated with violence. If there is an association, it is a relatively weak one—only 10% of the magnitude of the association between schizophrenia and violence, according to one estimate.

Most commonly, the offences committed are minor and include: common assaults (📖 p.IV.346); offences related to intoxication with alcohol or drugs; threats of violence; damage to property (📖 p.IV.350); theft (📖 p.IV.354); forging cheques or failure to pay; or sexual indecency (📖 p.IV.348). The victims in most cases are strangers to the patient.

Serious offences are recorded less commonly but include: GBH (📖 p.IV.346); arson (📖 p.IV.350); sexual assaults including rape (📖 p.IV.348); causing death by dangerous driving; and homicide (📖 p.IV.344). A small number of stalkers (📖 p.II.40) have also been shown to suffer from mania.

Other harms associated with manic states

- *Self-neglect* Overactivity preventing self-care
- *Reputational or financial damage* due to poor judgement
- *Vulnerability to sexual or financial exploitation* due to grandiosity and poor judgement.

Those in manic states not uncommonly enter into contracts unwisely. A psychiatrist may be called upon to report on whether the patient had the mental capacity (📖 p.IV.438) at the time to understand the nature and the implications of the contract they made, which may determine whether or not the contract can be enforced.

Depression & other affective disorders

The main disorder that causes depressive episodes is major depressive disorder, but such episodes can also occur in bipolar disorder (📖 p.II.67), dysthymia, cyclothymia, and secondarily in schizophrenia (📖 p.II.55), substance misuse (📖 p.II.56), PD (📖 p.II.58), stroke, and a wide range of other conditions.

These figures are for major depressive disorder, and mostly exclude depression secondary to anxiety-related disorders (most notably, mixed anxiety and

> ### Prevalence of major depression
> - General population: 6.7% (plus 1.5% dysthymia)
> - General psychiatric patients: 15%
> - Sentenced prisoners: 8% of men, 15% of women
> - Remand prisoners: 17% of men, 21% of women
> - Forensic psychiatric patients: approximately 5%.

depressive disorder, the prevalence of which among prisoners is 19–36%).

Comorbidity with other mental disorders
76% of people with major depression have one or more comorbid mental disorders, most commonly anxiety-related disorders (📖 pp.II.70, II.72) and impulse-control disorders (e.g. ADHD, 📖 p.II.77), followed by substance misuse or dependence (📖 p.II.56). Moreover, major depression often follows traumatic brain injury (📖 p.II.82). Depression secondary to PD, especially BPD (📖 p.II.61), is also seen in forensic settings.

Associations with offending behaviour
The association between depression and violence is predominantly the reverse of that of some other disorders: rather than depression being a risk factor for violence, witnessing or being a victim of violence, especially parental or intimate partner violence, is a risk factor for depression. Furthermore, the experience of custody following arrest or conviction for an offence is a risk factor for the onset of affective disorders.

However, in some circumstances, and especially in conjunction with other known risk factors for violence (e.g. alcohol abuse), depression c⁻ increase the risk of violence to others. For example, domestic killings not uncommonly committed by men with depression; it is likely th⁻ depression acts to lower the threshold for violence, whether in th⁻ of self-harm or harm to others. The trigger is often somethin⁻ done by the victim that provoked (📖 p.V.498) the depress⁻ when in other circumstances they would have been able to res⁻

The distinction between psychotic and non-psychotic depression is an important one. Women who become psychotically depressed can be at risk of killing their loved ones (especially children) as well as themselves, because they have come to believe that not only their own future but that of those they love is hopeless, and that the most loving response is so-called mercy killing (📖 p.IV.344).

Other harms associated with depression

- *Self-neglect:* lack of motivation to care for oneself, or others
- *Self-harm or suicide:* see 📖 p.II.137.

Depression is also relevant to forensic psychiatrists as a frequent consequence of victimization (📖 p.II.139) and of punishments such as imprisonment (📖 p.IV.364), and may form the basis of a claim for compensation (📖 p.V.514) in certain circumstances. Psychiatrists can be asked to assess the risk that imprisonment (or deportation or extradition, 📖 p.V.525) will lead to a deterioration in mental state, or other harm.

Post-traumatic stress disorder

In this context, 'trauma' means an exceptionally severe, life-threatening and distressing event, or a series of events that cumulatively are exceptionally severe and distressing. The relationship between such trauma and crime is complex. Post-traumatic stress disorder (PTSD) is one of the sequelae of trauma.

Prevalence of PTSD

- General population: 8% (lifetime)
- General psychiatric patients: 14–43%
- Sentenced prisoners: 4–21%
- Forensic psychiatric patients: 36–58%.

Women in prison appear to have particularly high rates of PTSD.

Diagnostic controversy

The diagnosis of PTSD requires, in essence, severe psychological disturbance following such trauma, involving involuntary re-experiencing of the trauma, hyperarousal, avoidance of stimuli associated with the trauma, and emotional numbing. Amnesia (📖 p.V.504) for the traumatic event is common, and usually dissociative in nature.

The diagnostic requirement of an objectively traumatic event generates a risk of circular thinking: that is, of regarding an event as objectively traumatic precisely because a person repeatedly and involuntarily re-experiences it. This is a particular risk in claims for compensation (📖 p.V.514), especially given the familiarity of the concept of PTSD amongst the lay population. Moreover, the nosological status of the diagnosis is still doubted by a few.[*]

The derivative disputed concept of complex PTSD (📖 p.V.546) is far less widely accepted than ~~si~~mple PTSD, which is the subject of this page. Complex PTSD, closely related to the competing ~~co~~ncept of borderline personality disorder (📖 p.II.61), is often associated with the kind of prolonged ~~phy~~sical, sexual or emotional abuse or neglect that forensic patients often suffered as children.

Comorbidity with other mental disorders

Comorbid drug and alcohol use is commonly seen in people with PTSD. The prevalence of PTSD in people with schizophrenia in forensic settings is higher than in general psychiatric samples. People with psychosis and PTSD tend to have more positive psychotic symptoms, heightened paranoia and more violent thoughts, feelings and behaviour. The relationship between psychosis, PTSD and violent behaviour is not fully understood.

Associations with offending behaviour

There is no definite causal link established between PTSD and offending behaviour. There, however, are a number of factors which are important in understanding offending behaviour seen in people with PTSD.

- *Hyperarousal*, resulting in a heightened emotional and physiological state may predispose to impulsive and reactive violence
- Psychological preparedness or *hypervigilance* is a phenomenon where the person with PTSD may be 'on the lookout' for threat or danger and correspondingly respond inappropriately to a stimulus as if it were a threat
- *Impulsivity* and *anger* are commonly seen in PTSD and may provide a mechanism through which violence is perpetrated
- *Flashbacks* may precipitate a violent response as a direct result of experiencing a threatening event
- The violent response may occur in a state of *dissociation*. Dissociation is a common feature of PTSD and violence may occur more frequently in this semi-conscious state
- Similarly, *nightmares* may result in violent actions during sleep or immediately on waking.

Combat veterans with a diagnosis of PTSD have been shown to be more likely to show reactive violence (as opposed to instrumental violence, 📖 p.II.21) than those without PTSD.

PTSD as a consequence of offending

The traumatic trigger for development of PTSD in forensic psychiatric inpatients may be the index offence in up to 70% of cases. PTSD is more likely to be a consequence if the offence was unplanned, if the offender is controlled and inhibited, and if the offender has no significant criminal history.

Treatment of PTSD caused by offending may have to be pursued alongside treatment of mental conditions that were (possibly causally) associated with the offending.

Relevance to forensic psychiatrists

PTSD, whatever its origins, may also be relevant to forensic psychiatrists when their patients face imprisonment (📖 p.IV.364) or deportation (📖 p.V.525), as it may form the basis of a claim that, in exceptional circumstances, the imprisonment or deportation would breach the patient's human rights (📖 p.IV.418) because of its impact on their PTSD and consequent risk of suicide or other harm.

In those forensic services that also treat victims of offending (📖 p.II.186), PTSD is the most common diagnosis.

Suffering PTSD after an injury or other major incident is one of the commonest reasons for claiming compensation for psychiatric injury (📖 p.V.514), which will require psychiatric evidence.

Anxiety disorders

Anxiety disorders include: generalized anxiety disorder (GAD); obsessive–compulsive disorder (OCD); panic disorder; phobias; and more broadly, adjustment disorders including grief reactions. Other disorders in which anxiety is a prominent syndrome (such as depression, 📖 p.II.69, and PTSD, 📖 p.II.70) are considered separately.

There is little evidence linking anxiety disorders with offending behaviour, although anxiety symptoms and disorders are prominent in forensic psychiatric inpatients.

Prevalence of anxiety disorders
- General population: GAD 3%, OCD 1%, panic 3%, phobias 1–9%
- General psychiatric patients: no data
- Prisoners: GAD 10–15% OCD 2.5–4%, panic 9%, phobias 1–3%
- Forensic psychiatric patients: no data.

Some studies have focused on the prevalence of neurotic illness as a single group, finding rates of approximately 10–25% in prisoners, well in excess of that in the general population. Anxiety disorders may be unusual in that rates in prison populations are not consistently found to be higher than the general population in all studies.

Associations with offending behaviour

There are no definite associations between a diagnosis of an anxiety disorder and offending behaviour. Anxiety states may be comorbid with other disorders more commonly associated with offending behaviour, but there is no evidence to suggest that the comorbid anxiety disorder *per se* affects the individual's risk of violence or other offending behaviour.

Severe anxiety may predispose to dissociation (📖 p.II.73), which itself may disinhibit the patient, allowing them to do things they would not otherwise do.

Other associations

Severe forms of anxiety disorder arising after injury or a major incident, particularly severe adjustment disorders and grief reactions, may form the basis of a claim for compensation for psychiatric injury (📖 p.V.514), in the same way as PTSD (📖 p.II.70).

Dissociative and conversion disorders

The current concepts of 'conversion' (of psychological conflict into the experience of physical symptoms) and 'dissociation' (from psychological conflict) have evolved from the historical idea of hysteria, which was first thought of as largely confined to women. All concepts incorporate two themes: the absence of organic pathology, and symptoms determined by the patient's ideas about illness rather than by biology or anatomy. Some sources, including DSM-IV (📖 p.II.109), define conversion and dissociation pragmatically by reference to their symptoms, with no reference to any underlying psychological conflict.

Prevalence of dissociative and conversion disorders

- General population: up to 33% in women, up to 25% general medicine
- General psychiatric patients: no data
- Prisoners: no data
- Forensic psychiatric patients: no data.

The prevalence data shown are from old (pre-1970) studies. The frequency of case reports indicates that the prevalence of hysterical or dissociative/conversion disorders has steadily declined since the late 19th century, and anecdotal evidence suggests that the current prevalence might be considerably lower than the figures shown.

The ICD10 conversion and dissociative disorders are:

- Dissociative amnesia, fugue or stupor
- Trance and possession disorders
- Dissociative identity disorder ('multiple personality disorder')
- Dissociative convulsions
- Dissociative anaesthesia and sensory loss (diplopia, blindness, deafness)
- Dissociative motor disorders (aphonia, ataxia, dysphasia, paralysis).

The upper three, affecting global mental function, are more often seen in criminal contexts; the lower two, affecting specific functions, are more often relevant in claims for compensation (📖 p.V.514).

DSM-IV includes fewer conditions, listing only dissociative amnesia, dissociative fugue, depersonalization disorder and dissociative identity disorder; all other conditions fall into a 'not otherwise specified' category.

Comorbidity with other mental disorders

Slater found, in a seminal 10-year follow-up study in the 1980s, that over half of patients diagnosed with dissociative or conversion disorders were eventually diagnosed with other neurological or psychiatric disorders, although some subsequent follow-up studies have not found this—and the finding may represent misdiagnosis rather than comorbidity.

Dissociative states are more common in patients with other mental disorders, specifically anxiety disorders (📖 p.II.72), depression (📖 p.II.69) and organic brain syndromes (e.g. after traumatic brain injury, 📖 p.II.82).

Dissociative symptoms, particularly mild degrees of depersonalization or derealization, are sometimes reported in normal individuals subjected to very great stress or anxiety, such as soldiers in the heat of battle.

Associations with violence

A substantial proportion of patients with dissociative symptoms have experienced or witnessed severe violence, leading to the suggestion that such experiences of severe violence predispose to dissociation. Individuals in a dissociative state are said to be released from acting as they might ordinarily do within their normal personality, and behaviour 'out of character' is itself suggestive of dissociation. However, it is unwise to assume that violence is related to dissociation without very clear other evidence or features to suggest it.

There is also some limited evidence to suggest, that experiencing 'trait' dissociation makes *future* violence more likely—that is, that having a dissociative disorder is associated with committing violent acts after the diagnosis is recognized.

Other associations with offending behaviour

Many people alleged to have offended claim *amnesia* for key events, including 10–70% of murder suspects. Such amnesia may be malingered (📖 p.II.87), or the result of psychosis (📖 p.II.54) or a sleep disorder (📖 p.II.83), but in many cases the condition in question is dissociative amnesia, often without a past history of a dissociative disorder.

Dissociate (or 'psychogenic') amnesia for offences is associated with offences committed in a state of high emotional arousal, where the victim is known intimately by the offender, and where the offender has drunk alcohol. The greater the degree of violence involved, the greater the likelihood of dissociative amnesia. Often the amnesia is patchy, with 'islands' of memory; usually, it begins with loss of memory of events close in time to the violent event or other cause of emotional arousal. Very commonly, it is complicated by intoxication at the time, raising the possibility of alcohol-related 'blackouts'. In addition, some defendants believe that by claiming amnesia they may escape conviction. For all these reasons, it is often extremely difficult to give a firm opinion on amnesia in legal cases (📖 p.V.504).

Some violent offenders describe depersonalization and derealization at the time of arousal and violence, or in response to extreme fear, which may then precede violence on their own part.

Somatoform disorders and chronic fatigue

These disorders, which are related to but distinct from the dissociative and conversion disorders, have no known association with violence or other offending behaviour. However, they may very occasionally be of relevance to forensic psychiatrists, such as when they form the basis for a claim for compensation after injury (📖 p.V.514).

Paraphilias

The term 'paraphilia' refers to a heterogeneous group of conditions in which the individual exhibits culturally atypical sexual behaviours that are longstanding and cause them or those around them marked distress, and also interfere with normal daily life. They tend to involve an inappropriate sexual target (e.g. pre-pubescent* children in paedophilia, animals in bestiality, or inanimate objects in fetishism) or inappropriate behaviours

---

* The DSM-IV definition of paedophilia specifies pre-pubertal children, i.e. those aged under 13 in most cases, whereas ICD10 includes 'early pubertal' children, i.e. many of those up to 15 or 16. There is a related term, 'hebephilia' for specific sexual attraction towards pubertal children.

for obtaining sexual gratification, as in exhibitionism, sadomasochism, frotteurism,[*] or voyeurism (see also 📖 pp.II.42–II.49).

Some argue that the definitional, subcultural (in that they may be perceived as normal by certain sections of society) and cross-cultural problems with the paraphilias are so great that they should be removed from official diagnostic manuals, at least until they are better characterized and understood. There is certainly a substantial risk of socially deviant (and often criminal) sexual behaviours being misdiagnosed as paraphilia if the doctor concerned does not adhere to a proper medical concept of mental disorder (📖 p.III.272).

Prevalence of paraphilias

- General population: 3% exhibitionism, 8% voyeurism, 5% paedophilia (0.5% in women)
- General psychiatric patients: 'rare' according to APA
- Prisoners: no data
- Forensic psychiatric patients: no data.

What data do exist are from Western countries. Rates differ considerably across cultures, mostly because of variation in sexual practices, the degree to which unusual sexual behaviours are defined as abnormal, and if they are, whether or not those abnormalities are regarded as a medical or psychiatric problem.

Paraphilias are generally thought of as disorders of male patients, but women do exhibit paraphilias too, albeit at a lower rate (perhaps 10% of the male rate). The most common paraphilias amongst women are paedophilia (36% of the male rate in one study), sexual sadism (29%), and exhibitionism (29%). Female patients do not differ from male in demographic, clinical or offence-related characteristics.

The Internet has made paraphilic pornography vastly more readily available than was previously the case. It is as yet unclear to what extent this has 'normalized' atypical sexual behaviours, and what effect, if any, this will have on the rates (or definitions) of paraphilias or of paraphilia-related criminal offences.

Comorbidity with other mental disorders

In general, patients with paraphilias often have comorbid mental disorders—for example, 93% of patients with paedophilia in one study had a comorbid mental disorder, most commonly a mood disorder and/or substance misuse. Approximately 75% of individuals with paraphilias who commit sexual offences (📖 p.IV.348) suffer from a PD, and one-fifth from psychopathy (📖 p.II.66). Paraphilias have been suggested by some authors to be more common in patients who also suffer from autistic spectrum disorders (📖 p.II.76), or from ADHD (📖 p.II.77).

---

[*] Non-consensual rubbing against another person in a sexual manner, e.g. on public transport.

Associations with offending behaviour

In most jurisdictions, the behaviours associated with certain paraphilias are in themselves illegal (e.g. bestiality, paedophilia, or frotteurism, which is not a specific offence but amounts to assault, 📖 p.IV.346, as may be consensual sadomasochistic practices in some jurisdictions). In other paraphilias, such as fetishism, the paraphilia may predispose the individual to the commission of other crimes; theft (📖 p.IV.354), in this case, such as of a woman's underwear from her washing line.

Other harms associated with paraphilias

Self-harm or accidental death, e.g. in sadomasochism.

Asperger's syndrome & other pervasive developmental disorders

People with Asperger's syndrome and other high-functioning autistic spectrum disorders are probably overrepresented in forensic populations. The autistic spectrum incorporates the triad of impairments of social interaction, communication and imagination. Learning disability is considered separately (📖 p.II.80).

Prevalence of autistic spectrum disorders

- General population: <1% (men) 0.3% (women)
- General psychiatric patients: no data
- Prisoners: no data
- Forensic psychiatric patients (high security): 1.5–5%.

It is likely that Asperger's syndrome is under-recognized in forensic psychiatric settings. When patients are diagnosed with the syndrome it is often the case that until that point they were believed to be suffering from schizophrenia (📖 p.II.54) and/or from PD (📖 p.II.58).

Some have postulated a link, or at least an overlap of features, between schizoid personality disorder and Asperger's syndrome.

The rates of offending in Asperger's syndrome are not conclusively higher than in the general population, although some studies suggest that people on the autistic spectrum commit more violent offences and criminal damage than the average.

Features of Asperger's that may predispose to violence

- Lack of concern for outcome
- Social naivety
- Lack of awareness of outcome
- Lack of empathy
- Misinterpretation of others' behaviour, e.g. as hostile
- Social or sexual rejection, bullying, or family conflict
- Comorbid drug and alcohol use
- Comorbid PD.

Associations with offending behaviour

The nature of offending in Asperger's syndrome relates in particular to:

- *Theory of mind* deficits, including a tendency to egocentricity resulting in lack of awareness of impact on victims, and of what is 'wrong' in social and emotional terms;
- Deficits in *social reciprocity*, which may predispose to sexual offences in particular (e.g. in an individual who wants sexual contact, without appreciating the complex reciprocal interactions that must occur between two potential partners in order for consensual sexual activity to take place); and
- *Restricted, repetitive interests* that may, for example, include fire-setting, or may lead to the commission of bizarre and sometimes persistent crimes without apparent ordinarily understandable motive (e.g. where the 'motive' is merely repetition of the act).[*]

Other reasons for offending in patients with Asperger's syndrome may be revenge for persistent bullying; explosive responses to stimuli or changes in routine; and susceptibility to exploitation and coerced involvement in criminal activity. Such offences can be extremely violent, even homicidal.

Attention deficit hyperactivity disorder

Attention deficit hyperactivity disorder (ADHD), attention deficit disorder, and hyperkinetic disorder (a more narrow definition) are some of the terms used for a syndrome characterized by persistent over-activity, impulsivity and difficulties in sustaining attention. The occurrence of the symptoms both within and outside the home, the presence of both inattention and over activity, plus the presence of conduct disorder (📖 p.II.79) are all associated with a more serious condition that is less responsive to treatment and which has poorer outcome. There is some overlap between ADHD and CD but they are different disorders.

Evidence suggests that inattentive and overactive subtypes of ADHD have distinct profiles. Those with the hyperactive-impulsive subtype of ADHD are characterized by extreme over activity, with oppositional and aggressive behaviours. Conduct problems are their most prevalent school-based difficulties and they have high rates of school suspension and special educational placement. Children with the hyperactive-impulsive profile are at risk of long-term antisocial behaviour problems and poor school adjustment.

Prevalence of ADHD

- General population: 5–10% during school age, 2.5% during adulthood
- General psychiatric patients: no data
- Prisoners: over 30% of young offenders (📖 p.V.458)
- Forensic psychiatric patients: no data.

The prevalence rate is four times higher amongst males than females.

---

[*]Nevertheless, despite the lack of an understandable motive for crime, patients with Asperger's syndrome often still have the (more narrowly-defined) legal intent (📖 p.IV.334) to commit the crime and may therefore still be convicted.

How do symptoms impact on risk of offending or violence?

Impulsivity, hyperactivity, and inattention in school can result in school failure, which is a further risk factor for offending. Impulsiveness may reflect deficits in executive functions (📖 p.II.99) of the brain, located in the frontal lobes. Individuals with these neuropsychological deficits will tend to commit offences because they have poor control over their behaviour, a poor ability to consider the consequences of their actions, and a tendency to focus on immediate gratification. Children with ADHD are also more likely than those without to have learning disability (📖 p.II.80).

ADHD symptoms are a common feature among individuals with early onset, persistent antisocial behaviour and the prognosis for antisocial individuals with ADHD symptoms is especially poor. Some will be diagnosed in adulthood with antisocial personality disorder (📖 p.II.60). In either case, the long-term risk of offending behaviour is high.

Other harms associated with ADHD

Impulsiveness is the most crucial personality dimension that predicts offending. Children with ADHD display a greater degree of difficulty, with aggression, oppositional and defiant behaviour, and conduct problems. The most common types of conduct problems are lying, stealing, truancy, and physical aggression. The symptoms of ADHD correlate with later violent behaviour and criminality.

Comorbidity with other mental disorders

The disorders most likely to be comorbid with ADHD are ODD, CD, mood disorders, anxiety disorders, and learning disorders.

What is the risk?

- Hyperactivity at age 11–13 years significantly predicts arrests for violence up to age 22, especially amongst boys who have experienced delivery complications
- Problems of attention and restlessness at age 5 more than doubles the risk for delinquency at 14
- Each comorbid condition further increases the risk of delinquency or offending.

Conduct disorder and oppositional-defiant disorder

Conduct disorder (CD) is a term used to denote a syndrome of core symptoms characterized by the persistent failure to control behaviour within socially defined rules. Conduct problems involve three overlapping domains of behaviour: defiance of the will of someone in authority, aggressiveness, and antisocial behaviour that violates other people's rights.

Oppositional defiant disorder (ODD) refers to a pattern of conduct problems characterized mainly by tantrums and conduct problems (typically occurs in pre-school years). ODD is distinct from CD and is less pervasive but is recognized as a possible developmental precursor of CD.

Prevalence of conduct disorder and ODD

- General population (lifetime prevalence): ODD 10%, CD 7% males, 3% females
- General psychiatric patients: no data but is one of the most popular reasons for referral to CAMH Services
- Youth detention: 90% of children in juvenile secure estate meet criteria for diagnosis of conduct disorder
- Forensic psychiatric patients: no data.

Conduct problems constitute a third to half of all clinical referrals to child and adolescent mental health services, and chronic conduct problems are the single most costly disorder of adolescence.

How do symptoms impact on risk of offending or violence?

By definition the antisocial behaviours indicative of CD increase the risk of juvenile and also adult offending. 40% of children with CD will go on to become young offenders (and 90% of young offenders had CD in childhood), whereas ODD is not particularly associated with offending behaviour.

Parental risk factors for CD include low monitoring, high conflict and inconsistent and harsh disciplining. Individual risk factors include soft neurological signs, impulsivity and ADHD (p.II.77). There is evidence that genetic vulnerability to impulsiveness interacts with abusive environments to cause an increased risk of CD in adolescence.

Aggressive children are unpopular because they have low levels of pro-social skills. This not only leads to social isolation (a risk factor for offending) but makes it more difficult for them to establish supportive relationships with non-deviant peers (a protective factor). Disruptive and aggressive adolescents may be similarly rejected by their peers. However, they are also more likely to associate with deviant peer groups during adolescence, which increases the risk that antisocial behaviour will be maintained.

Cognitively, individuals with CD exhibit hostile attributional bias, so that they interpret ambiguous social situations as threatening. With respect to affect, anger and irritability are the main mood states. Where there is a history of childhood maltreatment, this may lead to similar symptoms such as hypervigilance, aggression in response to any fear stimulus and fearful interpretations of others.

Other harms associated with ODD and conduct disorder

ODD can cause family disruption and school exclusion. ODD is also a risk factor for CD which is associated with delinquency and non-criminal rule breaking. Many conduct disordered youth are never considered young offenders because their illegal behaviours escape detection or may be below the threshold for criminal behaviour.

What is the risk?

There are different developmental trajectories (☐ p.II.30) for antisocial behaviour; and the development of CD is a significant marker for the development of so-called lifecourse-persistent antisocial behaviour.

A subgroup of individuals with CD will go on to develop ASPD (☐ p.II.60). Risk factors include early onset, wide range of symptoms, greater severity and frequency, range across situations (home, school, etc.) and hyperactivity.

In adolescence, the emergence of paranoid symptoms, and narcissistic or passive–aggressive personality traits are most associated with later antisocial behaviour and violence.

It may be that those who develop ASPD are either genetically more vulnerable, or have suffered more maltreatment, or both.

Learning disability

Intelligence is usually measured according to scores on IQ (intelligence quotient) tests. The IQ indicates the relationship between a person's 'mental age' and chronological age. The term learning disability (LD) refers to significant cognitive impairments (usually an IQ below 70) and significant impairments in social functioning or adaptive behaviours associated with everyday skills. For the diagnosis to be made, both of these impairments must be present before age 18.

The term 'learning difficulties' is often used for specific or generalized intellectual impairment that does not meet all of these criteria. Many people with dyslexia, autism, and a wide range of other conditions can be described as suffering from learning difficulties.

Prevalence of learning disability

- General population: 1.5%
- General psychiatric patients: no data
- Prisoners: 10% (up to 60% of male prisoners have learning *difficulties*)
- Forensic psychiatric patients: no data.

Prevalence rates for offending behaviour in patients with LD is higher than in the general population. International studies have shown a large range, from 2–40%, depending on methodological approaches.

People with LD, and to an even greater extent learning difficulties, are enormously over-represented in prison settings, as shown by the prevalence data listed. It seems likely that the same is true in secure hospital settings.

Reviews of high-security provision indicate offenders with LD have the longest duration of stay and are most difficult to discharge because of a lack of community resources.

How do symptoms impact on risk of offending or violence?

The main explanatory factor underlying the link between intelligence and offending may be the lack of ability to manipulate abstract concepts. People who are poor at this are likely to perform less well at school, and probably tend to commit offences because of their lack of ability to foresee the consequences of their offending and to appreciate the feelings of their victim. School failure, common in people with LD, is also linked to offending. Conversely, high intelligence might be a protective factor for offending.

People with LD are at higher risk for conduct disorder (📖 p.II.79) and ADHD (📖 p.II.77) in childhood and they are more likely to be rejected by their peer group. Deficits in verbal skills, memory, and visual-motor integration are also related to offending behaviour, independent of low social class and family adversity.

With regard to sexual offending, some individuals with LD may not have learnt the rules that define acceptable and unacceptable behaviour. A low level of social competence may result in acts that were meant to be friendly being seen as aggressive by others. Sexual offences may amount to inappropriate, impulsive expressions of emotion rather than premeditated violent acts (see also 📖 pp.II.42–II.52).

Violent behaviour in the LD population may be due to frustration, impulsivity or poor problem solving skills.

It is also likely that the increased prevalence of offending observed in LD is due to a greater likelihood of detection of crimes committed by this group. People with LD are vulnerable suspects (📖 p.V.453) and may also be disadvantaged by the criminal justice system because of a lack of appropriate support and legal representation from early stages in the process.

Other associations with offending behaviour

There is no significant difference in the frequency of violent or property offences between individuals with LD and those without. However, the proportion of individuals with LD convicted of sexual offences is six times that of those without. Moreover, 10% of people convicted of fire-setting have LD.

Low intelligence at age 3 significantly predicts officially recorded offending up to age 30.

Anecdotally at least, comorbid LD also increases the risk of offending associated with other conditions.

Who is at risk?

Sex offenders with LD have low specificity for age and sex of their victim and there is a greater tendency to offend against younger and male children. The characteristics of sex offences by those with LD are distinctive in that they are not carefully planned and typically the victim does not know the offender.

Acquired brain injury

Several studies and reports have suggested a link between acquired (i.e. traumatic) brain injury (TBI) and criminal behaviour. Any such association may not be causal, however: it is likely, for example, that individuals at risk of offending are also more likely to acquire head injuries.

Prevalence of traumatic brain injury

- General population: 5–15%
- General psychiatric patients: 17–43% (inpatients, including minor TBI)
- Prisoners: 50% in non-violent criminals; 100% on death row
- Forensic psychiatric patients: 22% in high security (60–70% have neurological impairment), 23–50% in other services.

Features of TBI that predispose to violence

Lesions in the frontal lobes can produce personality changes and can disrupt certain forms of planning and organization of behaviour (i.e. executive function, 🕮 p.II.99). This can result in disinhibition, which can be linked to violence. There is some evidence to indicate that damage to certain structures of the temporal lobes (i.e. the amygdala and hippocampus) is also associated with aggressive behaviour.

Certain factors that predispose to TBI, such as poor premorbid social functioning (🕮 p.II.23) and a history of alcohol and/or substance abuse (🕮 p.II.56), also predispose to violence.

Likewise, antisocial behaviour in itself may predispose to head injury which may result in increased risk of violent behaviour; this means that those most likely to suffer the adverse consequences of head injury may be those most likely to experience head injury. There are numerous such confounders in studying the effects of TBI on violent behaviour.

TBI is also associated with self-directed violence, including suicide. A significant proportion of patients who kill themselves deliberately (5.5% in one study) had acquired a brain injury within the past three years.

Post-concussion syndrome

This is a group of transient symptoms that occur in 30–80% of concussion (mild head injury) and many cases of moderate or severe TBI, and usually abate within 6 months. Independently of any permanent brain injury, it can predispose to violence. It typically comprises:

- Physical symptoms, especially headache, and also dizziness, photosensitivity, tinnitus, double vision, and insomnia
- Psychological symptoms, including irritability, anxiety and depression, restlessness, aggression, lability of mood, impulsivity, and loss of tolerance to alcohol or drugs
- Cognitive symptoms, including poor concentration, confusion, impaired judgement, amnesia (🕮 p.V.504) and other memory deficits

Associations with offending behaviour

There are a number of clinical hypotheses as to why traumatic brain injury may increase the risk of perpetration of violent behaviour (discounting the specific effects related to the site of a localized brain injury):

- Cognitive impairment affecting recognition of legal boundaries and motivation to adhere to laws
- Impulse control deficits
- Increased aggression, irritability or personality change
- Poor social judgement
- Increased vulnerability to involvement in criminal activity
- Comorbid antisocial PD/psychopathy
- Disinhibition.

Epilepsy and sleep disorders

Epilepsy is a group of disorders that are rarely associated with violence. Sleep disorders are similarly rarely associated with violence. However, both of these disorders are sometimes raised within defences (📖 p.IV.342) to criminal acts. Interest in epilepsy and parasomnias in forensic psychiatry is based on a historical association between the clinical phenomenon of automatism (📖 p.V.483) and supposedly inexplicable crimes. Malingering (📖 p.II.87) and dissociative disorders (📖 p.II.73) should also be considered when epilepsy and sleep disorders are raised as possible diagnoses.

Prevalence of epilepsy

- General population: 0.5–1% (point prevalence), 36% (lifetime)
- General psychiatric patients: no data
- Prisoners: 1–2%
- Forensic psychiatric patients: 5% (special hospital).

Prevalence of parasomnias

- General population: 2–25% depending on condition.

Comorbidity with psychiatric disorders

- Total prevalence of psychiatric disorders in patients with epilepsy: 20–30%
- Psychosis: 2–9%
- Depressive disorders: 20–60%
- Substance abuse: 20–50%.

There is no association between sleep disorders and mental disorders.

Violence and epilepsy

There is no general increase in violent acts associated with a diagnosis of epilepsy. However, epilepsy can be associated with complex behaviours outside ordinary conscious control which may occasionally result in violence. Violence in people with epilepsy is usually due to other risk factors, and it is probably the association with these that was responsible for the previous view that epilepsy itself was a risk factor for violence.

Ictal violence (that is, violence committed during a seizure) is rare. It is more likely in complex partial seizures than generalized tonic-clonic seizures. It is likely that most offending occurs in the post-ictal or inter-ictal period, often when there is also some external influence (such as pressure or suggestion from another person).

A potential confounding factor is that the very abnormality of the temporal lobes that may cause complex partial seizures may itself directly cause violent behaviour. Such abnormalities have been associated with the controversial diagnosis (📖 p.V.546) of episodic dyscontrol syndrome, in which there is an apparent lack of memory for explosive episodes of sudden uncontrollable violence. Possibly related to this is the equally controversial concept of 'explosive personality disorder'.

Assessment of link between epilepsy and violence

A neurologist should be involved in assessing a person with epilepsy alleged to have committed a violent offence. They should consider:

• The diagnosis of epilepsy should be confirmed with an electroencephalogram (EEG)
• Epileptic automatism should be established by clinical history and closed circuit TV-EEG monitoring
• Aggression should be observed by closed circuit TV-EEG monitoring
• The violent act should be characteristic of the patient's usual seizures
• There should be clinical judgement by a neurologist regarding the likelihood of the violence being a result of a seizure
• Any obvious motive, planning or premeditation should be considered
• Concealment of the offence
• Whether the offence is senseless or out of character.

Sleep disorders (parasomnias)

Sleep disturbance is a common component of many psychiatric disorders, but this is distinct from sleepwalking and other parasomnias such as sleep terror disorder and nightmare disorder. These disorders are more common in children.

Sleep disorders and violence

In adults, where violence occurs it is more common in males with a childhood history of parasomnias, including nocturnal enuresis. Sleep terror disorder and sleepwalking overlap and may be present in the same episode. A period of sleep deprivation, alcohol, marijuana and caffeine have been suggested as being associated with provoking sleepwalking.

Victims of crimes associated with sleep are usually known to the perpetrator. The sleepwalker may not appear to hear any cries from their victim or recognize their victim.

Whether the episode occurred in REM (rapid eye movement) or non-REM sleep may be significant. The notion that an individual in REM sleep is paralysed and therefore cannot be violent is no longer accepted.

The possibility of nocturnal epilepsy can further confuse the assessment, and may need to be considered as an alternative diagnosis.

Assessment of link between sleep disorders and violence

The following should be considered at assessment:
- Is there a history of childhood parasomnias?
- Was the violence preceded by a period of stress for the perpetrator?
- Did the arousal from sleep occur soon after sleep onset?
- Is there evidence of complex, goal-directed behaviour?
- Is the victim well known and loved?
- Was there any evidence of recognition of the victim?
- Was there a period of confusion following the attack?
- Is there amnesia for the event?
- Was there any obvious motive, planning, or premeditation?
- Was there any concealment of the offence?
- Was the offence senseless or out of character?
- Was the violence preceded by a period of poor sleep?

Organic disorders: dementia & delirium

Dementia is a syndrome characterized by global cognitive decline. Dementias can be subdivided into cortical (Alzheimer's disease, Pick's disease), sub-cortical (Parkinson's disease, Huntington's disease, Wilson's disease) cortical-subcortical (Lewy body dementia) and multifocal (CJD).

Prevalence of dementia

- General population: 5–10% (over 65 years)
- General psychiatric patients: no data
- Forensic psychiatric patients: 19–33% (over 60 years)
- Prisoners: 1% (sentenced prisoners over 59).

Prevalence of delirium

- General population: no data.

Comorbidity of dementia with other mental disorders

- Delusions and hallucinations (paranoid) in patients with dementia: 20–40%
- Anxiety and/or depression: 50%
- Cognitive deficits vary with dementia type.

Association between dementia and offending behaviour

Dementia is primarily a disorder of old age and people over 65 are under-represented as a proportion of all violent offenders (less than 0.5%) Behavioural and psychological symptoms of dementia (BPSD) and neuropsychiatric symptoms are numerous, and include agitation and aggression. This may include shouting and verbal insults but also hitting, biting, and other physical violence. These behavioural symptoms may occur in conjunction with other psychiatric and physical disorders. There is no confirmed association between dementia and serious violence. There are also no specific offences associated with dementia, although there is some suggestion that sexual offences may be more common in elderly people with dementia compared to those with other psychiatric disorders. Generally, minor offences are more common, if offending occurs.

Assessment

Anyone presenting with aggressive or offending behaviour (whether or not charged with a criminal offence) for the first time in older age should be assessed carefully to exclude dementia, especially if the offence is serious.

Likewise, in those with a history of alcohol abuse (📖 p.II.56), the possibility of delirium or alcoholic dementia should be considered, especially if such a defendant claims amnesia (📖 p.V.504) for an offence.

Management of offending behaviour in dementia

Despite the lack of association between violent crime and dementia there is an association between aggressive behaviour and dementia. The management should be considered based on individual needs and neuropsychiatric status.

- Non-pharmacological methods should be first line:
  - Psychological
  - Validation therapy (e.g. accepting without contradiction the factually incorrect statements made because of failing memory)
  - Structured social interaction
- Non-psychological:
  - Aromatherapy
  - Pharmacological
- If aggression is causing extreme distress then short-term (<12 weeks) treatment with antipsychotic (long-term treatment is associated with serious adverse events—including stroke and death):
  - In moderate to severe Alzheimer's disease when memantine is indicated then this is preferred treatment for agitation
  - If non-aggressive or low-risk agitation but memantine not indicated then citalopram or carbamazepine
- Longer term treatment—memantine, citalopram or carbamazepine:
  - Review treatment every 3 months with attempt at discontinuation.

Delirium

Delirium can be associated with a wide range of medical conditions, dementias, alcohol or drug intoxication, or withdrawal. The importance of delirium in offending behaviour is unclear but there is evidence that delirium can be associated with aggressive behaviour. The management of aggression in delirium will usually be by management of the underlying cause. Sedation should be avoided unless necessary to manage any immediate risk of harm to self or others. If pharmacological management is required then ordinary principles of rapid tranquilization should be observed.

Organic disorders

Other organic disorders of known aetiology have no general association with violence but, like dementia, may contribute to aggressive behaviour and even offending. Some organic disorders result in personality change and may be associated with changes in behaviour that could include offending behaviour. Alcohol, drugs and brain injury can result in organic personality change. Organic psychosis may be associated with increased criminality.

Malingering and factitious disorder

Both malingering and factitious disorder[*] involve the conscious, intentional feigning of physical or psychological symptoms[†] of illness. They can be contrasted with somatoform disorders, in which the patient is unaware of the psychological origin of their expressed symptoms.

Prevalence of malingering and factitious disorder

- General population: less than 1%
- General psychiatric patients: 0.4–0.8%
- Prisoners: no data
- Forensic psychiatric patients: no data.

Box 3.1 Common motivations for malingering

- Avoiding work and/or establishing grounds for benefit payments
- Obtaining compensation for negligence (📖 p.V.512), especially personal injury (📖 p.V.514)
- Avoiding criminal prosecution, conviction, or punishment
- Avoiding military service or similar social obligations
- Obtaining a prescription.

Where there is an external gain (such as in the examples in Box 3.1), the condition is labelled malingering and is not regarded as a mental disorder. Where instead the motivation is internal and is one of which the patient is apparently not consciously aware, even though they realize they are deliberately feigning the symptoms, the condition is labelled factitious disorder.

This distinction has been criticized as arbitrary and unhelpful. Establishing whether or not there is an external gain motivating the feigning of symptoms is extremely difficult and has low inter-rater reliability.

Some authors advocate a longitudinal approach to assessment, involving a prolonged admission, and others the use of instruments designed to exploit a presumed lack of technical knowledge of genuine symptoms or symptom combinations, such as the SIRS, the SIMS, and the TOMM (📖 p.II.104).

---

[*] Factitious disorder is often called Munchausen syndrome, especially if the feigned symptoms are physical. The feigning can include self-harm to mimic illness, such as causing wounds or infection. If the wounds, infections etc. are inflicted on another person, such as a child, the condition is referred to as factious disorder (or Munchausen syndrome) by proxy.
[†] Detecting that psychological symptoms are feigned is considerably more difficult than with physical symptoms.

However, some claim that lawyers can coach their clients to pass these tests, and partly for this reason the polygraph ('lie detector') is also used in some US states.

Comorbidity with other mental disorders

The presence of feigning does not rule out there being a genuine physical or psychological disorder. The data on the prevalence of malingering and factitious disorder are sparse and unreliable (partly because the conditions are intrinsically difficult to screen for or diagnose), and there are no available data on rates of comorbidity.

Claims of amnesia (📖 p.V.504) are relatively common among defendants accused of committing violent crimes and it is difficult to distinguish genuine versus simulated amnesia; the TOMM (📖 p.II.104) attempts to do this in a structured fashion.

Some authors have suggested that malingering is associated with antisocial personality disorder (📖 p.II.60) and psychopathy (📖 p.II.66), particularly malingered amnesia for an offence.

Associations with offending behaviour

There is no evidence to suggest that the presence of factious disorder or malingering is associated with subsequent offending, except insofar as the circumstances make malingering an offence in itself (e.g. benefit fraud, or in factitious disorder by proxy, harming the other person concerned).

Factitious disorder by proxy has become of niche importance in forensic psychiatry as a result of cases of mothers with the condition harming their children and being detected by CCTV on paediatric wards; and of cases of healthcare workers killing (usually elderly) patients in their care.‡

Malingering as a consequence of offending

Avoiding criminal responsibility, for example by appearing unfit to plead (📖 p.V.474), and avoiding punishment, for example by attempting to be transferred to hospital (📖 pp.IV.405, IV.410), are common motivations for malingering symptoms of mental disorder.

▶ Any forensic assessment considering these issues (📖 pp.II.90, II.113) should bear in mind the possibility of malingering in particular. It is important to recognize the difference between forensic assessment for legal purposes and therapeutic assessments: a motivation to malinger is more likely in the former.

---

‡ The most famous recent such case is that of Beverley Allitt, a paediatric nurse in Lincolnshire who killed four children and injured nine others, chiefly by injecting insulin or potassium chloride.

Chapter 4

Assessment in forensic psychiatry

The forensic psychiatric assessment

There are important distinctions ethically and legally between assessing a patient in a health context, and a defendant or litigant in a legal context; but whatever the context, and whoever is doing the assessment (an individual forensic psychiatrist, for example, or a psychologist and psychiatrist, or a psychiatric team), the clinical process should be similar.

See also the advice on assessment specifically with a view to providing reports (📖 pp.V.556–V.584), including the ethical requirement (📖 p.App. 4.651) to explain the context and purpose of the assessment, and the fact that there may be no therapeutic relationship or doctor–patient confidentiality.

Process

In a clinical context, the forensic psychiatrist and the MDT of which they are a part aim not only to determine a diagnosis but to reach an understanding of the patient and their situation (which may, even in a clinical context, include their legal situation) and to produce a plan for action. The individual forensic practitioner assessing in a legal context should pursue a similar process. This process may involve any or all of the following aspects:

- Understanding the context in which the assessment takes place, and adjusting as necessary by making special considerations (📖 pp.II.112–II.125)
- Obtaining information from an appropriate range of sources (📖 p.II.107), including the history as reported by the patient and relevant family members and others;* medical and other records such as education and social services files; and the doctor's own mental state examination and physical examination
- Performing or requesting specialized psychological tests (📖 pp.II.96–II.104), the nature of which will depend on the clinical issues at hand but might include special tests of personality (📖 pp.II.92), attitudes (📖 p.II.95), intelligence (📖 pp.II.99), or other aspects of psychological or neurological functioning
- Ordering biological or other investigations (📖 p.II.105), if necessary, including, for example, brain imaging and EEG investigations, and investigations directed at identifying general medical conditions that can affect brain function
- Reaching a diagnosis or differential diagnosis (📖 p.II.108), and an individualized formulation (📖 p.II.110)
- Assessing the risks of various possible harms (📖 pp.II.130–II.141)
- Constructing treatment (📖 pp.II.146–II.187) and risk management (📖 pp.II.190–II.204) plans.

Clinical records

Contemporaneous clinical notes should be kept that clearly record whether information from the interviewee is paraphrased or literally their words (which may be important not only medically but sometimes crucial legally). Occasionally, it may be appropriate to tape-record or even video-record part of an interview. Notes should also make clear what information arose from open questions (for example, 'Have you noticed any change in your

---

* Where the context is a legal one, gaining information from an informant may be subject to special rules if they are coincidentally witnesses, and may require legal permission.

thinking recently?') or closed questions (for example, 'Do you ever hear voices when there is no-one speaking?')—this may be important not only clinically but also legally, where the assessment is for a legal purpose.

Always be aware that your clinical notes can become part of legal proceedings, whether proceedings relating to the individual you have assessed as a defendant or litigant, or subsequent unpredicted proceedings such as an action in negligence (📖 p.V.512) or tribunal proceedings. Your notes may also be made available to the patient, or be disclosed during legal proceedings to others you might not expect, as the normal rules of confidentiality (📖 p.III.263) do not always apply. Clinical notes should therefore be constructed with precision and care.

Vignette: a forensic assessment

This short case example is aimed at illustrating some of the points made in the following pages

Responding to an emergency call made by neighbours, the police attend a house where they find Mr P near the body of a young woman who has been stabbed to death. Suspecting Mr P of killing her (i.e. of committing a homicide offence, 📖 p.IV.344), they arrest Mr P and take him to the police station.

At the police station, Mr P is seen by the forensic medical examiner (FME, 📖 p.V.452), who tells the police officer in charge of the custody suite that Mr P appears to have a mental disorder and is probably not fit to be interviewed (📖 p.V.452). The FME requests a Mental Health Act assessment (📖 p.IV.381).

Mr P is seen by a general psychiatrist, who diagnoses him with schizophrenia (📖 p.II.54). The psychiatrist and a second doctor recommend that he be transferred to hospital under a civil section of the Mental Health Act (📖 p.IV.383), and an AMHP (📖 p.IV.379) agrees to make an application, but the custody sergeant refuses to release him from the police station because of the seriousness of the alleged offence. Mr P is therefore remanded in custody (📖 p.IV.330) by the magistrates' court and sent to prison.

At the prison, he is seen by a Prison Medical Officer (📖 p.V.457) who notes the diagnosis of schizophrenia and informs the clerk of the court (📖 p.IV.312). When he is brought before the Crown court (📖 p.IV.320), the court requests a forensic psychiatric report (📖 p.V.556), and Mr P is therefore assessed (📖 p.II.90) by a forensic psychiatrist.

The forensic psychiatrist concurs with the diagnosis of schizophrenia, and finds that Mr P was probably suffering from psychotic symptoms at the time of the alleged offence. She passes her conclusions to Mr P's lawyer, who subsequently raises the issue of diminished responsibility (📖 p.V.491). A second forensic psychiatrist instructed by the prosecution agrees with the forensic psychiatrist instructed by the defence. At trial (📖 p.V.448), Mr P pleads guilty (📖 p.IV.330) to the offence of manslaughter (📖 p.IV.345) on the grounds of diminished responsibility and receives a hospital order (📖 p.IV.405). In the light of the forensic psychiatrist's risk assessment (📖 p.II.130), the judges also impose restrictions under section 41 of the Mental Health Act (📖 p.IV.412). Mr P is sent from court to a medium secure unit (📖 p.II.210) for further assessment and treatment.

Assessment of personality

What is personality?

Personality comes from the Greek word 'persona', meaning mask. There is no single definition of personality, but several theories of its nature and function. Some theories emphasize the social aspect of personality; how individuals perceive the world and interact with others within it. Other theories emphasize the individual nature of personality: the psychological structures and capacities of the individual such as affective traits, psychological defences, affective and arousal regulatory systems, plus cognitive biases and attributions.

Personality influences how an individual appraises and interprets the social world, and therefore affects how they tend to behave in given social situations. This can be psychiatrically significant whether or not the individual's personality is 'disordered': personality traits can affect the way that symptoms of mental illness are expressed, and how well an individual with mental disorder functions.

What is personality disorder?

PD (💷 p.II.58) is a disorder of identified aspects of those psychological constructs just described. The ICD10 (💷 p.II.109) definition emphasizes that PD is an enduring condition, developing and manifesting in childhood. It persists into the 4th and 5th decades of life, and is often accompanied by behaviours that interfere with optimal social functioning. DSM-IV (💷 p.II.109) requires evidence by very early adulthood.

Assessment of personality and PD

Personality and PD can be assessed by clinical interview combined with a wide range of sources of information, or by psychometric tests validated on large populations.

Clinical psychological assessment tends to suggest the presence of PD (or its absence) on the basis of personality structure as measured psychometrically, in terms of statistical variance from the mean, often without reference to functional consequences. Given that function can be determined by context, an individual may therefore appear non-disordered for many years until their vulnerability to dysfunction is exposed by a change of circumstance. Psychiatric assessment, on the other hand, requires evidence of dysfunction for a diagnosis to be made.

Assessment specifically for PD may be indicated where there is persistent behavioural and/or interpersonal disturbance in the absence of obvious cognitive impairment or psychotic disorder. More broadly, a personality assessment for will inform understanding of the patient, and assist with risk assessment, treatment planning and risk management.

Selection and use of personality assessment tools

There are a wide variety of psychology-based personality assessment tools, and each has its own strengths and weaknesses. The tools vary on the conceptualization of personality that underpins them. For example, the Eysenck Personality Questionnaire and the NEO-PI-R* are based on trait theories of personality; whereas the Millon assessment tools view personality as related to the degrees of various dimensions of pathology present.

Validity of PD assessment tools

There is also considerable debate about the validity of self-report tools specifically for PD, since many individuals exhibiting PD have very little accurate idea of how others see them. They will therefore complete the self-report instruments according to the distorted perspective from which they see themselves. There may also be motivations to complete the measure in a certain way determined by context, for example, if the outcome is to be used in a court report or to inform risk assessment. Some workers have therefore suggested that other informants should complete the assessment tools; however this also carries the possibility of bias, and crucially leaves out the subjective experience of the person assessed. It is therefore important to incorporate both self-report and other-report data within the assessment. Paper or computer based instruments can be helpful in reducing interviewer bias; and this may be of particular value in assessing individuals with likely antisocial or borderline PD, who may be antagonistic or hostile, and who may thereby distort the interviewer's perception of the individual.

Single versus multiple assessments

One-off assessments of PD are notoriously unreliable, and so either all individuals should be assessed more than once, or the limitations of a single interview acknowledged. If only a single interview is possible, the assessor must also use other sources of information, and should ideally talk to several informants. Assessment using different approaches and paradigms, for example those of psychiatry and psychology, can also aid validity and reliability, if they reach the same conclusion.

Measuring severity

There are at present no standardized assessments of severity of PD. It is reasonable, however, to assume that more severe forms or degrees of PD will result in more domains of social functioning being affected, as well as each domain being more severely affected. More severe PD is also likely to be associated with comorbidity with episodic, or enduring mental illness.

Personality disorder and risk assessment

As described elsewhere (□ p.II.58), most people with PD do not present a risk to anyone. However, there are subtypes of PD (□ pp.II.60–II.67) which are associated with significant risk of violence to others, and these will naturally be over-represented in forensic populations. Between 60–70% of forensic inpatients can be diagnosed as having a personality disorder, usually antisocial, borderline, paranoid, or narcissistic, and many of these patients will demonstrate traits of all four disorders.

---

*The abbreviation refers to the first three of the five factors the test is based on: neuroticism, extraversion and openness to new experiences. The other two are agreeableness and conscientiousness.

Psychopathy
Probably the most meaningful risk feature in PD is the degree to which the individual demonstrates psychopathic (📖 p.II.66) traits such as cruel, hostile or unempathic attitudes to others, especially the vulnerable. The Psychopathy Check List Revised (PCL-R, 📖 p.II.102) provides a measure of these traits.[*]

Normative scores

Most personality assessment tools have not been standardized on forensic populations. This may not necessarily be a problem, since deviance from non-forensic norms may be of importance in formulation. However, in clinical settings where treatment is being planned, standardized tests provide norms which are helpful in looking at outcomes, and the lack of appropriate normative data in forensic populations therefore reduces the opportunities for studying treatment outcomes with forensic patients.

Cultural factors

♦ Most personality assessment tools were devised and developed in the context of Western cultural values. They may therefore miss cultural values and attitudes that are of psychological salience to individuals from non-Western backgrounds. As a result it is not recommended that paper/computer based assessment tools be used with individuals from non-Western cultures. Such individuals need to be interviewed by professionals who are conversant with the values and beliefs of that culture, and who can also carry out interviews with other informants, also from that same cultural background. PD occurs in every culture, but it may have very different presenting features and different social ramifications in different ethnic/cultural groups.

Sexual attitudes and behaviour

The assessment of sexual attitudes and behaviour, coupled with assessments of mental state and personality (📖 p.II.92), will usually be done in order to give an opinion on treatment (📖 p.II.176) or on the risk of sexual violence or of sexual offending (📖 pp.II.132–II.137), or on whether a relevant legal defence applies (📖 p.IV.342). Reported deviant sexual fantasies or abnormally high levels of sexual arousal may prompt a request for specialist assessment, although deviant fantasies are also present in the non-offending population. Some sex offenders develop depression either in conjunction with their offending or in response to treatment; this must also be assessed.

Most sexual behaviour services will not assess or treat prior to conviction: the rate of improvement is often low because the acceptance required for treatment to succeed is inconsistent with seeking to deny or minimize the offence at trial.

---

[*] Strictly, the PCL-R is a diagnostic tool and not a risk assessment instrument, but it is frequently used as a component of violence risk assessment (📖 p.II.132) because of the strong correlation between psychopathy and risk of violence.

Assessing attitudes

The concept of 'attitudes' may be flawed because of its imprecise nature, but it has been the basis of most research and clinical assessment for some time, and there is no currently available alternative concept. The relationship of 'attitudes' to personality traits (📖 p.II.92) is complex. One view is that attitudes are more amenable to change than personality traits.

An assessment of sexual attitudes involves a clinical interview and collateral history, supplemented by standardized assessments such as the RSAS, EWT and ACS (see 📖 p.II.103 for the names and definitions of these tests). The aim is to understand the patient's *cognitive distortions* and relevant *schema* (see also 📖 pp.II.47, II.48).

Assessing behaviour

Behaviour is assessed using a combination of clinical interview, collateral history, official records including police and social services records, and direct observation.

Clinical interview

An interview for the purpose of assessing sexual attitudes and behaviour should cover:
- Sexual development and early sexual experiences
- Masturbation—frequency, fantasy, public/private
- Sexual partners—number, gender
- Consideration of paraphilia (📖 p.II.74) and deviant sexual interests
- Sexual preoccupations
- Strength of sexual arousal
- Violence in sexual relationships (actual and fantasized)
- Use of pornography.

Cognitive distortions

These are errors of thinking that tend to allow the individual to ignore others' perspectives (especially the victim's), and to justify their offending behaviour. However, it may be difficult to assess cognitive distortions in a way that is free from desirability bias: that is, not endorsing items that are obviously socially unacceptable. There is also a developing consensus that an analysis based solely on cognitive distortions is an oversimplification and that underlying core beliefs and possibly other motivations for sexual offending (📖 p.II.47) should be taken into account.

Schema

Schema (or schemata), derived from cognitive therapy (📖 p.II.165), have been described as implicit theories that potential offenders hold to explain the world around them. They may be considered to be underlying modes of thinking of which cognitive distortions are the superficial representations. Schema that have been described as motivating sexual offenders are described on 📖 p.II.48.

Pornography

❧ The use of pornography in general has not been shown to cause sexual offending. However, pornography depicting sexual violence has been shown to affect self-reported likelihood of rape or offending. More generally, the content of pornography preferred by an individual is an important guide to their sexual attitudes. Downloading child pornography is a major form of sexual offending against children (📖 p.II.44).

Psychological testing

Just as in clinical settings, psychologists often make use of psychometric tests, scales or instruments to evaluate psychological factors in the context of legal issues such as fitness to plead (📖 p.V.474), duress (📖 p.V.502), or mitigation (📖 p.V.506). Most such tests have been devised as aids to clinical judgement, and to measure outcomes following psychological interventions. The objective of most such tests is to obtain information about an individual in a standardized and valid way, based upon population studies.

Selection and use

There are a large number of tests available for use in clinical forensic psychological assessments. Any test used should one that is documented and reviewed in the scientific literature, and it should be accompanied by a manual describing the test's development, psychometric properties and procedure. It should be reliable and valid. The test should clearly be relevant to the clinical and/or legal issue addressed; and the standard administration recommended in the manual should be followed whether it is directed solely at clinical issues or ultimately at legal questions.

Note that some tests require the administrator to be trained, either in a relevant profession (e.g. a clinical psychologist, or a mental health professional more generally: for example, the PAS, 📖 p.II.102) or in that specific test (e.g. the MCMI, 📖 p.II.102).

> ### Cultural factors
> ⚠ Many psychological tests are standardized with Western populations and would not be appropriate for use with individuals from other cultures. When selecting a test it is therefore important to consider the population with which it has been standardized. Some tests are more culture-fair than others.

Reliability

The repeatability or reproducibility of results from a test or measure is referred to as its reliability. Specifically, in order to be deemed reliable, the test should:

- give consistent results each time it is applied to an individual (test-retest reliability), and
- when applied by different clinicians (inter-rater reliability).

There are several different statistical methods of measuring reliability, including correlation coefficients for test-retest reliability, Cronbach's alpha for internal consistency, and kappa for inter-rater reliability. Such reliability coefficients range from 0–1 and a test with a reliability coefficient of below 0.80 should if possible not be used clinically or in legal proceedings.

Validity

The validity of a test refers to whether it measures what it is designed to measure (and purports to measure). There are three main types of validity: content, criterion-related and construct validity.

- *Content validity* refers to the item content and how well it represents the behavioural or psychological domain to be measured
- Criterion-related validity refers to the effectiveness of the test as compared with results from a 'gold standard' test (the criterion): *concurrent validity* refers to how well the test results compare with those of the criterion measured at the same time, whereas *predictive validity* refers to how well the test results predict those of the criterion measured in the future (in the case of psychological tests, this might mean how well the test predicts the individual's future behaviour).
- *Construct validity* refers to how well the test measures a relevant theoretical construct or trait (e.g. how well the items in an IQ test each correspond to the known properties of intelligence).

Normative scores

Standardization is an essential part of psychometric test construction and development. It involves the test being administered to a representative sample of people for whom the test was developed. Standardized tests provide norms for several different populations.

Interpretation of results

Test scores should be interpreted with an appropriate comparative sample: that is, the scores obtained by the individual should be compared with those of an appropriate population (e.g. all forensic patients, or all violent criminals) in order to interpret it. For example, saying that Mr X has a PCL-R score of 15 carries little meaning; saying that this is well below the conventional cut-off score of 30 for a diagnosis of psychopathy is helpful; but saying that this places him in the 26th percentile of forensic inpatients, and that this means that 74% of forensic inpatients have a greater degree of psychopathy, is more useful still.

The score for a test should not be applied for a purpose for which the test was not developed. For example, a test designed to measure risk of violence after discharge from a forensic psychiatric hospital, such as the VRAG (📖 p.II.134), will not give meaningful results if applied to inmates of a young offender institution (📖 p.V.458).

Test data should be integrated and interpreted in relation to other sources of data. Scores should not be over-generalized or used in isolation. That is to say, the test results should be placed by the assessor in the context of the assessment as a whole. For example, a diagnosis of LD, or an explanation of that patient's behaviour, should not be based on an IQ score alone, but on that IQ score interpreted in the context of other assessment findings.

Disclosure of tests or test scores

Detailed descriptions of subtle psychological tests may undermine the validity of the test, as potential future test subjects may then be more likely deliberately to distort their responses. That said, the argument in favour of disclosure of some test items and raw scores is that it is difficult for another expert to evaluate the test findings in a legal context (for the purposes of cross-examination (📖 p.V.588) in court, say) if a certain amount of detail is not provided, and that this justifies the risk of the disclosed information becoming publicly available. Experts should be aware of the implications and ethical issues involved in disclosure or non-disclosure.

Problems in presenting test results in legal fora

Psychological tests are constructed by scientists, and used and interpreted by professional clinicians; each understands the strengths and limitations of any given test, including the limits of its interpretation and the importance of validating results by placing them in the context of a full clinical assessment.

However, when a test is used to come to clinical conclusions that are then applied to a legal question, and the clinician is subject to examination and cross-examination (📖 p.V.588) within an adversarial court process (📖 p.IV.314)—especially in front of a jury—there is much scope for deliberate lawyerly 'misunderstanding' of the test method, results and interpretation, especially in cross-examination. For example, a barrister might take individual questions within an instrument and question the expert witness on those questions, attempting to 'belittle' the test by a process of 'disaggregation', deliberately appearing not to understand that the items in the test must be taken as a whole. Resisting such techniques of deliberate misunderstanding can require much skill, and calmness, again especially in front of a jury, as well as discussion with the barrister on the same side, to advise what questions would enable a balanced understanding of the test to be communicated by the expert.

Psychological test domains

Brief descriptions of specific tests of each domain can be found on 📖 p.II.101.

Anger and violence Attitudes towards violence, and levels of anger are important to measure in both aiding risk assessment and general attitudes to offending. Measures in this area can be also useful in evaluating the outcomes of anger management groups and other therapies.

Blame attribution can be described as the way that a perpetrator accounts for their offending: for example, how much responsibility they take, and in what fashion. This is important both in how they are treated in the criminal justice system and in the assessment of future risk. This also gives some insight into how much remorse they feel for what they have done. Asking directly, for example, in a Mental Health Tribunal (📖 p.IV.309) or Parole Board (📖 p.V.459) hearing how much remorse an individual feels is unlikely to be useful or valid. Much more effective is measuring constructs that are relevant to remorse, but do not attempt to measure remorse itself. Indeed, remorse is a complex moral concept, whereas 'blame attribution' describes an individual's cognition in an area relevant to remorse.

Competency or capacity Individuals may be competent to carry out different sets of tasks. Fitness to give legal instructions, fitness to plead (📖 p.V.474), or competence to make medical decisions are most commonly relevant issues. There are a number of instruments that assess mental capacity (📖 p.IV.424) in the context of treatment, but most are derived from US populations and have not been standardized in the UK. There are no instruments relating to legal tests such as fitness to plead, although recent work in the UK suggests that a purely cognitive test will be inadequate for such tasks.

Executive function (EF) Consists of higher-order cognitive skills associated with the ability to engage in independent, goal-directed behaviour. Impairments in EF have been linked to dysfunction in the frontal lobes. EF can be broken down into different domains of functioning, e.g. verbal/ visual productivity, cognitive flexibility, inhibition, organization, and planning. Different tests tap into different domains of EF.

Intellectual/cognitive function An individual's intelligence refers to a variety of different domains including: an ability to solve problems, reason, apply previous knowledge to new situations, learn new skills, and abstract thinking. An IQ can be used to measure general intelligence. An IQ is a unitary measure and has a mean of 100 and a normal distribution. Other tests assess specific aspects of cognitive function, such as frontal lobe function, memory etc.

Malingering The term malingering (📖 p.II.87) is typically used to describe conscious fabrication or gross exaggeration of symptoms. 'Faking good' and 'faking bad' are possible forms of unreliability. There are three main areas of faking: cognitive deficits, amnesia, and psychiatric symptoms.

Memory Can be subdivided into: working memory (holding information in 'front of mind' in order to use it in the short term), registration (laying down new memories), short-term recall (recently-registered memories and experience), and long-term recall (permanent memory, nearly unlimited capacity). All tests of cognitive function implicitly test working memory, and many explicitly test registration and short- and long-term recall.

Personality Profiles should not be used in isolation, particularly not in relation to risk assessment (📖 p.II.130): this is a particular issue for psychopathy (📖 p.II.66) assessments. There are a number of instruments available for assessing personality, as listed on 📖 p.II.102. See assessment of personality (📖 p.II.92) for more details.

Premorbid functioning Various tests are available which estimate the level of intellectual or cognitive functioning before an illness or head injury. Most tests are based on vocabulary or reading ability. Any discrepancy between current and premorbid estimates will be highly significant, in that it will provide an indication of the degree of deterioration.

Sexual Deviancy This may be appropriate to assess in the context of risk assessment (📖 p.II.130), particularly risk of sexually inappropriate behaviour (📖 p.II.134). Sexual deviancy (📖 p.II.47) is usually assessed in terms of deviant erotic object choice, the association of sexual arousal with anger or hostility, and lack of empathy for victims.

Suggestibility and compliance These issues may be relevant in the assessment of retracted or false confessions (📖 p.V.479). Suggestibility refers to the extent to which, within a closed social interrogative interaction, an individual comes to accept and believe messages communicated during formal questioning; compliance to the tendency to go along with propositions, requests or instructions for some immediate instrumental gain, without accepting them. See 📖 p.II.123 for a fuller discussion of suggestibility and compliance.

The tests, GSS1, GSS2 and GCS (📖 p.II.102), were designed for use in relation to police interviews, but are applicable to any interview situation; it is not clear whether this includes giving evidence in court. Whereas the GCS is a self-report questionnaire, GSS1&2 involve reading a standardized story to the subject, asking them to remember all they can, asking them specific questions about the story, telling them forcefully that some answers were incorrect (whether this is true or not), and then repeating the questions. GSS1&2 give scores for 'yield' (responding with incorrect answers to leading questions) and 'shift' (changing answers after being told earlier answers were wrong). The GCS suffers from the lower validity of all self-report measures, whereas the association of elevated GSS1&2 with low IQ scores is also potentially problematic.

Traumatic experience There are various measures available that assess symptoms of trauma. However, in the forensic population it is common for individuals to have experienced multiple traumatic events and not all tools are good at accounting for complex trauma. Psychometric tests do not always distinguish between trauma as a consequence of earlier events and trauma as a consequence of offending.

Specific psychological tests

Key to tests

F	Test has a prominent functional/performance element
IS	Based on structured or semi-structured interview
QS	Questionnaire based on self-report
QI	Questionnaire administered by interviewer
P	Test has a prominent visual/pictorial element
R	Includes information from medical & other records
TP	Includes information from third-party informants
V	Test has a prominent verbal (word-based) element
*	Training in the specific test required

Cognitive: intellectual functioning

WAIS-IV	Wechsler Adult Intelligence Scales—4th edition*	QI,V,F,P
WISC-IV	Wechsler Intelligence Scale for Children—4th edition*	QI,V,F,P
WASI	Wechsler Abbreviated Scale of Intelligence*	QI,V,F
MMSE	Mini Mental Status Examination	QI,V,F
QT	Ammons Quick Test	QI,P
Raven	Raven's Progressive Matrices	QI,P

Cognitive: pre-morbid functioning

NART	National Adult Reading Test	QI,V
SGWRT	Schonell Graded Word Reading Test	QI,V
WTAR	Wechsler Test of Adult Reading*	QI,V

Cognitive: memory

WMS-III	Wechsler Memory Scales—3rd edition*	QI,V
CMS	Camden Memory Scales	QI,F,P
RBMT	Rivermead Behavioural Memory Test	QI,V,F,P

Cognitive: executive/frontal lobe functioning

BADS	Behavioural Assessment of Dysexecutive Syndrome	**QI,F**
DKEFS	Delis-Kaplan Executive Function System	**QI,V,F**
H-B	Hayling-Brixton Test	**QI,V,F**
Trails	Trails A&B	**QI,F**
Stroop	The Stroop Test	**QI,F**
WCST	Wisconsin Card-Sorting Test	**QI,F**
CAMCOG	Cambridge Cognitive Examination	**QI,V,F**
FAB	Frontal Assessment Battery	**QI,V,F**

Personality: dimensional

MMPI	Minnesota Multiphasic Personality Inventory[*]	**QS,V**
MCMI	Millon Clinical Multiaxial Inventory[*]	**QS,V**
MACI	Millon Adolescent Clinical Inventory[*]	**QS,V**

Personality: diagnostic

DIPD-IV	Diagnostic Interview for DSM-IV Personality Disorders	**IS,V**
IPDE	International Personality Disorder Examination[*]	**IS,V**
PAI	Personality Assessment Inventory	**QS,V**
PAS	Personality Assessment Schedule	**IS,V,R,TP**
PCL-R	Psychopathy Checklist Revised[*]	**IS,V,R,TP**
PDQ-IV	Personality Diagnostic Questionnaire—4th edition	**QS,V**
SCID-II	Structured Clinical Interview for DSM-IV, 2nd edition[*]	**IS,V**

General: diagnostic **SCAN** schedules for Clinical Assessment in Neuropsychiatry **IS, V**

Suggestibility and compliance

GSS1,2	Gudjonsson Suggestibility Scale version 1 or 2	**IS,V**
GCS	Gudjonsson Compliance Scale	**QS,V**

Sexual offending

MSI	Multiphasic Sex Inventory	QI,V
RSAS	Rape Supportive Attitudes Scale	QI,V
BRM	Burt Rape Myth	QI,V
EWT-V2a	Empathy for Women Test, version 2a	QS,V
Hanson	Hanson Questionnaire	QI,V
ACS	Abel Cognitions Scale	QI,V
QACSI	Questionnaire on Attitudes Consistent with Sex Offending	QI,V

Anger & violence

STAXI-II	State-Trait Anger Expression Inventory	QI,V
PI	Provocation Inventory	QI,V
NAS	Novaco Anger Scales	QI,V
WARS	Ward Anger Rating Scale	QI,V
MVQ	Maudsley Violence Questionnaire	QI,V

Competency

MacCAT-T	Macarthur Competence Assessment Tool for Treatment	IS,VF
CST	Competency Screening Test	QI,V
CAI	Competency Assessment Instrument	QI,V
IFI	Interdisciplinary Fitness Interview	IS,V

Post traumatic stress disorder, Trauma

CAPS	Clinician Administered PTSD Scale	QI,V
TSI	Trauma Symptom Inventory	QS,V
PDS	Post Traumatic Stress Diagnostic Scales	QS,V
IES-R	Impact of Events Scale, Revised	QS,V
DAPS	Detailed Assessment of Posttraumatic Stress	QI,V
TSI	Trauma Symptom Inventory	QI,V

(Continued)

CAPS	Clinician Administered Posttraumatic Stress Disorder Scale	IS
CTQ	Childhood Trauma Questionnaire	QI,V
IES-R	Impact of Events Scale, Revised	QI,V
PDS	Posttraumatic Stress Diagnostic Scale	IS

Blame attribution

| BAI | Blame Attribution Inventory | QI,V |

Fire-setting

FSAS	Fire-Setting Assessment Schedule	QI,V
FIRS	Fire Interest Rating Scale	QI,V
SDS	Severity of Dependence Scale	QI,V

Mood

BDI-II	Beck Depression Inventory—Second Edition	QI,V
BAI	Beck Anxiety Inventory	QI,V
GHQ	General Health Questionnaire	QI,V

Suicidal intention

SSI	Scale for Suicide Ideation	QI,V
BHS	Beck Hopelessness Scale	QI,V
SISQ	Suicidal Ideation Screening Questionnaire	QI,V
SADPERSONS	Screening questionnaire for suicidal ideation	QI,V
BSI	Beck Suicide Inventory	QI,V

Malingering

SIRS/SIMS	Structured Inventory of Reported/Malingered Symptoms	QI,V
TOMM	Test of Memory Malingering	QI,V
Many of the cognitive function tests listed here can also be used for malingering		

Instruments used for assessing risks are listed on 📖 pp.II.133–II.137. This list is not exhaustive: many others, more or less widely used, are available. Only those instruments more commonly encountered in forensic settings have been included.

Use of biological investigations

The purpose of conducting biological investigations in psychiatry is to identify any medical condition affecting brain function. Such investigations include brain imaging and EEG, plus potentially a wide range of blood and urine tests. Karyotyping and other genetic tests are not routinely performed.

Biological investigations are rarely specific to forensic psychiatric evaluation and the principles of such investigations are the same as for patients receiving general psychiatric care.* The factors commonly and specifically relevant to forensic psychiatric assessment are in the following section.

Indications for investigations

Forensic psychiatric inpatients may be investigated using biological techniques more frequently than in general psychiatry. This can occur because:

- There are higher rates of head injury in people convicted of violent acts necessitating brain imaging and EEG investigation
- There are higher rates of physical ill-health amongst forensic psychiatric patients including sexually transmitted infection and diabetes in particular
- Forensic patients often have comorbid drug and alcohol misuse, and therefore require urine drug testing and/or breath analysis to test for drug or alcohol use, as well as investigation for possible effects of chronic substance misuse
- Patients in forensic psychiatric services are more likely to be prescribed high-dose antipsychotic medication, resulting in the need for more frequent blood and ECG monitoring
- Forensic psychiatric patients are more likely to be prescribed clozapine, necessitating frequent blood test monitoring
- Forensic psychiatric patients are more likely to be required to undergo plasma monitoring of antipsychotic blood levels in order to test compliance with oral medication

Where a patient in hospital or a prisoner is facing a serious charge, the threshold for ruling out an organic cause of their condition should be low, because the criminal justice stakes are high. This can mean that no stone is left unturned when otherwise a 'wait and see' approach might be appropriate. Also, even subtle abnormalities of brain function can lay the foundation for a mental condition defence (📖 p.IV.342), most commonly that of diminished responsibility (📖 p.V.491) in relation to a charge of murder, and this again reduces the threshold for brain investigation.

---

*Further information can therefore be found in the *Oxford Handbook of Psychiatry*, or a textbook of general psychiatry.

Given the current poor state of knowledge about the biological basis of mental disorders, and the paucity of specific tests available, there is no place at present for routine biological investigation in the diagnosis of mental disorder or in assessing the cause or risk of violent behaviour.

▶Biological investigations should not be performed without a specific indication, such as suspicion of a condition that is diagnosable through the use of the test in question, or checking medication compliance by testing the blood level of the drug in question.

Presentation of the results of investigations

Caution should be exercised in reporting brain abnormalities to courts in relation to possible mental condition defences. This is because brain function does not directly map on to legal questions relating to criminal responsibility: the law asks questions that science cannot answer, and science answers questions that the law does not ask (i.e. they have different paradigms and constructs, ☐ p.IV.296). For example, a brain scan showing frontal damage, even combined with neuropsychometric tests suggesting impaired executive function (☐ p.II.99), may imply a disability in medical terms, but this might have little or no relevance for criminal responsibility when translated into the legal context (☐ p.IV.299). Whether or not criminal responsibility is affected is an ultimate issue (☐ p.V.543), and therefore for the court and not a psychiatric expert to decide.

Information gathering and liaison

A comprehensive psychiatric assessment takes into account not only information from the patient's history and examination, but also information from others who know the patient personally and/or professionally. This includes obtaining all relevant medical and other records wherever possible. Although this is often unnecessary and impractical in general psychiatric practice, it is the standard required in forensic psychiatric practice, and is essential for risk assessment (📖 p.II.130) in particular.

The following sources should all be considered, although a balance must be struck between the need for the information that a particular source might be able to supply, and the time or effort required to obtain that information.

From the patient, defendant, or litigant
- The history
- Mental state examination
- Physical examination
- Results of tests, investigations and psychometric assessments
- Letters, diaries, and other documents written by the patient (used with their consent).

From informants
- Collateral histories from family members
- Collateral histories from friends and colleagues
- Collateral histories from teachers, employers, and others who have known the patient professionally for a considerable length of time, such as former doctors and social workers

From records
- GP medical records
- Records from other psychiatric and general hospitals
- Reports written by previous psychiatrists
- Social work records from adult and child & family social services
- School reports, academic assessments and training records
- Police criminal record and police intelligence reports, including records held under the Multi-Agency Public Protection Arrangements (📖 p.V.468)
- Prosecution case summaries (for the current and also past cases)
- Witness statements (for the current and also past cases)
- So-called 'unused material' for court cases such as witness statements not placed in the prosecution bundle, or statements collected by the defence
- Court records, including judges' comments on sentencing
- Probation pre-sentence and other reports
- Housing and hostel records
- Employment records
- Reports from independent sector agencies such as voluntary work schemes, advice centres, support schemes etc.
- Court reports written by other experts.

Potential ethical problem

Where a defendant is admitted to hospital before trial, they are more likely to disclose legally-relevant information than they might be in prison, because they are in a therapeutic environment and have dropped their guard. For example, they might describe a clear thinking process during the alleged offence, and make it clear that they first experienced psychotic symptoms only in prison. It may be clinically appropriate to record this information in their medical records, as it relates to the onset and triggers of their psychotic episode—but the court might require disclosure of these records, which could then be crucial source of factual information to support the prosecution case. This situation may be unavoidable, and the patient should therefore be repeatedly warned about the possibility of disclosure to the court.

Potential legal problems

Witness statements are often an important source of information in the assessment of a defendant. They may record acts or statements made by the defendant, for example, that indicate their mental state at the time of an alleged offence. However, such statements will have been collected within a legal model (📖 p.IV.297) for legal purposes, and the clinician may wish to interview the witness directly, to ask more specifically about their patient's mental state or behaviour. There might be legal restrictions on doing so, however, and this should not be considered without first seeking the permission of the court, and the advice of a relevant solicitor.

A further problem arises when some of the information on which a clinical opinion is based would be inadmissible in court (📖 p.IV.318)—for example, because it lists previous offences. The clinician needs to take this information into account in order to reach their opinion (e.g. as part of a risk assessment), and may therefore need to include it in a section of their court report (📖 p.V.569), but should be careful to avoid disclosing the information while giving evidence in court* (📖 p.V.586) unless directly instructed to do so.

Diagnosis

The purpose of diagnosis is to categorize symptoms and signs, and to express them in internationally-accepted standardized terms that enable accurate, succinct communication. A diagnosis may also indicate the prognosis, and the response to treatment. Wherever possible, diagnoses are based on knowledge of the aetiology and pathology of the condition, but such knowledge is often lacking in psychiatry. As a result, most psychiatric diagnoses represent syndromes rather than diseases.†

---

* See also the vignette on changing your opinion (📖 p.III.250) in court, which addresses the dilemma of whether to disclose such inadmissible information.

† In more detail, psychiatric conditions range from those whose pathology and aetiology is relatively well-understood, such as dementia (📖 p.II.85) and other organic disorders, to those where it is not yet possible to choose between competing aetiological and pathological theories (e.g. personality disorder, 📖 p.II.58). The difficulty determining the aetiology and pathology of many

Diagnosis and forensic psychiatry

From the perspective of forensic psychiatry, what is usually most relevant is the certainty of a diagnosis, and its mental and behavioural manifestations; the extent to which it is known to be biologically determined is less relevant. However, the lack of objective biological criteria for most psychiatric diagnoses means that value judgements (📖 p.V.551) and other subjective factors may cloud the diagnostic process, something that must be guarded against, including through the adoption of values-based practice (📖 p.III.235).

Diagnostic classificatory systems

For psychiatrists there are two main diagnostic classifications: the World Health Organization's *International Classification of Diseases*, 10th edition, psychiatric section (ICD10 chapter V, 📖 p.App. 1.601) and the American Psychiatric Association's *Diagnostic and Statistical Manual*, 4th edition (DSM-IV, 📖 p.App. 1.601). The DSM-IV is preferred by some because it allows functioning to be rated, and makes dual diagnoses easier on its multiple axes,[*] and is often used in research, especially research into PD; the ICD10 is preferred by others because of its comparative lack of Anglo-American bias and its clearer system of numerical codes. New editions of both classifications are in preparation at the time of writing: ICD11 and DSM-5. The latter involves major revisions to several diagnostic areas, particularly PD, some of which are summarized on 📖 p.App. 1.616.

Caution in the use of classificatory systems in forensic settings

The DSM and ICD also have the advantage of setting out clear criteria for diagnoses, so that when one expert in a case makes a diagnosis according to the ICD or DSM criteria, others can be sure of how they have reached that diagnosis. However, these criteria are not a substitute for the exercise of clinical judgement in the individual case. The need for such clinical judgement can be ignored (sometimes deliberately) by lawyers drawn to the apparent simplicity of the criteria. Detailed cross-examination solely on the required criteria, aimed at undermining the expert's diagnosis by allowing the court or the jury to infer from the criteria alone that the defendant does or does not have the diagnosis, is inappropriate. Experts should not be drawn into such questioning.

Diagnosis, behaviour, and offence

▶ In forensic practice, it is important not to confuse diagnosis with behaviour, or with a criminal offence (or to attempt to treat the behaviour or offence, 📖 p.III.280). A man who sets fires (a behaviour) cannot be diagnosed with arson (a criminal charge). He may or may not be diagnosed as suffering from a mental disorder: but this requires careful assessment and cannot be inferred from the behaviour alone. It certainly cannot be inferred by reference solely to the offence, or offence narrative. To do so

---

conditions is presumed to indicate that those conditions arise from complex mixtures of genetic, psychological and social factors.

[*] Axis 1: clinical disorders and learning disorders; axis 2: personality disorders and intellectual disabilities; axis 3: acute medical conditions and physical disorders; axis 4: contributing psychosocial and environmental factors; axis 5: global assessment of functioning.

would amount to circular reasoning, and would also be outside proper medical practice. Even with a highly unusual behaviour which is also criminal (such as fetishistic sexual violence), and which is often assumed to indicate an underlying mental disorder, there is rarely a direct or simple relationship between mental disorder and complex behaviour.

Diagnostic tools

Day to day, psychiatrists rarely use structured clinical diagnostic tools, preferring to make diagnoses based on clinical assessment of signs and symptoms, albeit usually within the guidance framework of either DSM-IV or ICD10. However, there are structured diagnostic interviews for both psychotic disorders and PDs (e.g. the SCAN and the SCID-II, 📖 p.II.102). These have been devised to allow reliable diagnoses to be made for research purposes, but they may have utility in complex legal cases, especially where the presence or absence of any mental disorder is a matter of legal dispute. These tools require training in order to establish reliability in use by the individual clinician.

Formulation

Formulation is essentially a hypothesis about the causes, precipitants and maintaining influences of a person's psychological, interpersonal, and behavioural problems. It is different from a diagnosis in that it is more individualized and is theoretically driven, whereas diagnosis is intended to reflect an underlying pathology, or known pattern of symptoms and signs, as they occur in populations of individuals.

Formulation is of particular importance in forensic psychiatry because of the dual role of treating mentally disordered offenders, and helping reduce their risk to others. Because the relationship between mental states and action is complex, forensic clinicians need to make formulations which do justice not only to the treatment need but also to the patient's individuality and to the risk of harm they may pose to others. Formulations need to include both risk and resilience (protective) factors. Essential elements to consider in constructing a formulation include:

- *Salient developmental features:* here particular attention is paid to genetic vulnerability and exposure to fear/loss experiences in early years. A history of disrupted attachments and chronic fear experience is associated with an increased risk of developing mental disorders, especially PD, and is also associated with unempathic attitudes towards the self and others.
- *Any indication of early (pre-teen) antisocial values and attitudes:* early onset is a bad prognostic sign, as is any antisocial behaviour before the age of 10, or callous and unemotional attitudes in pre-teens (which are resistant to repair or reparation). Any indicators of positive response to care and attention or enduring attachments should be noted as resilience factors.
- *Later attachment history and adult relationship patterns* should be included in the formulation. Are adult relationships intense, unstable, conflicted and short lived (BPD) or distant, cruel, exploitative (ASPD)? Are any of these features relevant to the index offence?

- *Elements of impaired reality testing at the time of the index offence:* distinguish cognitive distortions from delusional beliefs. How much is the impairment a feature of this person's everyday world view, and how much is it situational? Do drugs and alcohol misuse play a part?
- *What the individual themselves makes of the offence:* is he shocked/baffled/in denial? What psychological defences is he using at the time of interview, and which might he have been using at the time of the offence? (NB. DSM-IV, 📖 p.II.109, allows for rating of psychological defences on Axis 4).
- *Risk factors for violence in this individual's case:* might they be relevant in in-patient settings and therapeutic relationships?

Common theoretical models used in formulations

Biopsychosocial

The classic psychiatric formulation, a two-dimensional table comprising biological, psychological and social factors that are deemed to predispose to the current or anticipated problems, precipitate them, perpetuate (maintain) them, and protect against them.

Cognitive-behavioural

A formulation based upon the CBT model (📖 p.II.165) of interrelated thoughts, emotions, sensations, and actions triggered by negative automatic thoughts and underlain by core beliefs. Like the biopsychosocial model it considers predisposing, precipitating, maintaining and protective factors.

Narrative

An individualized, largely unstructured formulation, though it may isolate and classify individual factors. It represents an individual's story from one perspective. It is personal to the formulator, and often seeks to explain a particular outcome, such as why a patient became ill or why they offended. The scenarios found in the HCR20 (📖 p.II.133) and other risk assessment instruments are examples of narrative formulations.

Psychodynamic

A formulation founded in psychodynamic or psychoanalytic theory, incorporating elements such as defences, drives, and internal objects.

Legal or criminal

A specific type of narrative formulation (though rarely described as such) constructed for use during trial (📖 p.V.448) and sentencing (📖 p.IV.361), comprising elements such as means, motive, intention (📖 p.IV.334), and opportunity.

Example case summary and narrative formulation

Mr Jones is a 23-year-old man charged with the murder of his stepfather. He was admitted to hospital from prison because of concerns about depression and suicide risk. In his early childhood, he was exposed to neglect and physical harm and taken into care between the ages of 4 to 6 years. He was returned to his mother's care but was exposed to further repeated physical violence from stepfather from the age of 8 years. He was antisocial at school from age 10 and was permanently excluded at 14 for violence. His first conviction was at 15 for criminal damage and he has multiple convictions for theft and criminal damage. Last year he assaulted his mother, breaking her arm, but she did not press charges. He has had no relationships with girls but does have one friend from school that he still sees. He is also in touch with his foster mother.

Resilience factors include intelligence and an absence of substance abuse history. *Risk factors* include early loss and fear experiences, mental illness, pre-teen antisocial attitudes, and a complex and angry relationship with his mother. His mother may therefore still be at risk from him; and therapeutic relationships with females should be carefully monitored. He is likely to be paranoid with male authority figures; male staff will need to handle him carefully and not rise to provocative behaviour.

Special issues in forensic assessments

A psychiatric assessment carried out within a forensic setting, particularly if it is for the purpose of a court report, requires that consideration be given to a number of special issues:

- The person being assessed should be informed fully about the nature and purpose of the assessment and that, if it will result in a report that may go to a court or to another part of the criminal justice system, the usual rules concerning confidentiality do not apply as in ordinary clinical situations. That is, in such situations the report is likely to be disclosed (📖 p.III.263) to individuals not involved in the care of the patient. If this is the case, they should also be informed that if they refuse consent to the assessment, a report may still be produced containing opinions based solely on other sources of information.
- Once fully informed, their consent (📖 p.V.540) to the assessment and the associated report must be obtained. This is so even where a court has ordered that a report must be submitted: if the subject refuses consent, a report should be submitted stating this. It might also include information from other sources, if appropriate (but see 📖 pp.III.265, III.277, and III.284 on the ethics of doing so).
- Consider the potential conflict in role between assessing a person for potential treatment only and having to testify or present a report to a court or tribunal. There are advantages and disadvantages to mental health professionals testifying about a patient they are treating. The professional may be the person who is in the best position to form an opinion; however the court assessment may adversely affect the subsequent therapeutic relationship.

- It is vital to consider the stage of the legal process the person is at when conducting the assessment as this will have implications for what the person might want to disclose, particularly if they are pre-trial (📖 p.IV.330); see also the caution on information-gathering during admission to hospital before trial (📖 p.II.108).

- Clinical method should essentially be unaltered by the fact that the assessment will be used to address one or more legal questions. However, it is likely to be necessary to concentrate upon particular clinical aspects in conducting the assessment in order best to inform the particular legal questions at hand. For example, a report answering a question about whether the defendant was capable of forming intent (📖 p.V.481) at the time of the alleged offence will focus on evidence from the patient and others of their mental state at the material time, as well as evidence of their usual mental functioning.

- Although caution should be exercised in gaining and interpreting information from the person being assessed, given that he or she may be involved in legal proceedings, this should not result in distortion of ordinary clinical procedure. It is inevitable that doctors ask patients direct questions which, to the lawyer, amount to leading questions. As a result vigilance should include attempts to check and confirm information, both within the interview and through access to other sources of information.

- The quality of a report to court is likely to depend crucially upon the care with which the clinical assessment and consideration of records and legal papers (e.g. the case summary and witness statements, 📖 p.II.107) is conducted. This will lay the foundation for the provision of a report, and determine its quality. Although a report may appear adequate at face value, any inadequacy is likely to be displayed clearly through the process of cross examination (📖 p.V.588).

- It is likely that interviewing the person being assessed about their family and personal history first will put them at their ease, enhance the reliability of information gained, and provide initial hypotheses about diagnosis (📖 p.II.108) and formulation (📖 p.II.110). This will assist when subsequently interviewing about matters directly relevant to the legal issues at hand (this may especially be the case with reports for criminal cases, 📖 p.V.569).

- Take into account any cultural or ethnic (📖 p.II.26) differences there may be between you and the person being assessed, and try to avoid being biased by assumptions based on such cultural factors. Supervision (📖 p.III.252) by an appropriately experienced colleague, or retrospective peer review[*], can be of great assistance in avoiding bias.

- Do not forget that individuals caught up in the criminal justice system, especially children and young people (📖 p.II.117) and those with learning disability (📖 p.II.80), can be highly vulnerable—whatever they are alleged to have done. Particular issues to watch out for as the assessing psychiatrist include suggestibility and compliance (📖 p.II.123)

---

[*] As is required, for instance, for all Home Office-accredited forensic pathologists in E&W, who must be associated with a group practice that undertakes regular peer review of autopsy reports to ensure freedom from bias.

Special issues in prison settings

The prison population has recently risen significantly in the UK and across the world, and the mental health needs of this group are high, as demonstrated in the prevalence data in this section. All forensic psychiatrists and many general psychiatrists are likely to assess patients in prison at least occasionally, and should be familiar with the process. In addition, some forensic psychiatrists work in prison psychiatric services (📖 p.II.217) and will assess and treat prisoners as a routine part of their daily work; this page focuses on psychiatrists who visit rather than work in prisons.

Prevalence of psychiatric disorders in prison population

- Psychosis: 10% men, 7% women
- Neurosis: 39% men, 75% women
- Personality disorder: 75% men on remand, 50% men sentenced
- Illicit substance use: 85% men, 69% women.

Reasons for assessing a prisoner

- In order to compile a court report (📖 pp.V.556–V.581)
- In response to a request for transfer to hospital (📖 p.IV.410)
- For statutory purposes such as preparing Parole Board (📖 p.V.570) reports.

Prior to a visit to prison

- Book the assessment at least 48 hours in advance via the prison healthcare department (or earlier, if the prison requires it)
- If the prison does not allow its healthcare department to arrange external visits, the legal visits service will arrange a visit, but will usually be unable to grant access to documents such as the IMR
- Be aware of the timings of the prison regime when requesting a visit at a particular time. For example, prisoners are usually confined to their cells while officers have lunch, during which time you will probably be asked to leave; if you arrive shortly before lunchtime you might have a long wait before being able to see the prisoner
- Review all the case papers and other relevant documents in advance
- Prepare your plan of assessment, including specific questions you wish to ask of the prisoner and records you wish to see
- Check the prison's identification and security rules beforehand to ensure you comply. Rules vary by security category and individual institution.

During the visit

- Arrive early as it may take 30–60 minutes to pass security checks
- Remember to take approved photographic ID, often a passport, driving licence or photographic Trust ID; some prisons require more than one
- Certain items are restricted e.g. mobile phones, Dictaphones, memory sticks, chewing gum etc. You may be allowed to leave these in lockers but it is worth checking prior to your visit
- Be prepared for a personal search (usually a rub-down or pat-down search as well as one involving an electromagnetic 'wand'), as well as searches and/or x-ray screening of your coat and bag, and being sniffed by a drug-search dog

- If appropriate, obtain information from the sources listed in
📖 'Sources of information', p.II.115 as well as from the patient/prisoner
- Ask the prisoner to sign a consent form for access to their medical records while you are with them, to facilitate viewing their prison records afterwards
- Remember that, with the exception of healthcare staff, it will usually be inappropriate to share confidential medical information (📖 p.III.263) with prison staff.

Assessment setting

Consideration needs to be given to the interview room. If it is on a prison wing, the room may be noisy or otherwise unsuitable. Even legal visit suites can be noisy and unsuitable for a clinical interview. It is usually best to arrange visits in the prison hospital wing.

More generally, prison is an inherently coercive environment. It is important to ensure that the prisoner is aware of the nature and purpose of the assessment (see 📖 p.II.112), of the limits on the usual doctor-patient confidentiality, and of their right to refuse to answer questions. Bear in mind that prisoners will often forget this and begin confiding in an empathic doctor: you may need to remind them of the limits on confidentiality.

Sources of information

- Inmate Medical Records (IMRs) held by NHS prison healthcare staff
- Electronic IMRs, if in use, such as EMIS
- Healthcare staff who know the patient/prisoner
- Prison officers who know the patient/prisoner
- Disciplinary and wing records (often a useful record of behaviour)
- ACCT or 2052SH forms, if in use (Assessment, Care in Custody, and Treatment; form 2052: Self Harm)—suicide and self-harm care planning documents

After the visit

- Ask to see the IMR and write that you have completed an assessment; include your contact details and, if appropriate, a summary of the clinical outcome of your assessment
- If conducting an assessment for a legal report, the notes made should usually refer only to the fact that an assessment has taken place and not to its legal implications, to avoid breach of court disclosure rules
- If you are concerned about a person's mental state, need for acute treatment, or risk of harm to themselves or others, liaise with the prison mental health team and document this in the ACCT (if in use).
- If you cannot usefully inform prison staff about an important and urgent clinical issue without breaching confidentiality (📖 p.III.263) or disclosure rules, this may nevertheless be permissible under the *Egdell* principle (📖 p.App. 3.635).

Special issues with women

Female offenders are a small minority among criminal rule breakers. In the UK in 2006, they constituted 8% of all offenders; and 5.5% of all those in prison. In a multicentre European study, women constituted 19% of the total prison population.

Women and violence

▶Only 20% of female offending constitutes violent crime. Women are most likely to be convicted of acquisitive offences, drug-related offences, or sex-worker related offences. Convicted women are more likely to receive non-custodial sentences than men for similar offences; at least in part because they are less criminal, less likely to reoffend, and because they are often responsible for dependent children. Some authors argue that the courts tend to 'pathologize' women offenders, on the basis that crime is 'not usual female behaviour'.

Differences between male and female offenders

Although there has been considerable interest in the difference between male and female offenders, in fact they are generally more alike than different. One key difference is that female offenders are more likely than male offenders to have sought mental health treatment prior to imprisonment.

Another key difference is in the rates of violence. In 2006, women accounted for only 5.6% of all violence against the person in the UK, and amounted to only 34 of the 567 sentenced homicide offenders. Women who are violent are therefore statistically unusual. Their victims are more likely to be family members, either partners or children. Some women commit acts of violence in partnership with a violent man; or fail to protect vulnerable children. In 2006, 32 acts of cruelty to children were committed by women as compared to 76 by men: these rates are in proportion to male and female rates of interpersonal violence.

Very rarely, abused women fight back, and even more rarely kill their abuser. The latter cases have presented particular problems for courts in applying the defences of diminished responsibility (🕮 p.V.491) and provocation or loss of control (🕮 p.V.498) fairly.

Mental disorder as a risk factor for violence in women

- In both sexes, previous violence or criminality (🕮 p.II.16), antisocial personality disorder (ASPD, 🕮 p.II.60) and substance misuse (🕮 p.II.56) increase the risk of violence. However, ASPD is comparatively less common in females
- In both sexes, paranoid psychotic disorders (🕮 p.II.54) increase the risk, but in females the risk is further increased where there is BPD (🕮 p.II.61) and unmet social needs (🕮 p.II.23)
- There is increasing evidence that psychosis is a greater risk factor for violence by women as compared to men
- Overall, violence by women tends to take place in the context of relationships with the victim; and assaults on strangers are very rare
- There is also some evidence to suggest that many violent women have been victims of violence both as children and adults (although this may also be true of male violent offenders; see also development of violence 🕮 p.II.30).

Mental disorder in female offenders

Prevalence studies of mental disorder in prisons have found similar rates of mental disorders in both sexes for most disorders, with the exception of ASPD, which is twice as common in men. BPD is particularly common in female prisoners.

Prevalence of mental disorder amongst female prisoners
- Psychosis: 14%
- Depression: 15–21%
- Personality disorder: 50% (ASPD 21%, BPD 20%).

As with male prisoners, a subgroup of female prisoners will require treatment in secure psychiatric settings: usually because they are psychotic, suicidal, self-harming or are otherwise hard to manage in the prison setting. Most female prisoners can be safely treated in medium secure (📖 p.II.210) services for women (📖 p.II.211), and only a tiny minority will require treatment in enhanced medium security (📖 p.II.210) or high security (📖 p.II.209). This latter group resemble their male counterparts in terms of their antisocial personality traits.

Assessing risk of violence in female offenders

Most risk assessment tools have been standardized in relation to male offenders, and their generalization to female offenders is of doubtful validity. The base rate for violence in females is so low, that predictive risk factors are much harder to establish.

The people most at risk of violence from women are their children. Studies of child homicide show that mothers and fathers are equally at risk; and that the majority of mothers had a mental disorder at the time of the killing. ⚠ Therefore when assessing the risk of *violence* in female offenders, it is crucial to consider whether she has children in her care.

▶ It should also be remembered that women who have been violent to others still have a higher risk of suicide or self-harm (📖 p.II.137) than of being violent to others again.

Special issues with children & youths

Forensic psychiatrists and child and adolescent psychiatrists may be asked to assess children and young people aged 10 (the lowest age of criminal responsibility, 📖 p.IV.338) to 17, if they present a risk to others and appear to suffer from mental disorder, substance misuse or learning difficulties. Young people most commonly pose a risk of harm to others (especially other young people) through violence, sexually inappropriate behaviour, fire-setting, or property damage (see also 📖 p.II.30). However, only a small minority persistently commit offences into adulthood (📖 p.II.30), or commit very serious offences; and, as with adult offenders, only a small proportion will come into contact with psychiatric services (Table 4.1).

This group has complex needs and vulnerabilities. They commonly present unique challenges due to poor engagement with services and the risks they pose. Common characteristics of young people referred to forensic psychiatrists are: difficulties in family and peer relationships, high levels of poverty, entrenched parental needs, history of school under-performance and exclusion, homelessness and experiences of living in or on the edge of social care.

Developmental approach to assessment

When assessing children and young people, one key difference from a standard psychiatric assessment of an adult is the need to recognize that they are still developing, and that future maturation (or its arrest) may impact on the treatment and prognosis of any identified conditions, or behaviours such as violence.

The *Youth Offending Team* (YOT, 📖 p.V.463) identifies the needs of each young offender by assessing them with a national structured assessment tool—ONSET or ASSET.

- **ONSET** is used with young people who have been identified as being at risk of offending, in order to help to prevent them from being drawn into the YJS. It is used to identify whether a young person would benefit from participating in a prevention programme, as well as to identify their needs and how best to address them, so as to reduce the likelihood of them becoming an offender
- **ASSET** is for young people who have offended. The information gathered is used to make a recommendation to the court on a suitable sentence. It will identify the activities that the young person will be required to complete as part of their sentence; identify whether work needs to be done with their parents/carers and identify how to protect the public. If a young person is sentenced or remanded to custody, the information gathered by ASSET is used by the YOT to assess whether the young person is vulnerable. This information is used by the YJB to decide upon the type of custodial establishment into which they should be placed.

There are various measures that are used by mental health professionals to assess both criminogenic and mental health needs in this population. For example, the Salford Needs Assessment Schedule for Adolescents (SNASA) can be used to identify psychosocial and mental health needs, and the Structured Assessment of Violence in Youth (SAVRY) is a measure of their risk of violence. The SAVRY is the youth equivalent of the HCR-20 (📖 p.II.133).

Table 4.1 Rates of mental disorder in children and youth

Disorder	General population (figures for 11–16-year-olds)	Prisoners (figures for 16–20-year-olds)
Any clinically recognizable disorder	12.8% (males)	90%
	9.6% (females)	
Conduct disorder	8.6% (males)	90% (males)
	3.8% (females)	
Emotional disorders (e.g. anxiety, depression)	5% (males)	41–67%
	6% (females)	
Suicide	8 per 100,000 (males)	20% (males)
Attempted suicide	3 per 100,000 (females)	30% (females)
	2%	

Table 4.1 (*Contd.*)

Disorder	General population (figures for 11–16-year-olds)	Prisoners (figures for 16–20-year-olds)
Functional psychosis	2 per 1000	8–10% (males)
		9% (females)
PTSD	No data available	4% (males)
		7% (females)
Drug dependence	25% (cannabis only): 16–19 years	52% (males)
		58% (females)
Hazardous drinking	24%	62–70% (males)
Medication (acting on central nervous system)	No data available	10% (males)
		40% (females)

▶11–15% of young males and 27% of young females receive help or treatment for psychological problems in the year before entering custody. Successful mental health intervention at that stage might help them avoid later imprisonment.

Children as witnesses
Children may require special measures when they give evidence, as discussed on 📖 p.II.121.

Special issues with witnesses

Occasionally, a forensic psychiatrist may be asked to assess a witness because they are thought to have a mental disorder that might affect their legal capacity to give evidence, or impair their credibility or reliability* as a witness. This is distinct from the more common situation of considering the same issues in a defendant, perhaps as part of a report that addresses their fitness during police interview (📖 p.V.452) and fitness to plead (📖 p.V.474) as well as their fitness to give evidence (📖 p.V.477).

Note that only impairments of credibility or reliability as a witness because of mental disorder are relevant; an expert should never find themselves in the position of attempting to bolster a witness's credibility (sometimes known as 'oath-helping'†).

---

* Credibility refers to whether a witness is thought by the court to be telling what they believe to be the truth; reliability refers to whether their evidence is accurate.
† Medieval courts treated statements by witnesses as proven fact if a fixed number of 'oath-helpers', often 12, stated before the court that they believed the witness to be telling the truth.

Competence of witnesses

Within criminal proceedings, to be fit to give evidence (📖 p.V.477) a witness must be able to:

- Understand questions put to them as a witness, and
- Give answers which can be understood.

Psychiatric evidence might be relevant to deciding whether a witness meets these two tests, but it is for the court to decide whether they are competent or not, and if so, how much weight to give their evidence (see also addressing the ultimate issue, 📖 p.V.543). One suggestion for the psychiatric assessment is to consider the two questions:

- Is the witness's ability to understand the oath impaired by mental or other disorder, and if so, how?
- Is the witness's ability to recall and recount what they have seen impaired by mental or other disorder, and if so, how?

Answering these questions may also require psychological assessment, including of cognitive function, suggestibility and/or compliance (📖 p.II.123).*
Conditions that might impair competence to give evidence include dementia, psychosis and learning disability.

The court will determine the competence of witnesses during a *voir dire* (📖 p.IV.319), based upon on a comprehensive psychiatric assessment addressed to these legal questions.

Reliability of witnesses

Even if a witness is considered competent to give evidence (or determined to be competent by the court), there may still be issues of reliability: that is, the weight that a jury might properly place on their evidence.

The assessment of a witness in relation to their reliability should involve a full psychiatric assessment. This assessment will then need to form the basis for considering whether there is any reason why the witness, as a result of mental disorder, might not give a reliable account to a jury. For example, fluctuating delusions might change the account they would give at different times.

Specific issues of reliability that are sometimes put to psychiatrists include the reliability of childhood memories (◆ especially memories of sexual abuse recovered after psychotherapy, 📖 p.V.546, that are subsequently alleged to be false), and the reliability of a witness or victim (such as a victim of rape or sexual assault) who acts in an apparently inconsistent way after the alleged offence. Unless the witness in question has a mental disorder that bears upon this issue, and you have special expertise in these areas, it may be more appropriate for the issue to be considered by a forensic psychologist or psychotherapist (📖 p.I.10).

---

* Although suggestibility and compliance have not yet been accepted by courts as relevant to the competence of a witness (as opposed to a defendant) in the UK or RoI, this may change; and in any case they may be relevant to considering their reliability as a witness or the reliability of police interviews with them.

Fitness to attend court

Mentally disordered witnesses and defendants may not be able to attend court to give evidence because of their mental condition. The court will usually expect evidence from a psychiatrist before adjourning or allowing the case to proceed in the absence of the witness or defendant.

Children and other vulnerable witnesses

Vulnerable witnesses include witnesses under the age of 17, witnesses suffering from a learning disability or other mental disorder, the elderly, or a witness whose quality of evidence, in the opinion of the court, is likely to be diminished by reason of fear or distress in testifying. The witness may well be competent to give evidence, and not considered unreliable in doing so, but require special measures to be applied. These may include:

- Allowing supporters to sit with them
- Using screens or video links to separate them from the defendant(s)
- Restricting public and media access while they give evidence
- Making proceedings feel less formal, for instance by removal of wigs
- Using communication aids such as computers or interpreters, and
- Granting anonymity, especially if there is a serious risk of intimidation.

Ethical pitfalls

Assessing the competence and reliability of witnesses is an area of practice where there are particular dangers not only of addressing the ultimate issue, but also of exceeding one's area of expertise (📖 pp.III.241, III.249, V.533) and allowing one's own values to affect one's opinion (📖 pp.III.274, V.551).

Special issues with victims

There are numerous psychological effects associated with being the victim of a crime. These include depression, anxiety, post-traumatic symptoms, increased paranoia, anger, and shame. The actual level of distress varies from person to person, and the victim's perception of the crime is important in determining their reaction to it. Factors that can impact upon the victim's ability to cope include their resources, vulnerability, degree of isolation and previous experience, if any, of being a victim.

Victims and the criminal justice system

Victim surveys (📖 p.II.18), both national and local, and smaller qualitative studies of the effects of crime on victims, are helpful in recognizing the demographics and the needs of this group. These studies have shown that whilst the likelihood of being a victim of a minor offence at some point during one's lifetime is high, the probability of being the victim of a serious offence is low. They also show that violent and sexual offences more often occur between people who know each other.

The relationship between the victim and the offender is important in terms of reporting of a crime. For example, victims of intimate violence are less likely to go to the police, as are juveniles who have been assaulted by their peers. Middle class victims are more likely to report offences.

Assessment of victims

It is uncommon for forensic psychiatrists to be directly involved in the assessment of victims. However, the following includes situations where a victim assessment might be performed:

- A forensic psychiatrist (not involved in assessing or treating the defendant) may assess the psychological needs of a victim in relation to risk assessment (📖 p.II.130), safety planning and treatment of the perpetrator
- In civil litigation (📖 p.V.509), the victim might be assessed when damages need to be assessed in cases of negligence (📖 p.V.512) of another health professional, or compensation (📖 p.V.514) for trauma in a claim for personal injury
- In family law (📖 p.V.510) proceedings, an expert might be required to carry out a competence or needs assessment on a child whose parents are undergoing divorce or other relevant proceedings
- As with witnesses (📖 p.II.119) there may be concerns about a victim's reliability in providing evidence in court, perhaps because of their suggestibility or compliance (📖 p.II.123).

What is not acceptable is to carry out an assessment of a victim in order to determine whether an offence was or was not committed against them. For example, it would not be reasonable to use apparent re-experiencing symptoms of PTSD (📖 p.II.70) to infer that the re-experienced events actually occurred.

Working with perpetrators generally means a high likelihood of having contact with the victims of their offences, as a large proportion are family members. Perpetrators are also likely to have been victimized (📖 p.II.141) themselves, and may experience high levels of post-traumatic symptoms, as well as so-called complex PTSD (📖 p.V.546).

Children and other vulnerable victims

►It is important for professionals who are assessing child victims to be aware in some detail of child development theory, in order to reduce the system-induced trauma suffered. Assessment of child victims is in any event more appropriately carried out by a child psychiatrist rather than an adult forensic psychiatrist.

Special measures

Special measures designed to reduce the stress of testifying for child victims (and to maximize their reliability as witnesses) include:

- The removal of gowns and wigs
- Video live-link systems that allow people to testify via closed circuit television
- The use of screens, and
- Pre-recorded videotaped evidence.

Other measures include the protection of certain witnesses from cross-examination by the accused and restricting the cross-examination (📖 p.V.588) of alleged rape victims about their sexual history.

In North America, following the success of the US argument that the use of such protective measures violated the defendant's Sixth Amendment right (📖 p.IV.304) to confront their accuser, an alternative approach to child witnesses was developed. Pre-court preparation programmes were designed in order to prepare children mentally and emotionally for their courtroom experience through support, familiarization, and encouragement.[*]

Suggestibility and compliance

Suggestibility

Suggestibility refers to the extent to which, within a closed social interaction, an individual comes to accept messages communicated during formal questioning. This could be in relation to a police interview or a clinical interview.[†] There are two main components of suggestibility: a tendency to incorporate into memory the suggestive information embedded in the question (yield), and a sensitivity to subsequent critical comments about one's earlier performance (shift). Research has indicated that it is difficult to fake suggestibility.

Associations with suggestibility

- Poor memory recall
- Low intelligence

---

[*] This demonstrates the difficult balance in justice that has to be struck between the right of the defendant to a fair trial, and the right of the victim not to be further traumatized by the trial process. The particular balance struck is likely to affect rates of reporting certain crimes, particularly rape (see 📖 pp.II.18, IV.348), as well as rates of prosecution and conviction.
[†] It could also in principle relate to giving oral evidence in court as a witness (📖 p.II.119), but there does not appear to be any specific literature on this.

- High emotionality and anxiety
- High social desirability
- Fear of negative evaluation
- Low assertiveness and self-esteem.

Compliance

Compliance refers to the tendency to go along with propositions, requests or instructions for some immediate instrumental gain.[*] The individual is fully aware that their action may be wrong. This is more common in a coerced-compliant confession (📖 p.V.479), when the suspect is confessing to something that they know that they have not done possibly due to external pressure.

Relevance to legal proceedings

A person's degree of suggestibility and/or compliance may be relevant in a psychiatric assessment in relation to the reliability of their testimony, whether they are the defendant, the victim or a witness. The main area of public concern in relation to these issues is that of rebutted (false) confessions (📖 p.V.479). In recent years there has been a rise in the use of expert witnesses (always psychologists, except where the person in question suffers from a diagnosable mental disorder, in which case psychiatrists and psychologists have worked together) to determine psychological vulnerabilities and to assist the court in considering whether those vulnerabilities rendered the confession (given how it was obtained) or other testimony unreliable. Such unreliability may determine the confession either inadmissible in front of the jury, or admissible but with expert evidence given to suggest that less than full weight should be given to it. The 'Guildford Four' and 'Birmingham Six'[†] cases are two notorious examples of psychological evidence being used to assist in overturning convictions based on confessions that were subsequently recognized to be unreliable.

The defendant's suggestibility and compliance are often raised in cases where a confession has been made but is later retracted. Suggestibility is associated with coerced-internalized confessions (📖 p.V.479), and can be more likely if the suspect is unsure of what they have or have not done.

Assessment of suggestibility and compliance

There are specific psychological tests (📖 p.II.99) that can be used to assess an individual's degree of suggestibility (Gudjonsson Suggestibility Scale, versions one, GSS1, and two, GSS2, 📖 p.II.102) and compliance (Gudjonsson Compliance Scale, GCS, 📖 p.II.102).

---

[*] This should not be confused with the related psychological concept of *acquiescence*, which is the tendency during psychological testing to respond to questionnaire items with the answer 'yes' or 'true', whatever the content of the question.
[†] Both cases concerned explosions in the UK caused by the Irish Republican Army, as part of a campaign designed to force the British to leave Northern Ireland. There was huge public pressure for convictions of those responsible; in the absence of safeguards such as those later enacted in the Police and Criminal Evidence Act 1984 (📖 p.App. 2.626), the police were able to pressurize suspects they believed to be guilty to give confessions that turned out to be false. The distinguished forensic psychiatrist to whom this handbook is dedicated, the late Dr James MacKeith, was, with Professor Gisli Gudjonsson, an important expert witness in the Irish bomb case appeals.

If there are concerns in relation to a defendant's or witness' level of suggestibility or compliance in a police interview, the expert should ask for copies of the police transcripts and interview tapes. When reviewing or listening to these, attention should be paid to leading or closed questions, the subject appearing to take on information originating in things said by the interviewer, and undue pressure by the interrogator. In the case of a defendant, the absence of a solicitor during questioning, or of an appropriate adult (📖 p.V.452) if needed, may also be relevant. Suggestibility and compliance are only relevant in cases concerning confessions if there is clear evidence that these psychological traits were in operation during the interview concerned.

Giving evidence in court

- If a vulnerable person is due to give evidence, then the assessment findings should be explained to the court, and it should be advised to ensure that questions are not leading or closed and no undue pressure is placed on the individual
- Through an application by a solicitor to the judge, the jury should be informed of the psychological factors that might make the individual's testimony less reliable
- Vulnerable individuals may well still be able to testify under the right conditions, with additional support as necessary (such as the special measures described for vulnerable witnesses and victims giving evidence, 📖 pp.II.119–II.123).

Risk assessment

Risk assessment versus harm prediction

What risk assessment is not

In other branches of medicine, harms (e.g. death during surgery, or the side effects of a drug) arise as a 'cost' of attempting to benefit the patient. Risk : benefit ratios reflect the risk of doing harm at the expense of pursuing welfare. That also applies in psychiatry: for example, giving anti-psychotic medication to treat psychosis with the risk of tardive dyskinesia developing, However, most risk assessment in psychiatry is directed at preventing harm arising from the patient's own (mentally disordered) behaviour: harm to themselves through suicide or self-harm, or harm to another, such as rape or assault or murder.

We all, relatives, society, the government, and (often) the patient themselves, wish harm to be prevented, particularly very serious harm such as homicide. This understandably strong desire, combined with a lack of understanding in the population at large about the nature of mental disorder and its consequences, tends to drive an expectation that it must be possible to predict when such a harm might occur: 'if we don't detain this man with command auditory hallucinations today, he will leave and kill his wife within a week', for instance.

However, a moment's reflection should make it clear that such detailed prediction of something as complex and multifactorial as human behaviour is impossible, and likely always to remain so. Outside the mental health field, nobody would expect to be able to predict, in normal circumstances, what another person will do at a particular moment.

What risk assessment is

What we are really saying when we decide to detain a patient under mental health legislation on the grounds of risk is more like 'the probability of this man, in his current circumstances and with his current symptoms, causing serious harm such as killing his wife, appears unacceptably high'.[*] Implicit within this formulation is a particular values based (📖 p.III.235) trade-off between preventing a feared harm by the patient, and harming the patient's interests, by restricting his liberty. Because harms cannot be predicted accurately, there will always be *false positives*: that is, situations in which action is taken against patients who would not have caused harm on that occasion—as well as *false negatives*, in which action is not taken and harm results.

This is not to say that there are no data at all, and that risk assessment consists solely of value judgements; merely that our best estimates of the data (the probability of killing his wife on Tuesday) are very poor estimates, and that we must use some element of value judgement to set these poor estimates against each other (the cumulative estimate of the probability of him killing his wife, and the estimate of the harm done to him by restricting his liberty by only allowing escorted leave, 📖 p.II.154, say).

---

[*] Other factors, such as the availability of appropriate treatment for his mental disorder, would still be necessary to justify detention under mental health legislation.

Risk assessment, therefore:
- Is imprecise and subject to great uncertainty
- Does not relate to specific events or times.

Instead, it relates to conditions, circumstances and situations, plus exacerbating and protective factors (e.g. 'in the presence of untreated command auditory hallucinations, if disinhibited by alcohol or drugs, with access to a suitable weapon, and if unsupervised by a trusted relative or professional, he would be at high risk of assaulting or killing the subject of those hallucinations, e.g. his wife').

Should we assess risk at all?

There is undoubtedly a great social and political demand for risk assessment (as well as for harm prediction), and for risk management (that is, acting to reduce the risk through the understanding of it garnered during the risk assessment: 📖 p.II.190). Moreover, some techniques of risk assessment such as some actuarial measures (📖 p.II.130) are right more often than by chance, and a few, used properly, do better still, such as the HCR20 (📖 p.II.133).

Psychiatrists may be tempted to eschew risk assessment altogether—it is time-consuming, controversial, can feel ethically dubious in certain circumstances, and often proves to have been wrong (in that someone assessed as low risk may cause harm, and vice versa—although the probabilistic nature of risk assessment means that by definition some patients adjudged 'low risk' will still cause harm, just a smaller proportion than of 'high risk' ones[†]).

However, what is the alternative? Psychiatrists must decide whether or not to act in one way or another with each patient they see. Are such decisions to be guided without consideration of possible harms at all (e.g. prescribing drugs without considering the risk and severity of side effects for this patient)? If not, how are such harms to be brought into consideration without some form of risk assessment procedure? For all the justified criticisms of the risk assessment techniques described in the rest of this chapter, risk assessment is inherent not only to medicine in general but to psychiatry in particular. It is unavoidable. Indeed, you do it even when you do not intend to do it. What matters is knowing not only the technical but also the ethical basis (📖 p.III.265) of what you are doing.

[†] This is one of the conundra of risk assessment: even when the probability of a certain harm at the level of the population or group is well known (e.g. it is well-established that 10% of patients with schizophrenia will commit assault at some point in their life), the probability of the harm at the level of the individual is very rarely well known (e.g. there is no current way of telling whether this patient with schizophrenia is one of that 10%).

Approaches to risk assessment

Human behaviour is determined by multiple internal and environmental factors, and assessing the risk of any given form of behaviour is therefore complex and difficult. Moreover, the research evidence available to inform practical risk assessment is substantially weakened by methodological limitations. Psychiatrists must therefore be cautious in attempting to assess such risks (including on ethical grounds, 📖 p.III.265), particularly where there is no intended or likely therapeutic benefit to the patient, such as in reports for criminal courts (📖 p.V.569). They must be even more careful to eschew harm prediction (📖 p.II.128) when assessing risks. They must be ready to demonstrate (for example, to a future homicide inquiry, 📖 p.V.471, or court in a negligence case, 📖 p.V.512) that they performed their risk assessment carefully and in accordance with recognized good practice.

How well can risks be assessed?

The empirical evidence on risk assessment is undermined by biases and confounding variables. Studies in clinical settings tend to over-estimate risk. This is partly because patients in clinical settings are at greater risk of perpetrating violence and inappropriate sexual behaviour than patients with mental disorder in general; also, the criteria for diagnosing some mental disorders actually specify such behaviours. Overall, the prospective accuracy (positive predictive value) of psychiatric risk assessments is poor: of those labelled as high risk, particularly high risk of violence, several will not cause the harm in question for each one that does.

Actuarial approaches

These are based on statistical estimates of risk in groups of people. They perform better in some controlled studies than do clinical judgements alone.[*] However, they have several flaws:

- They have a low positive predictive value, partly because of the low prevalence of relevant harms (e.g. serious violence in the case of the PCL-R, 📖 p.II.102)
- They are limited by their reliance on *static factors* (e.g. a record of previous violence) and limited use of *dynamic factors* (such as the presence of active psychotic symptoms) and therefore cannot measure changes in risk.
- The actuarial instruments currently available mostly ignore *protective factors* that reduce risk (for instance, a confiding relationship).

Group membership versus individual risk

A particular problem that bedevils the interpretation of actuarial risk assessments is that they inform you only about the aggregate risk of the group to which the patient belongs, and not about the patient as an individual. For example, studies that demonstrate that most 8-year-old boys presenting with acute abdominal pain have appendicitis, whereas most 80-year-olds with the same presentation have intestinal obstruction (due to bowel cancer, say), provide information about the aggregate risks of

[*] i.e. they have better receiver operating characteristics, and offer greater improvements in risk estimation over chance than does unstructured clinical judgement.

8- and 80-year-olds presenting with acute abdominal pain. This is useful, but insufficient: to decide what to do, you must also consider individual factors that show whether your patient is typical of the group, or in some way atypical. For instance, if the 8-year-old has a knife handle protruding from their right upper quadrant, you might not jump to the conclusion that they have appendicitis. Such individual factors must be added to the results of psychiatric actuarial risk assessments before they can be utilized.

Clinical approaches

These are based upon the judgement of an individual clinician or a team of clinicians, preferably from different disciplines; and can be unstructured or structured. In the latter case, the structure can act merely as an aide memoire (as in the case of the CRMT, 📖 p.II.139) or can incorporate some actuarial elements (e.g. the HCR20, 📖 p.II.133).

When used alongside an individual knowledge of the patient and their environment, structured clinical risk assessments like the HCR20 have been shown to improve the outcomes of clinical decision-making.

Risk assessment and the clinician

A range of approaches is needed. Psychiatry is a medical discipline concerned chiefly with the care of the individual patient: clinicians' judgements must take into account other factors as well as patients' membership of a group shown to be associated in aggregate with a particular risk.

Although risk assessment instruments focus almost exclusively on the risks of violence, sexually inappropriate behaviour, self-harm and suicide, the forensic psychiatrist must address a much broader array of risks, including:

- Absconding or escape
- Illegal drug use
- Medication non-compliance
- Self-neglect
- Exploitation
- Harm from others
- Relapse
- Others such as property damage.

Risk management (📖 p.II.189) requires more specific information than just a single number, or even a restricted range of numbers: it requires knowledge of the patient as a person, and the factors that increase or decrease the likelihood of certain behaviours in given situations.

Risk of violence

The law often appears to represent 'dangerousness' (📖 p.V.549) as if it were a largely stable and consistent aspect of a person. From the clinical perspective, however, the risk of harm is dynamic and depends at any given time on the interaction between the individual, their mental disorder (if any), and their circumstances. The aim of a risk assessment for violence is to evaluate those interactions so as to develop a management plan (📖 p.II.190) directed at minimizing the risk of violence.

What is violence?

For a discussion of the definition of violence from the clinical and epidemiological perspective, see 📖 p.I.21. Legal definitions are tied to specific offences such as murder (📖 p.IV.345), assault (📖 p.IV.346), rape (📖 p.IV.348), and riot or violent disorder (📖 p.IV.352).

Assessment of risk of violence

Specific prediction of violent acts is not realistic (📖 p.II.128). Although the risk of violence can be estimated, such assessments are inexact and no method is adequately sensitive and specific. Debate remains about the accuracy of clinical judgement alone (📖 p.II.130), but the integration of validated structured assessment tools into routine clinical practice will often be helpful. Because risk is dynamic, confidence in risk assessments is highest in the short term.

Relevant clinical and other factors

Most of these combine elements of group factors that are assessed by actuarial measures (📖 p.II.130), such as being an active substance misuser, with individual factors assessed by clinical judgement (📖 p.II.131), such as only misusing the substance when in the company of a particular friend.

Most important risk factor
- History of previous violent acts, including violence to people, animals and property, and with as much detail as possible on the nature and circumstances of each act (e.g. whether weapons were used, the relationship with the victim).

Biological factors
- Psychiatric disorder and specific psychiatric symptoms such as paranoia, persecutory ideation, command auditory hallucinations
- Intoxication or dependence (substance misuse)
- Response to psychiatric treatment.

Psychological factors
- Personality traits and other persistent psychological patterns affecting behaviour, such as sadism, callousness, affective instability and impulsivity, and especially psychopathy
- Personal resources such as planning, stress tolerance and problem-solving skills, ability to use tactics other than violence
- Personal and cultural attitudes towards violence
- Insight into any mental disorder (including compliance with treatment) and into the risk of violence

- Specific intent or plans to act violently, or motivation to do so (grievances, resentments etc.).

Social factors
- Developmental factors including experiences of childhood abuse or maltreatment, and age when significant violence was first used
- Social resources such as friends, relatives or employment, and especially intimate partners
- Opportunity to act violently, e.g. availability of potential victims, access to weapons and presence of other destabilizing factors such as drugs, and association with antisocial peers
- Monitoring or supervision by family, friends, psychiatric services, police, probation or other agencies.

Assessment tools

A variety of assessment instruments (see 📖 pp.II.133, II.136) have evolved over time. They tend to consider a range of static and dynamic risk factors (📖 p.II.130), the precise formulation of the factors depending on the development of the instrument, and often on the population on which it was normed or for which it was intended. Many of the risk prediction instruments overlap, for example the HCR-20, the SORAG and the VRAG include the PCL-R. Care must always be taken to ensure that the instrument is appropriate for use on the group to which the patient belongs. Most of the tools require specific training.

Violence risk assessment instruments

Structured professional judgement with actuarial information

- HCR-20 (Historical, Clinical and Risk management, 20-item scale):
  - 20 items in 3 domains (Historical, e.g. 'early maladjustment', Clinical e.g. 'negative attitudes', and Risk e.g. 'plans lack feasibility')
  - Includes emphasis on scenario planning based upon risk factors
  - See the scenario on 📖 p.II.141 for a worked example of using the HCR-20
- SDRS (Short Dynamic Risk Scale):
  - 8 items rating dynamic factors on 4-point scales e.g. hostile attitude, coping skills and consideration of others
- EPS (Emotional Problems Scale):
  - Rates 12-items on 5-point scales, e.g. anxiety, depression, self-esteem, verbal aggression, physical aggression. Validated for people with learning difficulties
- RAMAS (Risk Assessment Management and Audit Systems):
  - An integrated approach to risk assessment. This includes a Risk Assessment Checklist component
- OASys (Offender Assessment System):
  - Standardized process for the assessment of offenders jointly developed by the National Probation Service and Prison Service
- SARA (Spousal Assault Risk Assessment):
  - 20 item assessing risk of future violence in men for spousal assault

- VRS-2 (Violence Risk Scale- second edition):
  - Risk of violent recidivism in incarcerated offenders. 6 static and 23 dynamic factors.

Purely actuarial tools

- VRAG (Violence Risk Appraisal Guide):
  - 12 item actuarial tool including factors relating to antisocial behaviour, e.g. childhood behaviour problems, history of personality disorder, history of non-violent offending
- PCL-R (Psychopathy Checklist-Revised):
  - 20 item scale measuring psychopathy rather than risk assessment, but has been shown to have reasonable predictive power
  - PCL-SV is a screening version with predictive validity in institutional and community patients
- OGRS (Offender Group Reconviction Score):
  - A statistical reconviction scale used by probation officers in pre-sentence reports.

Child and Adolescent Tools

- ASSET & ONSET:
  - Structured risk assessment used by YOTs
- SAVRY (Structured Assessment of Violent Risk in Youth):
  - 24 items in 4 domains (historical, social/contextual, individualized/ clinical and protective factors)
- PCL-YV (Psychopathy Checklist—Youth Version):
  - A version of the PCL-R modified for use in adolescents. ◆ There are ethical controversies about its use (📖 p.III.265)
- EARL-20B (boys)/EARL-21G (girls):
  - 20 items (child, family, and responsivity) measuring risk of violence in children under 12.

Other instruments assess the risk of sexual violence. These are shown on 📖 p.II.136.

Risk of sexual offending

Most sexual offenders do not have a diagnosis of a mental illness, and only some are personality disordered. Hence, clinical or forensic psychologists, and probation services carry out the majority of assessments of sexual offenders. However, increasingly psychiatrists are involved in the assessment of sexual offenders where they are known or suspected to have a mental disorder. Assessments should incorporate all the components described as follows:

Clinical assessment

Probably the most widely used approach to psychiatrists' assessment of risk of sexual offending is clinical judgement (see 📖 p.II.131). A full history and mental state examination should be supplemented by particular focus on detailed psychosexual history including: history of being a victim in childhood; presence of violent sexual fantasies; sexual behaviour; attitudes towards women and attitudes regarding sex with children. Comorbid mental disorders should also be considered, particularly alcohol and drug misuse, LD, and PD. Research evidence suggests a link between psychosis and sexual violence. Mania associated with disinhibition may also predispose to sexual offending. An attempt should be made to assess the relationship between any mental disorder and sexual violence.

Structured clinical judgement

The risk of sexual violence can be estimated using structured clinical risk assessment tools (see ▢ p.II.131) for non-sexual violence. However, specific tools have been developed and include the SVR-20 (now modified and known as RSVP, ▢ p.II.133). This tool resembles the HCR-20 (▢ p.II.136) and requires consideration of more than 20 separate items, as well as incorporating formulation and risk management components. The risk factors for sexual violence, as with other risks, are often broken down into static and dynamic risk factors, usually considered by actuarial and psychological evaluation respectively.

Actuarial tools

Actuarial tools predict recidivism more accurately than unstructured clinical assessment (but see also ▢ p.II.128 on harm prediction). They address static factors, which produce a statistical probability of recidivism. This probability must be considered as the rate of recidivism in a group of people (convicted of a sexual offence) and not the probability of that individual reoffending. Unlike certain clinical instruments, actuarial tools do not include risk management components. The Static-2002 and Risk Matrix 2000 are the two most commonly used actuarial tools.

Psychological evaluation

Dynamic factors are those that change over time and have been the focus of sex offender treatment programmes. Those factors usually considered are: cognitive distortions; fantasies and deviant sexual arousal; sexual preoccupation; interpersonal relationships and intimacy deficits; anger, impulsivity and emotional dysregulation. These factors are considered at clinical interview but are also the focus of psychometric evaluation. The psychopathy checklist revised (PCL-R, ▢ p.II.102) is not specific to sexual offences but is one of the most reliable predictors of violent, sexual recidivism.

Penile plethysmography (PPG)

Penile plethysmography is a technique of assessing sexual arousal, heart rate and galvanic skin response in males in response to various visual and (especially in the US) audio* stimuli. It assesses sexual arousal by measuring penile girth. It is not a risk assessment tool but is a part of the clinical assessment of some sex offenders, and is occasionally used to measure treatment response. Its validity is open to question, at least when used in isolation from other assessment measures, partly because some offenders can use their own thoughts and images in order to avoid responding to the images portrayed to them (creating a false negative response).

---

* Audio rather than visual stimuli are often preferred because the former can be simulated, whereas the use of visual images of child sexual abuse requires such abuse to have taken place.

Polygraphy

The use of the polygraph ('lie detector') has been considered in the assessment of sex offenders. At present, however, it is only widely used in the UK as part of a trial of its effectiveness in supporting the management of risk of sexual offending (📖 p.II.199) in sex offenders.

Other issues in risk of sexual offending

Internet pornography offences (📖 p.IV.348) do not necessarily confer an increased risk of contact sexual offences. Assessment should concentrate on examining all other risk factors as described earlier in this topic.

Indecent exposure or exhibitionism (📖 pp.II.46, IV.348) is considered to be more predictive of contact sexual offending if the perpetrator exhibits in multiple places, pursues or touches the victim or displays an erect penis or masturbates.

Comparing assessment tools

A variety of assessment instruments (see 📖 p.II.136) have evolved over time. They tend to consider a range of static and dynamic risk factors (📖 p.II.130), the precise formulation of the factors depending on the development of the instrument, and often on the population on which it was normed or for which it was intended. Many of the risk prediction instruments overlap, for example the HCR-20, the SORAG, and the VRAG include the PCL-R. Care must always be taken to ensure that the instrument is appropriate for use on the group to which the patient belongs. Most of the tools require specific training.

The management of the risk of sexual offending is described on 📖 p.II.197.

Sexual behaviour risk assessment instruments

Structured professional judgement with actuarial information

- RSVP (Risk of Sexual Violence Protocol):
  - 22-item risk assessment for sexual violence in offenders over age 18 years. Based on structured professional judgement using formulation and scenario planning
- SVR-20 (Sexual Violence Risk—20):
  - 20 items assessing violence risk in sex offenders (11 items social adjustment, 7 sexual offences and 2 future plans). It is outdated and has been superseded by RSVP.

Purely actuarial tools

- RRASOR (Rapid Risk Assessment of Sexual Offender Recidivism):
  - 4-item screening instrument (any male victims, any unrelated victims, age less than 25, and prior sexual offences). Relies on file information. Superseded by Static 2002
- Static-99/Static 2002:
  - Actuarial assessment of static, unchanging factors validated to predict risk of sexual and violent re-offences in male adult sex

offenders only. Contains all 4 items from RRASOR plus items
concerning relationship history, violent offences, and stranger victims
- RM2000 (Risk Matrix 2000):
  - Uses static factors to predict risk (up to 15 years later) in men over
    18 with at least one conviction for a sexual offence. It is mainly used
    by the Probation and Prison Service
  - It consists of 3 scales (S- sexual reconviction, V- violent
    reconviction, and C –combination of both)
- MnSoST-R (Minnesota Sex Offending Screening Tool—Revised):
  - 16 items designed to assess risk of recidivism in incarcerated rapists
    and child sex offenders
- SORAG (Sexual Offending Risk Appraisal Guide):
  - 14 items designed to predict violent reoffending among sex
    offenders. It is a better predictor of general violence than other
    sexual offender risk measures.

'Conceptual-actuarial' tools

- Stable -2000/Stable-2007:
  - A 16-item actuarial scale of risk of harm from sexual offenders, with
    a method for combining the items scores into an overall evaluation
    of risk
- VPS-SO (Violence Prediction Scheme-Sexual Offender Version):
  - A scale incorporating a variety of dynamic (changeable) factors,
    again with a procedure for combining scores into an overall risk
    evaluation
- SONAR (Sex Offender Needs Assessment Rating):
  - 9-item scale measuring change in risk level. Includes 5 stable and
    4 acute factors

Child and adolescent instruments

- ERASOR (Estimate of Risk of Adolescent Sexual Offence Recidivism):
  - Uses both static and dynamic factors assessing risk of sexual
    offending in adolescents (historical sexual assaults, sexual interests,
    attitudes and behaviours, psychosocial functioning and treatment)
- J-SOAP-II (Juvenile Sex Offender Assessment Protocol, version 2):
  - A checklist to aid in the systematic review of risk factors associated
    with sexual and criminal offending. Designed to be used with
    boys aged 12–18 convicted of sexual offences or with a history of
    sexually coercive behaviour.

Risk of suicide and self-harm

Prevalence

In the UK, suicide accounts for the 3rd most lost life-years, after coronary
heart disease and cancer. The following figures are for the UK, or in some
cases England & Wales:

- General population: 11 per 100,000 per year
- General psychiatric patients: 15% die by suicide
- Prisoners and police custody: 28–60 per 100,000 per year; 9% attempt suicide
- Forensic psychiatric patients: no data.

Suicide accounts for 38% of deaths in custody. Half the suicides in English prisoners are amongst those on remand (📖 p.IV.330).

Risk factors for completed suicide

The identification of those at risk of completing suicide is important but despite much research, all the risk factors identified to date have low specificity and sensitivity, and immediate versus long-term risk cannot be distinguished. The factors include:

- Mental illness, especially major depression, bipolar disorder, alcohol or drug dependence, schizophrenia, and cluster B PDs
- Previous self-harm: 50% of those who die by suicide have made a previous suicide attempt
- Cognitive factors: hopelessness, impulsivity, aggression, dichotomous thinking, cognitive constriction, problem-solving deficits, over-generalized autobiographical memory, suicidal thoughts
- Reasons for hopelessness such as terminal illness, prospect of prolonged imprisonment, loss of a key relationship etc.
- Social isolation: being single, separated, or widowed
- Losses: personal (bereavement and divorce), financial, status
- Conflicts with other people
- Being male
- Stated intent: 2/3 of those completing suicide have informed someone of their intentions
- Older age (except in schizophrenia and drug abuse, where younger age at diagnosis increases the risk of completed suicide)
- Physical ill-health, especially chronic or painful illnesses
- Economic factors: unemployment or poverty
- Criminal history including early delinquent or assaultative behaviour and arrests for drunkenness (6% completed suicides had outstanding charges)
- Incarceration.

Assessment of stated suicide intent

- Conduct an unhurried, sympathetic interview
- Provide space for patient to reveal thoughts and self-destructive intent
- Explore historical risk factors and ongoing difficulties, including mood swings, impulsivity, aggressive tendencies
- Discuss precipitant, e.g. stressful life problems—particularly interpersonal, separation, illness of family member, court appearance, recent personal physical illness
- Explore protective factors (e.g. family or attitudes towards religion)
- Mental state examination for psychiatric disorder
- Specific questioning on current suicidal intent

- Direct questions concerning thoughts of suicide, specific plans, preparatory acts (e.g. saving tablets, gaining access to means)
- Homicidal thoughts as part of act—e.g. thinking of killing a spouse or child to spare them from (perceived) intolerable suffering
- Although assessment is particularly difficult if statements of suicidal intent are made repeatedly and interpreted as threats, it is important to take them seriously as the risk of completed suicide in those who have threatened suicide is high
- Consider whether the patient's self-description is coloured by illness or their situation, by obtaining a history from an informant
- Consider use of Beck Suicide Index (helpful in measuring changes in risk, but not absolute risk 🔲 p.II.104) or Clinical Risk Management.

Factors suggesting a greater risk of subsequent death
- Lethality of method
- Carried out in isolation
- Timed so intervention is unlikely
- Taking precautions to avoid discovery
- Preparations anticipating death
- Preparation for the act
- Communicating intent to others beforehand
- Extensive premeditation
- Leaving a note
- Not alerting helpers after the act
- Anger at failure of earlier attempt
- Admission of ongoing suicidal intent.

The management of the risk of suicide or self-harm is discussed on 🔲 p.II.199.

Other specific risks

The risk of a specific behaviour occurring in future is most often considered when that behaviour has occurred previously. In broad terms the principles of risk assessment for any act (see 🔲 pp.II.130–II.139) apply. Much of the research on violence risk assessment and management includes fire-setting and hostage taking within the general concept of violence.

The circumstances of a particular behaviour should be described, so as to develop a formulation of the pattern of behaviour and the circumstances in which it is likely to recur. The structure (if not the content) of risk assessment tools such as the HCR-20 can be used in assessing the risk of specific behaviours.

Fire-setting
Only a small proportion of acts of fire-setting (🔲 p.II.38) result in a conviction for arson (🔲 p.IV.350). The risk of fire-setting should therefore be considered routinely. There are no specific assessment tools for fire-setting. In young people, fire-setting has been shown to be associated with:
- Previous fire-setting
- Aggression, frustration, and boredom
- Lack of employment

- Parental mental ill health or inter-parental conflict
- Poor social skills
- Binge drinking
- Low levels of parental supervision
- Maltreatment or abuse.

Fire-setting by adults is associated with:
- Alcohol dependence
- ASPD
- Long-lasting enuresis in childhood
- Psychosis
- LD
- History of sexual abuse in women.

However, many individuals with such features will not set fires.

The meaning of the fire-setting to the individual is almost certainly the most important aspect of assessing and managing the risk of fire-setting. Common meanings include a source of revenge; an opportunity for self-harm or suicide; a way of controlling others; a source of sexual gratification; and a way of reducing internal tension. Assessments should also address the fire-setter's emotional state and cognitive distortions before, during and after the fire, and their reaction to having set it.

Hostage-taking

The taking of a hostage may be a component of an offence, or may occur after detention in prison or hospital in response to frustration or in an attempt to manipulate others. Assessment of the risk of hostage taking should incorporate a detailed functional analysis of previous incidents. There is no empirical basis for considering the risk of hostage taking but a structured clinical tool such as HCR-20 allows for formulation of different scenarios, with implications for risk management (p.II.195).

Unauthorized leave, absconding, and escape*

The risks of these behaviours occurring, and what might then occur if the patient did abscond or escape (including suicide and violence), require constant consideration in secure hospitals, taking up a large amount of a clinical team's time. The consequences of unauthorized leave, absconding or (especially) escape frequently include adverse media coverage no matter how carefully the risks were assessed. The management of these situations is discussed on p.II.200.

Factors found to be associated with absconding include:
- Young, male detained patients
- Previous absconding
- Diagnosis of schizophrenia
- Multiple previous admissions

---

*Escape involves a breach of physical security measures, such as climbing over a wall or cutting a hole in a fence, whereas absconding merely involves leaving the hospital without permission, and unauthorized leave failing to return on time.

- Longer total hospital admission
- Previous history of violence
- Season (more incidents in spring and summer).

So many patients exhibit these factors that formulations of past episodes, and current evidence relevant to these formulations, are essential to making decisions about leave (📖 p.II.154) or observations (📖 p.II.154).

Escape is, fortunately, sufficiently rare that no clear specific risk factors have been identified.

Victimization and exploitation

People with serious mental illness are at increased risk of being a victim of violent crime compared to the general population. People with mental disorder in prison are more likely to be victims of violence compared to prisoners without mental disorder. Both groups are also more likely to be exploited financially or sexually than others. However, vulnerability has to be considered individually, again based largely upon investigation of past experiences and circumstances of victimization.

Other risks

Other risks not specific to people in forensic psychiatric services include:
- Self-neglect
- Risks associated with driving or operating machinery
- Physical health complications
- Iatrogenic risks relating to treatment
- Risks of drug or alcohol use
- Risk of relapse
- Risk of committing non-violent crime.

Vignette: what is the risk?

This vignette describes the process of completing a violence risk assessment using the HCR20 (p.II.133). The process is similar for other structured risk assessment instruments.

Mr M is a 19-year-old man from Pakistan, who has been convicted of robbery (p.IV.354) from an older female stranger. He was referred by his solicitors for a pre-sentence psychiatric report (p.V.569), in which you intend to address the risk of future violence.

Mr M came to the UK aged 10 and was brought up by his maternal aunt. His parents live in Pakistan and he has not seen them for 9 years. He left school at 16 and has never worked. Just prior to his offence, he found out that his mother had been diagnosed with cancer.

Mr M has no previous convictions and this is his first time in custody. In prison he has undergone adjudications (p.V.456) for fighting on several occasions. He has never seen a mental health professional, nor ever used alcohol or drugs. He was in a longstanding relationship, but his girlfriend has left him and his family has disowned him on learning of his conviction for robbery.

Clinical assessment indicates that he has an average IQ, is mildly depressed, has low self-esteem and is concerned about his future. There is no evidence of impulsivity or hyperactivity. Mr M demonstrates limited insight into why he committed his offence, or into the impact on his victim. However, he says that he wanted to fit in with his peers (who are mostly negative influences).

Assessment using the HCR20 indicates no historical (H) risk factors in terms of history of previous offending, young age of first offence, substance use, psychopathy or major mental illness. However, there is a history of caregiver disruption (i.e. possible early maladjustment), and poor school achievement/employment problems.

On the clinical (C) scale, Mr M had limited insight into his offence but he did not demonstrate pro-criminal or antisocial attitudes, and he was willing to accept interventions offered to him.

As regards risk-management (R) factors, Mr M is currently in custody, which has probably increased the risk of mental health problems such as depression. The stress of the feared sentence is likely to be exacerbated by concerns about his mother's health. A past protective factor, the support of his girlfriend and extended family, has now been lost. Were he to be released into the community, this lack of support and his continued association with antisocial peers would be additional risk factors.

On the basis of this assessment, you conclude that there is at present a moderate risk of a further act of violence in the short term, should Mr M be released into the community. Your primary scenario, developed using the HCR20, is of a further impulsive assault or robbery, in the presence or under the influence of his friends, with the aim of impressing them, acquiring money, or expressing anger and frustration. You note carefully that his lack of a psychotic disorder or PD reduces the general validity of the HCR20 assessment (as the HCR20 was not developed for use on people with depression alone; see 📖 p.II.33), but that your clinical judgement based upon your own experience is that the findings are likely to be valid for Mr M. You go on to develop a risk management plan (📖 p.II.191) based upon your assessment and risk scenario, and taking into account the possibility of him receiving a custodial sentence (📖 p.IV.364), as well as the possibility of a community sentence (📖 p.IV.368).

If you are to have longer-term responsibility for managing Mr M (and perhaps even if you will not), your assessment will not stop there. There is a deeper question here: why did this particular young man commit this particular offence against this particular victim? Is the choice of an older female victim relevant, given what he had just learnt about his mother? These outstanding questions suggest the need for a narrative formulation (📖 p.II.111) of Mr M's offence. It might take some time, and possibly the involvement of a psychotherapist, to understand Mr M's behaviour in this way; but doing so might allow a higher quality of risk assessment, as well as (arguably more importantly) better ways to support and treat Mr M.

Risk assessment in non-clinical settings

Subjects who are not patients

Risk assessment, as performed by psychiatrists, is a procedure designed for use with patients. Clinicians' professional judgements are derived from experience with patients. The actuarial instruments (📖 p.II.130) sometimes used in risk assessment are 'normed' on patient populations: that is, they identify the group of patients, with one or more relevant factors, a patient most resembles. Both professional judgement and actuarial instruments are therefore *invalid* when conducted on people who are not patients—that is, people who do not have mental disorder. This may be particularly relevant to clinicians asked to assess the risk of offenders reoffending when they do not suffer from any diagnosable mental disorder; psychiatrists should decline such requests. In Scotland, conducting work on behalf of the Risk Management Authority (📖 p.V.469) may present this issue.

Assessments outside clinical settings

In general, it is often possible for a clinician to make an appropriate assessment of risk on a patient even when that assessment is conducted in prison or some other non-clinical setting. However, care must be taken to ensure that the non-therapeutic setting does not influence the process of information gathering (for example, by giving the patient an incentive to conceal relevant information lest it result in further punishment), nor distort the clinician's judgement (for example, by regarding the patient not as a person with a mental illness but purely as an offender who deserves punishment rather than assistance).

Assessments by non-clinicians

◆ The risk assessment procedures used in psychiatry presuppose a professional background on the part of the assessor. For example, consider item H9 on the HCR20 (📖 p.II.133), 'personality disorder'. The assessor not only needs specific brief training in the HCR20, in order to know the criteria for determining whether a particular diagnosis and level of severity are sufficient to score positively on the item. They also need the clinical skills to be able to obtain the information from the patient or other sources necessary for making a diagnosis of personality disorder; plus the professional judgement and knowledge required to decide which diagnosis, if any, is appropriate.

Clinical risk assessment instruments should therefore not be used by non-clinicians. However, there are other risk assessment instruments designed for non-clinical settings, such as OASys (Offender Assessment System; see also 📖 p.II.133), used by the probation (📖 p.V.462) and prison services (📖 p.V.456), and the ASSET and ONSET (📖 p.II.134) which are used in the Youth Justice System. Information from such instruments is routinely shared by these agencies through the Multi-Agency Public Protection Arrangements (MAPPA, 📖 p.V.468), which can create conflicts with the psychiatrist's duty of confidentiality (📖 p.III.263).

Treatment

Aims of treatment

The aims of treatment of MDOs are both similar to those of other psychiatric patients and also less straightforward. Both clinical and criminogenic needs (those needs that are associated with offending) must be addressed.[*] This introduces not only an additional focus of treatment but also an ethical dimension which is not present in the treatment of non-offender patients.

Lengthening and improving life

Forensic psychiatry has the same treatment aims as the rest of medicine:
• To lengthen life and postpone death by the successful treatment of disease, and
• To improve the quality of life, by ameliorating symptoms and/or rehabilitating (📖 p.II.213) the patient.

However, what does it mean to 'ameliorate symptoms' when talking about BPD (📖 p.II.61), for example? People with severe BPD experience episodes of extreme mood disturbance during which their need for psychological containment (📖 p.II.155) and their tendency to behave in ways that can harm themselves and/or others mean that detention in a locked ward and restraint (📖 p.II.156) may be required in order for any help to be given. This is generally thought to be acceptable even if the containment is the sole form of treatment, as long as it is rapidly effective in treating the acute problem. How, though, is the line to be drawn between this, and indefinite detention with no other forms of treatment being provided, for personality disorder traits or behaviours that are not improving? This might be legal within E&W, if not elsewhere (see 📖 p.IV.390), but does that make it ethical to regard it as an appropriate medical treatment (📖 pp.III.280, III.282)?

Risk reduction

In addition to the two core aims of psychiatry of lengthening and improving life, forensic psychiatry often has a third aim (see also 📖 p.IV.294):
• To reduce the risk the patient poses to others, or him- or herself.

To the forensic psychiatrist, this aim, and the risk management (📖 p.II.189) techniques it involves, presuppose a link between mental disorder and violence (📖 p.II.31) or other harms, which will sometimes be present (e.g. if a person attacks in response to command auditory hallucinations), but may well not be (e.g. if an offender has previously suffered from mania but is currently well; see 📖 p.II.143).

This aim is usually stated as being secondary to the first two; that is, if there is a link between symptoms of the disorder and offending, treatment of the former will also address the latter. However, where there is no treatment that will effectively meet the first two aims but that will meet the third, giving or withholding treatment may pose an ethical dilemma (📖 p.III.280)—such as, for example, when deciding whether to give an

---

[*] This does not contradict our advice that risk assessment should not be conducted by clinicians on non-MDOs (see 📖 p.II.143), but recognizes that, in assessing MDOs, there are often relevant factors which go beyond their mental disorder.

anti-libidinal drug (📖 p.II.161) to a sex offender with a PD that has not responded to psychological or social therapies.

For the forensic psychiatrist working in a MDT (📖 p.III.256), this third aim often raises an additional ethical dilemma. Other practitioners in forensic mental health, most notably forensic psychologists, sometimes use their professional expertise to address criminogenic needs in the absence of mental disorder (📖 p.IV.273), with the aim of reducing risk to others and minimizing reoffending. To what extent, if any, is it appropriate for a forensic psychiatrist to be involved with such clients?

Principles of treatment

Following the principles of the Reed Report (📖 p.App. 5.656), forensic psychiatric services are expected to work together with other agencies in order to provide care that is:

- Based upon the individual needs of the patient
- Provided in the community wherever possible
- Provided as close as possible to the patient's home
- Provided in the least restrictive or secure environment possible, and
- Aimed at maximizing rehabilitation and the prospect of independent living.

This relatively liberal approach is at odds with recent government policy, particularly in E&W.

Balancing benefits and harms

A further principle concerning decisions about treatment is that a decision to treat (or not) must take into account the severity and likelihood of the harms that the treatment might itself cause, and balance these against the magnitude and likelihood of the desired benefits. An example is the prescription of long-acting depot antipsychotic medication (📖 p.II.159): this may cause serious side-effects such as tardive dyskinesia which may be irreversible. Prescribing a treatment, no matter how well-intentioned, that causes more harm than good may not only be unethical (📖 p.III.247) but also result in disciplinary (📖 p.V.521) or even negligence (📖 p.V.516) proceedings—especially if the main aim is risk reduction.

Duty to patient and to society

Forensic psychiatrists are faced daily with striking a balance between their duty to their patient and their duty to society. The potential for conflict between the two usually cannot be avoided. What can be achieved is ethical insight into what you are doing and why (in any particular situation). What is not acceptable is ethical self-deception.

Treatment settings in forensic psychiatry

Taking account of the setting

Treatment interventions in forensic psychiatry must take into account the setting in which the treatment is to be delivered, and the impact this may have on its effectiveness, or on causing adverse effects. The legal context associated with a particular setting may likely also have an effect upon the administration and effects of treatment.

The chief settings in which forensic psychiatry is practised (📖 p.II.208) are:

- Secure hospitals
- Prisons
- Courts
- Police stations, and
- The community.

Different treatment options will be available in each setting, in terms of legal coercion (📖 p.II.149).* For instance, having assessed a person and found them to be acutely psychotic and competently refusing (📖 p.IV.390) treatment, it may be appropriate to order antipsychotic treatment under the Mental Health Act in a medium secure unit (📖 p.III.210). In prison, treatment cannot usually be given without consent†, so the antipsychotic could be given, but only voluntarily. In courts and police stations, giving an antipsychotic even with consent may be inappropriate in practice, because of the lack of trained staff or facilities to deal with side effects (such as acute dystonia in a neuroleptic-naïve young man).

Impact of the setting

Forensic psychiatry is often practised in settings that are essentially non-therapeutic, where the dominant culture is one of 'discipline', as with prisons (even a prison healthcare centre is still part of the prison). Here, the coercive nature of the institution, and any ongoing criminal proceedings, bear upon the interactions between patient (who is also a prisoner) and doctor in a way that may well be relevant to the patient's decision-making, perhaps negating their apparently freely given 'consent'. Even if legally their consent is still valid,‡ ethically the context alters the nature of the interaction and has to be considered when designing and administering treatments. This is one reason why it is normal medical practice in prisons not to compel patients lacking capacity to accept treatment under mental capacity law (📖 p.IV.424), unless the harmful consequences of not receiving treatment are severe.

---

* Moreover, the security of the setting can sometimes be therapeutic in itself by facilitating treatment: for example a patient with borderline personality disorder (BPD, 📖 p.II.61) may feel 'contained' in a secure hospital, lessening the manifestations of their disorder and enabling them to commence psychological work (see 📖 p.II.163). This is different from legally describing security as treatment in its own right (📖 p.III.282).

† The exceptions are the treatment of a patient under the common law rule in *Munjaz* (📖 p.IV.440) to prevent an immediate risk of significant harm, or of incompetent patients under mental capacity legislation (📖 p.IV.424).

‡ This was the ruling of the Court of Appeal for E&W in *Freeman v Home Office* (📖 p.App. 3.636).

In a different legal context, for example, offering a place in a sex offender treatment group (📖 p.II.176) to a prisoner on remand (📖 p.IV.330) awaiting trial on charges of indecent exposure (📖 p.IV.348) might result in them agreeing to participate not because of genuine informed consent and a desire to change, but in the hope of mitigation (📖 p.V.506) of sentence. This has not only ethical but also therapeutic implications, in terms of likely benefit from treatment.

Meta-analytic reviews of studies on the effectiveness of interventions for offending behaviour have indicated that, overall, community treatment is to be preferred wherever possible, although secure institutions may still achieve positive outcomes.

Impact of the setting on treatment for substance misuse

The impact of the forensic setting is particularly pernicious in treatment for substance misuse and dependence, where the primary treatment method involves motivational interviewing (📖 p.II.168), and an acceptance of the need to wait for the patient to be ready to reduce or stop their substance use (i.e. to be in the 'contemplative' stage, in the Stages of Change model). This is often in direct conflict with the assertive or even coercive treatment methodology of forensic services, making treatment for comorbid substance misuse particularly difficult for forensic patients. However, abstinence-promotion and relapse prevention programmes based on motivational interviewing have been effective in prison settings (📖 p.II.217), as have prison-based detoxification units.

Coercion and treatment

Definition: objective and perceived coercion

There are ethical and philosophical problems in defining coercion (📖 p.III.268). Research on coercion has addressed two forms of coercion:

- *Objective coercion:* measures such as detention in prison or under mental health law; restrictions on the use of the telephone, contact with friends, leave from hospital etc.
- *Perceived coercion:* the patient's own experience of lacking control or influence over what happens to them (cf. agency, 📖 p.III.268).

The latter is ethically and practically likely to be of greater significance.

Research has also demonstrated that clinical concepts are too narrow, in seeking to reduce coercion to a single measurable concept. The social science perspective involves seeing coercion as the product of the beliefs and expectations of, and interactions between, patients, staff, and society—though this concept is much more difficult to study.

Measuring coercion

Despite the foregoing, scales have been devised to attempt to measure the experience of perceived coercion, based upon patients' self-reports; as well as objective coercion, which includes coercive practices readily observed and recorded in the context of legal detention (such as the use of seclusion and restraint, 📖 p.II.156).

The most commonly used measure of perceived coercion is the MacArthur Perceived Coercion Scale (MPCS), which contains five true-or-false items. These items do not address coercion or perceived coercion directly but instead focus on control, decision-making, choice, freedom, and initiation of treatment, with the implication that perceived coercion emerges from these constructs.

Instruments such as the MPCS show that measured perceived coercion is not well correlated with legal status. This suggests that either the measure is too inaccurate, or that patients cognitively reconstruct their experience from that of 'being coerced', into (for example) 'being cared for'.

Prevalence of coercion

Studies describe significant levels of perceived coercion reported by patients, but no consistent association with objective coercion.

Using the MPCS, one study found that 10% of legally voluntary patients in two US psychiatric units felt coerced at admission, whilst approximately 35% of involuntary patients did *not* feel coerced. An investigation of psychiatric patients in the UK revealed that one third of voluntarily admitted patients felt highly coerced, whilst two thirds were not certain that they were free to leave the hospital. A Nordic study comparing rates of perceived coercion across countries and treatment centres found high scores on the MPCS in the majority of involuntary patients (74%), and in one third of voluntary patients.

It seems likely that the lack of coincidence of reported experiences of coercion and legal status is explained by contextual pressures which are not identified by the measures of coercion used. For example, perceived coercion may be greater than legal status would suggest on an open ward where the power relationship between the staff and patients, as expressed in arrogant or dismissive staff behaviour, makes patients feel unable to speak up for themselves. Conversely, the degree of perceived coercion may be less than the reality, for instance, on a locked ward or in a prison where staff are respectful and patients or prisoners are allowed to express their views, feel they are taken seriously, and have access to procedures for obtaining justice.

Domains of coercion

Coercion is located within many domains of the lives of those with mental disorder, and arises from multiple sources.

Patients report experiencing coercion within psychiatric institutions during their care and treatment, not only at admission. One study involving a narrative analysis of patient interviews identified coercion through:

- Not being allowed to go home or out
- The use of mechanical or personal restraint
- Being coerced to take medication
- Being threatened with sanctions, and
- Not being allowed to make decisions.

In another study between 24% and 40% of voluntary patients reported restrictions on leaving the ward, whilst up to 73% of involuntary patients reported such restrictions. Almost half of all involuntary patients experienced forced medication, compared with up to 28% of voluntary patients.

There is also evidence of increasing experience of coercion, and use of leverage, in the community: coercion may be an everyday aspect of community mental health work.

Clinical importance of perceived coercion

Aside from the ethical implications of coercing patients (📖 p.III.268), it is important in terms of its effect on treatment outcomes (📖 p.II.184). Insofar as perceived coercion has negative therapeutic effects, it is important for clinicians to understand how to minimize that perception; even insofar as its therapeutic effects are positive, it is important to consider when it is ethically appropriate to use coercion. If the effect of perceived coercion is to worsen treatment outcomes, this reduces the ethical justification for coercion and loss of liberty.

Factors associated with perceived coercion

- *Demographics* The evidence is mixed. Several studies have failed to find an association between perceived coercion and age, gender, ethnicity and social class; whilst others have found high levels of coercion correlated with older age and non-white ethnicity, female gender, higher levels of education, and single marital status
- *Psychopathology* Studies of the relationship between diagnosis or psychopathology and perceived coercion also present an unresolved picture. However, it is important to identify whether patients' reports of coercion have their basis in illness-related symptoms, and perceptual biases, or are derived from real events or circumstances
- *Procedural justice* This have been found to be negatively associated with perceived coercion. Patients who feel that they were dealt with unfairly or were not listened to tend to report higher levels of perceived coercion on admission
- *Information* Patients are often ill-informed about their legal rights, and in one ethnographic study there was a finding that information was often deliberately withheld from patients by staff. The provision of sufficient information has been found to reduce perceived coercion
- *Pressure* Perceived coercion is strongly correlated with negative pressure (threats and force designed either to press a patient into hospital admission or to persuade them of the negative consequences should they refuse), but not with positive pressure (persuasion and inducements brought to bear to convince the patient of a likely positive outcome). There is a strong association between negative pressures and perceived coercion when a police officer is involved in an admission; but a family member or friend pressurizing the patient to accept admission reduces perceived coercion. Clinical pressure, whether positive or negative (i.e. inducements or threats by staff) increases patients' perception of coercion on admission to hospital.

All such research highlights the importance of relationships and context.

Attitudes to treatment

Perceived coercion is associated with patients adopting more negative attitudes towards treatment, independently of whether it affects therapeutic outcome. Patients who feel coerced into admission are:

- Less accepting of medical accounts of their conditions
- Less satisfied with treatment, and
- More likely to hold negative views of their experiences.

Even when objectively coerced patients retrospectively acknowledge their need for hospitalization, they retain their negative opinions.

Future treatment
Patients' experiences of coercion make them less likely to seek treatment in the future. One study of mental health clients in California reported that 47% of respondents admitted to avoiding traditional mental health services for fear of being committed; and a recent study of individuals with schizophrenia spectrum conditions found that 36% reported fear of coerced treatment as a barrier to seeking help for a mental health problem.

It is unclear, however, whether perceived coercion affects patients' compliance with future treatment, once it has begun.

Clinical outcome
The relationship between patients' attitudes and clinical outcome is far from straightforward to address, and the currently available data on associations between perceived coercion and therapeutic improvement are scarce and inconsistent.

Two independent studies have found that patients with high perceived coercion scores are more likely to report little therapeutic gain, and to show less symptomatic improvement on the Brief Psychiatric Rating Scale and Global Assessment Scale; but others have reported that patients who viewed their admission as coercive had higher levels of functioning at discharge.

Therapeutic use of security

The aim of providing security is to minimize harm to the patient, and harm by the patient to others. The risk of harm to and by the patient, set against the degree and intrusiveness of the measures needed to minimize that harm, determines the level of security required. A balance often has to be struck between measures directed at avoiding harm and pursuing other therapeutic goals, which can sometimes be inhibited by security measures. For example, not granting leave to a patient may 'secure' them but may also inhibit their rehabilitation.

What defines different levels of security?
Security is not only defined by locks and fences. It comprises:
- *Environmental or physical security:* which refers to physical features of a service such as fences, locked doors, key chains and soft cutlery
- *Relational security:* which refers to the nature of the relationship with patients (albeit still a coercive one, 📖 p.II.149), defined by aspects such as pre-admission assessments, adequate trained staff, good communication, and meaningful activities
- *Procedural security:* which refers to practices such as searches, inspections, investigating and learning from incidents, staff pre-employment checks, plus other clinical governance arrangements and risk management approaches.

The contribution of each type of security varies between facilities and contexts. In some psychiatric settings (e.g. the community), relational security is the most important, and the others have little or no role.

Psychiatric institutional settings are usually categorized as follows:
- High, medium, or low* secure units (📖 p.II.209)
- Locked wards (e.g. psychiatric intensive care)
- Open wards (most general psychiatric wards).[†]

What security does my patient need?

This is intimately related to risk assessment of the patient (📖 p.II.89), and the risk management (📖 p.II.189) that it implies. The process of mapping the security need onto the risk management plan should be rational and as objective as possible, with acknowledgement of the ethical balance being struck between security (implying loss of liberty) and therapeutic objectives. In practice, the offence or alleged offence of any individual patient will often be the starting point for consideration of security level. Other considerations usually include the likelihood, imminence and severity of harm to others within any particular setting, the likelihood of escape from a given type of setting, and the likelihood and seriousness of the consequences of escape.

There is no objective, operationalized method for determining the ideal security level, nor generally-accepted criteria for each level:[‡] good practice is therefore for the MDT (📖 p.III.256) to strike the balance between security and therapeutic objectives after collective deliberation, with the least possible loss of liberty.[§]

Security levels set by the criminal justice system

Most forensic patients are admitted from court or from prison, and many are subject to restrictions (📖 p.IV.412) on discharge, leave or transfer. For these patients, the court or the Ministry of Justice (MoJ, 📖 p.V.464, or its equivalent in other jurisdictions) will make the final decision on the level of security; although they will be advised by the MDT, they are free to depart from clinical recommendations. In Scotland, Tribunals (📖 p.IV.414) can also make binding directions on change of security level, whereas elsewhere they can only recommend such changes.

---

* Whereas all high- and medium-secure units are within forensic services, some low-secure units are forensic and some are general (the latter with a different, largely non-offender, patient group).
[†] Many 'open' wards have locked doors some or even all of the time, in order to safeguard individual patients; although most patients may be allowed out whoever they ask, locking the door is likely to affect the ward culture, and the degree of perceived coercion (📖 p.II.149) experienced.
[‡] The ACSeSS (Ghandi, Eastman & Bellamy's Admission Criteria to Secure Services Schedule) attempts to define objective criteria for the use of each level of security. The criterion for high security is posing a 'grave and immediate danger' to the public.
[§] i.e. applying 'the least restrictive alternative', a principle set out in the Reed Report (📖 p.App. 5.656).

Transition between levels of security

Security need should be constantly assessed[*] and responded to in clinical management. This might mean increasing or reducing the frequency of observations, a form of relational security, for example; instituting searches even after escorted leave (procedural security); or moving the patient to a different ward (a change in physical security)—although the latter can impair continuity of care, and through the loss of staff who know the patient well, affect relational security[†].

Transfer can occur as part of gradual rehabilitation, usually involving a reduction in security, or to enable therapeutic interventions to take place in a safer environment (through an increase in security).

Observation

Although not usually thought of as a form of security, observation is a key relational tool for monitoring a patient's mental state and behaviour and for engaging them in a therapeutic dialogue. Standard 'levels' are:

- General observation (minimum level): the patient's location should be known at all times but they need not necessarily be within eyesight.
- Intermittent observation: the patient's location should be checked unobtrusively every 15–30 minutes. This level is appropriate for patients at risk of disturbed or violent behaviour or attempting suicide.
- Within-eyesight observation: the patient should be within eyesight and accessible at all times, including at night. This level is appropriate for patients at a high and imminent risk of harming themselves or others.
- Within-arm's-length observation: as per previous point, but with the observing staff in close proximity to the patient at all times. This level is appropriate for patients at high risk of acting very quickly if the opportunity arises (e.g. swallowing any small object within reach).

Leave outside the secure environment

Despite requiring a particular level of security, patients may nevertheless safely have periods of leave outside that secure environment, provided that the risks of them harming themselves or others, or absconding[‡] (□ p.II.200), are acceptably low. This may depend on:

- The stability of the patient's mental state
- Their insight
- Their rapport with staff
- Their engagement with treatment and rehabilitation
- Their motivation to abstain from drugs and alcohol
- Their past behaviour when on leave.

[*] One widely-used tool for such assessment is the HoNOS-Secure (Health of the Nation Outcome Scales, Secure version), which contains six scales for assessing a patient's need for security.
[†] This is one reason patients often remain at a security level for a time after they no longer meet the criteria for admission to that security level: transfer too soon would damage relationships with staff, impairing both relational security and those aspects of treatment that depend on therapeutic relationships with staff.
[‡] Absconding refers to leaving without permission when outside the secure environment, as opposed to escaping, which refers to getting out of the secure environment without permission.

Leave should only be granted with a specific therapeutic purpose in mind; it does not amount to parole.[*] Depending on the risk of absconding and subsequent harm, or of harm occurring during leave, the leave may be with one or more staff escorts, or unescorted. Permission for leave[†] is usually given by the clinical lead of the MDT (e.g. for detained patients in E&W, the Responsible Clinician or RC 📖 p.IV.379) and should always clearly state the purpose, destination, escorting arrangements (if any), transport arrangements (if appropriate), and other requirements such as abstinence from alcohol, or submission to urine drug testing on return.

How can an increase in security be therapeutic?

The use of security measures to manage the risk of harm can be unpleasant for the patient, necessarily limiting their freedom, may result legally in a deprivation of liberty (📖 p.IV.436), and therefore poses ethical dilemmas (📖 p.III.265). However, it may allow the reduction or stopping of sedative medication that was being used to control behaviour, which may in turn facilitate the use of psychological and social therapies. It can also provide a sense of containment, especially to patients with borderline personality traits (📖 p.II.61). This might mean, for example, that a patient can tolerate the development of insight into their offending behaviour, in the knowledge that they are being kept safe from reoffending; or that they can come to learn that their challenging behaviours can be coped with without rejection or abandonment. Some patients reduce or stop their aggressive behaviour merely through transfer to a higher level of security, because of this sense of containment.

Problems with the therapeutic use of security

- There are no clear rules on the level of security an individual requires[‡]
- There is an unavoidable tension between security (e.g. keeping out drugs) and therapy[§] (e.g. allowing patients to receive visitors)
- There are often disputes between services (📖 p.II.220) or within teams about the required level of security, during which there is a risk that the patient's needs, both secure and therapeutic, may be neglected
- Risk on admission may rapidly diminish with treatment, with difficulty in then achieving a rapid transfer back to a lower security level
- Substantial and/or prolonged use of leave may indicate an unmet need for lower security
- The facilities and policies of units at different security levels may not match, especially if they are at different hospitals (e.g. a patient's behaviour may be unmanageable at the lower-security unit but not deemed to meet the threshold for admission to the higher-security unit), sometimes leading to inappropriate use of longer-term seclusion (📖 p.II.158)

---

[*] Parole is the conditional release of a prisoner based upon a promise to observe certain restrictions (e.g. attending appointments with a supervisor, residing where specified, and not offending).
[†] Under Scottish mental health law, what is actually granted is a temporary suspension (📖 p.IV.392) of one or more aspects of compulsion, which is a broader concept than leave.
[‡] Though Scotland has a procedure under ss264-270 MHCTA for Tribunals to deem patients 'detained in conditions of excessive security' and to order transfer.
[§] Mental health legislation (though not human rights law, 📖 p.IV.418) defines 'treatment' widely so as to authorize the use of security measures, including seclusion (📖 p.II.157). However, this does not mean that security on its own amounts to treatment.

- Patients on the same unit often have different security needs, with patients complaining about the freedoms given to others
- The balancing of secure and therapeutic needs is difficult for MDTs, which often become overly biased towards pursuing one or the other.

Seclusion and restraint

Seclusion and restraint of patients occur in many psychiatric services including general adult and learning disability services, as well as forensic services. Both seclusion and restraint are most commonly required during the acute phase of an illness, or behavioural disturbance arising in severe personality disorder. They are contentious, and regulated under mental health law* and codes of practice. Although they often form part of a risk management plan (📖 p.II.190), they can also form part of therapeutic interventions, making a distressed patient feel safer and more contained. Whether experienced by the patient as unpleasant or as therapeutic, each amounts in law to treatment (📖 p.IV.390).

Prevention and de-escalation

Seclusion and restraint are possible responses to untoward incidents in forensic psychiatric units, but prevention of violent incidents (📖 p.II.191) is far better than responding to them, however well. Incidents can be made less likely by well-designed physical environments; sufficient staff, space and privacy; predictable routines; meaningful activities; and a sense of being respected and having a voice (which reduces perceived coercion, 📖 p.II.149). Observation (📖 p.II.154) of patients, and de-escalation techniques (using body language and speech to calm a patient, then helping them to find a non-violent solution to their distress or anger) are also preferable to responses such as restraint or seclusion.

Restraint

Control and restraint involves the physical holding of a patient to control their behaviour. In the UK, this is always achieved by staff; mechanical restraints such as bed straps are not used, although they are widely used in countries such as the US. Restraint may be used to manage a situation that is immediately dangerous to the patient or others, and to give medication (📖 p.II.159) if it is essential and cannot otherwise be given.

---

*For example, in RoI s69 MHA makes it an offence to restrain or seclude a patient unless it is necessary to prevent injury and complies with the MHC's rules.

Restraint should only be used as a last resort, when attempts at de-escalating or otherwise managing a situation have failed. There should be a plan for ending the restraint as quickly as possible, for example by giving the patient PRN medication while restrained, and aiming to end the restraint as soon as that becomes effective. Restraint should be:

- For the minimum time necessary
- Carried out by trained staff using approved techniques that do not cause pain
- Proportionate to the situation
- Carried out with no more than reasonable force
- Accompanied by monitoring of physical health
- Accompanied by a request for a doctor to attend urgently
- Used only when resuscitation equipment is available.

⚠ Restraint can be *fatal* for the patient, particularly if they are prone (face-down) and pressure is applied to their back, such as by a staff member sitting on them. To minimize the risk of death during restraint, the prone position should not be used, and one staff member should continuously monitor their airway and breathing.

Seclusion

Seclusion (usually the supervised solitary confinement of a patient in a bare locked room*) can be therapeutic and reduce harm to patients or others in hospital settings; but there are also allegations that it is harmful and traumatic. Attempts to reduce its use have produced mixed results; none has eliminated it altogether. Seclusion may be considered:

- When there is a need to contain severely disturbed behaviour and other methods have failed
- Only if absolutely necessary and not as a punishment or threat or because of staff shortage
- Only when satisfactory resources are available
- Only when the detaining hospital has a policy for seclusion.

During seclusion, there must be continuous observation of the patient's physical condition as well as their behaviour and mental state. There must also be regular reviews of their condition and the need for continued seclusion: usually at least 2-hour reviews by nursing staff, 4-hourly reviews by a junior doctor, and twice-daily reviews by a senior doctor. Doctors reviewing seclusion should address the following:

---

* It is distinguished from 'time out' by virtue of the locking of the room; whereas time out can occur, for example, in the patient's own room and not under locked conditions.

Factors to consider in seclusion reviews
- Physical health, including injuries from the original incident
- Food and water intake
- Mental state
- Interaction with staff
- Attitudes and beliefs, especially relating to staff and any victims
- Hostility, threat or violent behaviour.

Longer-term seclusion

Where a patient is already in the highest level of security, persistent severe violence can occasionally be managed only by repeated periods of brief seclusion, or even longer-term seclusion. In these exceptional circumstances, legislation, codes of practice and local policies may allow for such repeated and longer-term seclusion, subject to careful safeguards.

Physical treatments

Physical treatments other than medication play a very small role in forensic psychiatry.

Electro-convulsive therapy (ECT)

ECT may be used as part of the treatment of mental illness within forensic psychiatric settings as it is within general psychiatric settings. The chief indications (and NICE recommendations) are as follows:
- Severe treatment-resistant (or acutely life-threatening) depression
- Severe treatment-resistant (or acutely life-threatening) mania
- Severe treatment-resistant (or acutely life-threatening) catatonia.

The vast majority of ECT treatments are for the first indication.

Guidance for general use of ECT applies to patients within forensic psychiatric settings, although the complex nature of the presentation of many forensic psychiatric patients means that ECT is comparatively more commonly used for conditions other than depression, including for conditions outside the indications listed, especially in high secure (📖 p.II.209) hospitals, because other treatments have been tried and have failed.

Neurosurgery

♦ Neurosurgery for mental disorder (also called *psychosurgery*) is exceedingly rarely used, partly because of the controversial history of procedures such as lobotomy and prefrontal leucotomy.* Severe treatment-resistant mood disorders and very severe treatment-resistant obsessive–compulsive disorder are the only remaining indications, and then only if the patient is competent to consent to it (📖 p.IV.425) and actively requests it after all other treatments have failed.

Psychosurgery should be distinguished from similar neurosurgical procedures carried out in order to treat otherwise intractable severe epilepsy.

Other treatments

There are no other physical treatments that are recommended in forensic psychiatry. The use of complementary physical techniques such as acupuncture may be approved for limited indications (such as anxiolysis) in some local areas.

Pharmacology

Medication is the primary treatment for both psychotic disorders (📖 p.II.54) and mood disorders (📖 pp.II.67, II.69), the main types of mental illness encountered in forensic psychiatry. Medication is also used in calming violent or disturbed behaviour where other techniques such as de-escalation (📖 p.II.156) have failed.

Acutely disturbed or violent behaviour

Medication is considered when psychological and behavioural approaches are insufficient to manage a situation. *Rapid tranquilization* should then be used to assist in managing the risk of harm to self or others, and to help reduce the patient's distress. To avoid polypharmacy, wherever possible antipsychotics and other drugs used in rapid tranquilization should be the same as those regularly prescribed to the patient.

---

* The operation was introduced in 1935, at a time when most patients with chronic schizophrenia faced a life of incessant, debilitating symptoms and of indefinite detention in a mental hospital. The transcranial or transorbital section of the white matter tracts linking the prefrontal lobes to the rest of the brain, first termed leucotomy and later lobotomy, seemed to be a valid alternative to the other 'heroic' treatments available at the time: infection with malaria for general paresis of the insane, cardiazol shock therapy (a precursor to ECT), insulin-induced coma or barbiturate-induced 'deep sleep'. Moniz, who developed the technique, was awarded a Nobel Prize in 1949. However, from the mid-1940s onwards, as the procedure became common in the US, UK, and Scandinavia, it became progressively clearer that it deprived patients of their personality and a degree of humanity. It died out gradually as public opinion turned against it and as antipsychotic drugs became available in the late 1950s and 1960s.

Example rapid tranquillization protocol after de-escalation has failed
- 1. Oral treatment:
  - Lorazepam 1–2mg *or* promethazine 25–50mg
  - *or* if **not** on regular antipsychotic, olanzapine 10mg *or* quetiapine 100–200mg *or* risperidone 1–2mg *or* haloperidol 5mg
  - *or* buccal midazolam 10–20mg
  - Repeat once after 45–60 minutes
- 2. Intramuscular treatment:
  - Consult senior colleague and consider patient's legal status
  - Lorazepam 1–2mg (have flumazenil to hand)
  - *or* promethazine 50mg
  - *or* olanzapine 10mg (do **not** combine with IM benzodiazepine)
  - *or* aripiprazole 9.75mg
  - *or* haloperidol 5mg (high risk of dystonia, ideally only after ECG)
- 3. Intravenous treatment:
  - Diazepam 10mg over at least 5 minutes (have flumazenil to hand)
  - Repeat after 5–10 minutes up to three times
- 4. After any IM or IV drug, monitor temperature, pulse, BP, and respiration every 5–10 minutes for an hour and then every 30 minutes.

Local guidelines, or authoritative published guidelines such as those from NICE or the Maudsley Hospital, should also be consulted.

⚠ *Zuclopenthixol acetate ('Acuphase')* can be used for patients with psychosis who have not responded to repeated short-acting drugs. It has effects that last for up to 72 hours. ►It should *not* be used for rapid tranquilization because it takes at least 2 hours to have a significant effect. Because of the risk of dystonia, it should only be used with great caution in young men who have not previously received antipsychotics.

Violence and psychosis

Antipsychotic medication can have an indirect impact on violence by ameliorating symptoms that otherwise predispose to violence, such as command auditory hallucinations or perplexity. Second-generation antipsychotics, particularly clozapine, may have a superior impact on violence and aggression by inpatients. There is no known benefit of any particular antipsychotic medication on the risk of violence by community patients.

Depot or injectable formulations are used more frequently in forensic psychiatric settings, because of poor adherence to oral medication by many patients, and because the harms associated with relapse (such as renewed violence or offending) are often much more severe.

Personality disorder

No currently available drugs are recognized to treat PD itself effectively, but they can be used to treat or prevent comorbid mental illnesses that are more common in PD (e.g. mood disorders or transient psychotic episodes comorbid with cluster B PDs). Treatment should be focused on symptom domains rather than diagnosis:
- Cognitive-perceptual—consider low-dose antipsychotic
- Affective—consider mood stabilizer or antidepressant

- Impulse-behavioural—consider selective serotonin reuptake inhibitor (SSRI)
- Anxious-fearful—consider anxiolytic or SSRI.

Medication should not be used routinely but should always be considered for comorbid mental disorder including anxiety and depression.

Disturbed or violent behaviour in learning disability

LD itself does not respond to any currently available pharmacological treatment, but medication may be indicated for comorbid disorders such as psychosis, depression, or epilepsy. There is also some evidence to support the use of *carbamazepine* to reduce aggressive behaviour in patients with learning disability.

Anti-libidinal medication

Pharmacological treatments are a treatment option for some patients with paraphilias (📖 p.II.74), or those who commit sexual offences (📖 p.IV.348) or show inappropriate sexual behaviour (📖 p.II.197).

- *Medroxyprogesterone acetate* (MPA) and *cyproterone acetate* are anti-androgenic drugs that reduce testosterone, luteinizing hormone (LH) and follicle-stimulating hormone (FSH) levels. These drugs are used to reduce sexual drive, but have significant side effects related to their hormonal actions: depression, feminization, gynaecomastia, and weight gain. ⚠ These drugs should only be considered in conjunction with psychological treatment
- Gonadotrophin-releasing hormone (GnRH) analogues such as *triptorelin* are used to manage sexual deviance and hypersexuality. They are more potent than MPA and cyproterone but appear to have fewer side effects
- *SSRIs* are potentially useful in the management of sex offenders, particularly in managing sexual urges and fantasies, which bear a phenomenological resemblance to obsessive thoughts

▶Antipsychotics should not be used routinely as anti-libidinal medication.

Physical health in secure settings

It is known that the life expectancy of people with schizophrenia is, on average, 25 years less than that of the general population. More than half of this excess mortality is due to disease, rather than suicide or trauma. Beyond the reduced life expectancy, patients with mental disorders suffer much greater rates of physical ill-health and morbidity.

Why is there such a problem?

One study in an inpatient forensic psychiatric setting found:
- High rates of smoking[*]
- High rates of obesity
- Weight gain during hospital stay, and
- More than half having at least one diagnosed medical problem.

[*] In addition to lifestyle and cultural factors, it has been hypothesized that the nicotine in cigarettes directly ameliorates some of the neurological deficits caused by schizophrenia.

Additional factors may include:
- Little health awareness amongst patients
- Fewer opportunities for healthy living, especially for prisoners and detained inpatients
- Low detection rates for comorbid medical illness
- Poor compliance with physical health monitoring, and
- Iatrogenic harm from pharmacological (🕮 p.II.159) treatment (e.g. metabolic syndrome related to antipsychotic use).

Interventions

Health promotion should focus on information, advice, and resources aimed at addressing:
- *Smoking:* smoking cessation programmes have been shown to be effective although not specifically in psychiatric inpatients.
- *Nutrition* is a frequent problem in forensic psychiatric patients. There is conflict between allowing patients choice in what they eat and encouraging healthy eating. Regular meals may be poor quality and takeaways are often part of the culture of eating in secure units.
- *Exercise:* making opportunities available for exercise is the most challenging issue. Smaller forensic units may have limited facilities. Encouraging walking, organized sports, and use of internal gymnasia, may be the best ways to increase physical activity.
- *Weight loss:* requires support for increasing physical activity and dietary restriction. Psychological support for weight loss interventions may be required. Often, obesity will be associated with low self-esteem and vice versa, and the latter may need to be addressed in order for weight loss programmes to succeed.

Monitoring physical healthcare

A principle of equivalence should be applied, in that forensic psychiatric inpatients should be entitled to the same quality of physical healthcare as any person, despite their long periods of loss of liberty, during which they are administered medication and subject to coercion (🕮 p.II.149). This may be achieved by personal attention on the part of the forensic psychiatrist to maintaining and updating knowledge as a doctor. Some forensic services will have separate primary care provision by qualified general practitioners.

NICE and other guidelines have been developed concerning the physical healthcare of people taking psychotropic medication or with a diagnosis of schizophrenia. These guidelines clearly apply to many forensic psychiatric patients. Some typical key points are shown in Box 6.1.

Box 6.1 Recommendations for physical health monitoring

At baseline (e.g. at admission), and every 6–12 months thereafter:
- Calculate body mass index (BMI), and enquire about diet and exercise
- Enquire about EPSEs, akathisia, TD, and other possible side effects
- Perform a systems enquiry and physical examination
- Measure fasting glucose and lipid levels, urea & electrolytes, liver function tests, and thyroid function tests
- Perform an ECG and calculate QTc.

Psychotherapies in forensic psychiatry

Psychological therapies promote recovery from mental disorder, reduce distress, and aid psychological growth and resilience. There is an extensive range of therapies with these objectives, all of which have been shown to be effective for mental disorders, if the therapy is matched to the problem. Mild to moderate disorders may respond to psychotherapies alone; more severe disorders usually also need medical treatment.

In forensic mental health services, the situation is more complex. First, many, if not most, of the patients have severe long-standing disorders, with no good evidence for effective treatment. Secondly, 'treatment' is not aimed simply at making people feel better, but also at making people behave better; hence, some treatment goals are imposed on the patient in ways that do not usually occur in the psychotherapies. Lastly, most outcome studies in forensic psychiatry focus on criminal rule breaking as an outcome measure (📖 p.II.184); it is not always clear what psychological needs were addressed or benefited.

Psychological interventions divide into those that arise from clinical paradigms (administered by clinical psychologists, psychiatrists, and other therapists) and those that are strictly behavioural and related to offending and closely related factors (administered by forensic psychologists).

Prison interventions

Prisoners have access to a range of psycho-education and cognitive skills programmes in prison (📖 p.II.176). Some programmes address particular types of offending; some address generic cognitive skills. Traditional interventions by forensic psychologists in prison do not address mental disorders except the addiction programmes. It is likely, for example, that men and women with ASPD (📖 p.II.60) access these programmes, but they are not treatments for ASPD per se. The exception is the HMP Grendon programme which is specifically addressed to men with ASPD and mild degrees of psychopathy (📖 p.II.66).

Secure psychiatric settings

Secure psychiatric settings need to offer a wide range of psychological therapies. Traditionally the focus of forensic services has been on patients with psychotic disorders who offend; and the therapeutic emphasis has therefore been on medication. However, psychotic symptoms are rarely a sufficient explanation for offences, especially those which are unusually violent. Diagnostically, most forensic patients have both Axis I and Axis II disorders; and the latter will require treatment interventions in their own right.

Services for patients with complex needs (i.e. a combination of mental illness, substance misuse and personality disorder) are not yet widespread in secure psychiatric services, although in some areas they are being developed in community settings. Some of the prison programmes are available in a modified form for forensic psychiatric patients.

Ideally forensic patients need access to:
- Assessments from both psychology and medical psychotherapy
- Individual therapy from a range of practitioners. Individual work may be important for those who find it hard to engage or have highly avoidant attachment styles
- Group therapies that promote hope and pro-social function.

Technical indications for therapy in forensic psychiatry

There is good evidence that all the different psychological therapies are generally effective, in terms of distress and symptom reduction. However, in complex clinical cases, different techniques may be particularly effective for different problems on a case-by-case basis:
- CBT (📖 p.II.165) is useful for addressing conscious cognitive distortions and assumptions, including psychotic beliefs
- DBT (📖 p.II.166) may be helpful for affect dysregulation and impulsivity
- Psychodynamic (also called reflective) therapies (📖 p.II.170) allow for reflection on less conscious attitudes and relationships patterns. Empathy and perspective taking are best addressed in reflective groups
- Arts therapies (📖 p.II.169) may be especially useful for those who are alexithymic or socially avoidant or where psychotic thinking is still evident
- Structured group programmes (📖 p.II.171) addressing offence behaviours usually offer a mixture of cognitive and psycho-educational interventions. It is helpful to follow up such programmes with structured reflective groups that offer space to think about the meaning of offences and related affects.

Therapy planning in forensic practice

Ideally, each patient should be able to access therapies that address their diagnosis, psychopathology, index offence, and rehabilitation needs. Patients need a planned sequence of therapies that is linked to both mental health restoration and risk reduction. Therapies, once started, should not be abruptly terminated without good reason: such abrupt terminations are potentially risky because they may briefly raise the risk of violence in a disturbed individual.

Patients often need active encouragement from their teams to go to therapy. They commonly find it difficult at the beginning; and may actively rubbish or criticise the therapy (much in the way some patients resist medication). It is helpful if teams do not collude with this resistance; but instead sympathize with how difficult it must be, and emphasize the potentially good effects in rehabilitation terms. Inevitably patients will realize, and are often told, that discharge (including by a Tribunal) is likely to be affected in some measure by their level of cooperation with therapy. For many patients, this will be the first time they have taken their minds seriously, and it may well be an uncomfortable process at first.

Cognitive behavioural therapy

Cognitive behavioural therapy (CBT) was first developed by Aaron Beck in the 1960s. Treatment is based on the idea that disorder is not caused by events, but by the view that the patient takes of events. Individuals referred for psychotherapy often hold ingrained, negatively skewed views of themselves, others and the world. CBT is relatively short-term, collaborative therapy that addresses this by focusing on current problems, where the goals are symptom relief and the development of new skills.

Rationale

Behaviours and emotions are determined by the person's cognitions. Some pathological emotions are the result of 'cognitive errors'. Whilst underlying emotions are difficult to control, behaviour and cognitions are more easily controlled. If an individual can be helped to understand the connection between cognitive errors and distressing emotions, they can then develop techniques aimed at change. CBT aims therefore to 'change the way you feel by changing the way you think'.*

With respect to offenders, the assumption is that the foundations of criminal activity are dysfunctional patterns of thinking. By changing routine misinterpretation of events, offenders can modify antisocial aspects of their personality and consequent behaviour.

Techniques

The therapist aims to assist the client to: monitor cognitions; identify cognitive errors; understand maladaptive schema; explore strategies to challenge and change these and examine the resultant effects on behaviour. CBT makes use of behavioural, cognitive, and experimental techniques.

- Behavioural techniques include activity scheduling, graded assignments, exposure, response prevention, distraction, relaxation training, assertiveness/social skills training
- Cognitive techniques include psycho-education; reading assignments; identifying automatic thoughts; Socratic questioning; thoughts diary; role play; thought rehearsal; cognitive restructuring; and examining the evidence.

CBT in forensic settings

CBT is currently the predominant psychological method used for treating offenders in hospitals, prisons and the community. It may be targeted at an offence related issue (including criminal conduct or substance misuse), a symptom of a disorder, or the distress associated with current experience.

In summary, CBT in offender treatment targets the thoughts, choices, attitudes, and meaning systems that are associated with the antisocial behaviour and deviant lifestyles.

---

*This is a description of CBT as developed from Beck's original work. Some psychologists consider CBT more broadly as a family of therapies ranging from pure behaviour therapy and behaviour modification at one extreme, to metacognitive and schema-focused therapies at the other; and for these other therapies in the 'CBT family', the description of working primarily on thoughts is sometimes incorrect.

Until recently CBT was mainly used in prisons, primarily in group programmes addressing offending behaviour; and in particular anger management, sexual offending and addictions. Many of the accredited offending behaviour programmes (🕮 p.II.176) have a strong CBT emphasis, such as Enhanced Thinking Skills (ETS), Reasoning and Rehabilitation (R&R), and Sex Offender Treatment Programmes (SOTP). A main focus of the cognitive interventions is cognitive distortions (🕮 p.II.95) that are related to the offending and criminal thinking patterns (these are the dynamic risk factors, see 🕮 p.II.130). At a community level, CBT can help an individual to develop skills necessary in order to function appropriately outside forensic settings.

Some researchers have argued that cognitive behavioural approaches are not universally applicable to all groups of offenders, including the mentally ill. The effectiveness of rehabilitation depends on the application of treatment matched to the needs of the person. Often manualized programmes developed for the mainstream prison population need to be adapted to meet the needs of other groups, including mentally disordered offenders, women, and individuals with learning disabilities or from other cultures. The manual may be more appropriately labelled a guide for treatment (some are highly prescriptive, others less so). Meta-analyses show that CBT is effective in depressive disorders, including in offenders, but that its efficacy in psychotic disorders is less certain.

Principles for successful CBT treatment with offenders

- Interventions should use the cognitive behavioural and social learning techniques described in the rest of this section
- Patients should have some ability and willingness to think about their thoughts and feelings
- Reinforcements should be mainly positive, not negative
- Treatment interventions should be used primarily with high-risk offenders, targeting criminogenic need
- Where appropriate, community interventions are more effective than those in institutional settings

Dialectical behaviour therapy, mentalization-based treatment, and other psychotherapies

There are a number of psychotherapeutic interventions that chiefly address emotional arousal and distress in interpersonal relationships. Although they arise from different theoretical bases,* with the exception of MI they share an assumption that early childhood experience has a

---

*DBT is in essence a modified form of CBT (🕮 p.II.165), developed because CBT is often ineffective for borderline PD. MBT is a modified form of psychodynamic psychotherapy (🕮 p.II.170). IPT was developed as a 'control' psychological treatment for randomised trials, but found to be effective in itself. MI has a basis outside the psychotherapeutic tradition.

profound effect on how individuals learn to regulate negative emotions and soothe themselves. Technically, they share an emphasis on the here-and-now of the therapeutic process; and encourage patients to be consciously aware of their thoughts and feelings as they happen.

The interventions described in this section are not mutually exclusive and an individual might be offered various interventions at different stages of their rehabilitation.

Dialectical behaviour therapy (DBT)

DBT is a technique developed by Marsha Linehan that draws on theories of mindfulness, and of how an enhanced capacity to be mindful of one's own feelings and thoughts can help to reduce both emotional numbing/emptiness and overwhelming affect storms. It has been shown to be highly effective with people with BPD (📖 p.II.61), especially those who self-harm. It requires a trained therapist to work individually with the patient focusing on issues that come up during the week, using a treatment target hierarchy. The patient needs to participate in a manualized, modular group programme alongside the individual therapy. The four modules covered are: core mindfulness skills, interpersonal effectiveness skills, emotion regulation, and distress tolerance skills. The empirical evidence is that DBT is good for community non-forensic patients with borderline personality traits and reasonable social functioning.

There is less evidence for the general applicability of DBT to forensic patients; mainly because so many patients have comorbid conditions. The evidence base for DBT has not been established for patients who have complex disorders and poor social functioning. There are also risks to the therapist in offering exclusive intensive individual work with some types of offender. However, given its success in reducing impulsive behaviours, it should be offered to patients who have borderline psychopathology; and may be tried with other patients who demonstrate impulsivity. The psychoeducational component may be especially useful.

Mentalization-based treatment (MBT)

MBT is another approach to the treatment of borderline psychopathology, within which patients can experience hyperarousal in response to their own feelings or thoughts about others' states of mind. Empirically derived from attachment theory and other elements of psychodynamic theory by Fonaghy and Bateman, it has been shown to be effective in complex cases of BPD. Modified forms of MBT are offered to adolescents. Small-scale trials are also ongoing with ASPD. MBT promotes the capacity to think about one's own state of mind, and enhances awareness of others' minds, which in forensic settings is relevant to the development of empathy. At the time of writing, there are two pilot projects in England evaluating its efficacy but there is no evidence to support its use with forensic populations at present.

Interpersonal therapy (IPT)

This is a therapeutic intervention designed to address mild to moderate mood disorder. It has not been tested in groups with complex comorbidity or who are antisocial. It may be a useful adjunct to medication in depressed patients.

Psychological treatments for substance misuse

There is a wide variety of therapies for substance misuse, choice depending on context and setting. In the community, people with addiction problems may seek help from their GP or from specialist voluntary services such as Turning Point. Organizations such as AA and NA have a good record in supporting those who wish to be abstinent.

There are number of interventions available in prison for offenders with substance misuse problems. These include psycho-educational and cognitive therapeutic programmes. Services offering substance misuse interventions have historically worked in parallel with mental health services. There is a drive to bring these services together.

Few of these various interventions have been tested in secure forensic services, mainly because their patients are involuntarily abstinent. Psycho-educational interventions may be of value when patients are leaving secure conditions.

Motivational interviewing (MI)

MI is an approach based on the principle that all human behaviour is motivated. It was originally developed by Miller and Rollnick for use with people with substance misuse problems but has become increasingly applied to work with offending behaviour in the forensic population. MI is a directive and client centred approach designed to help individuals change their problematic behaviour by allowing them to explore and resolve ambivalence, which is thought to be the primary obstacle to change, as well as to see themselves as capable of and as instigating change. It acknowledges that people can see both the advantages and disadvantages of change as well as maintaining their current lifestyle. A key concept in motivational work is the Prochaska and DiClemente's Cycle of Change, the six stages of which are pre-contemplation, contemplation, decision, preparation, active changes, and maintenance or relapse. MI may often be the starting point to move an offender towards engaging in other forms of psychological intervention.

Arts psychotherapies

The arts therapies are those psychotherapeutic interventions that use arts media as the main form of communication. Also called the expressive therapies, they utilize creative processes to reduce distress, promote psychological recovery, and enhance individual resilience. Arts therapies are not about being good at art and do not require any artistic talent in order to be effective.

The central theoretical framework, based on repeated clinical observation, is that some types of symbolic and creative thinking may be spared in mental illness, and that enhancing such thinking can promote recovery. Using interventions based on the creative arts, in conjunction with other treatments, it is possible to:
- Assess patient psychopathology, and
- Promote growth, recovery and distress reduction.

The principal types of arts therapies are:
- Drama therapy
- Art therapy
- Music therapy
- Movement and dance therapy.

Therapies may be delivered in groups or individually. Although their efficacy is not well researched in adults (and there are practical difficulties in doing so), there is some evidence that symbolically expressive therapies improve mental health; both in physically and mentally ill patients.

Arts therapies with forensic patients

There are several reasons why the arts therapies may be helpful for forensic patients. In particular, levels of childhood abuse and neglect are high in forensic populations; and many patients have not had the opportunity to play creatively as children.

Arts therapies are indicated for patients who are cannot name and describe emotions (alexithymia). There are two groups of patients:
- The more chronically mentally disordered offenders who struggle to verbalize thoughts and feelings at all, and
- Those who are verbally articulate but affectless in their accounts of themselves and others (e.g. ASPD and sex offenders).

The intervention can help the patient to develop language in which to express their emotions.

The creative therapies allow the mobilization of affect through the use of imagery. This is a particularly useful technique for those patients who have both suffered traumatic events, and witnessed them. There are a limited number of descriptive studies which have shown benefits of these techniques for forensic patients.

The arts therapies often emphasize the therapeutic use of action which is controlled and creative. For patients whose actions have been very destructive and dangerous, and whose freedom to act is tightly controlled in secure settings, arts therapies can promote hope that actions can be creative. Similarly, for patients who have only used their imaginations in destructive ways, the arts therapies offer a different way of processing or coping with unpleasant thoughts.

Arts therapies can also be a useful method for introducing patients who are socially disabled to pro-social relationships. In being part of an arts therapy group, patients have the opportunity to create, individually or together; and sharing work offers the possibility of being a valued member of a group.

There are no known negative side effects of the arts therapies, nor any known contraindications. The same risks apply to the arts therapies as to any psychological therapy in forensic practice; that is, concerns about professional boundary violations (📖 p.III.247), deception or conning of the therapist, and poor therapeutic execution. Therapists require supervision in the usual way; and, because they are often single practitioners in a service, it is important that they do not become isolated from the rest of the clinical team in a secure setting.

Individual psychodynamic (reflective) psychotherapy

Individual psychodynamic psychotherapy has features in common with CBT (📖 p.II.165), MBT and DBT (📖 p.II.166), in that it is highly structured*, and improves the mentalization of negative affects. The additional technical aspect is the close attention by the therapist to the therapeutic relationship, and the feelings evoked during the process of thinking and reflecting in the sessions. The technique is based on evidence† that people unconsciously repeat interpersonal attachment patterns first learnt in early childhood. In forensic populations, insecure attachment patterns are associated with relationship dysfunction, poor affect regulation, and lack of empathic thinking.

Efficacy

In the general mental health field, there is a considerable amount of evidence that individual psychodynamic therapy is effective in patients with affective and personality disorders; and that it is highly valued by patients. Its effectiveness in the forensic setting is less clear; especially for ASPD or in moderately psychopathic patients. It is not indicated for patients who are acutely psychotic, although for more stable patients it may have some utility.

In forensic settings, individual therapy may be high risk as a first line of treatment for patients who have experienced prolonged abuse at the hands of caregivers. Such patients may become highly aroused and agitated in individual work; they may also behave in compliant or seductive ways

---

* It is a common misconception that psychodynamic psychotherapy is unstructured. It merely has a different structure, which focuses on the predictability of the therapeutic frame (the time, duration and location of sessions etc.), while allowing the patient freedom to select the material for discussion.

† There is admittedly little direct evidence for the processes of transference and counter-transference occurring in the way that psychodynamic psychotherapists describe; and the psychodynamic model of unconscious processes does not accord with evidence from neuroscience. However, the lack of evidence for the underpinning theory does not preclude the therapy being effective in practice (see 'Efficacy' 📖 p.II.170).

with therapists. Careful attention to the history may elicit warning factors; and it may be better for such patients to start with small group work, within which they can learn cognitive techniques and group skills.

Contraindications

There are no absolute contraindications to individual therapy. However, men and women with high levels of psychopathy may compete with, or con, the therapist; and the work is technically difficult (and should not be attempted by junior staff). The evidence for group therapy (📖 p.II.171) is stronger for these patients.

In the early stages of therapy, patients may become more aware of their distress and sadness at their situation. However, it is crucial that therapies are not stopped as patients begin to develop awareness of feeling. Patients should be aware of the possibility that they will feel worse before they begin to understand and manage their feelings better.

Confidentiality

Individual therapists need to work closely with clinical teams; and patients should be aware of this. This can give rise to problems in using dynamic psychotherapy in forensic contexts, in that some therapists assert that complete confidentiality (including from the rest of the team) is a technical requirement. Usually a compromise can be reached whereby limited confidentiality is offered, within which the patient is told that breach may be required if evidence emerges to suggest that either the patient or others are at significant risk of harm.

If the therapist extends their approach to confidentiality to excluding giving interpretations and formulations to the treating team then this will substantially limit the value of the therapy in terms of recommendations for release (or continued detention).

Group therapy

Group therapies are widely used in forensic work, both for staff and patients.

Benefits of groups

- Groups promote pro-social behaviours and attitudes, such as rule keeping
- Groups promote interpersonal skills and turn-taking
- Groups decrease shame and social isolation: both of which are criminogenic risk factors
- Groups educate patients about offending and its effects
- Groups promote hope and reduce hopelessness: a potent risk factor for suicide
- Groups are an efficient way of providing interventions to individuals with similar problems.

A working knowledge of group dynamics is essential for assessing relational risk in inpatient settings, and for managing forensic institutions.

Disadvantages of groups

- Poorly run groups may allow offenders to support each other's antisocial attitudes and beliefs (a risk factor for future offending). This may be a particular concern with young offenders
- It can be difficult for offenders who are avoidant, or who struggle with shame, to engage in groups
- Very anxious or antisocial offender patients may present a risk to others, and be destructive to the group process.

Group therapy in prisons

In the prison system, all psychological therapies designed to reduce risk are delivered in groups. Group therapy forms the basis of therapeutic communities (📖 p.II.173), and in England this form of therapy is offered at HMP Grendon, HMP Send, and HMP Dovegate. There is some limited evidence that inmates who complete treatment in prison therapeutic communities show reduced recidivism rates.

Group therapy in the community

For offenders with community penalties or those on licence (📖 p.IV.365), the Probation Service (📖 p.IV.462) offers a range of offender support and therapy programmes such as Think First, ETS, R&R, and the SOTP. These range from psycho-educational groups for alcohol related offences to manualized cognitive therapy groups for sex offenders and those who have assaulted others. There is some limited evidence that these programmes reduce recidivism (see 📖 p.II.184). The Portman Clinic in London provides out-patient group and individual psychodynamic psychotherapy to offenders. Originally focusing on delinquents, it now primarily offers therapy to sexual offenders and those with paraphilias.

Group therapy in secure psychiatric units

Psychological therapies in forensic psychiatric units are aimed at reducing either psychological distress or risk factors for future violence. Group therapy may therefore be targeted at an offence related issue, a symptom of a disorder, or at the distress associated with current experience.

Because many forensic patients have poor affect and arousal management skills, and deal with anxiety in antisocial ways, it is important for the groups to be highly structured in terms of time, place and content. Some groups have a set focus (e.g. CBT for psychosis); in others, the group members are responsible for the session content, i.e. the patients set the agenda. This is important technically in order to promote responsibility and agency. Therapists need to be active and confident.

There is good quality evidence that both cognitive and psychotherapy groups are effective in both reducing distress and increasing social functioning in patients with PDs and other complex disorders; so-called 'group factors' such as learning from each other are thought to be relevant. This is particularly so for patients with BPD. The evidence for efficacy in severe ASPD is less clear because patients who are very antisocial find it difficult to engage in groups or seek to exploit the other members and/or the therapists. Clinical experience suggests that groups work best when there is a mixture of psychopathologies. Patients with high levels of ASPD and no mental illness may be offered therapy in one of the five national

DSPD programmes[*] (three in prisons, two in high secure hospitals, 📖 p.II.209).

Given the increasing evidence of the efficacy of group therapies in offenders, all forensic psychiatric patients should have access to a group work programme. It is necessary that secure services offer programmes for PD in particular, and services in medium secure units need to link with community services.

Staff groups

All forensic staff working in long-stay residential psychiatric secure care should have access to reflective practice (📖 p.III.253) time to review their work with patients. This is because working with such disturbed patients has an emotional impact on staff; and emotional reactions to patients may be clinically relevant to understanding the patient and avoiding inappropriate responses. Reflective practice should be delivered in groups; and ideally involve all the members of a clinical multidisciplinary team. Group meetings are essential as a reminder to staff that reflection on the work is a professional necessity, not a personal luxury.

Therapeutic communities

The original therapeutic communities were set up in the 1960s as an alternative to the traditional disease treatment model of psychiatric care. Today, however, therapeutic communities are best considered as specialist programmes that provide psychological therapies in a highly structured format to groups of patients, usually with personality and/or mood disorders.

There is good evidence from at least one systematic review that therapeutic communities are effective at reducing distress and improving social functioning in patients with mild to moderate degrees of personality disorder, especially BPD. The therapeutic effect has been shown to be maintained at 6–12 months after finishing the programme, as well as offering significant reductions in costs such as healthcare consultations. TCs are most effective when the patient/resident completes the programme, and most benefits seem to be made after 12 months of treatment. Most programmes therefore offer a 12–18-month programme.

It is likely that TCs are effective in five ways:
- They offer psycho-education about mental states, social rules, and rule keeping
- They promote cognitive skills in the self-regulation of negative affects and a culture of curiosity about mental states
- They behaviourally reinforce pro-social behaviours and increase anxiety about anti-social behaviours. For example, most TCs make quick responses to rule breaking behaviour and require rule breakers to take responsibility for their behaviour
- They decrease social isolation and allow residents to make secure attachments to the programme and the community. This is of particular

[*] At the time of writing, the DSPD programme is under review and is expected to be terminated, but with most of the existing DSPD services continuing as Severe Personality Disorder services.

value to those who have had highly adverse childhood experiences resulting in insecure attachment patterns. Social isolation is a potential risk factor for violent offending
• They decrease shame about distress and offer new cognitive skills in managing distress.

TCs for prisoners and forensic psychiatric patients

In theory, the TC approach should have particular benefits for antisocial people; but by definition, antisocial people may be antagonistic to pro-social structures or seek to attack them. There is the further difficulty that, conventionally, voluntariness has been a key feature of entry into TCs; and may be a key therapeutic element.

A number of modified TCs have been set up in prisons in the UK (including HMP Grendon), Europe, and USA, with varying success. There has been particular success with TCs for offenders with drug-related problems, and for offenders with histories of serious violence. The different effectiveness of different TCs may also relate to their structure and style: for example, British 'democratic' TCs have less evidence in support of their effectiveness than do more coercive US 'concept-based' TCs for substance misusers. However, the therapeutic boundaries in prison/forensic TCs need constant attention and monitoring. Staff need to be trained and supervised in order to keep them 'on message' in terms of maintaining the therapeutic structure.

Systemic and family therapy

Systems theory asserts that interactions, relations, and context are of primary importance in understanding the behaviour of an individual. Instead of viewing family and other life contexts in terms of the patient alone, the therapist considers them in terms of their significant life contexts, and in particular interpersonal relationships. Systems therapy therefore includes both family systems therapy and work with couples.

In a forensic context, systemic therapists are informed by ideas of pattern and process in relationships. Systemic formulation includes consideration of the intergenerational transmission of attitudes and beliefs concerning violence, and of intergenerational and lifecycle experiences, as well as the context of the referral.

Systemic therapy can be used with different types of offenders in different contexts, for example with perpetrators of domestic violence, mentally disordered offenders and young offenders.

Within forensic psychiatry, systemic work can aid risk assessment, provide psycho-education to family members, facilitate reparation and provide the opportunity for victims to come to terms with their traumatic experiences. It can also deal with specific factors within the family system contributing to the offence.

Domestic/intimate partner violence

A significant majority of couples presenting for couples therapy report marital violence in their relationship. However, most therapists do not routinely assess the risk of violence within the relationship. Therapy should not be attempted with family members where there is still a high risk of further violence. When undertaking couples work there should be an agreement that both partners are committed to finding a way to live together safely.

There are a number of interventions available for perpetrators of child physical abuse. These include parenting programmes, parent support programmes, and family preservation models relying on crisis intervention and case management.

Mentally disordered offenders

The majority of patients in medium secure units suffer from schizophrenia, and victims of MDOs are most commonly family members. Family interventions have been shown to improve outcome and the management of this illness. Family therapy is not always available in MSUs, mainly due to a lack of appropriately trained therapists and resources.

Young offenders

Family therapy has been found to offer better outcomes compared to other modalities for young offenders. However, it is most effective with low-level offenders who are living at home and where the families are motivated. With high-risk young people, the family is less likely to engage and to be more fragmented, and the young person is more likely to be in custody or another out-of-home placement.

Multi-systemic therapy (MST) is used to treat youth offenders in the 11–17 age range. It is an intensive, family and community-based, individualized programme that targets social systems around the young person. A therapist works with a family or carer and aims to strengthen the protective factors known to reduce the risk of offending. It operates a 24 hours a day, seven days a week system and treatment usually lasts between 3–5 months, with around 60 hours of contact. MST is widely used in the US, and is also available in other parts of the world including the UK, Scandinavia, Australia, and the Netherlands.

Intensive fostering is a programme funded by the Youth Justice Board and Department for Education. It is an alternative to custody for children and young people whose home life is believed to have contributed significantly to their offending behaviour. The programme provides highly intensive care for up to 12 months for each young person, as well as a comprehensive programme for the family. The scheme is based on the Multi-dimensional Treatment and Foster Care (MTFC) model which has been used successfully with offenders for many years in the US.

Offender treatment programmes

Interventions for violent offenders

There are few examples of well-researched and evaluated specialist programmes for violent men, and even fewer for violent women or MDOs. Most interventions amount to short interventions targeted at a single factor (e.g. anger management), and longer multifactorial programmes that typically focus on cognitions, anger management, skills training, and relapse prevention. They are generally offered within prisons or by the probation service.

There are several specific interventions for young offenders (e.g. Aggression Replacement Training (ART), Equipping Peers to Help One Another (EQUIP) and MST, 📖 p.II.175). However these are not aimed at the most violent young offenders.

Interventions for domestic violence may be offered by prison, probation or specialist therapy centres. They may be based on a variety of theories (e.g. feminist theory of childhood experience), and generally utilize cognitive behavioural techniques. They may be offered to individuals, couples or groups.

Interventions for sexual offenders (📖 p.II.198)

The *Risk-Needs Model* (RNM) for sexual offender treatment proposes that intervention should adhere to three principles; risk, need, and responsivity. The risk principle states that higher-risk offenders should receive more intervention. The need principle states that treatment targets should focus on criminogenic need. The responsivity principle states that the style of treatment should be one to which the offender is receptive.

The *Good Lives Model* is a more holistic approach to intervention and was developed in response to critique of the RNM. It does not limit intervention to criminogenic need and uses a strength's based approach.

Components of treatment for both models may include psychological and pharmacological treatment. Psychological treatment programmes are the most common and include treating sexual interests, treating offence-related attitudes and cognition, improving social competence and relationship management, and improving self-management. Treatment may be offered by probation services or by specialist clinics which may utilize a different model (such as psychodynamic models).

Accredited Offending Behaviour Programmes[*]

Offending Behaviour Programmes are an integral part of the work carried out by NOMS (📖 p.V.464). They are accredited by the Home Office, and are provided within prisons (📖 p.V.456) and by the probation service (📖 p.V.462). There are over 40 programmes currently approved by NOMS' Correctional Services Accreditation Panel in E&W, including:
- Aggression Replacement Training (ART)
- Controlling Anger and Learning to Manage it (CALM)

---

[*] This section refer to the offending behaviour programmes run in E&W. Scotland has no national probation service; the criminal justice social work departments run by each local authority do not run a consistent programme. Northern Ireland's Probation Board runs substance misuse and violence reduction programmes, but not the full list of courses shown for E&W.

- Sex Offender Group Work Programme
- Internet Sex Offender Treatment Programme
- Drink Impaired Drivers Programme (DIDs)
- Offender Substance Misuse Programme (OSMP)
- Addressing Substance Related Offending (ASRO)
- Personal Reduction in Substance Misuse (PRISM)
- Enhanced Thinking Skills (ETS)/Juvenile Enhanced Thinking Skills (JETS; carried out by YOTs)
- One-to-One
- Think First
- Community Domestic Violence Programme (CDVP)
- Integrated Domestic Abuse Programme (IDAP).

Nature of the programmes

Psychological treatment programmes which have been developed for repeat offenders are generally based upon the belief that offending is caused by distorted cognitions about responsibility and agency, and a failure to utilize inhibitory and pro-social cognitions that might act to inhibit rule breaking. For general offenders, there is evidence that these programmes may reduce recidivism.

The prison programmes tend to focus on conscious cognitions, and not on unconscious affects. Such techniques may also not take account of the highly disorganized attachment patterns found in forensic patients that may either prevent their engagement in therapy, or result in attacks on the therapeutic process. Forensic patients usually need more long-term therapies which take into account the relationship with the therapist as part of the work. Finally, forensic patients may need therapies that help them to come to terms with the consequences of their offences, as well as offering therapeutic techniques that address risk reduction. They may need a portfolio of different therapies which are integrated with each other.

Nursing and the milieu

The recognition of forensic nurses as a distinct discipline is a contemporary development in mental health nursing. Forensic nurses primarily work with MDOs, although they may also work with families and victims. Just as with forensic psychiatry, exactly what constitutes 'forensic' nursing is disputed: some regard it as the application of general nursing principles to a specific group, but there is much to suggest the need for the application of specific 'forensic' skills. These include particular abilities in keeping boundaries, constant risk assessment, combining therapy with security, and understanding the ethical and practice aspects of working in what can be highly coercive environments. Forensic nurses work in both residential and community settings.

The term 'milieu' refers to the interpersonal environment of residential care. Other people form part of the environment that affects our mental state; and this is pronounced when people live together in closed groups. Forensic nursing in such milieux requires particular skills; because nurses and patients spend long periods of time together, and nurses can be forced towards a parental role of both care and control.

Qualifications and training

The basic qualifications for nurses in mental health are the general courses of the registered mental nurse (RMN; in RoI, registered psychiatric nurse, RPN) and the registered nurse for the mentally handicapped (RNMH). No specific qualification for forensic nurses exists.

There is a continued debate in the nursing profession as to how forensic nursing skills and competencies should be defined. General life skills and adult social competencies may be as valuable as clinical skills in managing forensic patients, which is important given that much nursing care is delivered by unqualified healthcare assistants or social therapists. Such staff need an adequate understanding of mental disorder, how it affects risk of violence, and how it may impact on staff.

What do we mean by 'milieu' in forensic psychiatry?

Early experiments in therapeutic communities (📖 p.II.173) emphasized the importance of the pro-social environment for making changes in patients' sense of belonging and autonomy. In forensic psychiatry, the milieu or the environment of long-stay secure care affects patients' behaviour and mental state. Both the physical security and the relational security provided by the nursing staff ideally help patients to feel more psychologically secure, less paranoid and more able to engage in treatment.

Nursing: processes and relationships

An important forensic nursing task is the development and maintenance of a secure therapeutic milieu, in which psychological and pro-social change is supported and encouraged. Relational security (📖 p.II.152) is an important part of this process because of its emphasis on observation and reflection on relationships, not only between the patients, but also between patients and staff.

There are challenges in maintaining a therapeutic milieu:

- Nursing staff are almost always responsible for the imposition of rules and day to day security measures (to some extent, even where there are separate security staff), which may cause conflict with patients
- Nurses are responsible for the immediate management of violence and aggression, to a greater extent than other staff groups, and are therefore more often victims of assaults
- Inpatient nursing staff may experience the highest levels of stress as a result of the constant fear of violence associated with managing people with a history of violence
- Nurses may over-identify with patients, and collude with them in boundary breaking (📖 p.III.247). This is a particular problem in services that treat PD (📖 p.II.58)
- Nurses may also avoid patients that they fear or dislike, and fail to enforce boundaries with them as a result

The development of relationships that are psychologically secure as well as physically secure (📖 p.II.152) requires close attention to the making and maintenance of professional boundaries (📖 p.III.247). Forensic nurses have to maintain a boundary between being personally supportive and encouraging, yet not compliant or bullied. This is difficult to do well for long periods of time; and non-nursing staff have a role in supporting the nursing staff in maintaining therapeutic boundaries.

When things go wrong

The word 'milieu' in French can also mean 'gangland' or 'underworld'. An anti-therapeutic milieu in secure settings is one where bullying, coercion, deceit, and denial flourish. This may involve staff bullying patients, staff colluding with patients, or both. All these behaviours have been reported in secure psychiatric settings (e.g. see the Blom-Cooper and Fallon inquiries, 📖 p.App. 5.655). Such antisocial milieux do not help patients become more pro-social and increase the risk of inpatient violence and attacks on staff. A forensic psychiatric milieu is more likely to become antisocial if:

- Nursing staff are expected to deliver care that they do not perceive as being therapeutic resulting in a perception that their skills are under-utilized or under-valued
- The nursing staff do not feel supported by non-nursing members of the MDT (📖 p.III.256), or are in active dispute with them.

Attention to team dynamics is essential in residential settings; and is best achieved through reflective practice groups and supervision (📖 p.II.252).

Other settings

There can be very different roles and issues for forensic nurses in:

- *Prisons* where there may be opposition to a compassionate approach to prisoners
- *Community settings* where the role may only be coordinating care; and
- *Court* e.g. diversion schemes (📖 p.II.216) where nurses and others may be expected to regard those they assess as defendants first and patients second.

Social work

Social workers are involved in a number of different contexts within forensic practice.

Social workers are regulated by the General Social Care Council and have completed a degree in social work. They have statutory duties under the Mental Health Act, and most social workers in mental health complete training in mental health and become approved by Local Authorities. In E&W, social workers used to have a special status under the MHA, as 'approved' social workers (ASW) who could apply for compulsory detention. Since 2008, however, the role has been recast as that of the Approved Mental Health Professional (AMHP, 📖 p.IV.379) which can be carried out by a range of professionals including OTs and nurses.

In terms of clinical experience, social workers in forensic mental health teams may come from a background in child protection, general adult mental health, or probation. Forensic social work posts usually require a minimum 3 years' experience post-qualification.

In the US there is a specialist role called 'forensic social work', and a national organization which supports social workers in all aspects of forensic sociolegal work. However, there is no equivalent in the UK; although the General Social Care Council may introduce this. The British Association of Social Workers has a 'Forensic Social Work' special interest group.

The role of the social worker

- They have statutory duties under the Mental Health Act in relation to applications for detention, consultation with relatives and carers, discharge, and supervision
- They are responsible for liaising with the local authority and other bodies about arrangements for care after discharge, including identifying and specifying suitable accommodation
- In forensic settings, they may also have a specific role in relation to the needs of past or potential victims
- They have mandatory duties in respect of child protection and safeguarding vulnerable adults
- Specific duties in respect of young offenders (see 📖 'Young offenders', p.II.175)
- They will be involved in the assessment and management of risk at all stages of the process.

Carers, children, and families

Social workers take the lead in contacting family members, gathering social histories, and keeping family members informed about patients' treatment, as well as in liaising with the local authority to arrange carers' assessments when necessary.

Some social workers have particular expertise in assessing the safety needs of children, and their carers' capacity to protect them. They may also have experience of working with young people in the care system ('looked after children') who may also be in contact with the forensic and criminal justice system. They will have a role in completing a family assessment, including advising whether there is any domestic or spousal abuse, and in identifying any potential concerns regarding child protection such as abuse or neglect. In most cases, however, this work would be performed by a social worker from the local children & family social services department, who would liaise with the forensic social worker.

Detained patients in forensic settings may have children; and it is the role of the social worker to liaise with Local Authority child protection services to ensure that any ongoing contact with the patient is in the child's best interest and is safely managed.

Young offenders

Social workers have a number of special duties with respect to young offenders, particularly in Scotland under the Children's Hearings (📖 p.IV.323) system, and in E&W in conjunction with Youth Offending Teams (YOTs). Prior to a young person going to court the social worker will meet them and their parents, and liaise with other agencies to identify the most appropriate intervention and placement.

Social work departments may undertake a range of non-custodial activities which are intended to rehabilitate young offenders but also to divert them from more severe custodial sentences. For example, some social work departments are involved with programs such as Intensive Fostering and Multi-Systemic Therapy (📖 p.II.175).

Occupational therapy

Occupational therapists are specialist therapists regulated by the Health Professionals Council (HPC). They have undertaken a basic training in the assessment of independent living skills and in the development and implementation of rehabilitation activities based on these assessments, such as personal independence skills, social activities and the development of educational and employment skills.

The British Association of Occupational Therapists and the College of Occupational Therapists recognize occupational therapy in mental health settings as requiring a special skill base. As well as providing opportunities for enjoyment, relaxation and social interaction, these activities can help to reduce the potential for tension and frustration amongst patients, can increase motivation, decrease isolation, promote good health, and aid relapse prevention.

In order to promote social inclusion and recovery (📖 p.II.213), it is vital to clarify and acknowledge the patient's aspirations and strengths, help the patient make their own choices, convey hope and optimism, and match these to opportunities. Occupational therapy has an essential role to play here.

Forensic occupational therapy

There is increasing recognition of the link between poor occupational performance, poor mental health, and increased offending behaviour. As a consequence there has been a rise in the number of occupational therapists (OTs) working with mentally disordered offenders. Forensic OT is a recognized subgroup of mental health work in OT; however, there is not as yet a 'forensic training', thus making it more difficult to define their role.

Most OTs who come to work in forensic settings will have had prior experience of working in mental health.

The role of the occupational therapist

- In inpatient settings, the OT will complete a series of assessments, primarily focusing on how a patient's current mental state impacts upon their ability to carry out independent living skills. A detailed history of a patient's routines, roles, and responsibilities may also be gathered to help build a picture of the individual's life
- Assessments may highlight both strengths and weaknesses which help inform goals set in collaboration between the patient and the OT
- The OT will have a role in motivating the individual in working towards these goals and increasing interest in developing life skills and purposeful occupation, including within the confines of an inpatient unit
- Risk assessment plays a major part in determining the opportunities open to patients within a forensic inpatient unit and the OT must, in conjunction with the MDT, carry out a full risk assessment when planning appropriate interventions, such as access to tool-use workshops
- Interventions focus on developing the individual's interests and building their abilities in carrying out independent living skills. Prior to discharge from hospital, interventions will also be focused on increasing responsibility and autonomy
- The OT will have a role in supporting an individual to find vocational work and employment opportunities after discharge
- In community teams, forensic OTs have a role in supporting patients to find work and activities to support their rehabilitation
- The OT evaluates interventions at regular stages, making adaptations where necessary and reviewing goals with patients, particularly prior to case conferences.

Model of Human Occupation (MOHO)

This is the most widely used occupation-focused model in occupational therapy practice internationally. It starts from the basic premises that occupation (not only work, but also leisure, self-care and domestic and community activities) improves health and well-being; creates a structure for life and organizes time; brings cultural and personal meaning to life; and is idiosyncratic. Most OTs use this model in their practice as it:

- Helps to prioritize the patient's needs
- Provides a holistic view of the patient
- Supports occupation-focused practice
- Offers a patient-centred approach
- Provides a good basis for generalizing treatment goals, and
- Gives a rationale for intervention.

Vocational rehabilitation

What is it?

Arising from work helping people with disabilities to access employment, vocational rehabilitation now addresses the needs of other populations including those with mental health problems. It has been described as a process that enables people with functional, psychological, developmental, cognitive and emotional impairments, or health conditions to overcome barriers to accessing, maintaining, or returning to employment or other useful occupation.

There are different methods of helping people access work:

- Prevocational Training—preparatory work prior to employment
- Supported Employment—employment in a standard environment with on the job support (Individual Placement Support, IPS, is a manualized intervention form of supported employment)
- Work schemes within secure units.

Barriers to employment in forensic psychiatry

The impact of severe mental illness on employment prospects is well known, in terms of:

- Stigma
- Discrimination
- Lack of support
- Concern over benefits
- Disempowerment
- Lack of skills
- Absence of recent employment
- Lack of freedom
- Restricted choice
- Low self confidence
- Lack of motivation
- The co-existence of an offending history.

People in secure hospital care generally have lower levels of education and employment experience associated with poor employment prospects.

Why is it necessary?

- 61–73% of people with severe mental illness are unemployed and lack structure or a daily routine
- Rates are even higher for people discharged from secure hospital care (up to 90%)
- Employment instability is associated with offending
- Employment can have an impact on many other factors related to quality of life including:
  - Increased income
  - Achievement of a valued social responsibility
  - Greater socialization
  - Increased self-esteem
  - Opportunities to use skills
  - Opportunities to give something back to the community
  - Provides an indicator of progress in recovery

- Offenders released from prison with mental health problems have high rates of unemployment, whereas employment reduces reoffending by between 30–50%

What exists?
- Individual schemes within secure hospitals
- Arrangements directly with employers
- Partnerships with charities
- Vocational rehabilitation provided by people from clinical and non-clinical backgrounds
- Sometimes linkage with the assessment and intervention done by the OT (📖 p.II.181).

Practice example
First Step Trust is a charity providing real work, training, and employment opportunities for people excluded from work because of mental health problems or other disadvantages. In addition to other projects they run work projects within secure hospital settings.

Does it work?
As with any intervention, there is a need to define the aim of that intervention. Vocational Rehabilitation as an intervention is difficult to evaluate as a large majority of people with severe mental disorder will remain unemployed.
- For people with severe mental illness supported employment (including IPS) is the most effective intervention for employment
- There is limited evidence on impact on symptoms, quality of life, or social functioning (conclusion limited by under-powered studies)
- The majority of evidence is from the US, not the UK
- There is no clear evidence for patients in forensic psychiatric settings.

Evaluation of treatment

Evaluation of whether treatment in forensic psychiatry has been effective may use one or more of a number of outcome measures (📖 p.III.221):
- Reduction in offending or risk of offending
- Reduced relapse or readmission rates
- Reduction in symptoms and distress
- Improvement in social and/or psychological functioning.

There has been a clear tendency to measure outcome primarily by way of recidivism rates alone, partly because it is relatively easily and cheaply measurable, and partly perhaps as a reflection of social priorities. However, this is partial and inadequate.

Reduction in offending
A period of great confidence in offender rehabilitation in the 1960s and 1970s was followed by a demoralization from 1975–81 when the view that 'nothing works' prevailed. In response, the mid 1980s saw the advent of the 'what works' literature, with meta-analytic studies of interventions.

This led to the development of an evidence-based practice approach to assessment, management, and treatment of offenders.

The principal measure of evaluation of effectiveness is reduced reoffending as measured by reconviction rates (📖 p.II.18), although there are several limitations with their use. Reconviction within 2 years is the standard across studies in E&W, but studies that continue beyond 2 years offer more information.

Evaluation studies typically compare the reconviction rate of a group of offenders who have participated in an intervention/treatment and those who have not participated. However there are inherent difficulties in implementing randomized controlled trials (RCTs) in criminal justice settings. The overall results of meta-analytic studies show that treatment or rehabilitation of offenders on average produces a 10% reduction in reconviction.

Violent offenders
Interventions for violence range from short programmes targeted at a single factor (e.g. anger management) to longer multifactorial programmes (including focus on cognitions, anger management, skills training, and relapse prevention). The most effective interventions target negative affect/anger, antisocial attitudes, and relapse prevention.

Sex offender treatment evaluation
A number of meta-analytic studies have found that cognitive behavioural treatment has a small but robust effect on reconviction rates for sexual offences. The combination of medical and psychological approaches seems particularly promising.

Domestic violence intervention evaluation
The literature generally concludes that there is either no, or only a small, effect of programmes on perpetrators of domestic violence. However, there are many methodological flaws with these studies and more multisite designs are needed.

Young offenders
The most beneficial interventions with respect to reducing reoffending in young offenders focus on criminogenic, rather than clinical, needs, and are structured and multimodal. Programmes that work directly with the individual should have a cognitive component that addresses attitudes, values and beliefs supportive of antisocial behaviour. There is some evidence for early prevention, parenting programmes, and systemic interventions, such as MST (📖 p.II.175), which address family, community and the wider risk factors.

Effective programmes
The literature suggests that, in order for an offender programme to be effective, it needs;
- A theoretical framework supported by empirical research
- To involve assessment to determine risk of future offending
- To target the criminogenic need
- To be structured, clear and directive

- High treatment integrity, i.e. the delivery of the programme is carefully planned and model-based
- More likely to be multimodal and skills oriented, with a cognitive behavioural focus, and
- More likely to be community based than in institutions.

It should be noted that the majority of offending behaviour programmes are still designed for white, adult, male offenders without significant mental health or learning difficulties. Although these programmes may be effective for mentally disordered offenders, there is a need for programmes to take account of both criminogenic and responsivity needs of different offender groups.

Mentally disordered offenders

It is only relatively recently that clinicians have begun to develop and measure treatment outcomes with this population. Relatively little is still known about what works, either in terms of reducing offending or ameliorating distress, in the treatment of MDOs. This lack of knowledge applies to all types of mental disorder. Various interventions for mentally disordered offenders are assumed to produce better outcomes but are not backed by a sound empirical base:

- Use of restriction orders (although uncontrolled studies suggest a low reconviction rate)
- Preferential treatment with depot medication
- Higher level supervision of offenders in the community

Difficulties with treatment research with MDOs

The evaluation of treatment programmes for MDOs is complicated by:

- Low base rates of outcome measures
- Difficulty in constructing RCTs
- The inherent complexity of treatment
- Inadequate measures of treatment
- Difficulty defining meaningful outcomes.

Treatment of victims

Who should treat victims?

There are major advantages in clinicians who treat offenders also having a role in the treatment of victims, in service terms. Forensic clinicians have an understanding of 'the offence event' and therefore have a major contribution to make to the treatment of victims. However, it is crucial that it is clear, in the individual case, who is being treated, and that there is no blurring of boundaries. Those treating offenders must have an understanding of the rights and needs of both the perpetrator and the victim, and must address both, but always from the perspective of their role with the patient. What understanding 'victimology' offers to those who treat offenders is a depth of understanding of the impact of their patient's offending on others, and acceptance of the importance of the victim perspective. Treating victims may often be an appropriate activity for a forensic service, but not in any way conjoined in the individual case with treating a perpetrator.

Victims' needs

The psychological effects of being a victim of a crime include PTSD (📖 p.II.70) and other traumatic stress reactions, depression, and anxiety disorders. There are both acute short-term reactions and longer-term effects.

Whether a victim seeks help is determined by their cultural background, expectations, and knowledge of what services are available, as well as by the severity of their post-traumatic symptoms. Apart from help with the psychological and emotional needs, victims may also need practical help, information and financial support. In E&W, the charity Victim Support offers this kind of assistance, free of charge. There are similar organizations in Scotland, Northern Ireland, and the Republic of Ireland.

Victim Support offers:
• Someone to talk to in confidence
• Information on police and court procedures
• Help in dealing with organizations
• Information about compensation and insurance
• Links to other sources of help.

In addition to voluntary services, some mental health services offer specialist traumatic stress services for patients with PTSD and related conditions.

Considerations in secure settings

Victims of offences may still be linked with the perpetrator on an ongoing basis. Working with perpetrators generally means a high likelihood of having contact with the victims of their offences, as a large proportion are family members. Victims may be attending care planning meetings or be involved in the interventions with the offender (e.g. systemic therapy). Careful consideration of the needs of the victims should be made in conjunction with the MDT, including social workers (particularly when children are involved). Victims of MDOs have rights to inquire about discharge planning through the Probation Service, and treating teams have duties to disclose information to victims in certain circumstances (📖 p.IV.442).

Perpetrators as victims

Perpetrators are also likely to have been victimized (📖 p.II.141) themselves, and may experience high levels of post-traumatic symptoms. A substantial number of offenders have been victims of crime, both as adults and children. Childhood abuse is associated with increased risk of developing personality and mood disorders in adulthood. Psychological intervention needs to consider the relationship between the trauma experienced and the index offence. The commission of the index offence may itself be traumatic, and there are recorded cases of PTSD arising from offending; especially family homicide. Suicide risk after family homicide remains high for perpetrators indefinitely.

Offender discharge/release into the community

Victim issues may sometimes determine that it may not be possible for an offender to return to their area upon discharge from hospital or prison; or there may have to be special restrictions put in place to protect the victim from contact.

Risk management

Risk management: general principles

Risk management is intimately related to risk assessment, and flows from it, even where some risk factors are not amenable to any management or reduction. This chapter should therefore be read in close conjunction with that on risk assessment (📖 p.II.127).

Treatment, risk management, and conflicting objectives

There is a substantial overlap between the goals and methods of treatment and risk management, but also a meaningful difference. The primary aims of treatment (📖 p.II.146) are to benefit the patient by improving quality of life or delaying death, whereas the aim of risk management is to minimize harm to the patient and to others. This will often simultaneously benefit the patient, at least in some ways (e.g. avoiding an incident of sexual violence and consequent prosecution and incarceration may improve the patient's quality of life during what would otherwise have been the period of incarceration), but it can also conflict with what is in the patient's interest, at least as they see them (e.g. giving an antipsychotic drug that reduces the risk of psychosis and the associated risk of reoffending, but that causes unpleasant akathisia).

The unavoidable ethical tension (📖 pp.III.265, III.280, III.282) between the interests of the patient and the interests of others determines that risk management must involve ethical reflection: that is, careful consideration of whether the measures proposed, and the impact they may have on the patient, can be justified not only in terms of the patient's own benefit but also in terms of the benefits to others as set against any disbenefit to the patient. There is an explicit ethical balance to strike.

Principles of risk management

The following list represents guidance, accepting that principles will sometimes produce conflicting results and trade-offs may be necessary.

- Separate out the various *apprehended harms*, and consider the risk of each individually
- Base the risk management plan on a careful risk assessment (📖 p.II.127). Even in an emergency, you can carry out a basic risk assessment in your own mind within a few seconds, such as whilst you are walking to the scene
- Apply the risk assessment, and particularly its actuarial (📖 p.II.130) elements, in the context of your personal understanding (e.g. your narrative formulation, 📖 p.II.110) of the patient
- In doing this, take into account the setting or context in which the risk management plan is to be carried out (e.g. inpatient ward, prison, hostel, or patient's home)
- If the risk assessment that can be carried out in the time or circumstance available is incomplete, make the continued gathering of further relevant information part of the risk management plan itself, and then update your assessment accordingly at a later stage
- Adopt the principle that the less comprehensive the risk assessment that is possible, the more measures should err on the side of caution, (e.g. emphasizing security) until a fuller risk assessment is completed

- Focus both on avoiding or preventing apprehended harms, and on a plan for dealing with them if they do occur
- Treat underlying causes (especially mental disorder) whenever these can be identified, not just the problem symptoms or behaviours
- Where there is a choice of actions to reduce risk, begin with those with the most positive, or least negative impact on the patient (for example, in a plan for managing the risk of violence, prioritize problem-solving counselling sessions above seclusion (📖 p.II.156)
- Only include actions that compromise the patient's freedom or that run contrary to their expressed wishes if they are *proportionate* and *justifiable* responses to the harms the plan aims to prevent, both technically and ethically
- Bear in mind the legal setting in which the plan will be carried out, and in particular whether any elements with which the patient does not agree are covered by a relevant legal power to act, e.g. under mental health (📖 p.IV.373) or mental capacity (📖 p.IV.424) legislation, and fall within local policies and codes of practice
- Ensure that the whole team knows and understands the plan, not just the individuals who compiled it. If there is conflict within the team, ensure that it is expressed and addressed, so that at least all members feel consulted
- Work collaboratively with other agencies in managing risk (📖 p.II.203)
- Review the plan, and the underlying assessment, whenever the situation changes materially, and in any event at appropriate intervals (e.g. at ward rounds or CPA meetings), and more often if the plan involves significant additional restrictions on the patient's liberty.

Specific risks relevant to forensic psychiatry

Specific management of the risk arising from each of the harmful potential types of behaviour is dealt with in individual topics of the handbook. These include:

- Risk of violence (📖 p.II.191), including specific scenarios such as hostage-taking (📖 p.II.195)
- Risk of sexually inappropriate behaviour (📖 p.II.197)
- Risk of suicide and self-harm (📖 p.II.199)
- Risk of absconding or escaping (📖 p.II.200)
- Other specific risks such as fire-setting or exploitation (📖 p.II.202).

Management of violence

Reviews of serious untoward incidents and the findings of homicide inquiries (📖 p.V.471), combined with established principles, have identified the following recommendations for the management of the risk of violence.

Preparation

- Structured risk assessment (📖 p.II.130) is clinically necessary and useful and should form the basis of the risk management plan
- Ensure you formulate (📖 p.II.110), not merely assess or attempt to quantify, the risk of violence—think explicitly about how and when the risks are likely to be emphasized in the patient's daily life

- *Keep in mind* the results of the risk assessment—both risk assessment and management are dynamic activities, not things to be ticked off as a job done and then forgotten about.[*]

Mental illness and violence

- In patients with mental illness and a history of violence, basic *symptom control* will often directly reduce the risk of violence (see also 📖 p.II.31)
- Do not accept *non-compliance* with medication or other key aspects of the care plan in someone who poses a significant risk of violence—keep encouraging and/or enforcing compliance every day
- Make use of the legal powers (📖 pp.IV.383, IV.412) available to ensure compliance with relevant aspects of the care plan
- *Intervene early* when relapse is reasonably foreseeable. The law[†] does not require the relapse to have occurred before the patient can be recalled (📖 p.V.467) or readmitted, as long as there is clear evidence that relapse (and increased risk of harm) is imminent if no action is taken
- Recognize that treatment and rehabilitation will often need to be *long term*. For some patients, a series of brief admissions is of much less value than a prolonged admission, and can even be counter-productive.

Substance misuse and violence

- Take substance misuse, including cannabis use, seriously. Sometimes substance misuse alone will be the additional reason that justifies readmission or recall; it can quite legally be the sole basis for recall if there is a clear history of relapse associated with the substance use.
- Whenever powers allow for the setting of *conditions* (e.g. under a restriction order (📖 p.IV.412) in E&W, or a community Compulsory Treatment Order (📖 p.IV.394) in Scotland), consider setting explicit conditions of abstinence and drug testing, with an explicit expectation that breach of the condition will lead to recall for inpatient reassessment.

General measures

- *Intervene early* when patients with a history of violence behave in a risky fashion, even if relapse is not imminent. Do not rely on extensive past knowledge of the patient—it may offer false reassurance

---

[*] The importance of 'good process' as the foundation of good clinical practice in a wide variety of domains can sometimes result in adherence to the formality of the process, in a relatively unthinking fashion. Good process provides a framework for thought, not a substitute for it.
[†] The definitions of 'mental disorder of a nature . . . which warrants . . . detention . . . in hospital for assessment [for] the protection of other persons' in the E&W MHA and in very similar terms in the NI MH(NI)O, and of 'mental disorder [causing] a serious likelihood of . . . immediate and serious harm' in the RoI MHA allow such early intervention. The Scottish requirement in the MH(CT)SA to demonstrate that it is likely that the mental disorder significantly impairs the patient's judgement makes early intervention slightly more difficult. See 📖 p.IV.384.

- Set *clear, operationalized criteria* for intervention and read..
  and write them into care plans. Make sure that patients know w..
  expected of them, and what those criteria are. Then stick to them
- General services should, when their risk assessment indicates a high
  risk of violence, make routine use of *forensic services* for advice
- *Share assessments* of risk openly and honestly with the patient, carers, and
  relevant services, within proper bounds of confidentiality (📖 p.III.263)
- Do not obsess about the 'correct' diagnosis with complex patients.
  Instead, focus on the treatment plan, risk assessment, and risk
  management plan, taking into account both or all the differential diagnoses
- Take *carers' concerns* about risk, especially changes in risk, seriously;
  investigate and respond to them
- Remember that the risk of *violence cannot be completely prevented*,
  (or even predicted, 📖 p.II.128), only made less likely.

Inpatients and violence

- On hospital wards, violence can be made less likely by well-designed
  physical environments; sufficient staff, space, and privacy; predictable
  routines; meaningful activities; and a sense of being respected and
  having a voice (see also 📖 p.II.151)
- Observation of patients (📖 p.II.154), and *de-escalation* techniques
  (using body language and speech to calm a patient, then helping them
  to find a non-violent solution to their problems) can reduce the
  chances of the patient becoming violent.

The management of specific violent incidents is described on 📖 p.II.193.

Managing acute behavioural problems

This refers to sudden changes in behaviour that pose an immediate
management problem. In all the situations described in this section, work
collaboratively with other staff, seek help from senior or other colleagues
and/or the police unless you (and the colleagues with you) are sure you
can manage the situation safely, and do not expose yourself, other staff or
patients to unnecessary risks.

On arriving at an incident

- Establish the nature of the incident before intervening, e.g. by telephone
  before arrival if time permits, or by speaking to other staff on arrival
- If time allows, gather as much detailed information as possible,
  particularly if the patient or patients involved are previously unknown
  to you
- If no colleagues are available to help, summon assistance before
  intervening (e.g. by pressing an emergency call button on a hospital
  unit, or by shouting if others are nearby, or by mobile phone)
- Clear the area of other patients and inessential staff.

Speaking to the patient

- Make it clear who you are, why you are there, and how you can help
- Be calm, clear, honest, and respectful

- Listen to what they say, and observe their body language—try to understand how they are feeling as well what they are thinking
- Empathize with their emotional state (this does not include agreeing with unreasonable things they might say or believe)
- Repeat information back to show you have understood
- Allow the patient to express themselves to you and to see that you understand before moving on to how to resolve the situation
- Be clear about what cannot be avoided or negotiated away (e.g. giving up a weapon, accepting PRN medication), and focus instead on aspects over which the patient can safely be allowed to exercise choice (e.g. whether to take medication orally or intramuscularly, whether to acquiesce quietly or to be restrained by staff)
- Show that you are focused on solving the problems the patient presents, in an appropriate way (e.g. acknowledging their distress over the refusal of another patient to lend them a cigarette, helping them think through whether and when they might be able to purchase a cigarette, promising to assist with requesting leave if appropriate to purchase cigarettes once the patient is calm and the situation is under control)
- If the situation cannot be made safe by such de-escalation techniques, consider restraining the patient (□ p.II.156) to prevent further harm.

Once the incident is under control

- In the immediate aftermath of an incident on the ward, consider an increase in the security level (□ p.II.155), the use of seclusion (□ p.II.157), or enhanced observations (□ p.II.154), if necessary
- Treat any acute aspect of mental or physical disorder that may have impacted on the situation (e.g. give food or fruit juice etc. if hypoglycaemic; offer PRN medication for acute psychosis)
- Even if the patient is calm, consider asking them to have a period of time out away from other patients if there is a risk of the situation re-escalating
- Consider calling the police (if they have not already been called), particularly if serious harm has been caused, or if there is an ongoing risk of further violence that cannot safely be dealt with
- Consider facilitating the prosecution* of the patient (□ p.III.287) if their violence amounted to a criminal offence
- Review the patient's *care plan*, if there is evidence of a link between the violent incident and their mental or physical disorder, their treatment, or the context of treatment
- Document the incident, your actions (and colleagues'), and your reasons for your actions, carefully in the patient's clinical record: this will both encourage clarity of thought, and provide a proper record available for future managerial inquiry, or legal scrutiny.

---

* This will usually require the victim to be willing to make a statement to police, but the police can accept evidence of the crime from others, and in exceptional circumstances (particularly cases of domestic violence) the CPS in E&W, the Procurator Fiscal in Scotland, and the NI Public Prosecution Service can prosecute without the agreement of the victim. The RoI DPP does not appear to have a policy allowing prosecutions without the victim's consent, however.

After the incident

The experience of dealing with acute incidents can often be traumatic for staff, the patient, and other patients who witness it, especially if serious injury or harm has been caused.

- Before staff leave after the incident, ensure that they obtain medical treatment for any injuries, and check whether they feel distressed in any way by the incident
- Ensure that an appropriate person (such as the relevant manager if they were not involved in the incident, or a more senior manager) offers staff the opportunity to leave work if they are too distressed to continue working safely, arranges cover, and arranges counselling if needed
- Apply the same principles to yourself—consider asking to go home if you are not fit to continue working, and consider requesting counselling through your Occupational Health department
- Ensure that you or someone else completes an incident report according to local policies (this is in addition to documenting the incident in the patient's notes)
- Request, and take part in, a debriefing and/or critical incident review after the incident, if one is necessary.

Hostage situations

A hostage situation is defined as an incident in which a perpetrator(s) holds one or more persons against their will in a location that is known to others. Hostage-takings and forcible confinement are rare within forensic settings. However, when they do occur they may cause significant psychological and/or physical harm not only to the hostages, but to staff and patients/prisoners who may be witnesses.

Forensic professionals may be asked to assess an individual who has taken a hostage during an index offence; or during a period of detention; or (rarely) they may be asked to advise the police during a hostage event. The taking of a hostage may be a form of intimidation, or may occur during detention in prison or hospital in response to frustration, or as an attempt to manipulate others towards some particular goal.

Assessment of risk

Assessment of the risk of hostage taking should incorporate a detailed functional analysis of previous incidents. There is no empirical basis for specific analysis of the risk of hostage taking. However, a structured clinical tool such as the HCR-20 (📖 p.II.133) allows consideration of formulation and management of different scenarios, including hostage taking.

Hostage negotiation

This is the most important aspect of any hostage crisis. Ideally this will be done by trained negotiators; and every forensic workplace should have identified personnel for the task.

Key issues are the separation of the roles of the commander (who has authority over the entire scene and all the personnel involved) and the negotiator (who communicates directly with the hostage taker). It is vital that these two positions are not held by the same person.

Factors to consider:

- *Motivation* Although hostage situations can vary greatly, it is important to understand the general motives of the hostage taker(s). In all hostage situations the hostage taker will want to obtain something. The target of the hostage taker is usually not the hostage but a third party, so that the hostages are 'bargaining chips'. With regards to MDOs, the specific reasons for the hostage taking may be illogical, and/or the hostage taker may be suicidal
- *Planning and resources* The level of planning of a hostage situation may have important implications. For example, if there was significant planning involved, the hostage taker's behaviour is more likely to be predictable than in circumstances in which the incident occurred spontaneously. The resources the hostage-taker has made available to themselves may also provide insight into the degree of planning
- When negotiating with a hostage taker, both parties need to demonstrate a *willingness to discuss the issues*. The negotiator should not make offers that will not or cannot be followed through
- The *longer the negotiations last*, the more likely that the outcome will be peaceful.

'Stockholm syndrome'

The Hostage Identification syndrome (or 'Stockholm syndrome') refers to the tendency in hostage-taking and similar situations for the victim to develop a psychological bond with their captor. This is more likely if significant time has been spent with the hostage-taker. This can develop into hostility towards the authorities trying to rescue them.

Role of the psychiatrist in hostage negotiation

- In most circumstances the psychiatrist would not be the negotiator. This is usually the role of a trained police negotiator
- In some settings, the forensic psychiatrist might be used as a consultant to the hostage negotiating team
- If the hostage-taker is a known patient, a psychiatrist who knows them may also know the factors that might have contributed to the incident, or which may bring it to an end
- Even if the patient is not known to the psychiatrist attending, they might be able to contribute useful knowledge and understanding to any discussion and decision-making, including risk assessment.

The termination phase

The termination phase of a hostage incident is brief and can have three outcomes:

- The hostage takers surrender peacefully
- The hostage takers are captured, harmed, or killed
- The hostage takers' demands are granted and they escape (possibly to be apprehended later).

Post-incident support and advice

Following an incident hostages, witnesses, and potentially the perpetrator are likely to experience stress reactions. There will need to be a debriefing concerning the incident, and potential critical incident stress management planning.

Managing problematic sexual behaviour

Exactly what amounts to such behaviour is socially defined and contextual: for example, commenting approvingly on a person's sexual attractiveness might be problematic on a ward but acceptable at home amongst friends. In addition to legally-defined sexual offences, problematic sexual behaviour in psychiatric contexts often includes:

- Exposure (not necessarily of genitals)
- Inquiries about other people's sexual behaviour
- Requests for sexual activity
- Remarks on sexual desire or use of inappropriately sexualized language
- Comments on the appearance of other people
- Use of pornography
- Prostitution or use of prostitutes
- Development of inappropriate sexual relationships (e.g. between a patient and a staff member, or between a prisoner and a prison officer).

Special patient groups

- Disinhibition secondary to mania, psychosis or neurological disorder
- Convicted sex offenders with comorbid mental disorder
- Socially inappropriate behaviours associated with LD
- Hypersexuality in people with dementia.

Approach to management

Management should be based on an assessment (📖 p.II.134) and formulation (📖 p.II.110) of the risk of problematic sexual behaviours and of their motivation (📖 p.II.47). For example, offenders with 'avoidance goals' (who recognize offending is wrong but use inappropriate coping tactics in high-risk situations) require a different psychological approach to those with 'approach goals' (who deliberately set out to commit a sexual offence).

- Multidisciplinary (and often multi-agency) approach
- Identification of the problematic behaviours including related factors such as mental state, substance use, environment, and cognition
- Gather detailed background information (often from multiple agencies)
- Thorough analysis of the nature, frequency and circumstances of behaviours, e.g. with antecedents, behaviours, consequences (ABC) model
- Targeted intervention based on the formulation with measurement of the intervention's likely impact on nature, frequency and severity.

Interventions

Many of the interventions described here are only appropriate for convicted sex offenders.

Pharmacological

- Treatment for any underlying mental disorder
- Specific anti-libidinal medication (📖 p.II.161) may be helpful as an adjunct to psychological treatment if the person has high levels of sexual arousal, masturbation, and preoccupation with sexual fantasies, which is interfering with their daily life; likewise, SSRIs can assist treatment of offenders with paraphilias (📖 p.II.74).

Psychological treatment programmes (📖 p.II.176)

- The *risk, need, responsivity theory* for managing sex offenders, the principles of which are that treatment is matched to the offender's risk of reoffending, that criminogenic needs are identified and targeted and that interventions are tailored to the individual's strengths
- Relapse prevention models of managing sexual offending focus on identifying high-risk situations that could lead to reoffending and on identifying and eliminating dynamic risk factors. Relapse prevention models arise from risk, need, responsivity theories and have evolved to incorporate related areas such as cognitive distortions
- The Good Lives Model of sexual offending is a strengths-based approach. It relies on the assumption that human beings are goal-directed and motivated to seek primary goods. These can be states of mind, activities, and experiences, and increase well-being if achieved. The focus is on enabling the offender to lead a different kind of life (the 'new me'): achieving their goods without recourse to offending
- The Sex Offender Treatment Programme (SOTP) is delivered in prisons. This group cognitive behavioural programme is usually provided by prison staff and psychologists. It includes the core (medium risk offenders), adapted (low IQ/LD offenders), extended (high-risk offenders), better lives (pre-release based on Good Lives Model) and healthy sexual functioning programmes. The main aim of SOTP is to reduce rates of reoffending. These programmes are allocated based on risk assessment and whether offenders are serving a long enough sentence. Other treatment programmes are often completed in addition, such as Enhanced Thinking Skills (ETS)
- Probation services deliver programmes for sex offenders who receive short or community sentences. The iSOTP programme exists for internet offenders. These interventions have not been subject to such extensive evaluation (📖 p.II.184) as standard SOTP
- Hospital-based treatment groups for people with comorbid mental disorder or LD tend to be based on the SOTP interventions but are adapted for these groups
- Multisystemic therapy (MST, 📖 p.II.175) is being evaluated for young sexual offenders.

Other

- Legal sanctions (📖 p.IV.361) can be used to manage risk of sexual offending
- Local volunteer projects for supporting sex offenders in the community have developed since the 1990s. They focus on social isolation and loneliness as risk factors for reoffending. These projects also offer social support and reintegration with the goal of reducing reoffending

- Some probation services and psychiatrists have begun using *polygraph* ('lie detector') tests to enhance openness and compliance with risk management programmes, based on the premise that subjects believe most lies would be identified. The E&W Ministry of Justice is currently evaluating the effectiveness of this approach with offenders in the West Midlands; the 3-year trial is due to complete in 2012. Polygraphs are used more widely with sex offenders in North America.

Managing the risk of suicide & self-harm

General psychiatrists tend to possess particular expertise in managing the risk of suicide and self-harm, and may be consulted if necessary.[*] However, it is sufficiently common in forensic psychiatric services for forensic staff to need to be familiar with its management, both in isolation, and as part of the phenomenon of attempted suicide after homicide. Forensic psychiatrists may also be asked to advise on suicide in the context of deaths in custody (📖 p.V.471).

Working with patients who want to harm or kill themselves

- Treat the underlying mental disorder
- Include measures related to suicide/self-harm risk in the care plan
- Ensure ready access 24 hours a day in case of suicidal ideation (e.g. a crisis line, or staff on site)
- Offer psychological support as part of crisis resolution, such as short-term counselling or problem-solving counselling
- Consider admission to hospital if in the community, movement to an observation cell if in the police station, or transfer to the healthcare wing if in prison
- If the risk is acute, consider observation (📖 p.II.154) by appropriate staff.

Safety measures in hospital, prison and the community

- Minimize availability of means of suicide or self-harm so far as this is appropriate, and possible in the setting (e.g. design wards to obviate points from which a ligature could be suspended; remove sharp objects from areas to which the patient has access)
- Make use of special ligature-free cells or rooms where available
- Refer high-risk prisoners to the Listener scheme and/or request that they be placed on the ACCT (Assessment, Care in Custody and Treatment) system
- Observe medication being taken, to prevent stockpiling for overdose
- In secure units, search visitors, patients after leave, and rooms as necessary to prevent means of suicide or self-harm being acquired.

---

[*] Useful information may also be found in the *Oxford Handbook of Psychiatry*, or a general psychiatry textbook.

Dealing with suicide attempts and self-harm

- Take immediate life-saving measures as necessary—for example:
  - With colleagues, support the weight of someone who has hanged themselves, and cut them down
  - Remove ligatures from around the neck
  - Assess their airway, breathing and circulation, and resuscitate if necessary
  - Monitor pulse, temperature, BP, especially if their consciousness is impaired
  - Give oxygen if available, if there has been a period of asphyxia or significant blood loss
  - Consider activated charcoal after overdose; do not induce vomiting
  - Transfer to A&E for assessment unless this is clearly unnecessary
- Assess the situation rapidly and determine what has taken place (in particular, if an overdose is suspected, establish what has been taken and how much, including by asking the patient if conscious and/or searching the immediate area for bottles, packs, etc.)
- Transfer patients who have swallowed objects or inserted them into the anus, vagina, or other orifices to A&E for investigation and specialist removal, which may involve surgery
- If transferring to A&E, send a summary of diagnosis, current mental state, legal status, risks, and management plan with a suitable member of trained staff who should accompany the patient
- If not transferring to A&E, ensure frequent monitoring of the patient on the ward as appropriate (e.g. mental state, plus pulse, BP, temperature after overdose), and consider investigations as needed (e.g. urea & electrolytes, liver function tests, or specific drug levels after overdose)
- Only suture wounds or treat other injuries if you are confident that your skills are sufficiently good and up to date, a cosmetically sensitive area is not involved, and no deep structures (nerves, tendons, blood vessels) might be affected
- As with other incidents, consider a debriefing session for staff and other patients after the situation has been made safe—you and your colleagues and patients may have been affected emotionally by the incident. 🕮 p.II.195 for more details.

Absconding and escape

Managing the risk of absconding or escape* begins with a risk assessment for absconding or escape (🕮 p.II.140) that incorporates an individualized understanding of the patient. This should take account of the patient's general characteristics (e.g. young male patients with psychotic disorders are at particular risk of absconding), and of the features that may place them at higher risk at certain times (e.g. after conviction and the perception of a long period of detention; when the opportunity to escape or abscond arises, such as when attending court or a general hospital for medical treatment; or when experiencing persecutory delusions about staff).

*Escape involves a breach of physical security measures, such as climbing over a wall or cutting a hole in a fence, whereas absconding merely involves leaving the hospital without permission, and unauthorized leave failing to return on time.

The risk of absconding or escape does not refer to a harm in itself (other than potentially to the reputation or legal liability of the ward, service or individual clinician) but to the harms that might follow, either to the patient or to others. Hence, assessment of the risk of subsequent harm should contribute to the level of management of the risk of absconding or escape.

Risk management interventions

With respect to absconding, the key risk management intervention is the granting or withholding of leave (📖 p.ll.154) of one form or another, or setting the terms of that leave (such as the number of escorts, the duration, or the destination), whereas with respect to escape it is the use of an appropriate level of security (📖 p.ll.153) and of observations (📖 p.ll.154).

In deciding on how to act, in addition to the risk assessment described, the following tips can be of assistance. Risk management plans incorporating such measures were found to reduce absconding rates by 25% in one group of hospitals.

- Two studies of incidents of absconding have suggested that the peak time is early afternoon, around 3pm when the nursing shifts change. Avoiding scheduling leave for this time, and increased vigilance during handovers, may reduce the risk of absconding
- Similarly, the first few days and weeks after admission, after renewal of detention or receiving other bad news, or after transfer to another ward or unit are periods of increased risk of absconding or escape
- Periods of leave and their terms should be planned in advance (taking into account factors such as those already listed), and matched to the staff available on the day
- Every period of leave should be logged when planned, when the patient and escorts (if any) leave, and when they return
- A description of the patient and their clothing on the day, and any contraband items signed out to them (such as mobile phones) should be made before they leave
- Escorting staff should have a means of summoning assistance while out on leave, such as a two-way radio or mobile phone with relevant numbers pre-set
- Leave terms should be relaxed only gradually (e.g. increases in the duration of leave, or reductions in the number of escorts)
- Staff should have a method of contacting patients on unescorted leave, such as a mobile phone given to the patient for the period of leave
- Particularly during unescorted leave, staff on the ward should be actively aware of when the patient is due to return, and should have a predetermined protocol to follow if they do not return on time. The earlier absconding is detected, the greater the chance of locating the patient quickly
- Wards should have up-to-date photographs of the patient and information about next-of-kin and contact information of any known associates or locations they are likely to visit on leave.

After a patient has escaped or absconded

Without delay, the staff member detecting the incident should:

- Notify the police, giving them the description of the patient and their clothing, a brief risk assessment and information on their mental state, their legal status, the time and location where they were last known to be, and any other relevant information (such as addresses where they might have gone)
- Inform senior colleagues, who will:
  - Consider sending appropriately trained staff to a location where the patient is thought to be, if it is safe to do so
  - Consider informing potential victims
  - Make plans for managing the patient on their return (e.g. admitting them directly to a more secure ward, if appropriate)
  - Request a post-incident debriefing.

Managing other specific risks

With other risks, such as the risk of fire-setting or other non-violent forms of offending, the general principles of risk management (📖 p.II.190) apply, as they do with the risks considered in other topics in this chapter.

Fire-setting

When a patient is assessed as at significant risk of fire-setting (📖 p.II.38):

- A functional analysis of previous incidents of fire-setting should be undertaken in order to understand the motivation and risk factors, as well as any relationship there may be with mental disorder or concurrent mental state
- There should be regular room searches to ensure there are no materials in patients' rooms that could be used to set fires, e.g. newspaper, boxes, reports, etc. (the absence of matches or a lighter is not necessarily of relevance in that they might still be acquired, or a fire might be set utilizing an electric socket)
- Smoking and the use of lighters should be supervised.

Following an incident of fire-setting on a ward, depending on the severity and the damage, other patients may need to be moved and this is likely to increase distress and other risks, such as escape (📖 p.II.200). Both staff and patients will need to be debriefed.

In the community, programmes run by the Fire Service (such as 'FACE UP' in E&W) can help some patients to recognize the harmful consequences of their actions and to change their behaviour.

In general, psychological (especially group) work on self-esteem and assertiveness can reduce the risk of future fire-setting for many patients.

Exploitation or victimization

Where an incident of apparent abuse (physical, sexual, material, financial or emotional abuse, neglect, discrimination, or institutional mistreatment) indicates that a vulnerable adult, such as a psychiatric patient, is at risk of exploitation or victimization, the care team in E&W and Scotland have a duty to follow the so-called Safeguarding of Vulnerable Adults (SoVA) policy in force in their local area. Details vary from one area to another, but in essence the care team must report the potential for abuse of a vulnerable adult to the local SoVA team, usually based in the social services department of the local authority, and must cooperate with them in devising a multi-agency safeguarding plan.

In E&W and Scotland, there are also legal powers (📖 p.IV.440) to remove a vulnerable adult to a hospital or other place of safety, and in Scotland to ban people who may be endangering them from having contact with them.

Working with police & other agencies

Psychiatrists and other mental health professionals working in forensic settings will often need to work with the police and other non-health agencies as part of a risk management plan, particularly where the patient is in, or is planned to be in the community. This raises both technical and ethical issues and challenges (📖 p.III.258).

General principles

Whatever the legal or administrative structure, if any, under which you are working with other agencies, the same general principles apply:

- Remember that, although you may be cooperating on a specific issue, health services and other agencies (especially criminal justice agencies) explicitly adopt different goals (📖 p.IV.294), which may in practice conflict with those of a forensic health service. For example, when working with the probation service (📖 p.V.462) to prevent your patient reoffending, your aim will be to promote the patient's welfare, whereas the probation service's may be to protect the public from them, which might lead them to use more coercive methods
- The legal and ethical duties that apply to your normal clinical work continue to apply when working jointly with other agencies. Most notably, you continue to owe your patient a duty of confidentiality (📖 p.III.263), and you cannot disclose confidential information about them to partner agencies unless you have their consent, or one of the statutory or public interest exceptions (📖 p.III.263) applies
- The duty to cooperate with justice agencies does not alter the ethical and legal duties you owe to your patient, including in relation to confidentiality. Always remember that other agencies are not subject to the same duties as you, and may use your information or assistance for purposes that would amount to breaches of your duty to your patient. Always satisfy yourself as to what will be done with your information or assistance before acting
- In preparing documents for inter-agency working, always do so in the light of your duty of confidentiality to the patient; bear in mind that the basis for breach of confidence is not 'need to know' but 'significant risk of serious harm to the public' (the *Egdell* principle, 📖 pp.III.264, App. 3.635).

Multi-Agency Public Protection Arrangements (MAPPA)

These arrangements provide a mechanism for agencies in E&W, Scotland and NI to work together in the management of the risk of harm to others posed by certain offenders, including certain mentally disordered offenders. The arrangement, and the categories of offenders who are covered, are described on 📖 p.V.468.

However, joint working with other agencies with offenders not covered by MAPPA is still possible under informal or ad hoc cooperation arrangements, guided by the principles set out in 'General principles', 📖 p.II.203.

Multi-Agency Risk Assessment Conferences (MARAC)

In a fashion similar to the MAPPA, inter-agency working to protect vulnerable individuals, particularly victims of domestic violence, has now become commonplace, and most areas of the UK now have a standing Multi-Agency Risk Assessment Conference (MARAC) for discussing and co-ordinating agencies' safeguarding (📖 p.II.202) and other plans.

Forensic psychiatric services

History of forensic service development

The origins of what are now called forensic psychiatric services are found first in the provision of secure residential care for people with mental illnesses who committed serious offences; and second in concerns about the mental health of prisoners.

Madness has been seen to be associated with unpredictable violence since Roman times. However, until the 19th century, families were largely responsible for the care of their dangerous relatives. Long before the development of forensic psychiatry (🕮 p.I.11) as a subspecialty, special facilities were created to manage mentally disordered offenders. Chiefly because of the effects of the Criminal Lunatics Act 1800 (🕮 p.II.216), two new wings of Bethlem Hospital were opened in 1816 to accommodate high-risk patients who needed long-term supervision in a secure setting. In 1853, Broadmoor Hospital (🕮 p.II.209) was built to accommodate over-crowding in the Bethlem units, 3 years after the Central Mental Hospital in Ireland, which took offenders as well as other patients.

People with mental illness who offend

In Victorian times, mental healthcare focused on 'asylum', in the sense of indefinite residential detention, safe from the rest of society. It was envisaged that all patients would live in the hospitals for the rest of their lives; thus many of the early residents of Broadmoor would not now be seen as needing high secure care. The concept of different levels of security need arose in the wake of the closure of the asylums, and increasing understanding of mental disorders as treatable.

Two further high secure hospitals in England were opened in the 20th century, along with the State Hospital in Scotland. The development of Regional Secure Units (RSUs, 🕮 p.II.210) in the UK was recommended by the Butler inquiry (🕮 p.App. 5.654) in 1974; it and other contemporaneous reports also recommended increased provision for prisoners with mental health needs, court diversion, women patients, offender patients from different ethnic backgrounds, and offenders with personality disorders.

Mental health needs of prisoners

Professional concerns about the risk posed by the mentally disordered proceeded in parallel with public health concerns about the mental well-being of prisoners. Prisoners who became mentally ill in prison needed to be transferred to forensic services that could be secure enough to prevent most escapes. In part, the development of improved mental health services was driven by the results of epidemiological studies that showed very high levels of mental illness and personality disorder in prisons, most notably the ONS studies (🕮 p.App. 5.655).

Mentally disordered men and women in hospitals who posed a risk to others were managed exclusively by general psychiatrists until the subspecialty of forensic psychiatry emerged in the 1970. Thereafter, forensic psychiatrists took over the management of higher-risk patients, while leaving general psychiatrists to care for a large number of patients who still posed a significant risk of harm to others.

Current services

Services for forensic patients in the UK and Ireland are now divided into prison services, community services and residential secure services (see ☐ p.II.209). Prison services (☐ p.II.217) are provided by NHS/HSE in-reach teams, who are able to liaise with other health services to facilitate care. There are still concerns about lack of access to secure beds and delays in transfer. Community services may be provided by general psychiatric services and/or community forensic teams (☐ p.II.214). These services typically liaise closely with probation and substance misuse services.

An important development has been the diversion (☐ p.II.216) of mentally disordered people who have offended away from the prison system; and into mental health. However, there are concerns about the lack of access to inpatient care; and the stigma that offender patients still face.

People with mental disorders who pose an ongoing significant risk of violence are usually managed in prison or long-term secure care. Patients with high and medium security needs tend to be managed by specialist forensic psychiatric services, where the professional staff have particular experience and training. Patients with lower security needs, and who require rehabilitation into the community may be managed by community forensic teams; but also by general psychiatric services.

There has been a marked contraction of the numbers of high secure beds since the RSUs opened (though this is not the case in RoI, where all medium and high secure services remain at the Central Mental Hospital). They now mainly serve patients who are grossly behaviourally disturbed, and/or whose offences are so severe as to warrant long-term detention.

There has been a huge expansion in the number of medium secure beds in the NHS; and also in the independent sector, accommodating those service needs that cannot be met by the NHS. Several of these units offer specialist rehabilitation for special groups of forensic patients (☐ p.II.211), such as sex offenders, young people, and female offenders, and those with learning disability or autistic spectrum disorders.

Conclusion

The development of services for people who commit crimes while mentally disordered has often occurred in response to high-profile disasters, and associated public anxiety about the risk of violence that those with mental disorders may pose—rather than rational needs assessment (☐ p.II.222). However, most people with mental disorder do not commit violent crimes (see ☐ p.II.31); and most prisoners who need mental health services are serving sentences for non-violent offences.

A good example of how service development can be driven by publicity, rather than evidence-based policy, is the development of the former DSPD services (☐ p.II.211) in E&W. Over £140 million was spent developing services for the needs of 2,000 men who were thought to be at especially high risk of violence. The programme has been alleged to have been inefficient, and much less effective at risk reduction than community substance misuse and rehabilitation programmes; much of the hospital programme appears likely to be scrapped in the current review.

The structure of forensic services

Forensic psychiatric services in the UK and Ireland fall largely into two groups. First, those services that provide 'inreach' into parts of the Criminal Justice System (CJS), which may either be specialist forensic or general services. Second, specialist forensic secure versions of general psychiatric services.

Inreach into the CJS

The CJS, as described in more detail on p.V.448, comprises the main institutions shown in Box 8.1. Each has its own forensic psychiatric service, although the exact nature of those services varies between (and within) jurisdictions. In some areas, these 'forensic' services will be provided by general psychiatrists and general psychiatric teams.

> ### Box 8.1 CJS institutions and their forensic psychiatric services
>
> - Police stations: Police liaison CPNs (p.II.216)
> - Courts: Court diversion teams (p.II.217)
> - Prisons & YOIs: Prison inreach & inpatient service (p.II.217).

A further key component of the CJS is the Probation Service (p.V.462). Probation services often run behavioural group programmes for offenders; some forensic psychiatric services offer similar groups, particularly psychology-led behavioural programmes for sex offenders, and these may be organized jointly with the probation service and/or accept referrals from it.

Secure psychiatric services

General psychiatric services comprise the following main components:
- Hospital wards, including psychiatric intensive care units (PICUs)
- Outpatient clinics
- Community services (e.g. CMHTs).

Each has its forensic equivalent: secure hospital wards and secure ICUs, described on pp.II.209–II.213; forensic outpatient psychiatry and psychology clinics; and Community Forensic Teams (p.II.214).

Pathways of care that allow patients to move between different forensic services, and between general and forensic services, are both essential and a frequent source of intra-professional conflict. Common issues are described on p.II.220.

Parallel or integrated services?

After regional forensic and local secure services were first recommended in the Glancy and Butler reports (p.App. 5.654) in 1974, a prolonged debate ensued as to whether (or to what extent) forensic and general services should be integrated with each other, or operate in parallel.

This referred in practice to questions such as:
- Should it be possible for patients in high security (p.II.209) to be discharged directly to general services, or should they spend the last part of their secure admission in a medium secure unit (p.II.210)?

- Should general inpatient wards expect to receive patients from forensic services before discharge, or should forensic services manage them until they are ready for discharge to the community?
- Should forensic inpatient services discharge their patients to the care of general community teams, or should Community Forensic Teams (📖 p.II.214) be established?
- Should low secure wards be within general services, forensic services, or both?
- Should forensic services cater for all patients who pose a sufficient risk of harm to others (including those with personality disorder), or only those with psychosis?

Different services in different places have answered these questions in different ways. In some parts of E&W in particular, forensic services span the whole spectrum, including community teams; in Scotland and RoI, by contrast, forensic services are largely confined to central secure hospitals. In recent years, there has been a tendency for forensic services to expand; it remains to be seen how the current round of financial cuts in most areas will affect this trend. However, this has not created a fully parallel model: instead, a partially parallel model has evolved in many areas,[*] in which patients can move between forensic and general services at lower security levels, depending on their needs and the risks of harm they pose.

Secure hospital settings

A secure hospital or unit, whether part of a forensic or general service (see 📖 p.II.208), is one with the capacity to detain patients who pose a significant risk of harm to others, restrict their movement and activities, and prevent escape. Security level (📖 p.II.153) is a function of physical architecture, procedures and relational factors such as numbers of staff; and is defined in some cases by government specifications. There are three main levels of security offered: low, medium, and high.

In 2006, there were 1496 admissions to forensic secure hospital wards in E&W, including those in the independent sector: far lower than the number of admissions to general psychiatric wards. There were 4500 forensic secure beds, compared with over 31,000 general psychiatric beds. The duration of admission to forensic secure beds was considerably longer than general admissions: the mean duration of stay (averaged across all levels of security) was 5 years. Over 25% of patients in forensic secure settings were detained for 10 years or more.

High-security hospitals (Special Hospitals)

In E&W, Broadmoor, Ashworth, and Rampton Hospitals provide high secure care. There were in 2007 approximately 800 high secure beds in E&W, all in the NHS, predominantly housing male patients who have committed (or were at very high risk of committing) acts of severe violence to others. These include services for women and people with learning disability or deafness who need high secure care at Rampton Hospital.

[*] This is the case in the NHS and HSE. However, many psychiatric units in the independent sector tend to blur the distinction between forensic and general services and patients.

The State Hospital at Carstairs covers Scotland and NI, and provides approximately 140 high secure beds with special services for people with learning disability, in addition to a number of medium secure beds. The Central Mental Hospital at Dundrum, Dublin offers 105 beds at all levels of security, including high security.

The key criterion for high secure care is posing a *grave and immediate* risk of serious harm to the public (including healthcare professionals). In practice, the high secure services take mentally ill prisoners whose level of risk of serious harm to others is assessed as high; and patients from medium secure services who are too high risk in that context to be managed safely there.

Medium security (Regional Secure Units)

The majority of forensic mental healthcare is provided in medium secure units. There are clear guidelines for the quality of medium secure units in seven domains, issued by bodies including the E&W Department of Health, and the Royal College of Psychiatrists' Quality Network. These address:

- Safety and security
- Clinical and cost effectiveness
- Governance
- Patient focus
- Accessibility and responsiveness of care
- Care environment and amenities
- Public health.

In 2007, there were approximately 3600 medium secure beds in total across the UK & Ireland, with approximately 35% provided in the independent sector.

There are no widely accepted criteria for medium secure care, partly because medium secure services in different areas take different patient groups, depending on the capabilities of their local high and low secure services. The E&W DoH has described medium secure units as catering for 'high-risk' mentally disordered offenders, and set out many standards that medium secure units in E&W must attain. In practice, patients may be admitted from prisons; from low secure services or general adult services and from high secure settings. Medium secure services have an important role in the long-term rehabilitation of patients who have spent long periods of time in high security.

Women's Enhanced Medium Secure Services (WEMSS)

WEMSS aims to replace physical security with enhanced procedural and relational security measures to the maximum extent possible. There are 46 beds in three WEMSS units across E&W, in London, Manchester, and Leicester. They were developed in response to two observations:

- Many women in high secure hospitals had not committed offences that would warrant detention in high security, but
- Their behaviour was too disruptive to the environment of standard women's medium secure wards for them to be transferred there.

Low security

Services that amount to more than a general psychiatric ward with a locked door, but that do not meet the specifications for medium security, are loosely described as 'low secure', or sometimes 'minimum secure'. A survey in 2006 found 1583 beds in 137 low secure wards across the UK, roughly the same as the number of general PICU beds (1242 beds in 170 wards), but this may be a significant underestimate.

Low secure wards may provide step-down care from high or medium security; longer-term care for the most chronically disturbed patients in general services; and care for lower-risk patients transferred from prison. They may also provide 'readmission capacity' for patients in specialist community forensic care, where medium (or high) security may not be necessary; some low secure units have a higher turnover of patients than medium secure units, therefore making urgent readmission more feasible in practice. Many low secure wards are indistinguishable from locked rehabilitation wards, and indeed some rehabilitation wards now describe themselves as 'low secure' despite being outside forensic services.

Special provision in secure settings

Personality disorder and DSPD

The Dangerous and Severe Personality Disorder (DSPD) programme was launched in E&W in 2001 to provide services specifically for people who present a high risk of committing serious sexual and/or violent offences as a result of severe personality disorder, defined as having diagnoses of two or more PDs, plus a high score on the PCL-R (📖 p.II.102). The capacity has been shared between two high secure hospitals, Broadmoor and Rampton, and two category A (📖 p.V.456) prisons, HMP Frankland and HMP Whitemoor, with each unit having 70–80 beds. At the time of writing, the future of the DPSD programme is in question, and Broadmoor Hospital has redesignated its former DSPD unit as a Severe Personality Disorder unit; it seems likely that only the prison units will be retained.

There is no equivalent to the DSPD system in Scotland, NI or RoI, although the TBS system in the Netherlands and the Sexually Violent Predator services (📖 p.III.280) in California and some other US states offer relevant comparisons.

Women's services

Women comprise one in eight of the UK forensic psychiatric population, twice their proportion of the prison population.

For Scotland and NI, secure psychiatric wards for women at all levels of security are provided at the State Hospital, Carstairs in addition to medium secure facilities for NI at the Shannon Clinic; for RoI, the Central Mental Hospital provides secure care for women.

The Women's Enhanced Medium Secure Services (WEMSS, 📖 p.II.210) in E&W were developed specifically for women thought to require enhanced levels of intervention and treatment in medium security and for whom most medium secure units were not adequate. The Primrose DSPD Unit at HMP Low Newton was set up alongside the DSPD programme for men, to deliver more effective interventions for severely disordered female prisoners.[*]

Learning disability services

Specialist forensic LD services cater for individuals with significant impairment of intellectual functioning (evidenced by assessment using a standardized measure of intellectual functioning), significant impairment in adaptive functioning, onset of impairment in both of these in the developmental period, and possible additional mental disorders. There are both medium secure and high secure hospital facilities for this population across the UK and at the Central Mental Hospital in RoI, but there is a lack of community services. There is also little provision for those in the borderline range of intellectual functioning who have deficits in social skills; this group tends to be overlooked by general and forensic psychiatric services. If an individual is not deemed suitable for healthcare disposal, then a sentence in prison may result, raising concerns.

Autistic spectrum disorders (ASDs)

Offenders with ASDs often find themselves in generic forensic secure settings, or LD settings if they are low functioning, given the lack of provision for specialist services in this area. This often presents major problems, especially for generic forensic services, because their staff usually lack the necessary skills for treating such patients and because ASD patients do not usually sit easily alongside other forensic patients within the community of a ward. This problem is exacerbated by a tendency to sentence individuals with ASDs under mental health law, as opposed to giving prison sentences. However, there are a few independent sector providers in E&W that cater specifically for patients with ASDs.

Brain injury services

As with individuals with LD and ASDs, individuals with brain injury are often treated in mainstream forensic services or non-forensic Acquired Brain Injury (ABI) units. There are a limited number of forensic specialist services for people with complex physical, cognitive, and functional difficulties that typically follow brain injury, who are demonstrating socially inappropriate behaviour and need medium or low security. Those that exist at the time of writing are in the independent sector, in E&W.

Deaf services

Deaf and hard-of-hearing patients suffer a greater lifetime prevalence of mental disorder (40% as against 25% by one estimate), but can struggle in mainstream psychiatric services, because of the oral nature of many therapies, and because the vast majority of staff are unable to communicate using sign language, and lack awareness of aspects of deaf psychology

---

[*] Like the DSPD programme for men, the Primrose Unit is under evaluation and may not continue in its present form. Similarly, the WEMSS service will be evaluated for effectiveness at some point in the future; some in the field have claimed that its benefits over ordinary women's medium secure wards, if any, do not justify its additional costs.

and culture. Three specialist general psychiatric services for deaf patients cover the UK between them. In addition, at least three independent sector hospitals provide specialist secure units for deaf people.

Adolescent forensic services

In E&W, which has extensive (and controversial) facilities for the detention of children (📖 p.V.458), a small number of specialist secure psychiatric units have been developed for adolescents. These aim to divert some adolescent mentally disordered offenders from custody. They often face difficulty in transferring patients to appropriate facilities, particularly community facilities, when they reach 18 years of age.

Scotland, NI, and RoI have no secure inpatient units specifically for adolescents, who must therefore be treated in general psychiatric units.

Rehabilitation & recovery in secure services

The Rehabilitation and Recovery Model

The rehabilitation and recovery model is an approach to treatment which argues that individuals with mental illness can be rehabilitated back into society and make a recovery that does not necessarily require the complete relief of symptoms, but which recognizes the person's individuality and personal aspirations. The recovery model emphasizes treating the person as a whole, and as an individual, not as 'a diagnosis' or 'an offence'. Just as people can live with physical disabilities and have a good quality of life, so too can many people with mental health problems.

This model emerged in E&W as deinstitutionalization resulted in more individuals, many with quite severe continuing symptoms, living in the community. Interest in the model grew because traditionally informed services were perceived to be both exclusive and stigmatizing of psychiatric service users.

Core principles of the model:

Some of the principles of the recovery model can be in tension or conflict with the elements of coercion (📖 p.II.149) common to much forensic treatment; this can lead to compromise of some of its core principles, which are:
- Recovery is the ultimate goal of rehabilitation and all interventions must aid this process
- Patients should be helped to re-establish normal community roles and reintegrate into life in the community
- Personal support networks should be developed
- Quality of life should be enhanced by attention to the individual's personal goals and values
- All individuals have the capacity to learn and grow
- Individuals accessing services have the right to direct their own affairs, including those that are related to their mental illness
- All individuals should be treated with respect and dignity

- There should be a consistent effort to avoid using diagnoses to label and discriminate against service users
- Culture and ethnicity play an important role in recovery as sources of strength and enrichment for the individual and services
- Interventions should be person-centred; and strength and resilience focused
- Interventions should actively encourage and support the involvement of the individual in normal community activities, such as school and work, throughout the rehabilitation process.[*]

Barriers to implementation of the model

- The belief that medications are the only effective treatment to mental illness
- Not enough trained staff to treat patients through psychosocial Rehabilitation and Recovery
- In forensic settings, patients' liberties and many rights have been removed and there may be legal restrictions that prevent re-integration into the community
- Courts may impose mandatory requirements on the individual to receive treatment or complete intervention programmes, thus removing the ability of the individual to make their own decisions and choices
- Risk assessment and risk management may lead to interventions that increase social exclusion.

Community forensic services

Historically, forensic psychiatry was an almost exclusively institutionally-focused subspecialty, originating in the prisons and the high secure (special) hospitals and later extending to a network of medium and low secure units established around the country. The prevailing model was that patients were detained in hospital until their risk to themselves and others was deemed to be sufficiently low for them to be discharged to general psychiatric services in the community. Small numbers of patients discharged from medium and low secure units to the community were kept on as outpatients by their inpatient forensic consultants, but these were seen as the exception rather than the rule. Some services avoided providing community follow up entirely.

However, the greater resources given to forensic services from the early 1990s (driven by political and public concern over the risks to the public thought to be posed by mentally disordered patients) allowed for some experimentation in service models, and forensic services began to develop explicit and more substantial community forensic services.

Advantages & disadvantages of community forensic teams

Specialized services allow staff to develop more specialized skills, and confidence in working with high-risk patients and with the criminal justice system.

---

[*] This may be particularly difficult to achieve with some forensic patients in that risk management may conflict with this objective, and stigma may make reintegration more difficult.

Such services may promote their staff obtaining expertise in techniques such as motivational interviewing and cognitive-analytic therapy, which would not be cost-effective for generic staff. Moreover, having earmarked budgets for such services can permit staff to maintain the small caseloads necessary for intensive work with certain mentally disordered offenders. In summary, there is advantage in concentrating the care of high-risk patients within a specialist community forensic team (CFT).

However, a parallel system of services for often-unpopular patients can encourage stigmatization of those patients, allow general staff to feel relieved of responsibility for them, and can lead to pressure for all similar unpopular patients to be referred to, and accepted by, that service. Moreover, the recruitment of knowledgeable and highly-motivated staff to a specialist service can result in the 'de-skilling' of general services.

Whether the advantages outweigh the disadvantages can depend on the threshold for accepting patents into the CFT in a local area, and the degree to which the CFT offers consultation, support and joint working to other local community teams.

Community forensic service models
- The *integrated model:* staff with special training in forensic psychiatry work within general community mental health teams (CMHTs) or assertive outreach teams (AOTs).
- The *parallel model:* specialist community forensic teams (CFTs) exist separately from CMHTs and AOTs.
- An *intermediate* between these two models, such as one in which specialist forensic psychiatric staff have their own team base but are managed jointly with CMHT staff.
- The *outreach model:* inpatient staff working at the regional secure unit (RSU) provide community psychiatric services to their discharged forensic psychiatric patients, maximizing continuity of care at the expense of having enough community patients per team to develop into a full CFT.

A survey in 2007 found that there were around 40 CFTs in E&W. The majority operated a parallel model and all services offered risk assessment and management; around half also offered anger management and CBT. Very few offered treatment for personality disorder, substance abuse, or sex offending.

How is a CFT different to an assertive outreach team?
The intention of AOTs is to work intensively with a small number of patients, with the aim of improving their compliance with treatment and their motivation to participate to the extent that they can be returned to a CMHT within a reasonably short time. In this respect, they are the community equivalent of a psychiatric intensive care unit (ICU). Like ICUs, AOTs focus on patients with mental illness and substance misuse, and dislike being 'clogged up' with patients with personality disorder whom they perceive as unlikely to change. In contrast, community forensic teams:
- Expect to treat patients with personality disorder (☐ p.II.58), comorbid substance misuse and challenging behaviours (☐ p.II.193), and to have the expertise to deal with them effectively

- Expect treatment to last much longer, and a minority of patients to remain in their care indefinitely, sometimes for regular contact and review of risk and mental state even after all options for treatment have been exhausted, and
- Expect to deal regularly with other agencies such as probation services (📖 p.V.462), prisons (📖 p.V.456), and the police (📖 p.V.449), and to take part in the multi-agency public protection arrangements (MAPPA, 📖 p.V.468); and are skilled in negotiating the issues of consent (📖 p.III.284), confidentiality and disclosure (📖 p.III.263) involved in doing so.

Diversion services

It has been possible for mentally disordered defendants before the criminal courts[*] in the UK and Ireland to be 'diverted' from the usual process of trial and punishment since time immemorial. Until the passing of the Criminal Lunatics Act 1800,[†] arrangements were haphazard, and defendants acquitted because they were found insane (📖 p.V.489) might be committed to hospital or asylum, or cared for by their families, or left to their own devices. The Act required defendants found insane to be detained by the court 'until his Majesty's pleasure be known', and in practice resulted in their indefinite committal to Bethlem Royal Hospital and, later, Broadmoor Hospital (📖 p.II.209).

The principle of diversion having been established in statute and government circulars, the diversionary options available to courts (and the police) have steadily grown, and now include those listed here. These now include options for diverting patients without discontinuing legal proceedings.

Pre-court diversion

On arrest, the police may take an apparently mentally disordered person to hospital or another approved place for assessment (📖 p.IV.400).

At the police station, the police (or a doctor or Forensic Medical Examiner) may request a mental health assessment. If admission is recommended, the custody sergeant[‡] may release the person, after which they may be admitted either voluntarily or under section (📖 p.IV.383), in which case there will be no criminal prosecution. Alternatively, they may bail (📖 p.IV.330) them to hospital, whether or not they have also been sectioned, in which case the person may be charged and prosecuted at a later date.

The *prosecutor* (📖 p.IV.448) has discretion to drop charges at any stage of the process, and may do so in order to allow a person to be admitted to hospital.

---

[*] Those before the civil courts might sometimes be protected from being sued (for breach of contract, for example), or be held incapable of suing others (in which case the Official Solicitor may be able to act on their behalf, see 📖 p.IV.438), but there is no diversion into a separate psychiatric system by the court.
[†] The Act was introduced 4 days after the trial of James Hadfield, who had attempted to kill George III but who was acquitted by reason of insanity. The authorities were worried that he might try again to kill the King and passed the Act to ensure his detention despite his acquittal.
[‡] In Ireland, the member of the Garda Síochána in charge of the police station.

Diversion from court

Before or during trial, a court can remand (💷 p.IV.330) a defendant to hospital for assessment (💷 p.IV.403) or treatment (💷 p.IV.405), and may suspend the legal proceedings until the assessment is complete. If the assessed mental disorder renders the defendant unfit to plead or stand trial (💷 p.V.474), they may be admitted to hospital, released, or supervised in the community, and the prosecution may be discontinued, or suspended until they become fit to plead.

Upon conviction, a court may also remand the defendant to hospital for psychiatric assessment and compilation of a pre-sentence report (💷 p.V.462). It can also, in many circumstances, sentence (💷 p.IV.405) the defendant to detention in hospital instead of punishing them (or in addition to punishing them, in the case of hospital directions and hybrid orders, 💷 p.IV.408).

Diversion from prison

If prison staff believe that a prisoner is mentally disordered and requires treatment in hospital, they can request transfer to hospital (💷 p.IV.410). Different rules apply depending on whether the transfer is before or after sentence.

Court diversion psychiatric teams

Since 1989, when the first pilot schemes were established, many criminal courts across the UK and Ireland have had access to specialist psychiatric teams that can perform brief psychiatric assessments on the spot, and arrange admission to hospital on behalf of the court, subject to the court's agreement. Some of the courts that do not have a diversion team can 'cross-remand' defendants to another local court that does.

One Home Office review showed that psychiatric diversion teams can quadruple the rate of detected mental disorder, and reduce the time from arrest to admission by a factor of seven.

There are no generally accepted standards for the composition and functioning of such teams; and, depending on local resources, they vary from a lone CPN giving oral advice to magistrates, to multidisciplinary teams that can produce instant, authoritative written psychiatric reports and arrange admissions to acute and secure units without delay. Teams with efficient full-time administrators as well as clinicians with good relationships with local services have been shown to be far more effective than those without.

A related development is the attachment of specialist liaison CPNs to larger police stations, where they can conduct initial psychiatric assessments and advise police officers and FMEs (💷 p.V.452) on diversion.

Prison psychiatric services

The prevalence of mental illness, personality disorder, substance use, and suicidal or self-harming behaviour are all high in prison settings (💷 p.V.456), and much higher than the general population (e.g. the rates for psychosis are 7–14% in prison as against 0.4% in the general population, 💷 p.II.54).

In the UK,[*] the NHS took over responsibility for providing healthcare in prisons in 2000, with the aim that prisoners would have access to services of an equivalent standard to those in the community. This has helped the development of common standards of care, and continuity of care planning when patients are detained or released, though most accept that services are not yet equivalent.

Prison medical services in both the UK and Ireland aim to identify mental disorder in prisoners as early as possible, and to offer treatment in the prison where possible, and transfer to hospital where necessary.

Reception screening

On arrival into custody, new prisoners are, in most prisons, interviewed briefly using a standardized instrument, to identify any obvious mental health needs. The focus at this stage is on the risk of suicide and self-harm, and on giving prisoners the opportunity to tell staff about conditions they may have and medication they may have been prescribed.

First night centre and induction wing

The first week in custody is an especially high-risk period for suicide. The first night centre and induction wing are two initiatives designed to make the experience less stressful for new inmates. However, they are not provided in all prisons.

Primary care services

The provision of primary care services varies greatly from one institution to the next, with some provided by directly-employed prison GPs (often locums), and others by local general practices. Prison psychiatric nurses provide a significant amount of primary care through wing-based triage, clinics and crisis intervention. It is often difficult to maintain continuity of care between prison and the community, particularly as 50% of prisoners were not registered with a GP before going to prison.

Secondary care services

87% of prisons had a psychiatric in-reach team in one survey. Of those that did not, most were lower security prisons that only take inmates who have previously been screened in prisons with such services (in theory, though sometimes prisoners are transferred without adequate medical consultation). Prison mental health in-reach teams are usually designed to resemble CMHTs. Prisoners receive an assessment, including care-planning, an allocated CPN or care coordinator, and treatment. In-reach services were originally designed to focus on severe and enduring mental illness; however, teams are often overwhelmed with referrals for a much wider range of mental health problems.

---

[*] In Ireland, health care in prisons is provided by the Irish Prison Service, which contracts doctors and dentists to provide primary care on a part-time basis; agreements exist for referral to psychiatric services provided by the HSE.

Drug treatment services

A large proportion of prisoners have serious substance misuse problems. Many prisons now offer a methadone maintenance programme. As with community services, prison drug treatment services need users to be motivated to change, whereas prison mental health services assertively encourage treatment even in unmotivated patients, and these different models make it difficult for teams to work jointly with the same patients. Clinical drug treatment services are supplemented by non-clinical counselling services, known in prisons in E&W as CARATS.[*]

Prison inpatient services

98% of prisons in E&W have some inpatient healthcare facilities but less than half of these have psychiatric beds. There is approximately one bed for every 53 inmates on average. The prison inpatient healthcare services provide multidisciplinary input to prisoners with more severe mental health problems. Not all require hospital transfer: some recover within prison.

Compulsory treatment in prison

Prison healthcare units do not count as hospitals in the UK,[†] and inpatient treatment cannot be enforced there under mental health legislation. However, in law compulsory treatment can be given to incompetent patients under mental capacity legislation (☐ p.IV.424), and in emergency situations a common law power (☐ p.IV.440) can be used to treat prisoners in order to prevent significant harm occurring—although there are major practical obstacles to using such powers in prisons, which means that in all but the most severe emergencies, patients refusing treatment remain untreated until transferred to hospital.

Transfer to hospital

For the most seriously ill prisoners, the prison setting is inappropriate and prisoners are transferred to hospital (☐ p.IV.410) for treatment. In law, any person who could have been admitted compulsorily from the community can be transferred to hospital, but in practice the threshold is much higher because of the limited number of available secure beds.

---

[*] Counselling, Assessment, Referral, Advice and Throughcare Services.
[†] The Irish MHA does not appear to rule out designating prison healthcare units as 'approved centres' under the Act, but no prison units have been so designated by the Mental Health Commission.

Relationships between services

Although often conceived of as separate systems, patients often need to move within forensic services and between forensic and general psychiatric services, or between hospital and prison services. This includes transfer in the following situations:

- When the risk of harm to others posed by a forensic service patient has declined (e.g. through treatment) and they can safely be managed in lower levels of security or an open rehabilitation environment
- When a forensic service patient has been discharged to the community, and either there is no local CFT (📖 p.II.214), or they have been managed by the CFT for a period of time and their risk of harm to others is now deemed acceptably low
- When a prisoner cared for by a prison inreach team (📖 p.II.218) is released from prison and requires aftercare (📖 p.IV.398) in the community
- When a prisoner cared for in a prison healthcare centre (📖 p.II.219) requires transfer to a psychiatric hospital*
- When a general service patient is convicted of an offence and ordered to a secure hospital by a court, or diverted (📖 p.II.216) into a secure hospital, or
- When a general service patient's behaviour cannot be safely managed on a general psychiatric ward or PICU, and they require care in a secure environment (📖 p.II.152).

Given the frequency with which patients need to move between services in this way, it is unfortunate that a variety of historical, commissioning and other factors often combine to produce misunderstanding and discord between forensic and general services, with each raising obstacles to the transfer of the other's patients. It is therefore worth the while of clinicians in all types of service to:

- Make personal contact with clinicians in other services wherever possible, ideally before needing to discuss potentially contentious cases, so as to build trusting relationships
- Discuss and agree policies and protocols for common scenarios, such as those described here, setting out the mechanisms for assessment, transfer and return of patients, and for joint working where appropriate
- Discuss disagreements with colleagues and managers at an early stage to ensure that opinions are reasonable and well-grounded, and be ready to consider changing one's opinion if it is unsupported by others
- Have rapid access to mutually agreeable dispute-resolution mechanisms, such as 'pathways' meetings (at which representatives of various services meet to discuss patient placements and transfers) or binding arbitration procedures.

---

*Although the commissioning of prison healthcare services in the UK by the NHS has improved transfer processes considerably, in many areas (especially in E&W, and most egregiously in London), there are major disjunctions and delays, which have led in a few cases to adverse outcomes in prison and subsequent negligence proceedings (📖 p.V.516) involving the hospital concerned.

Future service development

All health and social care services change over time, in response to a multitude of factors including political priorities (nationally and at the local managerial level), varying political philosophies, the state of the economy and available financial resources,[*] the availability of resources such as suitably trained staff, and the needs of the local population. Forensic psychiatric services are no exception. Senior clinicians, especially those with explicit management responsibilities, will periodically be involved in service development.

Needs assessment

Rational planning of future services must include an assessment of the needs of the population being served—e.g. MDOs in a specific geographical area. However, although needs assessment (□ p.II.222) may attempt to be objective, it is dependent upon the values underlying both the method of assessment adopted and assumptions made.

Service evaluation

Assuming that what is planned is not an entirely new service where none currently exists, an equally important step is to evaluate the existing service, including what works well and how it may be failing. The evaluation should use valid outcome measures (see □ 'Outcome measures', p.II.221) and consider the following domains:

- Inputs such as the service's human and financial resources, its capacity, its structure, its protocols, its information systems, and relevant constraints such as government policy
- Processes such as specific clinical interventions and their frequency and duration, the relationships between clinicians and patients, the movement between service tiers, the service's pathways, waiting lists and bottlenecks, the continuity of care, and efficiency
- Outcomes, such as reduced reoffending (not a health outcome, but often considered by service commissioners), reduced patient symptoms and distress, and increased social (re)integration

Outcome measures

For the purposes of service evaluation and development, outcome measures must examine outcomes at the population level, not the level of the individual patient. They should ideally:

---

[*] This is an especially acute concern at the time of writing in the UK and RoI, and has led to an increase in debate about the most appropriate and most cost-effective service structures. Although financial pressures pose major problems for psychiatric as for other health services, debate about more efficient service provision often stimulates innovation (the closure of the asylums and development of 'community care' is a notorious example). A particular debate at the time of writing concerns prison psychiatric services (□ p.II.217): with the vast majority of severe or enduring mental disorder being treated in the general community, is it still appropriate for the main response to severe or enduring mental disorder in prisoners to be transfer to an inpatient psychiatric unit instead of treatment within the prison community? Another cost-driven innovation in the NHS in England is the current introduction of service-line accounting and payment by results, which appears likely to lead to major recasting of hospital and community services, once the new approaches expose the actual costs and efficiency of each individual service.

- Be multidimensional (e.g. combining clinical, social/rehabilitation, humanitarian and public safety variables)
- Examine multiple perspectives (e.g. patient, carer, society), including the value of the outcome from each of those perspectives (e.g. reduced distress may be more valuable to the patient and carer than to other members of society who do not know them personally)
- Collect data longitudinally (i.e. over time) as well as cross-sectionally
- Be standardized and published, to allow peer review and replication
- Take costs into account, within a model of cost effectiveness

Existing outcome measures—used, for example, when evaluating treatment (📖 p.II.184), rarely live up to these demanding criteria.

Needs assessment

Need implies and requires the ability to benefit. Needs assessment can be 'individual', being clinically based, or population based, as part of service planning (📖 p.II.221). Most service design in the last 20 years in the UK has been based, usually explicitly, upon a rational approach of 'needs assessment'. Needs assessment may appear objective, but is heavily value-laden.

Population needs assessment should involve:

- A clear definition of the population assessed, with determination of the level of need required to infer 'forensic caseness', in both qualitative and quantitative terms (e.g. does a mentally disordered offender have to have had a conviction to be defined as such? At what level of offending do they cross the threshold of forensic caseness?)
- A clear decision as to whether the definition of forensic caseness is based upon data relating to the patient alone or upon which service will properly respond to his need (forensic or generic service)
- A clear definition of 'need' (e.g. is the need for health, social care, or other well-being, or for reduced offending? Should unmet needs, where there is currently no evidence based intervention, be included?)
- An agreement on whose need is to be responded to: that of the patient or society, or some balance between the two?
- A rigorous, transparent method of measuring incidence and prevalence (📖 p.II.18) of need.

Methods of population needs assessment

Needs assessment can never be definitive and must rely upon a variety of sources of data, with judgement taken by viewing a variety of 'perspectives on need'. Available data can include:

- Survey (either those currently being treated or population surveys)

- Rates under treatment ('met need')
- Social indicators (use of sociodemographic indicators to 'predict' likely need)
- Key informants (use of views of stakeholders)
- Community forum/opinion

Needs assessment in relation to (alternative) responses to need is closely related to cost benefit and cost effective analysis.

- *Cost benefit analysis* identifies money cost set against an assumed money value of the outcome achieved, thus effectively giving a money value to a range of outcomes and deciding which intervention(s) to adopt based upon rating and ranking of 'net values'
- *Cost effective analysis* identifies a given outcome required, without attaching any value to it, and identifies the different costs of alternative ways of achieving that outcome.

Limitations and considerations of needs assessment

- Lack of objectivity—no needs assessment is policy-neutral. Its results are dependent upon the values underlying both any particular method of assessment adopted and the data applied within it. This is inevitable, but it is crucial to identify such influence when interpreting any particular needs assessment
- Ability to benefit is intimately linked to outcomes (📖 p.II.221); and desired outcome may be in dispute and difficult to measure.
- Needs assessment amounts to taking a judgement upon available data, or the data selected for use
- Only 'perspectives' on a given need can be achieved. The final decision as to what is the identified need is arrived at by way of judgement, based upon effectively weighing more than one perspective on a given identified need, each perspective arrived at by its own method. If only one perspective, and method, is utilized then the need identified will be biased in terms of the method adopted
- There are various social constructions of need, with each potential definition being rooted in the philosophical, moral and temporal contexts within which it sits. Within mental healthcare, social attitudes heavily influence the need definitions adopted
- Government definitions have limited the concept of need to 'a need that can be responded to by intervention'—that is 'ability to benefit'. If there is a valid health need but no remedy it is seen as pointless to identify it as such, except as a basis for research aimed at identifying an effective therapeutic response.

Special forensic issues with needs assessment

- Forensic mental health needs assessment is fraught with values problems beyond those which are present in most health domains, because of the dual purpose of forensic mental health services in being directed at both patient and public benefit. This gives rise to the fundamental question 'Whose need is being responded to?'. The needs of each may often be in conflict (e.g. the most effective rehabilitation of an offender patient may require granting a leave programme (📖 p.II.154) which puts the public more at risk than a more cautious leave programme)

- Needs assessment is often pursued in terms of QALYs ('quality-adjusted life years'). However, forensic mental health needs involve not only a QALY element but also potentially a LALY ('liberty-adjusted life year') element, where the two may be in conflict (e.g. the patient will improve in their mental health by treatment but will also experience two years of loss of liberty). Ethical tensions (📖 p.III.245) may arise in responding to both
- Although needs assessment is separate from service response, identifying alternative responses involves comparing service solutions—such as comparing treatment within hospital and within the healthcare services of a prison. This is a matter of policy
- Law can infer a service response in the absence of need. For example, a hybrid order (📖 p.IV.408) served by an MDO who has benefited adequately from hospital care, and who cannot properly then be transferred to prison without loss of health, cannot be released because of his underlying prison sentence, forcing the hospital to continue detaining and 'treating' him despite the lack of a continued health need.

Services outside the UK & Ireland

Countries outside the UK & Ireland fall into two main groups as regards their forensic psychiatry services:

- Countries that offer therapeutic services to mentally disordered offenders, run either by specialist forensic psychiatrists or by general psychiatrists, and
- Countries that offer no therapeutic services to mentally disordered offenders, and in which forensic psychiatry is confined to expert testimony.

Countries with forensic psychiatric services

Most of Western Europe (e.g. Germany, the Netherlands, and Scandinavian countries), some of Eastern Europe (e.g. Russia, Bulgaria), and culturally Anglo-Saxon countries (Canada, Australia, New Zealand) have forensic psychiatric services, where mentally disordered offenders are offered treatment. In some countries, this service is offered within prisons; others have a system of secure residential clinics as in the UK. Transfer of prisoners with mental illness to psychiatric hospitals in Europe is often problematic owing to disputes about diagnosis or concern regarding the level of security required. Only in Scandinavian countries are almost all prisoners with psychosis transferred out of prison.

In these countries (as in the UK), forensic psychiatrists may not only treat patients, they may also give expert testimony in a variety of settings. In criminal court, they may be invited to give expert opinion because they have expertise in working with MDOs. Occasionally, they may be invited to give expert testimony about cases that involve defendants known to their services.

Countries without services

In countries where there are either no public health services, or where because of lack of resources services are poor, adequate mental healthcare may only be available to the wealthy (e.g. most of Eastern Europe, India, Africa). Mentally ill people who commit offences are likely to be imprisoned; and prisoners are unlikely to have access to anything but the most basic healthcare.

In these countries, forensic psychiatry is the practice of medico-legal psychiatry: the provision of expert testimony on a range of issues (📖 p.V.532). Forensic psychiatrists in these countries may or may not have experience of working therapeutically with mentally disordered offenders. The key professional issues are how to ensure quality of testimony; and the maintenance of the ethical standards (📖 p.II.227).

There are other countries that do not offer any provision for mentally disordered offenders because of a lack of acknowledgement of the issue. Politics may play a role: in some states, dissidents without mental illness may be labelled as disordered and imprisoned (e.g. in the former Soviet Union, or allegedly in China[*]): this represents an abuse of psychiatry (📖 p.IV.442).

The United States

The US provides some therapeutic services for prisoners, usually in the form of psychiatric clinics in prisons and courts. Its state hospitals also provide some limited secure provision for mentally ill people who commit offences.

Nevertheless, forensic psychiatry in the US is defined as medico-legal activity only. There is extensive professional guidance and literature about forensic psychiatry in this context, including a rich professional literature on the ethical obligations of psychiatrists who give expert testimony, some of whom in the US call themselves 'forensicists' in order to differentiate the ethics of testimony from the ethics required in medical practice (see 📖 p.III.245).

Of particular interest is the claim by many academics in US forensic psychiatry that the sole duty of a forensicist is to the court, and not to the person whom they are evaluating. This position has been criticized by many European psychiatrists who feel that it is incompatible with basic principles of medical ethics (📖 p.III.247). The US counter-argument is that all citizens, including professionals, have a duty to assist the justice process, which trumps duties to individuals. Many US forensic psychiatrists also take the view that it is ethically unwise to offer expert testimony about a defendant whom the psychiatrist has treated, as often occurs in the UK.

[*] For example, as a mechanism for the suppression of the Falun Gong religious movement.

The ethics of forensic psychiatry

Chapter 9

Ethical decision-making

How to use this part

Clinical ethics is concerned with how we put values into practice in our clinical work. The word 'ethical' is a description of a type of reflective process and discussion. There is rarely a 'right' answer, but there may be more than one justifiable answer.

In this, and the following pages, we will be looking at types and specific examples of ethical dilemmas in forensic psychiatry, and at ways in which ethical decision-making can be approached. Ethical dilemmas arise almost daily in clinical medicine; and especially in psychiatry both because the status of some mental disorders is not clear, and because psychiatrists are given unusual legal powers to treat patients against their will.

Forensic psychiatrists meet multiple and complex ethical dilemmas in clinical practice for three main reasons:

- They must negotiate the interface (📖 p.IV.299) with criminal justice and other agencies (📖 p.III.258), and potential conflicts of ethical duties
- Psychiatrists have dual responsibilities, involving a duty of clinical care to the patient, and a duty to the state, in terms of pursuit of justice and/or the protection of others
- The forensic psychiatrist can have other roles, as a professional witness and/or an expert witness as a doctor. Likewise, the patient themselves may also have other roles, as a defendant (or witness, 📖 p.II.119, or victim, 📖 p.II.122) as well as a patient.

Ethics as distillation

In summary, clinical ethics is about understanding the 'ethical nuts and bolts' of a particular situation, what consequences, rights, and duties are in play and what is implied ethically by making one choice rather than another. We might call this making decisions with 'ethical insight'. It involves distilling out the ethical elements and then making a justifiable decision. Good ethics is therefore about good process, not a single right answer or there having occurred a good outcome.

Practice makes better

Occasionally through the handbook case vignettes are presented, many of which raise ethical dilemmas that are common in forensic psychiatry. When you read the theory offered in this part of the book, we suggest that you look to see how it can be applied the vignettes, or to cases you have encountered yourself. There are many approaches to ethical reasoning (📖 p.III.231); the purpose of this part of the handbook is to assist the practitioner to develop high quality ethical decision-making, using accepted approaches.

Raising ethical consciousness

Reading this part is also intended to make the reader more aware of ethical dilemmas in daily forensic practice. It is a common error for doctors to mistake ethical decisions for clinical ones; that is to mistake a 'should' ('normative') statement for an 'is' (or 'positive') statement. A key test question is usually: I *can* do this clinically, but *should* I?

Ethics and law

This part of the book is also intended to make clear the distinction between legal and ethical approaches to dilemmas. It is common for professionals faced with an ethical dilemma to ask, 'What does the law say? Finding out the legal position may offer *an* answer, it may even contribute to determining an ethical answer: but it may well not itself be *the* ethical answer. At most the law offers an answer that may be capable of ethical justification. Alternatively, law and ethics may be in conflict; or the law may be silent on an issue, such as whether there is a duty to disclose to the court a report which was commissioned by the defence. Similarly, the law cannot tell you whether you should let a patient have unescorted leave when all members bar one of the clinical team support the decision.

Ethics and data

Good ethical decision-making is dependent upon reliable empirical evidence, or facts. Empirical data, however, only usually helps with thinking about the consequences of alternative courses of action; it cannot of itself assist towards constructing an ethical analysis of a dilemma.

Diligence in ethics

Neither the process nor the outcome of ethical decision-making is usually straightforward. An apparently simple answer is likely to be wrong; or at least to have missed out important facts or perspectives. Good-quality, ethical decision-making often takes time: yet anxiety will often impel people towards quick (and often ethically suspect) solutions. If you are in an ethical dilemma, take your time, talk to others, gain different perspectives, and make notes of your thinking and discussions, not just the decision arrived at. Put simply, 'show your workings': doing so is likely to enhance both the quality and clarity of your thought, and at a later stage (perhaps at an inquiry) may demonstrate the soundness of your reasoning to others.

Approaches to medical ethics

What is and is not medical ethics

Medical ethics is concerned with making good quality ethical decisions in everyday clinical work. It focuses on distilling out the ethical essence of a situation and is more about acquiring and applying reasoning skills and a type of intelligence than it is about being sure about what is the right or wrong thing to do.

Moral philosophy is the study of how we decide what is 'good' and 'bad'; and medical ethical decision-making is about deciding what to do in terms of 'good' and 'bad' in a practical way. Essentially medical ethics is about maximizing clinician insight into the ethical implications of alternative decisions and 'biting the ethical bullet'.

The need for medical ethics

It has always been recognized that healers have increased power and authority within social groups; first, because of their specialist knowledge; second, because of their value to the group in terms of health and welfare preservation; and third, because they have to relate to others who are vulnerable. With increased power comes increased responsibility.

Early practitioners in Greece wrote about the behaviour of doctors and how they should conduct themselves. Some early writings became known as the Hippocratic Oath, and have persisted as a marker of professional medical identity to the present day (although the oath has no formal status and is only actually taken as an oath per se by a handful of medical graduands).

For centuries there was no practical ethical guidance for doctors. As the medical and surgical professions grew and developed, it was widely assumed that the word 'ethical' meant the same as 'good'; and that because medical practitioners sought to bring about good health consequences for their patients, it was assumed that the doctor's view was always right: 'doctor knows best'.

Elaboration of the need for medical ethics

In the post World War II period, there were two massive cultural challenges to this tradition. The first arose in response to the civil rights movement, which challenged insults to individual choice and dignity. Within this movement the medical profession was seen as treating 'patients' as second-class citizens, who could not be trusted to make decisions for themselves; much as white patriarchies were seen as oppressing people of colour and women. A number of seminal legal cases were brought at this time which challenged medical authority, arguing that patient autonomy should be privileged over medical beneficence.

The second challenge to the presumption 'clinically right is ethically right' arose as a result of the Nuremberg trials of Nazi doctors, and the disclosure that doctors had taken part in murder and cruelty to the vulnerable in the name of 'medical practice'. 45% of the medical profession in Germany were members of the Nazi party, and many applied their medical clinical skills to the euthanasia programme, research on live humans without consent, and selection for murder in death camps. Revelations of these practices led to a sea-change in the direction of travel of medical practice, and its regulation, which continues still.

The development of codes

The Nuremberg Code of Medical Ethics has been revised and expanded. There is now a World Medical Association (WMA) declaration of the ethical duties of doctors (📖 p.App. 4.653) with substatements addressing various specific issues, such as research, boundary violations and the influence of drug companies in medicine. For psychiatrists there are a number of particular statements that apply.

Internationally, most doctors are bound by a variety of professional ethical codes, which are enforced by their licensing authorities. In the UK, doctors are registered and licensed with the GMC, which gives ethical guidance to doctors in the form of Good Medical Practice. This is continually being reconsidered and revised.

The status and role of codes

Codes (see 📖 p.III.241) offer general statements which, in turn, represent a particular ethical 'solution' to types of dilemmas. They are not a substitute for ethical reasoning but offer an aid and input into that reasoning. They are written in very broad terms and do not purport to give unambiguous answers to all potential ethical dilemmas.

Psychiatrists are bound by the principles of Good Medical Practice (📖 p.App. 4.649) and also by the guidance given by the Royal College of

Psychiatrists (Good Psychiatric Practice) (📖 p.App. 4.649). UK forensic psychiatrists are the only English speaking professional group who do *not* have a Code of Ethics. There is a specialist ethical code, for example, for forensic psychiatry within the USA, the AAPL Code (📖 p.App. 4.651), which offers guidance on many of the problems specific to the discipline.

The 'ethical consult'

In the US there is burgeoning use of specialist bioethicists as 'advisors' to clinicians (via 'the ethical consult'). There is a risk that this can undermine the ultimate responsibility of clinicians for making not only technical but also ethical decisions in regard to their patients. In the UK emphasis is placed upon clinical ethical decision-making being part and parcel of clinical practice ('the raspberry that ripples through the ice cream'). An increase in Clinical Ethics Committees (CECs) in hospitals throughout the UK enhances rather than undermines this, since CECs operate essentially as aids to good ethical thinking by clinicians and not as substitutes for clinician based ethical decision-making. By contrast Research Ethics Committees do sanction research, based upon detailed protocols. The boundary between the functions of CECs and of Research Ethics Committees is sometimes less than clear, especially where research and audit overlap.

Schools of ethics

Ethical reasoning is generally distinguished into those accounts that say that what matters are the *consequences* of decisions, and those that say that *intentions* matter most. Each account has a long history in moral philosophy. A background assumption to each account is that there are moral rules that should not be broken; and that challenges to those rules need to be justified in terms of either positive consequences, or positive intentions, or possibly both.

The four principles

A popular (and dominant) account in medical ethics appeals to both principles and consequences. It states that doctors should pay attention to four principles or duties:[*]

- A duty to respect patient *autonomy*
- A duty to bring about good consequences: *beneficence*
- A duty not to cause harm: *non-maleficence*
- A duty to respect *justice*: to treat people fairly, but also engage with the legal system appropriately (doctors do not have an option on respect for criminal law, for example).

Faced with an ethical dilemma, the doctor considers these duties as a framework for determining what is a (not necessarily *the*) right action. Although the four principles are not hierarchically sequenced, there is a general acceptance amongst philosophers that respect for autonomy is most important; this is especially true within the practice of psychiatry.[†]

[*] The proposed Mental Capacity (Health, Welfare and Finance) Bill for NI (📖 p.App. 2.624) is explicitly based on the Four Principles.
[†] This philosophical view poses a considerable challenge not only to the views of some forensic psychiatrists, but also to at least some of the principles of mental health laws (📖 p.IV.377), which are emphatically not founded primarily on respect for autonomy.

Utilitarianism This holds that you should act in ways that maximize the benefit for as many people as possible. Intuitively this is appealing for doctors, but it can easily lead to 'the ends justify the means'. Also, it involves a calculus which weighs different types of outcomes for different individuals, inferring value judgements. However, it has an important place in medical ethics, especially in policy-making and risk assessment.

Deontology This holds that you should act according to principles that could apply universally. Most famously it was explicated by Kant, but drawing on Judeo-Christian thinking (e.g. the Ten Commandments). It has appeal insofar as it privileges human intention, but can give no guidance on what to do when principles conflict. Another important aspect of Kantian thought is the injunction that we should never treat others merely as means to an end. The school is important for questions concerning autonomy and responsibility; and research ethics.

Liberal individualism This is a rights-based theory, within which respecting others' rights is deemed the proper basis for resolving ethical dilemmas. This appeals to lawyers as it is rule-based. It offers little guidance however on what to do when rights conflict; nor is at all clear that a 'right' is meaningful if no other person will respect it.

Communitarianism A theory developed in response to extremes of individual rights-based theory. It argues that we are connected to each other through common values and goals; and that privileging individual autonomy risks losing sight of the extent to which we are social animals. To some extent, Anglo-Saxon criminal law assumes this position; an offender offends against the large group or state, and in criminal law it is the state (and not the individual) that charges and prosecutes the offender on behalf of everyone, not the victim.

Ethic of care Also known as relational ethics, this theory argues that to do the right thing, one must understand the network of relationships that affect the patient; including the doctor. This theory has gained wide appeal among nursing staff, because it takes account of the feelings of carers. It has real relevance for psychiatrists and psychotherapists.

Virtue ethics This holds that you should be as much like the character of a good doctor as you can be. The assumption is that being the good doctor will give rise to ethically reasonable decisions (without recourse to reasoning and without having to deal with conflicts between different ethical approaches). This is particularly appealing in psychiatry, where personal qualities are often crucial to therapeutic success. In other spheres of medicine, virtue may matter much less: a morally dubious surgeon's lack of virtue, for example, does not affect their technical expertise in the way that it can affect a psychiatrist's.

Values-based practice (see 📖 p.III.235) This is a contemporary account that sees ethical dilemmas in mental health as representing clashes of values between different players, each of whom only see their values from their own perspective. Better understanding of each other's values may therefore help resolve dilemmas. It is appealing because it addresses MDT problems (see 📖 p.III.256), and because it offers a way to think about respect for diversity without collapse into relativism; though problematic in forensic psychiatry where it is hard to see how a good psychiatrist can respect an antisocial patient's value system. It also suggests relying upon 'good values practice' rather than law to protect patients' rights.

Comparing theories

All these theories have something to offer, at different times and in different situations. In many ways, together they offer ways in which we remain conscious of appropriate complexity in our ethical discussions.

Different ethical decisions may be defensible using different models and through resolving conflict between duties in different ways, each justifiable in its own right.

Values-based practice

Values-based practice (VBP) is a theoretical skills-based approach to dealing with ethical dilemmas in mental health practice. It is based upon the work of Professor KWM (Bill) Fulford. VBP theory suggests that many ethical dilemmas arise in mental health practice because of clashes of values perspectives between different players that are not fully explored and acknowledged. It emphasizes resolution of ethical dilemmas by way of a process of reflection on values that are in tension; and not seeking simplistic answers in terms of law, local policy or clinical facts. All perspectives are important, especially those of the service user.

A values-based approach in practice

A VBP approach emphasizes:
- Awareness of the facts and values relevant to the case
- Awareness of the different perspectives of the different players, especially in relation to risk of harms
- Respect for the different value perspectives
- Reflection on and discussion of these different perspectives
- Resolution.

VBP in forensic settings

Some suggest that values in forensic psychiatry contradict values in general psychiatry and medicine; especially where there is conflict between values relating to a doctor's duty to society as a whole and values relating to care of patients as a doctor. This conflict is acutely observed within the role of forensic psychiatrist as expert witness (📖 p.III.245). or where there is a balance to strike between the right of the patient to liberty and the right of society to be protected from the patient.

In clinical forensic settings, VBP may add to the quality of discussions between staff and patients, particularly in relation to risk assessment and management. Anxiety about risk is often high; and can push professionals towards taking decisions quickly and without reflection.

> *Example:* Mr King is detained in a medium secure unit following a violent offence 3 years ago. He has a diagnosis of schizophrenia and has no current symptoms. He was psychotic at the time of the offence. He has limited insight, does not accept responsibility for the offence, but has engaged in all treatment. He and his family believe that he should be allowed leave into the community. There is division within the clinical team about this decision.

Process

Different values perspectives will often result in different contributions to discussion. Mr King's view emphasizes the value to him of his freedom; and does not 'see' the value of risk reduction. Some clinicians emphasize the values of harm and risk avoidance and focus on issues of denial, insight, and victim empathy. Those who advocate taking the risk of giving leave may place a greater value on patient engagement and rapport. Mr King's parents may place value on other factors that mitigate risk, for example, interpersonal factors, sense of humour and subtle factors only apparent to family. The MoJ (📖 p.App. 3.464) may solely value public safety.

Respect

Respect in VBP means allowing all voices and points of view to be heard. This is often best done by creating reflective spaces for discussion, where professionals and service users can find common points of reference, as well as clarify areas of difference, especially in relation to risk. Adopting this approach may be particularly helpful for decisions regarding high-risk patients, where anxiety can easily cause conflict between teams.

One team member or agency may well value rehabilitation more highly than public safety by comparison with another. What is crucial, however, is that there is agreement on the available data on which a decision might be based, so that any difference of values being applied by different individuals is made evident. The alternative of one party selecting different facts in support of their value judgement is unhelpful. The basis of any disagreement must be made apparent, being honest about the values applied. Within teams, it is worth noting that there is often strength in acknowledging uncertainty, or being open about values, particularly when it is expressed by senior staff, since this is likely to allow less experienced colleagues to do likewise.

Resolution and review

Resolution includes recording discussions and the way that different perspectives have been considered. A plan of action is agreed; and this can be recorded, as well as dissenting views. The recording and rationale of a values based approach to risk based decisions allows risks to be taken in a way that clinical teams can feel comfortable with, and that can readily be scrutinized. Later review is also an essential part of resolution.

Limits of VBP in forensic psychiatry

Many VBP principles may be difficult to apply in forensic psychiatry.

- Some values may be difficult to respect—a person who has values supportive of violence, or a person who places little value upon the safety of others
- The values of individuals may be trumped by political, social or legal values—social or political risk aversion can prevent adoption of VBP
- Circumstances of a case may overwhelm any proper attempt at values resolution—high profile offences may prevent any consideration in the manner described
- Expert evidence resulting in a mentally disordered person receiving treatment may be easier to reconcile with values held as a doctor than may expert evidence resulting in indeterminate or extended custodial sentences (see 📖 pp.IV.364, V.549)
- Values other than objectivity may have no place in the courtroom (however unrealistic this may be as an aspiration).

Relationship between law and ethics

The law is a set of rules, devised to regulate relationships between individuals, and between individuals and the State, or society as a whole. There are two main divisions of law; civil and criminal (see 📖 p.IV.329). The civil law deals with wrongs that the parties may have done to each other: breach of duty or contract, for example. In contrast, the criminal law regulates the relationship between the individual and the larger community or state to which he is affiliated. Hence in the US, it is the State that charges and prosecutes an alleged offender; and in the UK, it is the Crown. Criminal charges arise when harm has been done by one party (or parties) to another: the philosophical assumption being that when harm is done to one, it is done to the community as a whole.

The law, as a set of rules, evolves over time and changes according to circumstance, in common law jurisdictions (📖 p.IV.306) by way of either statute or case law. Although there are some aspects of law that are clear and explicit, often it may be impossible to know exactly what the law is on a given question (see 📖 p.IV.304); within a common law jurisdiction, what the law is will therefore be determined subsequently by the court, effectively with retrospective application. The law is the codification of a social consensus about an issue, which effectively will commonly express a particular value, or balance between competing values; only rarely, though, does it address questions of value explicitly.

Ethics[*] or morality is also about the relationship between individual parties, and about the relationships between the individual and the wider social group. Ethical statements tend to include the words '*ought*' or '*should*'. So, for example, under mental health law, it may be legally possible to detain someone: but the ethical question may be: should you?

Ethical questions usually deal with matters of conflicting moral value, e.g. it is good to tell people the truth, but if I tell this patient the truth, he may become angry and violent. Should I tell him the truth? The law cannot provide a general answer to this question, although it might set specific rules requiring truth telling (or truth concealment) in specific situations, such as when a patient makes a subject access request under the Data Protection Act (📖 p.App. 2.622).

Because laws reflect the wishes of society, or at least its rulers, at a given time, it is possible for laws to be ethically incoherent and unjust. Consider both the Nazi eugenics laws, and the South African apartheid laws. The Nazi laws allowed doctors to end the lives of those who were disabled; but ignored the basic ethical question of whether one should ever deliberately end the life of another. The apartheid laws, which categorized all subjects as White, Black, Coloured, or Indian, determined where people in the Black (and to a lesser extent, Indian and Coloured) group could live, work and travel, and even with whom they could interact, and in what circumstances. However, they did not address the fundamental ethical conflict between these policies and the idea of every life having equal value.

Law follows ethics

It is a good rule that the law should follow ethics, rather than the other way around. Law should have justice as its central value: justice for all, applied fairly and transparently, with equal access. However, if you have an ethical dilemma, the law may be able to help you with guidance about what acts are socially permissible: but it is unlikely to be able to tell you what you should do.

Mental health laws and *mental capacity laws* give powers to certain professionals to detain people for assessment and treatment or to act in their best interests. Because the state should not in general detain individuals who have not broken any law (a tenet of human rights law, 📖 p.IV.418), there need to be special powers to detain those who are ill,[†] and might benefit from detention. Mental health legislation empowers professionals to detain: it does not impose a duty to do so (see 📖 p.IV.377). It cannot answer questions such as, 'How should I balance my patient's personal interests against the public interest in being protection from someone at high risk of violence?'. For a discussion of this vexed issue, see 📖 p.III.242.

---

[*] The term 'ethics' can also mean the philosophical study of morality, and the specific moral codes adopted by a professional group. In much of this handbook (e.g. 📖 pp.III.239–IV.301) the latter meaning of ethics is adopted, but in this topic the reference is to general morality.

[†] Not only patients who are mentally disordered: for example, there are powers to detain people with certain infectious diseases for treatment, and to remove persons in need of care and attention (📖 p.IV.440) from their home for treatment.

Chapter 10

Professional duties and personal integrity

Professional guidelines and codes

A professional is someone who 'professes' an identity or role by virtue of specialist knowledge and commitment to that role. Most professionals gain their identity through prolonged study, examination of their competence, and practice. Once accredited (e.g. through GMC registration and licensing) the question is then how best to maintain, and 'revalidate' professional skills, so as to offer a proper quality service to those who benefit from professionals' skills. Accreditation and revalidation relate to both technical competence and ethical practice, which are intertwined (persisting with poor technique cannot be ethically justifiable; and ethical decision-making is part of clinical practice, see 📖 p.III.233).

Maintenance of professional identity is achieved by:
- Continued development of professional knowledge and skills, and
- Adherence to professional standards, and guidelines as to how to maintain the professional role in all circumstances (or as to how it can reasonably be modified in particular circumstances). Guidelines give an indication of what the good professional is expected to do, or how he or she is expected to behave.

Guidelines are authoritative statements by the bodies that issue them, and in this context cover both clinical and ethical matters. An unjustified failure to follow guidelines may contravene good ethical practice, and might also be relevant in any legal proceedings.

Technical protocols versus ethical codes

Guidelines vary in their nature, from detailed instructions on how to perform a specific clinical procedure, to very broad statements of principle about professionals' ethical duties. Many guidelines fall between these extremes; some combine elements of both. The former sort may be referred to as a protocol, and the latter (if they contain a number of coherent ethical statements covering the same area) as an ethical code, but these terms are not always used consistently.

Clinical guidelines and protocols

These are usually based on meta-analytic reviews of published evidence about the medical treatment of disorders. In the UK, the National Institute for Health and Clinical Excellence (NICE) regularly publishes treatment guidelines which may be helpful in allocating treatment resources and determining policy. The DoH defines clinical guidelines as 'recommendations on the appropriate treatment and care of people with specific diseases and conditions within the NHS'.

Guidelines help healthcare professionals in their work, but they do not replace their knowledge and skills. However, because guidelines rely on aggregate data, they may be of limited use in individual cases, and may conflict with the professional duty to make the care of patients one's first concern. Where there are published clinical guidelines, it is good practice to consult them; and to record the reasons for not following them in any particular case. Even clinical guidelines may infer value judgements (e.g. NICE makes a value judgement, based on cost:benefit analysis, 📖 p.II.223, in deciding whether to approve a particular treatment).

Ethical guidelines and codes

Ethical guidelines in medical practice represent codification of professional consensus. They are informed by the medical ethical literature, as well as by developments in medical law.

The main source of ethical guidelines for doctors in the UK is *Good Medical Practice*, published by the General Medical Council, and updated regularly (📖 p.App. 4.649). Separate advice is available on consent, disclosure, privacy of information and professional misconduct. Departures from these guidelines can form the basis of charges of impairment of fitness to practice. The medical defence societies also provide information about ethical guidance, as well as legal guidance and support.

Codes of ethics in psychiatry

There has been debate over many years as to whether psychiatry needs a particular frame for ethical decision-making: because psychiatric patients are especially vulnerable to abuse because of the effects of many mental disorders on capacity and volition (📖 p.II.20); because there are historical precedents for abuse by way of spurious or unsupportable psychiatric diagnoses (such as sluggish schizophrenia, 📖 p.IV.422), inappropriate treatments, and unethical research; and because mental health law gives unusual power to doctors to override a competent patient's refusal of treatment.

The World Psychiatric Association (WPA) publishes codes of ethics (📖 p.App. 4.653) for psychiatrists; with particular emphasis on research ethics. The American Psychiatric Association (APA) and the Australian & New Zealand College of Psychiatrists (ANCP) have codes of ethics for their members.

In the UK, the Royal College of Psychiatrists publishes Good Psychiatric Practice (📖 p.App. 4.649); although this is not the basis for regulatory review and is not a Code as such, it does set out some of the expectations of psychiatrists.

Codes of ethics in forensic psychiatry

There is no UK or Irish code of ethics specifically for forensic psychiatrists. In relation to expert testimony, there is some advice in Good Medical Practice. In addition, the Royal College of Psychiatrists produces updated versions of specific psychiatric advice, entitled Good Psychiatric Practice (📖 p.App. 4.649), relevant in particular to writing reports (📖 p.V.555) and giving evidence (📖 p.V.585). However, these contain little specific advice about forensic practice.

The American Association of Psychiatry and Law's ethical guidelines (📖 p.App. 4.651) are also useful in this regard. The key requirements are not to go beyond one's competency; always to practise honestly; and not to become aligned with any one side of an adversarial debate. The expert's duty is to assist the court and not assist a legal cause.

Ethical dilemmas in clinical forensic psychiatry are not adequately addressed by current guidelines; particularly in regard to dilemmas concerning the role of the psychiatrist in the pursuit of public protection or the role of the expert witness (📖 p.V.532), and related concerns about doing patients harm (although some argue, in the latter regard, that individuals assessed for risk in relation to non-therapeutic sentencing are not patients, and the clinician is not a doctor but a 'forensicist' (📖 p.II.225).

Legislative codes of practice

There are codes of practice which suggest how to apply legislation, most notably mental health law (📖 p.IV.373). These are not ethical codes, though they may contain matters of ethical substance. Good professional practice may take account of codes of practice, which (like other professional guidelines) should be followed unless there is a justifiable reason for not doing so.

Guidelines, codes, and law

Guidelines, ethical codes, and legislative codes of practice do not themselves have the force of law, but may be referred to within legal proceedings in determining the outcome of cases according to legal rules. They offer the courts explicit though not incontestable descriptions of clinical standards across a wide range of medical practice. However, British and Irish courts are not always uncritically swayed by such guidelines and may question their authority and status as embodiments of customary care; although they may become increasingly significant in determining legal cases.

Professional codes and managerial policies

Medical ethics must be distinguished from hospital or national policies which may have ethical implications which can be in conflict with professional ethics. Hospitals themselves often develop policies which are ethical in nature or in their implications (e.g. policies concerning participation of clinicians within MAPPA, see 📖 p.V.468) and there is room for conflict between the policies of hospitals and professional ethical codes of practice. Similarly, direct government instructions or 'circulars', coming down to clinicians through managers, can conflict with professional or individual values and codes, the conflict being made acute where the clinician holds a contract of employment under which he or she can be disciplined for disobeying managerial orders.

A duty to prevent violence?

Most psychiatrists accept that they have a duty to treat patients (📖 p.II.146) who pose a risk of violence to others in such a way as to manage and minimize that risk (📖 p.II.191). However, outside the profession it is commonly assumed that psychiatrists have a much more stringent duty, to *prevent* patients acting violently to others. This is contentious, in regard to both ethics and law (📖 p.V.519).

✏ The argument for a responsibility to prevent violence

Most philosophical accounts of responsibility state that each adult is responsible for their own actions; and no adult is normally responsible for the actions of another. To become the responsibility of another, a person must either:

- Be mentally incapable (📖 p.IV.424) of making their own decisions, or
- Be in the legal custody of the other person.

The latter of these conditions almost always applies to forensic psychiatric inpatients (the custody being detention under mental health law). Therefore, it is argued, forensic psychiatrists are responsible for their patients' behaviour whilst they lack capacity or are detained, or perhaps even if they are merely subject to legal restrictions in the community.

This certainly appears to have been the UK government's view during the past two decades; at least, this is one interpretation of the system of formal inquiries into the actions of services (📖 p.V.471) whenever a patient commits a homicide in E&W. Most forensic psychiatrists can expect to be the subject of such an inquiry in a working lifetime.

The relationship with the mental disorder

Where a patient is in a grossly disturbed mental state and therefore lacks capacity, doctors must act in their best interests (📖 p.III.277); few would dispute that this could include a duty to prevent them from acting in harmful ways towards others. However, most forensic psychiatric patients do not lack capacity, or criminal responsibility (📖 p.IV.338) at the time of committing serious violence or homicide (and most violence is committed by people without mental disorder).

It can therefore be argued that it is unreasonable to hold a psychiatrist responsible for the behaviour of their patient when the patient is capable or criminally responsible, or where their behaviour was not directly related to mental disorder or to a failure of psychiatric care.

The relevance of risk assessment

Forensic psychiatrists specifically assess the risk (📖 p.II.127) of their patients being violent, and construct risk management plans (📖 p.II.190). It could be argued that by doing so they take on additional responsibility for such violence if it occurs.

However, risk assessment is a very imprecise process (see 📖 p.II.130), and one incapable of predicting violence (📖 p.II.128). Only by detaining a very high proportion of forensic patients indefinitely could there be effective prevention of violence in the community by those patients (as opposed to merely reducing the risk of it) using current risk assessment and management techniques. Even if this could be justified on financial and human rights grounds (📖 p.IV.418), it would not prevent all violence by patients, merely displace some from the community to hospital wards.

A general duty to others

Most philosophical accounts of a 'good life' include duties to others as well as duties to oneself, and responsibility for oneself. This is often couched as a reciprocal relationship between an individual and society; if we as citizens seek protection and benefit from being a member of group, we have to acknowledge duties to that group. These duties may in some cases be purely moral, with no prospect of legal sanction if they are broken, but they are significant nonetheless.

A specific example of such a duty is the expectation that doctors will use their professional knowledge and skills to improve the health of society at large, where they are able to do so. Vaccination programmes are a good example of where this works well.

What is less clear is how doctors contribute to public health, if 'health' is expanded to include public safety,* and other citizens' (i.e. patients') liberty may be restricted in that pursuit. One way to look at this has been to argue that where there is no knowledge there is no duty; but as a doctor acquires more knowledge of a dangerous situation, they then have an enhanced duty to do something (although whether this is as a citizen or a professional is debateable).

For example, in relation to child protection and the safeguarding of vulnerable adults (📖 p.II.202), doctors are expected to participate fully in child protection or safeguarding procedures, even where this may mean breaching the confidentiality of another patient (📖 p.III.264). The ethical justification is that the duty to a child or vulnerable adult outweighs any duty to a less-vulnerable patient who is more able to protect themselves.

Doctors can owe a duty to those who might be harmed by their patients. However, what is important is determining the ethical justification of that duty, as doctor or citizen; and its limits in a given situation, by balancing the duty to others against the duty owed to the patient.

Conclusion

Both general duties as a citizen, and specific professional duties, combine to require forensic psychiatrists to do what is reasonable in the circumstances to minimize the risk of their patients being violent, which might include treatments, risk management measures, and sharing information where appropriate (e.g. under the MAPPA, 📖 p.V.468). However, this is a limited duty. The argument that forensic psychiatrists have an absolute duty to prevent all violence by their patients is unsupportable.

Competing interests and role conflicts

Competing interests

Competing interests arise in medicine in situations where a doctor is aware of duties, loyalties, or ethical principles that are in conflict one with another. Major kinds of competing interest include:

- Where one ethical duty conflicts with another in a clinical setting (e.g. where to give adequate pain relief will bring about death, the so-called 'doctrine of double effect').
- Where a doctor has a personal interest in a situation which conflicts with their professional duties, so that their opinion may not be as objective as it should be (e.g. a doctor may conduct research funded by a pharmaceutical company that makes an antidepressant, and regularly lecture on the relative merits of different antidepressants; or may be over-cautious in granting leave to or discharging patients, out of fear for their career should a patient cause serious harm to others).

---

* A lack of public safety can result in injury (damage to health), but to include public safety itself (and therefore crime prevention) as an aspect of public health is excessively to medicalize society.

- Where the doctor has strong personal values which are relevant to a professional setting that are likely to affect their judgement (e.g. professional jealousy when reviewing another colleague's work for a grant application or for publication; if the reviewer has strong personal feelings about the colleague, or the colleague's work, then they may not be neutral in their review). For this reason, doctors are often asked to declare competing interests, so that any potential bias is known about and appreciated.

Competing interests also include situations in which there is frank conflict of interests. Consider a doctor working for a pharmaceutical company who discovers that it has concealed data that would alter the outcome of a clinical trial. They then have a conflict between their contractual and professional duty to their employer to keep the data confidential, and their professional duty to maintain good medical knowledge, protect potential patients, and not to collude with deception. Note that it would be in their personal interest not to disclose the information.

Role conflicts represent another way of conceiving competing or conflicting interests. The professional role is only one of a number of roles we may have in our lives. The doctor may feel constrained not to assess a defendant solely for non-therapeutic penal sentencing purposes but as a citizen may feel duty bound so to do (see 📖 p.III.261).

Role conflicts and competing interests in forensic psychiatry
Risk versus rehabilitation
In psychiatry (both general and forensic), there is an ever present concern about how to set the balance between risk management and public safety, and proper concern for the patient's welfare and need for recovery. Increasingly, psychiatrists may now have a personal interest in not being criticized by any (imagined) inquiry; and these anxieties may impact on their clinical decision-making, and consciously or unconsciously affect how they set the balance between public protection and patient welfare.

Therapist versus expert for court
The most common situations in which role conflicts arise are in legal contexts. It is not uncommon for forensic psychiatrists to be asked to give expert testimony in relation to their own patients. They may be in the best position, in terms of knowledge, to do so; but their natural concern for their patient may hinder their ability to be objective.

For example, a doctor who has built up a working relationship with a patient in the community who is later accused of murder may be more ready to support a plea of diminished responsibility (📖 p.V.491) than a doctor with no previous knowledge of the defendant. Similarly, a doctor who has been treating a patient for PTSD may not be completely objective in writing a report for a compensation claim (📖 p.V.514) against someone alleged to have caused the PTSD.

Hence, because the expert's duty to the court may conflict or compete with the duty to make the care of the patient one's first concern, treating psychiatrists are advised not be experts for their patients.

Professional versus expert witness, versus advocate
There is a similar potential for role confusion when forensic psychiatrists give evidence at Mental Health Tribunals (📖 p.V.592). Technically they

appear as professional witnesses (📖 p.V.534) having knowledge of the patient. However, they also provide the Tribunal with expert opinion (📖 p.V.532) about whether the legal criteria for continued detention are fulfilled, including in relation to risk. This situation can be further complicated ethically, in that in some jurisdictions the psychiatrist can elect to represent the detaining hospital (thereby allowing him or her to cross-examine witnesses and put forward argument on behalf of the hospital), although the hospital's interests may directly oppose those of the patient.

Professional versus contractual duty

Psychiatrists may experience conflict between professional duty and contractual duties to their employer, such as when their employer requires them to participate in multi-agency information-sharing regimes such as MAPPA (📖 p.V.468) but they feel that disclosure of certain information would be an unjustifiable breach of confidentiality (📖 p.III.263).

Resolution of role conflicts

As with other examples (e.g. 📖 pp.III.263, III.265) of ethical dilemmas, communication and reflection are important tools for managing, if not resolving, role conflicts. What is crucial is adopting justifiable and transparent process of resolution and a justifiable resolution, clearly articulated as such. It is also worth considering whether conflicts may sometimes be more apparent than real; and whether they are clearly personal or legal.

Professional roles and relationships

Professional roles

The scope and nature of the psychiatrist's professional role is set out in:
- General professional ethical standards for doctors[*] (see 📖 p.III.241)
- Specific professional ethical standards for psychiatrists[†] (see 📖 p.III.241)
- Duties under mental health law
- Duties agreed in their contract and job plan.

The roles and duties of a psychiatrist originate therefore from a mixture of regulatory expectations, professional expectations and employment law. Employers cannot[‡] require employees to carry out actions that would breach their professional duties, if these are clearly and unambiguously relevant to the decision at hand.

---

[*] In the UK, the General Medical Council's several *Good Medical Practice* booklets; in RoI, the Irish Medical Council's *Guide to Professional Conduct and Ethics*.

[†] In the UK, the Royal College of Psychiatrists' several *Good Psychiatric Practice* booklets; in RoI, the College of Psychiatry of Ireland (which split from the UK Royal College in 2009) has not yet produced its own guidance on psychiatric ethics.

[‡] Although this may be the legal position, in practice clinicians may be highly vulnerable to pressure from employers.

All practitioners need to be familiar with the duties and guidance from all these sources. Some of the key duties are:

- To make the care of your patient your first concern
- To practice skilfully and competently
- To keep those skills up to date
- Not to practise in an area beyond your competence
- To be mindful of ethical professional guidance
- To act in ways that uphold the good standing of the profession.

The role of the psychiatrist

A professional relationship is one which draws on the professional's skill and knowledge in order to benefit patients. In their professional role, the psychiatrist will carry out the duties listed in 'Professional roles', 📖 p.III.246. Other duties include:

- Maintaining good working relationships with colleagues and others
- Involving and respecting carers of service users as appropriate
- Participating in teaching and training as appropriate
- Contributing to service improvement through audit and research where possible.

Roles and boundaries

Professional boundaries are determined by the values and behaviours that mark out a doctor's professional identity. Professional identity and boundaries may be set out in codes of practice and ethical guidance (📖 p.III.241) about how a good professional should behave.

Boundary violations (📖 p.V.519) are situations in which a healthcare professional crosses the boundary between their professional and personal identity; promoting their personal values and feelings, and abandoning the professional stance. Boundary crossings may range from the mild and common (e.g. giving a patient a little too much personal information) to the severe and generally unusual (e.g. having a sexual relationship with patients). The severe type of boundary violation usually results in professional or disciplinary proceedings (📖 p.V.521).

Mental health professionals are especially vulnerable to professional boundary violations, because of the emotionally intimate nature of their work. It is not possible (or desirable) to be completely impersonal in mental health work, and so the boundary between the personal and professional is always under strain. This is especially so in forensic work, where staff may have powerful emotional responses to their patients and their offences; or where patients detained for substantial periods of time may exert strong pressures on staff to breach boundaries.

To reduce the risk of boundary violations, all therapeutic work should be discussed in supervision (📖 p.III.252); and it is good practice to reflect on the tension between the personal and professional demands of mental health work in reflective practice (📖 p.III.253).

Professional roles and relationships in forensic psychiatry

Forensic psychiatrists have the same duties within their professional role as do other doctors and psychiatrists. There are two main areas where they may have specific duties:

- In long-stay residential secure care, where much of the care will be delivered by MDTs, there is a particular duty to maintain good professional relationships with other clinicians, such as psychotherapists, psychologists and nursing staff

• In medico-legal work, forensic psychiatrists need to be thoughtful about the type of relationship they have with individuals they evaluate for legal proceedings. Some professionals argue that these are non-therapeutic relationships which are necessary for the proper administration of justice; others argue that doctors cannot have non-therapeutic relationships when they are in professional roles, or that they necessarily utilize therapeutic skills and methods of communication in order to assess for legal purposes (see 📖 pp.III.261, III.265)

It is important to be clear with patients assessed for medico-legal work about the purpose of the assessment and to whom it will be communicated (see 📖 pp.II.90, II.112). Because such assessments are often not primarily for the patient's benefit, it is advised that forensic psychiatrists do not confuse the clinical and expert witness (📖 p.V.534) relationships, especially with patients they are treating (a role conflict, 📖 p.III.244).

Acknowledging uncertainty

Making good judgements

The ability to make good judgements is a skill that we work on throughout our lives; both in our personal and professional lives. It involves awareness of the nature of the question to be addressed, thoughtfulness about context, and discernment of cognitive and emotional bias. Judgements typically become more complex and difficult as we progress through our careers, as well the decisions to be taken becoming more important or serious in nature.

A key feature of medical decision-making is the application of both evidence-based and values-based reflection (📖 p.III.235). Empirical data are often crucial to determining exactly what question is being asked, albeit that most decisions also involve the application of value judgement.

It is therefore essential that doctors are clear about not only what they know, and with what level of confidence, but also what they do not know. In certain circumstances (e.g. where consent to assessment (📖 p.II.112) has been refused by the patient, or an agency has refused to disclose records about the patient), there may be much that the doctor is aware they do not know. It is usually unwise and unsafe to guess, and certainly guessing is no part of 'assessment'. This should be obvious; but a lengthy medical training sometimes leaves juniors with the feeling that they have failed if they admit that they do not know the answer to a question. This might apply to examinations, but has no application in professional life, within which learning can only be achieved by acknowledging both ignorance and uncertainty.

Value judgements are applied not only in weighing one outcome against another (e.g. where different courses of action are being compared) but also in determining what level of probability of outcome is acceptable. Put simply, values are placed upon different outcomes each potentially having a different probability of outcome, where one outcome might be more highly valued than another, but where the probability of each occurring is different. Clearly, different deciders might be differently 'risk averse' such that, for example, two deciders might both agree upon which of two options they value the more highly yet, because the probability of each occurring varies, and because the two deciders are differently risk averse, they might choose different options.

Decision makers sometimes maintain the view that they always make decisions 'wholly rationally' as a means of feeling confident that they have done their best. However, there is evidence to suggest that it is wiser to acknowledge that there are always likely to be gaps and errors in our reasoning. Better decisions may arise from taking uncertainty seriously than going for a simple, certain (and almost certainly wrong) answer.

Clinical uncertainty in forensic psychiatry

Clinical forensic psychiatry requires decision-making in conditions of uncertainty for a number of reasons:

- There is a lack of robust evidence about the efficacy of many treatments in forensic psychiatry; and current practice is often based more on consensus and traditional practice than being evidence based
- There is uncertainty about the reliability and validity of risk assessment (📖 p.II.129). Such uncertainty can provoke anxiety, especially when civil liberties are at stake; or when there are major conflicts of values perspectives between team members, or between different agencies which have to work in concert with one another (e.g. within MAPPA, 📖 p.V.468).

What is crucial, however, is acknowledgment and agreement of what data are available, with transparency about evidence and the values being applied. Sometimes one person, or agency, will emphasize or ignore particular facts so as to justify their particular position. This is empirically unsound and potentially dishonest and unethical. Where there is disagreement about risk assessment, not only the fact, but also the basis of any disagreement must be made apparent.

Within teams acknowledging uncertainty and being open about conflicting values can promote cohesion, particularly when senior staff do so, since this is likely to allow less experienced colleagues to do likewise.

Uncertainty in expert witness practice

In medico-legal practice the adversarial process (📖 p.IV.307) can tend to push experts into expressing greater levels of confidence in their opinion than they might express, for example, in a clinical discussion. That is, the adversarial process tends to polarize evidence.

This emphasizes the importance of acknowledging areas of uncertainty or lack of knowledge in relation to expert testimony (📖 p.V.532), and to be honest in terms of the degree of certainty with which a view is held. Indeed, the duty to the court (📖 p.V.538) specifically requires that an expert sets out areas of uncertainty in his opinion; and failure to do so risks making the whole of one's testimony appear unreliable. Research evidence from the US suggests that juries tend to believe the testimony of experts who express themselves 'about 70% confident' of their opinion over those experts who say that they are 'certain' of their view.

Failure to acknowledge ignorance or uncertainty can lead to an expert straying outside his or her areas of competent expertise, with potential for professional fitness to practise proceedings (📖 p.V.522).

Changing opinions or reports

Proper changes of opinion

In both clinical and medico-legal settings, it is essential to be prepared to change your opinion if new information comes to light that is relevant, or if a new and more appropriate way of formulating existing information into an opinion becomes apparent. Good quality opinions include acknowledgments of uncertainty (📖 p.III.248); and therefore it is both empirically rational and professionally ethical always to be open to appraising fresh information or evidence, or to acknowledge that a different way of analysing available information from the one you have adopted and which has now been demonstrated to you is more appropriate. To do so also shows evidence of intellectual integrity and commitment to objectivity, which are goals of high value in their own right, but evidence of which is also likely to inspire confidence in patients, fellow clinicians, and judges.

Where a previous opinion has been expressed in writing, for example in a report to a court or tribunal, in making changes to one's report, the change should be made transparent, including explaining the rationale for the changes made.

When not to change your opinion

In medico-legal practice, solicitors may ask you to change the opinion set out in your report, because it does not support their case or because it undermines their case (see also 📖 p.V.566). It is clearly wrong to change your opinion in either circumstance. In relation to reports, the only valid reason for changing an opinion is if new evidence or facts have come to light, or been admitted into court. Your duty is to the judicial process and not to the side that has instructed you.

Alternatively, lawyers may request not that you change your opinion but that you remove certain data from the report that you have collected (usually through a clinical interview or interview with informants). Again, circumstances in which this request might reasonably be acceded to are rare. If the data in question are wholly irrelevant to your clinical opinion, and wholly irrelevant to the legal question(s) to which your opinion is to be applied then there may be a basis for removal. However, such circumstances are rare, and great caution should be exercised in acceding to the request. Indeed, there is Court of Appeal ruling indicating that such behaviour by an expert is usually wholly improper. This holds even if, for example, a report is requested for one legal purpose, not used for that purpose but then a request is made for data to be removed so that it can be used to address a different legal issue from the issue to which it was originally directed (e.g. a report not used in relation to trial per se might then be thought of as useful in relation to sentencing). What matters is the use to which it is now intended to apply the report, and whether the data, though not relevant to the original legal purpose of the report is relevant to the new purpose.

When not to give an opinion

Hopefully rarely, instructing solicitors may state that they are seeking an expert opinion that will state or support a particular position, for example after having received an unhelpful report from another expert. Experts should never take instructions on this basis. To accept instructions on such a basis would be prima facie evidence of misconduct in expert testimony and potentially grounds for complaints to the GMC.

Disclosure by the author of a report

Your report technically belongs to those who instruct you; and they are at liberty not to disclose it if the rules of procedure relevant to the case at hand allow this (not applicable to family proceedings concerning children, and largely only applicable to the defence in criminal proceedings).

Where a report is not used, there is a duty of confidentiality upon the author not to share the contents of the report (including the opinion) with anyone else without the consent of the instructing solicitors. However, disclosure may be lawful where it is deemed to be in the public interest, for example in order to reduce 'a significant risk of serious harm to the public' (*W v Egdell*, 📖 p.App. 3.635); or where it is deemed in the public interest that the report be disclosed in the public interest for the administration of justice, for example in relation to proper sentencing of a defendant (*Crozier*, 📖 p.App. 3.634) (see 📖 p.V.540). However, the process may be uncomfortable and you are advised to seek legal advice before doing so.

Vignette: changing your opinion in court

You are asked by the defence to assess a defendant charged with murdering a man whom he had met once previously and who he alleges sexually assaulted him immediately prior to his killing him.

You assess him and diagnose schizoid and avoidant personality disorder (📖 p.II.58). You also note his uncertain sexual identity, with a tendency towards homosexuality, but you have no evidence of deviant sexual behaviour (📖 p.II.197).

While you are giving evidence, the jury is asked to leave and the prosecution indicates to the judge that they have new evidence: substantial quantities of sadomasochistic pornographic material on the defendant's computer. However, this is ruled inadmissible (📖 p.IV.318) because it was not disclosed to the defence within the relevant time limit. The new evidence significantly affects your assessment of the risk of inappropriate sexual behaviour (📖 p.II.134), in your opinion, and also bears on your evidence in support of his pleas of diminished responsibility (📖 p.V.491) and loss of control (📖 p.V.498).

Do you continue to give evidence after the jury returns as if nothing has happened, or do you ask to stop and change your opinion, even though explaining why will mean disclosing inadmissible information and therefore possibly the collapse of this trial and the need for a retrial?

Supervision, peer review and reflective practice

As a trainee or career junior doctor, you should have access to regular supervision from trusted senior colleagues. Generally, this will be the consultant for whom you work; although it need not be. As a senior you should be exposed routinely to peer review, including of expert witness work.

Supervision

The purposes of supervision for the junior are to allow them to learn more about the profession on which they have embarked, and to develop their professional identity. It is therefore important that they feel able to ask the supervisor questions, and to explore uncertainties; especially about ethical dilemmas in psychiatry. A supervisory space should not be a test of knowledge but an opportunity to reflect upon practice, both technically and ethically.

However, a supervisor will ideally be a good source of feedback about performance and will contribute to the trainee's overall evaluation. It is therefore important that the trainee feels comfortable with their regular supervisor; if they do not, it may be sensible to ask for regular supervision elsewhere, from an additional supervisor. It is important to discuss this with the tutor or educational supervisor.

Clinical supervision is particularly important in psychiatry because psychiatric practice is emotionally and personally demanding in ways that other branches of medicine are not. Psychiatrists are over-represented amongst doctors with mental health problems, substance misuse problems and as subjects of fitness to practice hearings (🕮 p.V.522).

It is therefore very important for the trainee to take their own mind and feelings seriously; and regularly to consider the impact of their professional work on their personal life, and vice versa. Emotional detachment may be valuable in emergency medicine and surgery, but is neither entirely possible, nor necessarily desirable, in psychiatry. Using supervision to reflect on these issues is a key professional competence in psychiatry, as is training towards later supervising others as a senior psychiatrist. Balint groups should be available for all trainees, designed to help the exploration of emotional reactions to clinical work.

Peer review and support for the consultant

None of the foregoing ceases to be relevant when a trainee takes up a consultant post in psychiatry. Mentoring during the early years of appointment is highly valuable and regular peer group discussion should be available to (and taken up by) all psychiatrists. This will become even more obviously important in the UK once revalidation and re-licensing is in place. Within forensic psychiatry discussion of medico-legal aspects of the work will be important, even for those psychiatrists who do little court work, since all psychiatrists give evidence to Mental Health Tribunals, and even this gives rise to major challenges (see 🕮 pp.V.567, V.592).

Expert witness work (🕮 p.V.531) is frequently 'reviewed' by lawyers and courts and sometimes opposing experts, but this alone would be inadequate, particularly given the clinical, medico-legal and ethical potential pitfalls of the work. All forensic psychiatrists conducting any medico-legal work should include that work in their regular peer review and support arrangements.

An additional reason for this is the risk of 'baseline drift': that is, of becoming systematically biased towards the defence or prosecution cases.* This risk is considerable in forensic psychiatry, with its scope for value judgement, or the intrusion of personal values (📖 p.V.551) into professional opinions.

Reflective practice

This has been described as the capacity to reflect on action so as to engage in a process of continuous learning, and as a defining characteristic of professional practice. It involves attending critically to the values and theories which inform professionals' actions, by examining practice and gaining insights that lead to personal and team development.

Whereas supervision and peer review are usually one-to-one activities, reflective practice often most beneficially involves group discussions: although not essential, the group discussion introduces several perspectives on work and may help question and challenge assumptions that have caused problems. Psychiatrists who work in MDTs (📖 p.III.256) should encourage the team to participate as a whole in a reflective practice group, if it does not do so already.

Various formal models of reflective practice exist: in essence, they all provide techniques for asking oneself to recall significant events and outcomes in recent practice; to evaluate them critically; and to consider what might be done differently in the future to improve those outcomes.

---

*The risk of baseline drift is recognized in forensic pathology, for example: in order to join the Home Office list of accredited forensic pathologists, the pathologist must practice within a peer group and participate in peer review.

Conflicting ethical values

Working in multidisciplinary teams

As the practice of medicine becomes more complex, there has been a need for different types of expertise to deliver best quality care. Doctors are required to work effectively in teams with other colleagues as a matter of good medical practice, as defined by the GMC. Breakdowns in team functioning can lead to impaired patient care and increased risk. It is therefore essential that all psychiatrists understand, and respect, the different professionals who also offer care to patients who use mental health services. This is particularly true in forensic psychiatry, where it is certainly not possible for the doctor to deliver all aspects of patient care. The team is the repository of both technical and ethical decision-making.

Multidisciplinary team (MDT) members and their roles

Most MDTs consist of a psychiatrist, psychologist, nurse, occupational therapist, social worker and possibly a creative/forensic psychotherapist (e.g. music/drama and/or arts therapist).

The *psychiatrist* typically manages the diagnostic and pharmacological treatment of the patient. They are usually also the responsible clinician (RC, 🕮 p.IV.379) or equivalent, although in E&W this role can be taken by any member of the MDT who is suitably qualified and experienced. The RC is legally responsible for the treatment and management of detained patients; and for making sure that all involuntary treatments are lawfully given. Consultant psychiatrists are usually in the position of being the MDT leader; which requires leadership skills of communication, consultation and confidence of authority.

The *clinical psychologist* in a team has specialist experience of the assessment and treatment of psychological disorders and distress. Clinical psychologists undergo a three-year doctoral level training in all aspects of clinical work, in addition to their basic undergraduate degree. Clinical psychology training is highly competitive. In addition to clinical training, clinical psychologists in forensic services may have additional clinical or research experience in different settings. Clinical psychologists in forensic services usually have expertise in risk assessment; the use of specialist psychological tools and treatment programmes that involve psychological techniques such as cognitive and behavioural therapies. Psychology services also include assistant psychologists who are professionals, who typically have an undergraduate degree but have not yet managed to get a place on a clinical training, and/or trainee psychologists, who are currently completing the doctoral course.

The MDT may also include *forensic psychologists*, and trainee forensic psychologists, who train in various forensic settings, such as prisons, probation or secure hospital settings, and so have wide experience of assessing offenders, and delivering offence based interventions. However, forensic psychologists have not completed a clinical training; and therefore may have less experience with mental illness and its management.

The *nurses* in forensic mental health services have different roles depending on the service setting. Qualified nurses have a specialist mental health nursing qualification; and generally have management roles in relation to unqualified nursing staff, such as healthcare assistants. Healthcare assistants may have an undergraduate degree (such as psychology) but do not have further qualifications.

Community teams include nursing staff whose role is to make good therapeutic relationships with patients; and often act as a liaison between the patient, the patient's carers, and the rest of the MDT. They also work closely with the psychiatrist in relation to medication delivery.

In secure residential settings, nursing staff (📖 p.II.177) are responsible for the day-to-day care of the patient. They will also be responsible for managing the security requirements of inpatient settings. They often have enhanced understanding of the patient's mental mechanisms and mental state; however they are also subject to increased stress and anxiety because of their close and prolonged contact with forensic patients. Both psychiatrists and psychologists in forensic MDTs are expected to be able to support the nursing role; and to work closely with senior nurses as part of the management of the service.

The *occupational therapist* (📖 p.II.181) is trained to understand both the effects of mental disorder on work and creative function; and to offer interventions that promote recovery. They typically work closely with both psychologists and nursing staff, especially in inpatient settings.

The *social worker* (📖 p.II.180) in a forensic MDT may or may not have specialist forensic experience. They typically have a degree in social work; then acquire mental health experience.

Forensic psychotherapists consist of a range of professionals, such as creative therapists (drama, music or arts therapy; see 📖 p.II.169), medical psychotherapists or psychologists.

Disputes within teams

All groups of highly experienced professionals are likely to disagree about the management of complex cases at times; and it must be remembered that dissent can be healthy in a group. Often the person who is dissenting holds a very important piece of information that needs consideration (however uncomfortable). All members of MDTs need to be thoughtful about the potential for blaming all of a team's difficulties on one person (scapegoating).

It is important that teams have some framework for managing disputes to prevent them becoming personal and angry. Use of reflective practice time (📖 p.III.253) is beneficial; especially for teams dealing with complex patients. The Department of Health recommends mandatory reflective practice time for services managing patients with personality disorder (📖 p.II.58), especially forensic ones. Professionals who know the team and the work but who are independent of the team (such as forensic psychotherapists or other senior professionals) may be useful here.

Working with other agencies

Agencies commonly encountered

Psychiatry inevitably involves working with many different professional groups and intellectual communities, because it relates to different social worlds.

As a healthcare service, forensic psychiatry needs to relate to other social care and welfare services, for example:

- Other branches of medicine
- Social care services (including child protection)
- Housing agencies
- Charities and other voluntary bodies.

However, forensic psychiatry also interfaces with non-welfare related justice agencies, whose purposes, cultures, and ways of working are very different from those of welfare agencies. Forensic teams therefore also relate to:

- Lawyers (solicitors, barristers and judges)
- Courts and tribunals (📖 p.IV.308)
- Prisons (📖 p.V.456)
- Probation services (📖 p.V.462)
- Police and other criminal investigatory bodies (📖 p.V.449)
- Prosecution agencies (📖 p.V.448)
- The Ministry of Justice (and equivalents in Scotland, NI and RoI, 📖 p.V.464)

Finally, forensic psychiatrists in the three UK jurisdictions are expected to participate directly in public protection, and the public management of any risk posed by forensic patients. This is usually under the auspices of the MAPPA (📖 p.V.468). This raises major legal and ethical challenges.

What does 'working with' agencies mean?

Many of the earlier listed agencies will be involved in the life of any single forensic patient. Some will be able to assist in their rehabilitation and recovery; others will have no interest in the forensic patient's welfare, but be concerned solely with public safety (their only interest in the patient's welfare will arise from what linkage their might be between his mental disorder and risk of harming others).

'Working with' usually involves establishing professional cordial relations and channels of communication. Discussions may be had; if so, notes of them should be kept and checked by both parties.

Written reports about the patient's condition, treatment and prognosis may be requested by any of the earlier listed agencies. As with any other report (📖 p.V.558), nothing should be committed to paper unless and until the author has established:

- What is the possible purpose of this report?
- Who will see it?
- Can the recipient guarantee its confidentiality?
- What are the specific questions that need addressing?
- Has the patient agreed to this report being written?
- If the patient has refused permission, is this a case where it may be possible to justify writing a report without consent?

It is important to remember that just because someone important sounding asks for a report, or some feedback, does not mean that it has to be given. If in doubt seek advice (if you are a junior, seek this from senior colleagues).

Special ethical problems 'working with' justice agencies

As has been noted elsewhere (📖 p.III.263), the main ethical tension in working with other agencies is in relation to privacy and disclosure of confidential information about forensic patients. Other agencies have different professional agendas and ethical obligations from health agencies; and may be insistent that psychiatrists help them to deliver these, even if to do so would mean that the psychiatrist breaches his obligations.

There is ethical guidance for NHS employees about confidentiality in general (2006); and in relation to MAPPA. The GMC also provide guidance about confidentiality obligations. However, there is often little specific advice about how much information to disclose or in what detail; nor is there defining guidance on whether public safety interests trump duties of confidentiality.

The core ethical basis for breach of confidence within health service provision is on a 'need to know' basis, where the need to know is defined in terms of needing to know in order better to effect the patient's health and welfare. It has become customary, however, to use the term also in relation to non-welfare, that is justice, agencies, in relation to the objective of public safety. This is profoundly misguided. The only justification for breach of confidence where the purpose is not the patient's own welfare is where breach is in the public interest, on the *Egdell* principle (📖 pp.App 3.635, III.263), that is, where without breach there would be a significant risk of serious harm to others.

There is a danger that, where health and justice agencies work closely together, including sitting in rooms together discussing an individual, the proper boundaries around function, and information, will become blurred or lost. Also, rather than reports into MAPPA by healthcare professionals being written specifically for the MAPPA purpose, with information that should not be share excluded, existing health originating reports will be offered (if only because of time constraints). This must be resisted.

Notably, the police rarely share all relevant information they have relating to an individual within MAPPA. Health agencies should be similarly cautious.

It is better to conceptualize relationships with justice related agencies not as 'working with' but as 'working alongside'.

Working with other public bodies

Other public bodies commonly met in forensic psychiatry

As described elsewhere (📖 p.IV.299), forensic psychiatric practice inevitably involves working at the interface with different social systems that are given power and resources to protect public welfare. On preceding pages, we have described the agencies that forensic psychiatrists may encounter clinically. Here we describe the public bodies that they are likely to have to encounter professionally.

An 'agency' provides a service to citizens. In contrast, a 'public body' is a group, usually set up by parliamentary statute and principally funded by government, to contribute to the process of government.

There are over 700 non-departmental public bodies working in E&W alone. They are affiliated with government departments, but operate at a remove, so as to encourage independence.

Forensic psychiatrists may be invited to advise or work with:
- NHS/HSE provider bodies, such as Hospitals[*] and Foundation Trusts
- NHS/HSE commissioning bodies, such as PCTs, Health Boards, etc.
- The Law Commission or its equivalents[†]
- The Parole Boards
- The Care Quality Commission or its equivalents[‡]
- Advisory committees such as the Sentencing Advisory Panel and Victims' Advisory Panel.

What does 'working with' with public bodies mean?

As with other agencies (📖 p.III.256), 'working with' usually involves establishing professional cordial relations and channels of communication. Written communication should be kept and where discussions are had, notes should be kept and agreed by both parties.

The psychiatrist working with these bodies will usually do so in an advisory/expert capacity, either as an individual or as a representative of a medical body, such as the Royal College of Psychiatrists. They will usually be invited to provide general advice and advice. Individual clinical material is unlikely to be involved; although where this is the case, the usual advice about confidentiality should be observed (📖 p.III.263). Where service related research is commissioned there may be issues which arise about interpretation of the findings if conflict arises between the service researcher and the commissioner of the research and this may present ethical problems for the researcher.

Problems relating to commissioning of services

In those countries that maintain a split between commissioners and providers of health services (chiefly NI and E&W), there are particular problems concerning confidentiality of clinical information. In some circumstances, commissioners conduct 'micro-commissioning' of specialist services for named individual patients, including some forensic patients. Commissioning staff may then request detailed information about patients, or seek to approve detailed care plans for patients themselves, including adopting their own risk assessments.

Such practices are ethically problematic for a number of reasons. First, the commissioning staff do not have the same clinical or ethical duties to patients as psychiatrists do, so there may be conflict between what is in the patient's best interests and what is in the commissioner's interests. Psychiatrists operating as Clinical Directors, or Medical Directors, may be particularly affected by such potential conflict.

---

[*] Scotland has abolished the commissioner/provider distinction for secondary care, and it has never existed in RoI; in these countries, the same bodies usually both plan and provide care.
[†] The NI Law Commission, the Scottish Law Commission, and in RoI the Law Reform Commission.
[‡] e.g. The Health Information and Quality Authority in RoI.

Second, the commissioner may not be competent to carry out these assessments; yet they are the chief source of funding for the psychiatrist's employer and to criticize them may adversely affect career prospects.

Faced with potential conflict, or significant concerns about the uses to which a commissioner might put confidential information, it would be wise to seek advice from the doctor's defence organization, or directly from the GMC, and to present that advice to the commissioner with which the doctor is in dispute. The ethical duties owed by doctors to patients may override legal duties under doctors' employment contracts, when they conflict

Working in non-therapeutic contexts

A therapeutic context is one in which the forensic psychiatrist is working as a doctor addressing the clinical needs of an individual patient. A non-therapeutic context is one in which there is no individual doctor–patient relationship; and where the psychiatrist is invited by some agency, public body, court or tribunal to provide information, with or without an opinion, that is not directed at any benefit of the individual who is the subject of the information or opinion but at some other social purpose. This can arise either because the doctor is giving information not about an individual 'patient' but in the aggregate, albeit to a health or welfare body (📖 p.III.256), or because they are giving information and opinion about an individual but to a non-health related agency (📖 p.III.259).

Examples

A forensic psychiatrist who gives advice to the Care Quality Commission about services for mentally abnormal offenders is working in a non-therapeutic context in that they are using their professional expertise to assist a public body (📖 p.III.259) in circumstances where no individual patient's welfare is considered.

A forensic psychiatrist who discusses a patient's clinical condition with a social worker or housing officer in an effort to find the patient housing is working in a therapeutic context, in that the patient's welfare is a key aspect of the discussion. In a therapeutic context, the UK General Medical Council advises doctors that they must 'make the care of my patient my first concern'.

A forensic psychiatrist giving evidence in relation to diminished responsibility (📖 p.V.491) within a murder trial, for either the defence or prosecution, is not acting therapeutically, even though the evidence is about an individual, because the purpose is a justice one and not a therapeutic one. Giving evidence about risk of harm to others to a court in relation to imposition of an indeterminate sentence is clearly not therapeutic in nature or purpose.

Even giving evidence in favour of a criminal court making a hospital order (📖 p.IV.405) under mental health law is not a therapeutic act, even where the defendant is the doctor's patient already, because the purpose of the court is sentencing, albeit therapy may be facilitated by imposition of a hospital order. Particular ethical issues arise in relation to assessment for, and giving evidence about, either verdict (📖 p.V.543) or sentencing (📖 p.V.547) issues.

Argument with the therapeutic-non-therapeutic distinction

It is often argued that that there cannot ever be a 'non-therapeutic' context for doctors; and that there is always an overriding medical duty to any potential patient. This implies that the doctor must never act so as to intend to cause a potential patient harm.

Consider the following example. An indeterminate sentence (📖 p.IV.364) may be passed in most jurisdictions for the purpose of public protection, if the judge decides the offender is 'dangerous' (📖 p.V.549). A forensic psychiatrist may be instructed by the Crown or the defence to assess the defendant and give an opinion on their risk. Clearly evidence stating, or inferring that the defendant is dangerous may influence the judge towards imposing an indeterminate sentence, which the defendant is not likely to see as being in his interest. Some would argue that a doctor should never provide any testimony that might harm an individual's interests. On this argument, any doctor who gives evidence for the prosecution has improperly abandoned medical duties.

Counter-arguments

If psychiatrists were never to work in non-therapeutic contexts, then public bodies and courts would not be able to benefit from their expertise. The professional knowledge that doctors have is acquired for the public good as a whole; and not just for individual advocacy. The process of either health and welfare provision or of justice may be threatened without such information; in a way that constitutes the potential for harm, or loss of welfare, to the body of citizens.

A further argument against working solely within an individual therapeutic model is that the doctor may have more than one individual's welfare to consider. A common example is where a psychiatrist considers that a mother may pose a risk to her baby. The mother will be distressed to be separated from her child; but the doctor cannot avoid putting the child's interests above the mother's, even if the baby is not their patient and so the situation is not simply one of competing interests between two of their patients.

Finally, some argue that the core of forensic psychiatric practice is the pursuit of public safety. Hence, if psychiatrists do not participate in non-therapeutic work they will deny society the benefits of their conducting risk assessments.

It is also argued that good-quality risk assessment benefit patients; because preventing the commission of an offence, prevents a patient suffering the harmful consequences of any such offence for him. Although some would argue that preventing a patient from harming others is in their interests, this is not a principle which is applied to any other citizen without a mental disorder, and is therefore discriminatory.

Conclusion

If what psychiatrists do may cause people harm, they need to be open and honest about it. They also need to be as objective and transparent as possible in collecting information and coming to their opinions.

Confidentiality and disclosure

The medical duty of confidentiality is based on the principle of respect for autonomy (📖 p.III.275); that people should have control over their personal information as a matter of principle. It also recognizes that, in medical treatment situations, people need to share information with doctors that could make them vulnerable to social shame or criticism; and that they would not otherwise share such information, which could harm their health or that of others (e.g. in the case of an infectious disease). For both reasons there is said legally to be not just a private interest but also a public interest in keeping confidentiality.

Article 8 of the ECHR (📖 p.IV.420) gives individuals rights to a private life, which includes privacy of healthcare information. Under the law in the UK and RoI, medical information is protected by the Data Protection Act; and express consent is required from a patient before private medical information can be disclosed. It is accepted that members of clinical teams and service providers will share information with each other in order to provide good quality medical care, on a 'need to know' basis; including for purposes of audit and service evaluation. However, in effect, a patient's medical information is their property, and may not be disclosed without consent.

Consent to disclosure is not usually difficult to obtain. Patients may request that information is not shared with certain family members; and such requests should generally be respected. Patients may themselves access any part of their medical record, unless to do so would present a serious risk to someone else.

Disclosure and risk

The duty of confidentiality has never been synonymous with secrecy; and breaches of confidentiality are nearly always justified in terms of either harms averted or benefits gained. The UK General Medical Council takes the view that it is permissible to disclose medical information to the police for the 'prevention, detection and prosecution of serious crime'. In the case of possible harm to others, GMC guidance states that doctors 'should' disclose information if it is necessary to protect a person from *death or serious harm*. The GMC also offers guidance about contacting licensing authorities about drivers (📖 p.IV.439) whose medical conditions put them at risk of causing harm to others and who refuse to disclose the relevant information.

In all cases, it is advised that doctors should try to obtain consent for disclosure from their patients; if only to let them know that there is a risk issue that is of concern. In many cases, patients may be happy to give consent to disclosure; especially if the limits of disclosure are made clear.

If the patient cannot be persuaded to inform the licensing authority, or if the doctor has evidence that they are continuing to drive, the doctor must disclose their medical condition to the authority, and let the patient know that they have done this.

Disclosure without consent or in the face of refusal

Harm to others

If the perceived risk of serious harm to others is great, and disclosure is likely to help to avert that harm, then disclosure of a patient's information may be permissible, even if they have refused, or if necessary without their knowledge. The test is that there must be 'a significant risk of serious harm to others' (*W v Egdell*, 📖 p.App 3.635). In all cases, there is an expectation that all such disclosures, especially without the patient's' knowledge, will be discussed with senior colleagues and with those in charge of information governance and management within the organization. Justification for such decisions needs to be recorded in writing. *Egdell* also sets the bar high for the right of a clinician to disclose information, and so is also a basis for keeping confidence in most cases.

There is a general expectation that doctors will take an active role in public protection; and will contribute to crime detection and prevention. For example, doctors are now required to inform the police if a patient is admitted to hospital with gunshot or stab wounds (unless if self-inflicted).

Legal proceedings

Similar issues relate to confidentiality in regard to reports prepared for criminal court proceedings on the instruction of the defence. Although such reports cannot be disclosed by their author to anybody other than the defence solicitors, there can be circumstances where that rule can legally be breached, mainly in relation to sentencing.

In the case of *R v Crozier* (📖 p.App 3.634) a defence-instructed psychiatrist disclosed his report against the wishes of the defence to the court, on the basis that the court had a legitimate interest in seeing it in relation to sentence. As a result the court substituted a hospital order with restrictions (📖 p.IV.412) for a determinate prison sentence (📖 p.IV.366). The defendant subsequently failed in an action for breach of confidence.

Otherwise, a court can, in certain circumstances, require disclosure of medical information, against the wishes of both patient and doctor.

Sharing information with justice agencies

Current guidance and case law has implications for forensic psychiatric practice, since most patients will (on paper) pose a high risk of causing some harm to others in the long term. Hence, questions concerning the extent to which there can be valid disclosure of personal information (e.g. in MAPP arrangements, 📖 p.V.468) may regularly arise. Many community forensic patients may be regular suspects in criminal investigations; and mentally disordered patients will often be the focus of violent crime investigations. It is important therefore to inform forensic patients early that it may not be possible for them to enjoy the same degree of confidentiality, with regard to personal information, as non offender patients.

Vignettes: do I disclose?

Mr P has made good progress in the medium secure unit (📖 p.II.210). He has been compliant with his depot medication (📖 p.II.159), and has been conditionally discharged (📖 p.IV.413) to live in a hostel for ex-offenders with mental illness. A level 2 MAPP meeting (📖 p.V.468) has been called at which Mr P is to be discussed. He consents to you disclosing his diagnosis, his current care plan and a few details of his history.

At the meeting, a police officer is present, who listens to your report, and then says 'He sounds like a Mr P who we interviewed on several occasions in relation to the murder of two prostitutes three years ago. The murders have not been solved. If this is the same guy, then he also has a long history of domestic violence, but his ex-partner wouldn't press charges. Can we come and interview him again?'

Mr P's social worker has accompanied you to the meeting. She suggests that Mr P's latest risk assessment (📖 p.II.127) should be circulated to the meeting to assist in deliberations. She also raises the question of whether on the basis of the police officer's information Mr P should be recalled to hospital (📖 p.V.467), and advises you to contact the Mental Health Unit at the Ministry of Justice (📖 p.V.464).

Should you agree to the police officer's request and the social worker's suggestions? The discussion earlier in this topic and elsewhere in this chapter should help you decide.

An alternative scenario

Consider Mr Q, a middle-aged man who has been admitted to a low secure ward (📖 p.II.211) after having been convicted of ABH (📖 p.IV.346): he had assaulted his wife during an episode of depression (📖 p.II.69) complicated by narcissistic and antisocial personality traits not amounting to personality disorder (📖 p.II.58).

During the admission, he begins to show choreiform movements that worsen progressively. A neurological examination suggests Huntington's disease, which is confirmed by genetic testing. In hindsight, you realize that his depression was probably an early presentation of the Huntington's disease, and that he may well have been predisposed to violence by the condition.

The geneticist informs you that there is a high probability that some of his children are carriers of the disease or will go on to develop it themselves. Both his daughter and one of his sons are planning to start families with their partners.

Mr Q refuses consent (📖 p.III.278) to disclosure of his condition to his children, and you are satisfied that he has the capacity (📖 p.IV.424) to do so.

Should you breach confidentiality (📖 p.III.263) and make the disclosure to his children, in their interests and those of their potential children? Is your decision affected by the possible relationship between his condition and his index offence and risk of violence (📖 p.II.132)?

Ethical risk assessment & management

An ethical analysis of risk assessment

Risk assessment is a form of consequential analysis: not a prediction of future events (📖 p.II.128) but an assessment of the likelihood of various scenarios in which harm might occur within a given period of time. If a person with mental disorder is assessed as being likely to cause serious harm in the near future, then others may believe it is their professional duty to intervene to reduce that likelihood; and failure to do so may lead to professional criticism, as in the Barrett inquiry[*] (🕮 p.App 5.624).

For this reason, some psychiatrists may wish to avoid risk assessment altogether, but risk-taking is unavoidable in psychiatry (🕮 p.II.129) as in the rest of medicine, and choosing to take such risks while being wilfully blind to their nature and magnitude is neither ethically nor legally defensible.

However, actions that reduce the likelihood of an offender causing harm may result in conditions that the offender perceives as harmful, such as loss of liberty through detention in secure conditions (🕮 p.II.152). The offender may also perceive himself to be wronged: for example, if professionals fail to inform them, or even deceive them, about disclosure of confidential information (🕮 p.III.263). Even the very fact of being known to have been the subject of a forensic risk assessment, whatever the result, can stigmatize patients.

The question of consent

Doctors may not take actions that could harm a patient without seeking their informed consent (🕮 p.III.275), and can act in the absence of consent only where there is a specific legal power to do so. If a patient has consented in full knowledge of how their interests might be harmed, there is no ethical dilemma in carrying out a risk assessment, and for this reason some advocate seeking consent to risk assessment (🕮 p.III.284). This is, in effect, to treat risk assessment[†] as a technical clinical procedure, akin to CBT (🕮 p.II.165) or, say, colonoscopy.

In many situations in forensic psychiatry, either it will be reasonable not to perform the risk assessment if consent is refused, or there will be a legal power that clearly overrides a patient's refusal of consent. However, scenarios such as that presented in the box that follows pose serious problems, and in those many psychiatrists will proceed with risk assessment on the ground that the benefits to others (e.g. staff and other patients in hospital, or in this case Mr E's children and potentially the children of others) outweigh the possible harm to the patient:

---

[*] The details of this case were more complicated than suggested in the text; for example, the patient's RMO had believed at the time that he was not at high risk of causing serious harm.
[†] 'Risk assessment' here refers to a formal process, particularly when carried out by a team using a structured instrument such as the HCR20. If the term is used in the more general sense of 'reaching an opinion on the risk the patient poses', especially a single, personal opinion, then it is not meaningful to seek consent for the forming of that opinion; but consent might be needed before acting on that opinion as part of a risk management plan, or disclosing it to others.

Mr E is suspected by the police of a contact child sexual offence, but is not prosecuted due to lack of evidence. He is treated informally on a general psychiatric ward for a transient psychotic episode related to an established diagnosis of borderline personality disorder. His treating team wish to assess his risk of sexual offending in order to assist social services in deciding whether (and subject to what conditions) he should return to live with his children. However, he refuses consent, fearing that the result might adversely affect his contact with his children. The MDT decide that they have no choice but to conduct the assessment nevertheless, using information already available to them.

Transparency and joint enterprise

If harm is to be done to the patient (or potential harm to be risked) because the interests of others have been allowed to override the patient's interests, then it is essential that clinicians are honest with themselves and colleagues about this; and that they are open about it with the patient. It may be debatable whether it is acceptable for forensic psychiatrists, as doctors, to act against the patient's interests in this way; it is certainly not acceptable for them to deceive the patient about doing so and to claim that they are acting covertly for their benefit.

Being open about this process risks damaging the therapeutic relationship with the patient; but the risk of serious long-term damage to the relationship from a covert approach is far greater, should the patient subsequently learn of how they have been deceived and harmed. Moreover, building a long-term relationship based upon openness facilitates approaching risk assessment as a joint enterprise with the patient, within which their different values perspective (📖 p.III.235) is acknowledged and respected despite being overridden.

Reporting the results of assessment

Once a risk assessment has been performed, a further ethical dilemma may arise in having to decide whether to disclose it to others, and in particular whether to include it in a court report if its conclusions are against the patient's interest as he is likely to perceive it. There may be a specific legal duty to disclose it (e.g. in response to a subpoena, 📖 p.III.264) or to include it in a report (📖 p.V.555) in certain circumstances. Otherwise, as with the decision to perform the original risk assessment, there should only be disclosure, or inclusion, if there is a compelling reason to override the patient's interest in favour of the interest of others.

Organizational liability and the 'tick-list' mentality

Situations within which a patient's interest in not undergoing risk assessment may be overridden must be considered on a case-by-case basis. It is not acceptable to adopt a blanket policy of risk assessment, particularly if coupled with disclosure, solely in order to discharge or limit the corporate responsibility of the organization.

Philosophy and ethics of coercion

Legislation in the UK and RoI allows involuntary treatment for mental disorder even where the patient retains the capacity (📖 p.IV.424) to decide for themselves, and without reference to their best interests (📖 p.III.277). This remains ethically contentious, especially given that healthcare is otherwise increasingly directed towards enhancing patient autonomy (📖 p.III.275), and because of the impact of coercion on treatment (📖 p.II.152).

What is coercion?

The starting point is that coercion is the use of force on another person in order to change their behaviour, whether that amounts to physical force or the use of threats, rewards, intimidation or other measures (i.e. objective coercion, 📖 p.II.149). However, this ignores a number of subtleties, not least the fact that the coercion noted by an 'objective' observer may be very different to the coercion perceived by the subject.

Is coercion identical with legal compulsion in mental health settings?

There is a considerable quantity of evidence that involuntary legal status is a poor gauge of perceived coercion (📖 p.II.149). In any case, significant variations in the terms of legal coercion between jurisdictions renders the identification of coercion with legal status inadequate; legal criteria for commitment are too diverse to provide anything approaching a uniform definition of even objective coercion.

Definitions of coercion by involuntary legal status also fail to do justice to, the complexity of a construct that has been the subject of much philosophical debate. Many philosophers defined coercion as a state-sanctioned imposition on personal autonomy, a forceful intervention justified under certain social conditions and contracts; whereas to more recent commentators, coercion is viewed as the narrowing of an agent's rational choices within interpersonal negotiations.

The relationship of coercion to agency

Agency, to a philosopher, is a person's capacity to act: to make choices and then to impose those choices on the world. Coercion in psychiatric settings, whether related to legal status or other factors, usually significantly impairs the patient's sense of agency, but coercion fails to explain the full effect on that sense of agency. In addition, the social status of being a patient (particularly a psychiatric patient, and especially a forensic psychiatric patient) itself affects patients' agency, both by limiting the choices the patient believes they are able to make as a patient, and by limiting the choices other people will respect[*].

There is a related debate about the degree of agency that should be ascribed to someone who is the subject of coercion. Does being coerced remove their agency altogether; or does it act through agency, by altering the choices the subject would otherwise make? These questions have relevance for the closely related ideas that the presence of coercion negates mental capacity (📖 p.IV.424), and that a lack of capacity precludes the possibility of coercion. In relevant practical terms, does the offer of

---

[*]For example, a shopkeeper might refuse to sell an expensive item to a patient, wrongly believing them to be unable to pay, or to lack the capacity to make legal contracts.

'leverage' (e.g. an inducement such as the offer of a hostel or flat, or even money) leave the patient with more agency, despite the experience of perceived coercion—or somehow with less?

Perspectives on coercion

Not only is legal status inadequate as a measure of coercion, so are instruments which purport to measure perceived coercion (📖 p.II.149). A social science critique of the 'clinico-ethical' paradigm represented by, for example, the MPCS (📖 p.II.149), is that it attempts to reduce patient experiences that do not exist in isolation but which depend upon interaction with others and the environment to a delineated, quasi-clinical concept, which is externally imposed upon the patient's experience. That is, much is lost by defining the experience in a manner which allows it to be measured. Sources and domains of coercion are better measured qualitatively by patient's stories, which can capture subtlety of experience.

When is coercion justified?

How this question is answered depends to a great extent to the ethical value placed on individual autonomy versus that placed on paternalism (e.g. improving the objective health of the patient, or protecting society from harm by the patient).

Coercion into treatment is generally motivated by concern for the welfare and safety of the individual, or of others, with any loss of individual agency, justified by way of an overall ethical calculus addressing both individual and social risks and benefits. There is a policy assumption that the liberty costs of legal coercion are outweighed by welfare benefits to patients or society. This assumption of net ethical gain emphasizes the importance of determining whether such coercion actually results in improved mental health outcomes (see 📖 p.II.152).

Clinical situations raising ethical issues

Concepts of mental disorder

In clinical settings, forensic psychiatrists use the same diagnostic systems as all other psychiatrists, most notably the ICD and the DSM (📖 p.II.109). Like other psychiatrists, they work in MDTs (📖 p.III.256) and therefore require some familiarity with the concepts of mental disorder used by other mental health professionals. However, forensic psychiatrists, to a greater degree than other psychiatrists, also work alongside professionals from other agencies (📖 p.III.258) concerned neither with health nor welfare, which have their own, conflicting contructs (📖 p.IV.296) of mental disorder. The use of some of these constructs, if only for the purpose of translation (📖 p.IV.299), can involve an ethical tension.

Models used by mental health professionals

The *medical model* of mental disorder assumes that it represents the presence of disease that can be treated by medical interventions (particularly medication) and thereby relieved or even cured. This works relatively well for mental illnesses such as depression (📖 p.II.69), but less well for axis II disorders such as personality disorder (📖 p.II.58) and autism (📖 p.II.76), which have to be treated as if they were congenital diseases.

Psychologists use a variety of *psychological models* of mental disorder (e.g. cognitive behavioural, 📖 p.II.165; mentalization-based, 📖 p.II.166; systemic, 📖 p.II.174), all of which treat individuals as having a greater or lesser degree of a particular trait, dimension or difficulty. The concept of 'abnormality' exists, but relative to an ultimately arbitrary cut-off on each dimension, rather than a disease category.

Social workers' training focuses on the amelioration of individuals' social deprivation: not only disease, but also poverty, and various forms of material and political inequality. Social work models do not grant mental disorder any special status relative to other forms of deprivation, and are ready to see some forms of mental disorder (e.g. ASPD, 📖 p.II.60; or hebephrenic schizophrenia) as purely social constructs employed in order to disadvantage politically unpopular groups (in the way that the concept of sluggish schizophrenia was misused in the Soviet Union, 📖 p.IV.422).

A more recent arrival is the *model of human occupation* (see 📖 p.II.181) used by occupational therapists. Occupation is seen as an important aspect of a fulfilling life for every person, irrespective of whether or not they are mentally disordered; the aim is to empower all people to occupy themselves in a way that is meaningful and fulfilling to them.

Many practitioners from each of these disciplines aim to combine the strengths of these different models insofar as they are compatible. Unifying models notably include the *biopsychosocial* model, which eschews a clear statement of what mental disorder *is*, in favour of a multifactorial treatment of how it arises.

All of these models, from the ethical perspective currently under discussion, have one particularly attractive feature: their clear, unambiguous focus on the welfare of the individual patient. They explicitly hinder the harming of the patient (e.g. through detention; see also 📖 p.III.265) in the interests of others, such as potential victims.

Moral and legal concepts of mental disorder

In contrast to mental health professionals, the philosophical starting points for most legal and criminal justice professionals are morality (doing what is 'right') and justice (📖 p.IV.297; in this context, treating people according to what is fair, due or owed). From this perspective, mental disorder is as irrelevant as hair colour or height, except insofar as it alters what is the fair or 'right' response to the mentally disordered criminal.

This allows courts, for example, to harm individuals' interests or welfare, perhaps by forcing them to pay substantial damages to another party, or by punishing them through a prolonged period of imprisonment, because this harm is justified by that individual's moral transgression, and/or by fairness, in that the harm to them is outweighed by the benefit to others (such as when a person with highly infectious tuberculosis is compulsorily isolated and treated in the interests of public health, despite not being morally blameworthy). It is proper for a society to adopt this approach, but it is not ethically acceptable for a doctor to so, because of their competing duties to their individual patient.

Symptoms, behaviours, and causes

A related problem is misidentifying the aspect of the patient to which the doctor should respond, and treating their symptoms or behaviour (as a court would 'treat', i.e. punish, that behaviour), as opposed to treating the underlying mental disorder*. This may sound obvious, but when there is a characteristic and close relationship between a behaviour and a disorder—such as between violence (📖 p.II.31) and ASPD (📖 p.II.60), or between incompetent stalking (📖 p.II.41) and LD (📖 p.II.80)—or, conversely, when the underlying disorder is difficult to identify and/or intractable, it becomes difficult to see past the behaviour to treat the disorder.

This problem is exacerbated in forensic psychiatry because people are often referred purely because of their behaviour: for example, sexually inappropriate behaviour with children, or fire-setting. The referrer wants the behaviour abolished, and will not necessarily easily accept that the psychiatrist can only treat any underlying mental disorder (if there is one†), which might or might not affect the behaviour. This problem is particularly acute if the behaviour is not shown during the psychiatric assessment (for example, during a period of assessment on a medium secure ward), but is expected to recur after discharge.

A practical consequence of this is that it is very important to recognize and acknowledge uncertainty (📖 p.III.248) from the outset, and to be open with referrers and patients about what might and might not be achieved by the assessment or treatment that is being offered.

---

*This problem is not unique to doctors: a social worker, for example, should likewise identify and ameliorate the underlying social deprivation, not the behaviour.

†In extreme cases, diagnoses may be wrongly applied or even defined based upon behaviour alone; for example, a sexually deviant behaviour may be defined as paraphilia (📖 p.II.74) merely because it conflicts with social values, in the absence of distress or interference with daily life.

Values and diversity in forensic practice

Respect for values and diversity of values

People who suffer with mental illness and disabilities that impair their autonomy are potentially vulnerable to being neglected, not taken seriously or exploited. The rehabilitation and recovery movements of the 1960s and 1990s respectively emphasized the importance of respect for the values and experience of psychiatric patients, no matter how disabled or treatment resistant they may be. Such approaches are consistent with principles of biomedical ethics that emphasize respect for autonomy (📖 p.III.275).

A key aspect of such principles is respect for the diversity of experience and identity in human psychological experience. Critics of psychiatric services often argue that mental health professionals who have never been mentally ill, or do not otherwise share a patient's experience, cannot fully appreciate their point of view or values. Respect for diversity entails thinking about stereotypes that may be operating in mental health systems; and which may affect professional judgement.

Diversity in psychiatry

Psychiatrists are often asked to comment on unusual behaviours (📖 p.III.273). However their assessment of behaviours may be affected by their own cultural mores, or stereotypes concerning what is 'normal' behaviour. Stereotypes may operate in relation to:

- Sex role: 'normal men do not dress like that'
- Gender role: 'normal mothers never hate their children'
- Age role: '69-year-olds will be unable to participate in workshops because they are too old'
- Professional role: 'civil servants do not hit their wives'
- Ethnicity: 'that black man is psychotic, he must have schizophrenia'— not asking about abnormal mood, or life events (see 📖 p.II.26)
- Religious roles: 'Christians do not commit suicide'; 'all devout Muslims reject European value systems'
- Educational status: 'she has no qualifications, so she must be stupid'
- Health status: 'patients and their relatives will be unable to understand professional views'.

It should hardly need saying that it is both polite and clinically wise to treat each new client or patient as an individual and not make assumptions about their experiences, hopes and aspirations. It is equally offensive to assume that this person will not share any ordinary human wants, wishes and needs because they differ in terms of skin colour, sex, or experience.

Respect for diversity of values in forensic psychiatry

This can be complicated in forensic psychiatric practice because many service users have antisocial beliefs and attitudes, which conflict with the values of their communities (📖 p.III.237). Alternatively many service users may not share the values of their treatment teams or the Ministry of Justice e.g. in relation to taking medication that might reduce risk.

For many forensic patients, being 'different' has meant being criminal or antisocial. It may also have been a means by which to survive traumatic and frightening experiences. Building therapeutic relationships with forensic patients usually requires an empathic understanding of both the patient's antisocial stance; and how difficult it feels to give it up. It is also important to take into account potentially conflicting views and beliefs of family members as they may play a key role in the treatment of the patient. Their value systems may differ from that of the patient.

Autonomy and self-determination

Autonomy means 'self-rule': being able to reflect on the past, consider the present and plan for the future in an integrated way. It may be thought of as divisible amongst thought, will and action; a person may lack autonomy of action (e.g. be in a wheelchair) but still have autonomy of will and thought. Autonomy is similar to the philosophical concept of agency (💷 p.III.268).

Mental disorders sometimes impair autonomy; in some cases (e.g. relapsing schizoaffective disorder, or incipient dementia), the first sign may be relatives noticing that the patient is 'not themselves'. When people recover from illness, we often describe them as 'back to their old self', and it might be said that the purpose of treatment is therefore to restore autonomy.

Impairment of autonomy is of particular relevance in forensic psychiatry because it can be related to:

- A reduced ability to behave pro-socially and in accordance with the law
- Impairment of mental capacity (💷 p.IV.424), and
- A reduction in (or loss of) criminal responsibility for one's actions (💷 p.IV.338).

Forensic psychiatric evidence may be called to help the court distinguish a person whose autonomy has been impaired from someone who has chosen to act unlawfully.

One of medicine's ethical aims (for example, under a principles approach, 💷 p.III.234) is to respect and promote patients' autonomy. This can be a complex issue in forensic psychiatry, because patients' autonomous choices and values sometimes involve exploitation of others or disregard for rules. Respect for one person's autonomy or freedom of action must be balanced against respect for that of others (e.g. their potential victims), and considered in the relevant social context. For example, it might be appropriate to restrict a patient's freedom of action in a secure psychiatric unit in a way that would be unacceptable in the community.

Consent to treatment

The requirement of consent is based on the right of an individual to determine what shall be done with their body or mind. The principles of autonomy and self-determination (💷 p.III.275) are fundamental to this right. The primary focus of consent in mental health is treatment for mental disorder. The law on consent to treatment (💷 p.IV.390), and capacity law (💷 p.IV.424), are considered separately.

Patient autonomy

It is an established principle that competent (📖 p.IV.424) adults and older children (📖 p.IV.428) can refuse medical treatment (📖 p.III.278), except where there are specific laws to the contrary. Examples of such laws include compulsory isolation and treatment for infectious diseases in the interests of public health, or compulsory treatment for mental disorder (📖 p.IV.388) in the interests of patient health or safety, or public safety.

Principles of consent

- Consent, or refusal to consent, to treatment must be voluntary; it must not be based on coercion or undue pressure
- The individual has the mental capacity (📖 p.IV.424) to consent
- The consent (or refusal) is informed, based on knowledge of the purpose and nature, risks and likely benefits of the proposed treatment and the alternatives.

Process of obtaining consent

- Explain purpose of treatment
- Explain details and reliability of diagnosis
- Explain all options for treatment including no treatment
- Explain the likely benefits and chances of success of each option
- Explain possible risks and side effects of each option
- Give the name of the doctor responsible for the treatment
- Point out that consent can be withdrawn at any time.

Methods of giving consent

Express consent involves the patient making an unambiguous statement orally or in writing that they consent to the proposed treatment. Often this will also involve the patient and doctor signing a consent form, but note that legally the form is merely a record of consent being given at a particular time, a piece of evidence only, which is open to contradiction by another piece of evidence. The consent can be withdrawn any time.

Implied consent is deemed to have been given when the patient acts in a manner consistent with having given consent, such as holding out an arm for an injection. In general, implied consent will only be considered sufficient for minor procedures, or procedures with very few risks or side-effects.

Inferred consent is a term used by some authors for the fiction that consent has been given by an unconscious patient when a treatment is proposed that they are known to approve of, or that a reasonable person would consent to in similar circumstances. This only applies to uncontentious treatments and circumstances, such as changing a patient's bed sheets; it would extremely unwise to rely on 'inferred consent' in a situation in which there is (or could be expected to be) any dispute about the correct course of action. The safest course of action with unconscious or other incapacitated patients is to apply mental capacity law.

Consequences of treating without consent

Unless there is a specific law authorizing treatment without consent in the current situation (such as a detention under a valid mental health order or 'section' that includes a power to treat), then a doctor who treats a patient without their consent is acting unethically, may be liable in law for negligence (📖 p.V.516), and may have committed a criminal offence such as battery (📖 p.IV.346).

Treatment without consent

Incapacity to consent

It is an ethical and legal requirement to obtain valid consent (📖 p.III.275) from a patient before carrying out any medical intervention. However, many patients seeking help have lost the capacity to consent, because of their physical or mental disorder. At least 30% of patients in general medical in-patient settings, for example, lack capacity to make treatment decisions, and this number is likely to be greater in old age services, intensive care and palliative care.

When treating patients who lack capacity, the following ethical principles must be observed (as reflected in capacity law, 📖 p.IV.424):

- Treatment should be in the patient's *best interests*, not those of other parties (although in the case of public protection, forensic psychiatrists not uncommonly override the patient's interests: 📖 p.III.265)
- Even though the doctor or MDT will make the final decision, the patient should participate in the decision-making process as far as is possible
- Any wishes expressed in the past when the patient had capacity,[*] and any knowledge of their settled values and beliefs, must be taken into account in determining their best interests
- Relatives, friends and any other appropriate people[†] should be consulted before a decision is made, if possible (but only in order to ascertain the patient's values and likely views, not to ask the relatives for permission to treat)
- Treatment should be provided in a manner that least restricts the patient's rights and future freedoms.

The law is essentially the same whether an incapacitous patient accepts or refuses treatment, but the latter situation presents additional ethical, practical and emotional difficulties (📖 p.III.278).

Mental illness and incapacity

Where a patient lacks capacity because of mental disorder, there will often be a power to treat them under mental health law (📖 p.IV.373) as well as under mental capacity law (📖 p.IV.424). Where there is freedom to choose either power (though local guidelines will usually constrain the choice), the system that provides the greater protection for the patient's interests should be chosen. In practice, this usually means mental health law, which allows for external review of clinicians' decisions by Tribunals.

---

[*] If expressed in written form, these wishes ('advance statements') may be binding in certain circumstances in some jurisdictions: see 📖 p.IV.430.
[†] Certain people can sometimes make treatment decisions on behalf of the incapacitous patient that bind the doctor, in some jurisdictions: see 📖 p.IV.432.

Ethical history

Capacity law's provisions for treating those who lack capacity arose primarily from two sorts of poignant human story:

- Those with serious (and sometimes terminal) illnesses who wanted to make sure that they had the treatment they wanted and could refuse what they did not want, and
- Those who lacked capacity to consent to or refuse treatment on a long-term basis and needed someone to make treatment decisions for them.

The latter group were sometimes known as 'involuntary informal' patients because they lacked the ability to consent to treatment (which could not, therefore, be described as 'voluntary') but could not be detained under mental health law, as they were not refusing treatment. They are now treated indefinitely under mainstream capacity law.

However, capacity legislation does not provide legal safeguards for those whose liberty is adversely affected by their treatment, for instance by being kept indefinitely in nursing homes.* The Bournewood case (p.App. 3.631) provided a high-profile example of the distress (at least to carers and families) that can result, and prompted the development of special safeguards for treatments that involve a deprivation of liberty (p.IV.436).

When patients refuse treatment

Capacity to refuse treatment

It is a key aspect of respect for autonomy of all people that their decisions about their own welfare should be respected. However, doctors have (given their tradition of paternalism) often found it hard to accept patients' refusal of care, especially when refusal appears to be life threatening.

---

*Except for those patients who previously had capacity and had the foresight to issue an advance statement (p.IV.430) covering this situation, or who appointed (or had appointed for them) a donee (p.IV.432).

Capacity law (📖 p.IV.424) presumes all people to have capacity, until the contrary has been shown. A person with capacity may legally refuse all treatment* no matter what the consequences,† and no medical treatment can be forced on a patient with capacity. Making a (medically) unwise decision is not evidence of lack of capacity.

However, treatment refusal, especially if it could lead to death, often does trigger capacity assessments. About half the capacity assessments carried out by liaison psychiatrists are for treatment refusal.

Refusing treatment for physical illness

The majority of patients who refuse treatment in general hospitals are males over 60, many of whom have mild cognitive impairments. Only a minority, however, lack capacity.

Some of those who lack capacity may be treated under mental capacity law (📖 p.IV.426). If the patient is actively and physically refusing treatment (e.g. pulling out cannulae, or fighting off staff), it is important to try to address the high emotions involved, and to calm the situation. Research suggests that involving family members and friends is often effective, both because they may be able to calm or persuade the patient, and because staff will feel easier about what they have to do if they have the support of those who know the patient well.

Patients with capacity have the legal right to refuse treatment and this must be respected, no matter how uncomfortable this may be for professional staff. It is permissible however to try and find other ways to care for them that they can accept. Many patients who are refusing treatment actually change their minds after a psychiatric consultation, whether they have capacity or not. This rather suggests that many 'refusals' are really explained by poor communication by medical and surgical teams; and a lack of understanding of how anxiety may be manifest in mild anger and aggression.

Refusing treatment for mental disorder

People with mental illness who are detained may or may not lack capacity to make treatment decisions. Studies of psychiatric patients in the UK have found that between 30–60% of inpatients lack capacity. Many of the 40–70% of patients with capacity are treated against their will under mental health legislation, which allows compulsory treatment of such patients' mental disorder (with variation between jurisdictions: RoI does not allow compulsory treatment of capacitous patients; Scotland only allows such treatment for a short period; and E&W and NI allow it long-term, subject to a second opinion—see 📖 p.IV.390).

---

* Although there may be other legal powers that enable treatment to be enforced despite their capacitous refusal, particularly under mental health law (📖 p.IV.373), but also public health and welfare laws (📖 p.IV.440).
† Such as in the English cases known as Miss B (📖 p.App. 3.630) and Re C (📖 p.App. 3.633).

Ethical problems

These current legal positions reflect different balances between the duty to respect individual autonomy (📖 p.III.275) on the one hand; and a duty to promote the welfare of mentally disordered patients, and to prevent risk of harm* to themselves and others.

The ethical dilemma becomes more controversial when considering the long-term compulsory treatment of incapacitous individuals who wish to refuse treatment; and/or where treatment has no proven efficacy or consists mainly of preventive detention (see 📖 pp.III.280, III.282). Typically this applies to patients with severe personality disorders, who have capacity but present a risk to others. The DSPD programme (📖 p.II.211) in E&W raised exactly this issue, particularly in the cases of prisoners who are transferred to hospital (📖 p.IV.410) under the programme shortly before the end of determinate sentences (📖 p.IV.366), and who therefore experienced a much longer period of incarceration than they would otherwise have done, for compulsory treatment they did not wish to receive and which has not been shown to be effective.

The controversy is still sharper in relation to sex offenders thought to pose a high risk of harm to others through recidivism. In the US, over 40 states have enacted Sexually Violent Predator laws.† These allow people convicted of violent sexual offences (📖 p.IV.348) who have a 'mental abnormality' (📖 p.IV.296) such as a personality disorder to be detained indefinitely in a secure hospital on the grounds of risk of harm to others (📖 p.III.265). The California SVP programme at Coalinga State Hospital, amongst others, explicitly countenances indefinite detention for the 75% of its inmates who refuse the intensive psychological treatment on offer. Although no equivalent programme currently exists in the UK or RoI, the removal of the exclusion of sexual deviance as a ground for detention under the Mental Health Act in E&W might have cleared the way for such a programme in the future.

What should we treat?

Doctors make diagnoses, and treat the pathology that causes symptoms and signs of disorder. Where this is not possible, symptomatic relief, including the relief of distress and pain, is still a reasonable treatment goal (📖 p.II.146). Psychiatrists are no different from other doctors in this respect.

However, forensic psychiatrists may be explicitly asked to treat the offence, i.e. to inhibit or abolish those factors in the patient that increase the risk of offending, particularly violent or sexual offending. Forensic patients detained in secure settings (📖 p.II.148) are often unable to move on and regain their freedom until their risk to others is seen to have been adequately reduced, no matter how mentally well they may be.

---

* There is an implicit assumption by society that all mentally disordered people pose a risk of harm to others, or at least to themselves, when in fact very many pose no such risk at all.
† Also known by the names of the victims of sexual violence whose high-profile cases led to the passing of the laws, such as Megan's Law and Jessica's Law in California.

There is some social support for this approach, as evidenced by the fact that there is mental health legislation (📖 p.IV.373) that makes it possible. What is at issue is not whether continued detention in the absence of current symptoms is lawful but whether it is ethically justifiable for doctors to assess and treat for risk in the absence of any direct benefit to the mental health of the patient (see 📖 p.III.265).

Treating disorders, not behaviours

It can be argued that, once psychiatrists have improved a patient's mental health, their professional job is over; according to this argument, the management of a patient's risk is socially important, but not a medical matter. However, if the risk of harm arises directly from mental disorder then clearly it is justifiable for psychiatrists to manage the risk arising in that way. However, it is not the role of forensic psychiatrists to manage the risk of harm arising from ordinary criminogenic factors. Where offending arises from a combination of mental disorder and criminogenic factors then their role becomes less clear. Consider the following example.

> Henry kills his best friend in an unprovoked assault. On remand, he is found to be psychotic and transferred to secure services. A diagnosis of paranoid schizophrenia is made, Henry is convicted of manslaughter on the grounds of diminished responsibility, and is given a hospital order with restrictions. Henry recovers quickly on antipsychotic medication and is soon symptom-free. After 2 years in hospital, during which he has been perfectly well, and has not been violent or behaved inappropriately, his clinical team requests transfer to a less secure unit. Both the Ministry of Justice and the receiving hospital refuse, saying that Henry's risk to others is still not understood, and this justifies his continuing stay in a high security setting.

The court accepted that Henry was less criminally responsible because of his mental illness; and sent him to hospital because he needed treatment for it. The fact that he was psychotic around the time of the offence, and that his behaviour has improved with antipsychotic treatment (although this could also be a result of the secure environment) suggests that his psychosis was an essential factor in the killing.[*]

The logical corollary of this is that, once the treating team can be confident that his schizophrenia is well-controlled, he can safely be discharged, even though this means he will return to the community long before he would have done had he received a prison sentence (📖 p.IV.364). To satisfy the objection from the MoJ that the risk is still not understood merely entails a review of the aspects of his mental disorder in the absence of psychosis that might cause unprovoked violence or contribute to future offending[†]. Not all of these will be amendable to treatment.

---

[*] Though this is some way from saying that it was *the*, cause of it.
[†] Which in practice would have been started soon after admission, not after two years of stability, as in this example.

The offender/patient confusion

In practice, the objection by the MoJ to discharge is likely to persist despite such a review. Even if not stated explicitly, despite the court's reasons for making a hospital order, it is very easy for the index offence and the harm to others that resulted to loom so large in the minds of the police, MoJ and MAPPA (📖 p.V.468) partners, all of whose primary responsibility is public protection, that they persist in regarding Henry as a criminal of bad character, who should not be released until he has been punished (📖 p.IV.297) sufficiently. Using detention in hospital for this purpose is both wrong, and a waste of a scarce resource.

Double jeopardy

Failing to resist the imperative of punishment, for example by colluding with the shift from a mental health to a criminogenic paradigm via accepting that there are still some risk factors, leads to what is effectively double jeopardy for Henry. Having complied with treatment and made a good recovery, he will face a new (and non-psychiatric) enquiry into the motives for his offending, with a direct impact on his liberty. The central question changes from 'How ill is Henry now?' to 'How risky is Henry now?'. Since the strongest risk factor for future harm is past harm, Henry will be at risk of never being able to demonstrate that he poses little risk, merely by virtue of his index offence.

An ethical position

Forensic psychiatrists have a duty (📖 p.III.246) to treat patients fairly and with respect. Even where treatments are aimed at risk reduction rather than health benefits,[*] there must be some connection with mental disorder (as, for example, with psychological treatments for ASPD, 📖 p.II.60); some argue persuasively that such treatments are only ethical if there is some hope of health benefit. Pressure from other parts of the criminal justice system for measures to be taken for other purposes such as punishment must be resisted.

What counts as treatment?

The problem of deciding what to treat (📖 p.II.280) is inherently linked with the question, what is treatment? Both questions are especially sharply focused with patients whose sole diagnosis is personality disorder (📖 p.II.58) or psychopathy (📖 p.II.66). There may be no medical or psychological treatment that can be offered that will reduce the patient's distress, or reduce the risk of them harming themselves or others. Is there any other form of treatment that it may be right to offer?

---

[*] And especially where there is 'double effect' in ethical terms, i.e. where the treatment involves risking unwanted effects such as diabetes and obesity with atypical antipsychotics.

Forms of treatment

Consider a patient with an amputated limb after a road traffic accident, or a terminal illness such as cancer, or a highly infectious condition such as tuberculosis. The following might be offered in health and social care settings:

- Medical treatments, including antibiotics or chemotherapy
- Surgical and related treatments, such as resection of a primary tumour, or the fitting of a prosthetic limb
- Psychological treatments, such as counselling from a Macmillan nurse
- Habilitation or rehabilitation: the (re)acquisition of useful skills, such as walking using a prosthetic limb
- Personal care, such as assistance to wash or dress
- Social care, such as a residential home, or a 'home help'
- Secondary preventive treatments, such as dressing wounds
- Palliative treatments, such as analgesics
- Preventive detention, such as segregation in an isolation ward.

These represent a variety of different types of intervention, with different aims, carried out by different professionals. Which of them is it appropriate to call 'treatment'? By analogy, within forensic psychiatry what types of intervention directed at someone with personality disorder can properly be called 'treatment'? In the mental health setting, which of the interventions listed would it be ethical to administer compulsorily, without consent (📖 p.III.271) or even in the face of a competent (📖 p.IV.424) refusal of consent (📖 p.III.278)? Would the answer be different if the primary aim was non-therapeutic, such as public protection? What if the only aim was public protection? Crucially, can preventive detention amount to treatment if there is no discernable benefit to the patient?

The legal definition of treatment

As described on 📖 p.IV.390, the legal definition of treatment varies between jurisdictions in the UK and RoI. However, in all jurisdictions it is broad, and includes everything listed in 📖 'Forms of treatment', p. III.283, down to and including social care; moreover, secondary prevention and palliation are accepted as forms of treatment if their intention is to ameliorate the disorder in question.

However, in E&W the definition is the broadest: 'medical treatment the purpose of which is to alleviate, or prevent a worsening of, the disorder or one or more of its symptoms or manifestations'. Any treatment under the direction of the responsible clinician counts; it does not have to be treatment for the 'core disorder', and can include treatments aimed at helping the patient cope with or work around the symptoms of their disorder. In the case of a detained patient with severe borderline PD (📖 p.II.61), these definitions would presumably cover secondary preventive or palliative treatments given in the face of a refusal of consent, such as training in victim empathy, or a mood stabilizer at a low dose[*]—as might the law in Scotland, NI and RoI.

However, would the E&W definition allow the detention itself to be considered a 'treatment', if while in secure conditions the patient did not

---

[*] The former might not alter the patient's personality traits itself, but would hope to prevent or minimize the consequence of victimizing others; and the latter would be palliative insofar as it reduced distressing mood swings for the sufferer.

show the violence (a manifestation of the disorder) that they showed when in the community? If so, mental health law in E&W would allow indefinite administrative detention—that is, detention that is justified neither by a criminal offence* nor on health grounds. This legal 'treatment' goes far beyond any medical or psychological notion of treatment.

The intention and the likely effect of treatment

Further, in E&W and RoI there does not even have to be any likelihood of benefit: treatment must merely have the *purpose* of alleviating, or preventing a worsening of, the disorder or one or more of its symptoms or manifestations. (The definition in RoI is that treatment includes, but is not limited to, 'the administration of physical, psychological and other remedies . . . intended for the purposes of ameliorating a mental disorder'.) This presents the psychiatrist with a further ethical problem: even if there is no evidence base for an intervention with this type of patient, it can still be given compulsorily. Even if it has been tried for this patient before, and has repeatedly failed, the patient can continue to be detained for it to be tried again, as long as it is an 'appropriate treatment'.† In RoI, patients with personality disorder alone cannot be compulsorily treated at all, which mitigates the effect of the broad definition of treatment somewhat, but in E&W it applies to all patients with mental disorder.‡

The position in Scotland and NI is less clear: the definition of treatment is not based upon intention, but neither is there any requirement to show a likely benefit, so the exact ambit of the law will not be known until it is tested in court.

Consent to risk assessment

Consent to examination, investigation and treatment is essential in all areas of medicine, albeit with exceptions in the absence of capacity, or under the terms of mental health legislation. However, the status of risk assessment as an investigation per se, or as a prelude to treatment, is uncertain. If there is a therapeutic intention and context, is it part of assessment for treatment, or should it be considered distinct?

---

* This same definition of treatment applies to patients detained under the Act's civil provisions (📖 p.IV.388), as well as to those ordered to hospital by a criminal court. If this interpretation is correct, the E&W Act goes even further than the Sexually Violent Predator statutes in the US (📖 p.III.280), which at least require the commission of an offence before they apply.
† Exactly how the courts will interpret 'appropriate treatment' remains to be seen; they might hold that treatment cannot be appropriate if there is no likelihood of benefit.
‡ By contrast, under the law in E&W before 2008, compulsory treatment of patients with personality disorder (or milder forms of learning disability) was only permissible if it was likely to alleviate or prevent a deterioration of the condition; this was known as the *treatability test*.

The ethics of consent to risk assessment therefore relates to:

- Situations where there is no right to assess without consent: for instance, where the assessment is explicitly solely for risk assessment purposes (e.g. to assist with sentencing, 📖 p.IV.361), and not carried out under mental health or mental capacity law
- Situations where risk assessment is part and parcel of clinical assessment directed at therapeutic purposes with an informal patient, where consent is again required, and
- Clinical situations governed by either mental health or mental capacity law, again where risk assessment is part and parcel of clinical assessment directed at therapeutic purposes.

By conducting risk assessment without consent, the person assessed lacks the opportunity to weigh the harm or benefit to them of engaging in the process. The issue is particularly important in forensic psychiatry because of the potential impact of risk assessment on the individual's liberty. They may not even suspect that assessment which is presented (perhaps intended) as solely directed at the possibility of treatment in hospital might be used judicially for the purpose of sentencing.

Any consideration of the ethics of risk assessment (📖 p.III.265), and of the ethics of the context of the risk assessment (such as a court's assessment of dangerousness, 📖 p.V.549) must therefore include consideration of the ethics of assessing risk in the absence of consent.

Seeking consent to risk assessment

If it is decided to seek consent to risk assessment, then the same ethical rules as for consent to treatment (📖 p.III.275) apply. That is, the patient must have capacity to consent (📖 p.IV.424); they must be appropriately *informed*; and they must not have been coerced to consent.

A key ethical difficulty for any psychiatrist or psychologist relates to how a risk assessment might in the end be used, and therefore to what information they should give the patient. For example, although the expert intends the risk assessment to support a recommendation for a hospital order (📖 p.IV.405), it could in fact be used by the court to justify an indefinite sentence of imprisonment (📖 p.IV.364). For consent to risk assessment to be valid, the patient must be informed about such undesired but foreseeable possibilities.

Informed consent to risk assessment

Depending on the circumstances, if consent to risk assessment is sought, some or all of the following information should be given to the patient.

- This assessment will include an assessment of your risk of harming others
- This assessment may be used by the court to assist in determination of your dangerousness
- This assessment may result in the imposition of a restriction order or indeterminate or extended sentencing even if that is not my recommendation
- This assessment may be helpful for you to avoid further offending
- This assessment may help healthcare professionals or other agencies support you in managing risks to yourself.

Consent to risk management

Although consent is not usually sought for risk management in so many words, in many ways the position is more straightforward than for risk assessment. Each risk management intervention, such as giving an antipsychotic to reduce command auditory hallucinations to kill, or disclosing information to the police (📖 p.III.264) about a patient's plans to abuse children, will clearly require either specific consent, or a legal power allowing it to be carried out in the absence of consent or in the face of a refusal (📖 p.IV.278).

Consent to research

Obtaining informed consent from research participants is central to ethical research practice. Ethical frameworks for medical research were developed following exposure of abuse experienced by human research subjects during World War II. Local research Ethics Committees (LRECs) were formed in the UK in 1968. Institutional Review Boards (IRBs) in USA have similar functions, backed by Federal law, to regulate medical research and to ensure adherence to regulation.

In 2001 the Department of Health developed Research Governance Frameworks, and ethical approval for all research must be sought from local RECS using this framework. Applications for such approval must include evidence of how researchers will approach participants; how they will obtain consent, the information they will give participants, and how confidential data will be kept securely.

Participants in research must be free to make their own informed decisions about taking part in research. Participants must usually have capacity (📖 p.IV.424) to give consent. Where potential participants cannot consent but the research is deemed appropriate and in the interests of the participants by the ethics committee, permission to proceed may be granted, subject to conditions (📖 p.IV.427).

Participants should be able to exercise free power of choice over consent and refusal. Special considerations apply when carrying out research with detained patients, or prisoners, in order to ensure that consent is indeed free, and not influenced by any power over the patient's future placement or situation that he perceives the researcher might have. Participants should have sufficient knowledge and understanding of what is involved in the research, so that they can make informed decisions. Fully informed consent may not always be possible, as by definition the subject under research is poorly understood; but the legal position is that participants need to be informed about any potential significant risks of serious harm that any reasonable person would want to know.

Researchers have to comply with legal frameworks and regulation (outlined earlier). They also have to balance a range of competing interests, such as the aims of the research, what they consider to be in the best interests of research participants and the interests of formal and informal gatekeepers.

In practice

- Whenever possible, the investigator should inform all participants of the objectives of the investigation

- The investigator should inform the participants of all aspects of the research or intervention that might reasonably be expected to influence willingness to participate
- The investigator should, normally, explain all other aspects of the research or intervention about which the potential participants enquire, or a reasonable person might wish to know
- Failure to make full disclosure prior to obtaining informed consent requires additional safeguards to protect the welfare and dignity of the participants
- Investigators should realize that they are often in a position of authority or influence over participants who may be their students, employees, clients, or patients. This relationship must not be allowed to pressure the participants to take part in, or remain in, an investigation
- The payment of participants must not be used to induce them to risk harm beyond that which they would risk without payment in their normal lifestyle
- If harm, unusual discomfort, or other negative consequences for the individual's future life might occur, the investigator must obtain the disinterested approval of independent advisors, inform the participants, and obtain informed, real consent from each of them
- In longitudinal research, consent may need to be obtained on more than one occasion.

Consent in vulnerable groups

Children, older adults, people with a range of physical and mental health problems or LD:
- Children under 16 are not automatically assumed to be competent to give consent. However if a child can be judged to understand what participation in research will involve then parental consent is not necessary (see 📖 p.IV.428). There is a distinction between consent, which is a legal term, and infers fully weighing up the decision based upon adequate information; and assent, which falls short of this and amounts simply to agreeing to take part. Children need to assent even if parental consent is given
- Consent from parents, guardians, or other representatives is generally necessary in relation to research with children and adults who lack the capacity to give consent for themselves
- When research is being conducted with detained persons, particular care should be taken over informed consent, paying attention to the special circumstances which may affect the person's ability to give free informed consent.

The prosecution of patients

The shift in attitudes

Historically, people with mental disorder were prosecuted just as other members of society when they were alleged to have offended, with the only variation in procedure being that they could be acquitted on the grounds of insanity (📖 p.V.489).

During the 19th and 20th centuries, however, the idea that mentally disordered persons should be diverted (📖 p.II.216) from the criminal justice system into hospital gradually took hold, and by the late 20th century it had become commonplace for the police, prosecutors and courts to stop proceedings for all but the most serious charges, and to take people they thought to be mentally disordered to hospital for assessment. Police officers and prosecutors became reluctant to charge or prosecute people they thought to be mentally disordered, believing that it was inappropriate and/or that the prosecution would be very unlikely to succeed because they would be unfit to plead (📖 p.V.474) or would be unable to stand up to cross-examination (📖 p.V.588), although in most cases this is a misconception.

In the UK at least, there was a general move towards extended (📖 p.IV.367) and indeterminate (📖 p.IV.365) sentences of imprisonment based upon public protection (as opposed to the usual principle of pro-portionality, 📖 p.IV.363), under the New Labour governments from 1997 to 2010. Some mentally disordered offenders, particularly those with personality disorder, were caught up in this cultural shift, receiving more punitive sentences as a result.

When is it appropriate to prosecute?

At the extremes, the decision whether to prosecute[*] a person with mental disorder is straightforward: a floridly psychotic patient arrested for a minor offence (e.g. breach of the peace, 📖 p.IV.353) could be diverted and escape prosecution without controversy, whereas most would accept that it is appropriate that a patient with antisocial personality disorder (📖 p.II.60) who is alleged to have seriously assaulted or killed should be pros-ecuted, provided that there is the possibility of psychiatric treatment in concert with the prosecution. In between, though, how are the welfare of the patient and society's interest in justice (📖 p.IV.294) to be balanced?

The harm to the victim

One obvious consideration is the seriousness of the offence, and in par-ticular the severity of the harm to other people that resulted. Victims have a legitimate interest in seeing the person who harmed them tried and, if appropriate, punished: this is one of the key goals of the criminal justice system (📖 p.IV.294). This includes staff working with the patient, for instance when they are the victims of assault; and fellow patients.

The nature of the mental disorder

Another consideration is the patient's mental disorder, and the likeli-hood that if prosecuted they would be fit to plead, or would be acquitted because of one of the mental condition defences (📖 p.IV.342). Diversion of a patient is more appropriate if any prosecution would be likely to fall on these grounds.

---

[*] This section discusses charging & prosecution as if there were a single decision, made by the clinical team. In practice, the clinical team, the victim, the police and the prosecutor will make a series of decisions: whether to report the alleged offence; whether to arrest the patient; whether to charge them; and whether, finally, to prosecute. Box 12.1 summarises the factors weighed up by the Crown Prosecution Service in E&W in making its decision.

Prosecution as a component of the care plan

In some cases, such as where the risk assessment (📖 p.II.127) indicates a substantial risk of future violence, it will be appropriate explicitly to consider prosecution as an element of the patient's care plan, and objectively to determine what offending behaviour they exhibited. This is most likely to occur with patients with personality disorder (📖 p.II.58), where (in combination with treatments such as group CBT, 📖 p.II.171), the patient experiences consistent consequences to their behaviour, such as prosecution for offending behaviour.

Box 12.1 Crown Prosecution Service guidelines on the decision to prosecute

- Is there enough evidence to prosecute this defendant?
  - Enough for conviction to be more likely than acquittal
  - Takes into account the quality of the available evidence, e.g. the credibility of witnesses
- Is prosecution required in the public interest?
  - How serious is the offence?
  - What are the views of the victim?
  - Would the court be likely to give only a minor punishment?
  - What are the alleged offender's circumstances—e.g. many previous convictions/repeat offender? Mentally disordered?
  - Is an out-of-court disposal (e.g. conditional caution, 📖 p.IV.361) more appropriate?

Part IV

Law relevant to psychiatry*

*Part IV (Chapters 13–16) deals in detail only with topics from criminal law, mental health law, and mental capacity law. Practical applications of some areas of civil law are also covered in Chapter 19. For an authoritative treatment of these or other areas of law, you should consult a legal textbook or a professional lawyer.

The interface between psychiatry and law

Goals of the psychiatric & legal systems

The relationship between psychiatry and law is at the heart of forensic psychiatry. Whether practising clinical forensic psychiatry or providing psychiatric evidence to a court or tribunal, an understanding and knowledge of the different goals of the legal system, and the way the law asks and answers questions in the service of those goals, is crucial.

The aims of medicine & psychiatry

As discussed elsewhere, the aims of treatment (📖 p.II.46) in medicine are, essentially, to maximize the quality and duration of patients' lives, both individually and at the population level. Psychiatry shares these aims, but adds a third, the reduction of the patient's risk of harming themselves or others. Wherever possible, risk reduction is done in the interests of the patient themselves, and with their consent, although occasionally forensic psychiatrists override the patient's interests in order to protect others (see the discussion of ethical risk assessment & management on 📖 p.III.265).

The legal, criminal justice and youth justice systems

Whereas medicine and psychiatry focus primarily on the welfare of the individual patient, criminal justice is concerned with the interests of society as a whole. Three interlocking systems, with subtly different aims, should be distinguished:

- The *legal system*, comprising the civil, criminal and other courts and tribunals (📖 p.IV.308). Its sole aim is the administration of *justice*,[*] through making decisions about competing claims by different parties, including the state
- The *criminal justice system* (CJS), comprising the criminal courts, the police, prosecution service, probation service, prison service, and government departments overseeing these (e.g. the Ministry of Justice). Its aims are the prevention, detection and punishment of crime
- The *youth justice system* is that part of the CJS that deals with children and young people (up to 21 years old in some cases). Like the rest of the CJS, it aims to prevent,[†] detect and punish crime, but it aims to do so in a way that promotes the welfare and developmental needs of the child or young person. (This aim can be seen clearly in the Scottish Children's Hearings system (📖 p.IV.323), but is less obvious in E&W, which is more punitive.)

---

[*] The term 'justice' has many competing interpretations. On this page, it is used in the sense of the fair allocation of benefits and harms between competing parties, such as when a court decides who should compensate whom for what, or who should be punished for what. Another major sense, also found in this handbook (such as in the discussion of the justice model (📖 p.IV.296) and in relation to sentencing (📖 p.IV.361) refers to doing what is 'right' by reference to a moral standard.

[†] In E&W, the Crime & Disorder Act 1998 makes the prevention of offending the 'principal aim' of the YJS.

Psychiatry and law: a two-way relationship

The relationship between psychiatry and law is bilateral. Psychiatry is used by law to assist in answering the law's questions, as when psychiatrists testify (📖 p.V.586) as to whether a defendant was capable of forming the requisite intent (📖 p.IV.334) for a particular crime; it also uses legal processes to therapeutic ends, as when a psychiatrist decides as part of their risk management plan (📖 p.II.190) to recommend a restriction order (📖 p.IV.412) in a report on disposal (📖 p.V.569). In all these situations, the forensic psychiatrist must be alive to the differences between their own goals and ways of thinking (📖 p.IV.296) about the patient, and those of the other agencies (📖 p.III.258) they deal with as they negotiate the psycho-legal interface (📖 p.IV.299).

Is forensic psychiatry converging on the CJS?

Early in the development of forensic psychiatry (📖 pp.I.11, III.206), the discipline approached public protection essentially as an adjunct to, or knock-on effect of, the treatment of patients. This amounted to the 'rescue' approach to forensic psychiatry; that is, achieving diversion from the justice system into mental healthcare services (sometimes with discontinuance of the justice process) of those with severe mental disorders.

Increasingly, however, society has demanded to be kept safe from the people it fears, and has therefore increasingly expected forensic psychiatrists to manage and contain the risks posed by mentally disordered offenders whether or not with they can offer benefit to the patient through treatment. These forces cause forensic psychiatry to converge on law's public protection functions—as distinct from law and psychiatry converging with the common purpose of welfare-based rescue.

Manifestations of convergence

Convergence can be seen in:

- A developing shift in the clinical balance adopted between the goals of treatment of the patient and protection of the public
- The widening of definitions within mental health legislation so as to allow detention of those who may not benefit from treatment, and
- The increasing involvement of forensic psychiatrists in the administration of risk-based sentencing.

Convergence also implies the potential for movement away from the core objectives and values of medicine.

Accepting or resisting convergence

Forensic psychiatry in the UK has, in the past decade, experienced an internal schism in its identity and values. Some have held steadfastly to the rescue approach to the discipline, resisting involvement in social functions that amount solely to risk management of the mentally disordered. Others have accepted, even embraced, the risk agenda on the basis that forensic psychiatrists are best placed in society to assess risk arising from the mentally disordered and owe a duty to society to assist; some have even defined forensic psychiatry so as to include the notion of 'treating violence'.

Legal and psychiatric constructs & models

Law and psychiatry as two 'lands'

Law and psychiatry are like two neighbouring countries, each with its own purposes (📖 p.IV.294) and languages, and each with its own districts and regions, expressed in the various branches of the law and in psychiatric diagnoses and diagnostic categories. Travelling from one to the other involves translating (📖 p.IV.299) the language of one into that of the other, creating many opportunities for confusion and distortion of meaning.

The problems in the relationship between psychiatry and law are very different from those between (say) forensic pathology and law, where the law is interested only in matters of fact (e.g. the nature of a wound and therefore how it was probably inflicted). Psychiatry deals with constructs apparently similar to those of law; for example, volition (📖 p.II.20) in psychiatry and intention (📖 p.IV.334) in law. Although these are distinct constructs, they are sufficiently close for the difference between them often not to be apparent to psychiatrists and lawyers. This can lead to mutual misunderstanding and, for the psychiatrist, ethical tension (📖 p.III.272).

Constructs from purposes

The constructs used in a discipline derive from its core purposes. The core purpose of medicine is the amelioration of disease, illness and suffering (see 📖 p.II.146). Hence, although medicine investigates disease in order to understand it, ultimately it does so with the purpose of treating it and increasing the welfare of the individual patient. In contrast, the law pursues justice, an abstract concept concerned with what is fair, due, or owed, implicit in which is the idea of balancing the interests (or welfare) of one party against another, or the state.

The differences between often apparently similar legal and psychiatric constructs flows from their different purposes. Compare and contrast psychosis (📖 p.II.54) within psychiatry and insanity (📖 p.V.489) within law, each of which involve a loss of reality testing, the ability to recognize the true nature of actions. Similarly, 'abnormality of mental functioning' within diminished responsibility (📖 p.V.491), although appearing almost medical, is distinct from anything medical. Psychiatry defines[*] psychosis by its symptoms and aetiology, so that it can be reliably identified by different doctors, and classifies it into separate diagnoses (📖 p.II.108), so as to make a prognosis and facilitate appropriate treatment, not to determine whether the psychotic defendant should be found unfit to plead (📖 p.V.474).

To the criminal law, however, the concepts of insanity and diminished responsibility exist only to allocate criminal responsibility justly, in different ways (should Mr X be held responsible and punished for assaulting or killing Ms Y?); and it defines unfitness to plead in order to determine whether a fair trial is possible. Since the consequence of insanity is to

---

[*] The fact that there can be competing definitions in some cases reflects only imperfect knowledge of the condition in question: all agree that, once the condition is better understood, a consensus will form around a single definition.

remove responsibility entirely, whereas that of diminished responsibility is merely to reduce it, the law adopts different and essentially inconsistent definitions for the two legal defences (a 'defect of reason' to define the mental disorder component of insanity, as compared with the much looser 'abnormality of mental functioning' for diminished responsibility).

Disputed models

The picture is complicated further by the fact that psychiatrists and lawyers often disagree about the model their field should adopt (see also p.IV.295). For example, there is a lively debate as to whether the criminal law should be interpreted, and judicial discretion used, purely to do what is *fair* or just overall, regardless of the consequences for the individual offender; or to focus on what is proportionate or just for that one offender, i.e. their '*just deserts*'; or to include taking account of the *welfare* of the offender; or to *deter* the offender and others from offending.

A homeless teenager convicted of their twentieth minor theft, might be sentenced (p.IV.361) to a fine under the justice approach, a community order with a residence requirement under the welfare approach, or a short sentence of youth detention under the deterrence approach. This is relevant to mentally disordered offenders in that, for instance, lawyers advocating the welfare approach will be more in favour of diverting (p.IV.216) them to hospital than those advocating a pure justice approach.

Conversely, lawyers often experience frustration when faced with psychiatric experts with differing opinions as to whether a patient suffers from, say, schizophrenia or a transient paranoid psychosis, conditions which might have different legal consequences. From their perspective, psychiatrists' nuanced disagreements, significant to them in relation to prognosis or treatment, appear incomprehensible and irrelevant.

Autopoesis versus reflexivity

These terms refer to law's openness, or otherwise, to adopting the concepts used in other disciplines.

Family law is relatively reflexive; it adopts relatively loose concepts and process, and can accommodate a wide range of types of expert evidence and constructs, even at the cost of apparent imprecision and some risk of different courts faced with the similar facts reaching different decisions.

Criminal law, however, is highly autopoetic; it employs only its own strictly defined concepts, within a strictly observed discourse, which greatly inhibits adoption of the concepts or methods of other disciplines, and which can seriously distort the meaning of concepts given in evidence. This is because it is preoccupied with ensuring that its procedures (such as the rules of evidence, p.IV.317) are scrupulously fair to defendants and prosecution.

The use of information

History versus evidence

Psychiatry and law, because of their different purposes (p.IV.294), regard information in quite different ways:

- To a court, any piece of information is *evidence*, to be admitted or excluded, deemed truthful or false, and given greater or lesser weight, all according to the rules of evidence (⌨ p.IV.317). All such evidence contributes to an overall verdict of guilt or innocence, or in favour of one or other party

- To a psychiatrist, however, the same piece of information forms part of the patient's *history*, to be taken into consideration with much less concern about whether a particular piece of information is itself is 'true' (although some assessment of the reliability of the source must still be made). Rather what is looked at is the overall pattern of information (e.g. of symptoms) and whether, overall, it is sufficient to make a particular diagnosis (⌨ p.II.108) or formulation (⌨ p.II.110), within which it is to be expected that some symptoms will be absent or there will be symptoms inconsistent with the diagnosis*

- The process amounts to consideration of whether the information available is sufficient, taken together, to infer the diagnostic (or other) conclusion, rather as with a jigsaw puzzle, in terms of whether there are enough pieces of a particular picture to be convincing that the picture is really there. Such an approach infers that the combination of pieces of evidence can be mutually reinforcing in terms of the weight to be attached to each piece. Hence validation in medicine is very different from truth finding in law.

Methods of gathering and selecting information

These also differ between law and psychiatry. Courts will only consider evidence that is put before them by the parties,† and which is deemed 'admissible'; it will then test each piece of information adversarially. A forensic psychiatrist will actively seek out information from the patient, corroborate or contrast it with that given by the others, and will look at anything available in an investigative fashion.

Implications for forensic psychiatrists

These differences have several consequences for forensic psychiatrists.

- Clinical data collected by the psychiatrist, and contained within a court report (see ⌨ p.V.555) can have not only medical but also legal relevance, including to guilt or innocence; some of which may be admissible and some not. In order to ascertain what weight to give that evidence should it be disputed, the court will wish to know the expert's status (e.g. consultant, trainee), post, relevant qualifications and experience, which should be stated in the report

- For the same reason, the sources of any information used by a psychiatrist should be made clear (patient, informant, records, etc.), so that the court can apply its own approach to what it holds to be true

- There may be disparity between the information that a psychiatrist would use in determining a diagnosis or formulation and that which is admissible within the relevant legal proceedings. This can cause

---

* However, if numerous or significant, they challenge the psychiatrist to question whether the perceived pattern (diagnosis, formulation) is correct, or the whole explanation.
† This is only true in countries such as the UK and RoI; in civil law jurisdictions (⌨ p.IV.306), judges and magistrates often actively conduct investigations.

ethical tension for an expert in court (e.g. where he is told that certain information cannot be considered by the court). There may be information that they are aware is inadmissible (📖 p.IV.318) as evidence but which may be diagnostically or clinically highly relevant. Reports should make clear how conclusions have been derived from information, including inadmissible information, but that information should be contained in a separate section of the report that can be withheld from disclosure if necessary

- Information contained within court proceedings, for example witness statements, can be used as data by the forensic psychiatrist (by analogy with informant information in ordinary clinical practice); however, witness evidence may be contradictory, such that the expert has to make conditional statements ('if the court believes A then the diagnosis of X is reinforced, if B then it is undermined')
- Information received from the criminal justice system should be given great weight if it has been considered and accepted by a court, because it will have been tested against the rules of evidence and been subjected to attempts by one or more parties to disprove it (so convictions should weigh more heavily in a risk assessment (📖 p.II.127) than allegations, for example).

Negotiating the interface

The forensic psychiatrist unavoidably straddles the two 'lands' of psychiatry and law (📖 p.IV.296). The effective forensic psychiatrist is able to spot when the different constructs and models (📖 p.IV.296 from each are in play; and is strict in keeping to their proper role when having to work across the border, such as in aiding the law by translating from the language of psychiatry into that of the law. Identifying the interface facilitates the keeping of proper boundaries in psycho-legal practice.

Where is the interface?

In situations such as giving evidence at a tribunal (📖 p.V.592) or writing court reports (📖 p.V.555), the interface is obvious. However, it is also present in many seemingly purely clinical tasks—for example, when sectioning (📖 p.IV.381) a patient (or deciding whether to discharge from a section), when the clinical facts must be set against the legal criteria for detention; or when drawing up a treatment plan, constrained by knowledge of what has been approved on a second opinion certificate (📖 p.IV.391). The relevance of legal constructs must therefore be borne in mind throughout clinical psychiatric practice.

Translation

For there to be dialogue between psychiatrists and lawyers, each must be prepared to understand and work with the constructs of the other, translating between the two where necessary. In strongly autopoetic (📖 p.IV.297) branches of the law, and perhaps all law, a perfect translation is impossible. For example, no legal concept could adequately capture the subtle variation (between individuals, and over time) in the behavioural manifestations of depression (📖 p.II.69), because legal constructs are one-dimensional and binary in nature, such as 'did the defendant act without any control by the mind or in a state involving loss of consciousness' (as in automatism, 📖 p.V.483)?

Minimizing errors in translation

Although a perfect translation may be impossible, the effects of the inherent mismatch between concepts may be minimized where:

- Lawyers ask psychiatrists clear legal questions, especially when giving instructions (📖 p.V.558)—e.g. 'please explain how the defendant's diagnosis might or might not amount to a "defect of reason" as opposed to 'please give a report on the defendant's mental condition'
- Psychiatrists understand how the law will wish to use the answers they give, i.e. to determine justice, not to achieve what is in the interests of the defendant (who may coincidentally be a patient under treatment)
- Psychiatrists recognize the limits of their professional expertise and role, and do not attempt for example to address the ultimate issue (📖 p.V.543).

Interpretation

Deciding how the law applies to particular facts and expert opinion is the core of jurisprudence (📖 p.V.542), and an issue that leads to frequent disagreements between lawyers (📖 p.IV.297). Ultimately, courts decide. However, often clinicians have to operate at the interface with law (e.g. in recommending detention under mental health legislation) without knowing how the law would view their own interpretation of the law.

Mental health law (📖 p.IV.373) allows wide discretion to clinicians in deciding whether or not to use its powers, because of the broad definition of some of its key concepts, such as the mental disorder (📖 p.IV.381) or appropriate treatment (📖 p.IV.390). This leaves clinicians free to import their own (mis)understandings of the law, and their own ethical values (📖 p.III.245), into their psycho-legal decision-making.

Such decision-making (for example whether to recommend compulsory detention, or whether a patient retains capacity to refuse treatment) amounts to interpreting what the law is in relation to this particular patient as if a lawyer, but with interpretation then open to review by a tribunal or court. In all such activities, the psychiatrist is not only ethically and legally responsible for their clinical treatment of the patient (e.g. in the law of negligence, 📖 p.IV.512), but also has an ethical duty to promote the patient's autonomy (📖 p.III.275) and respect their human rights (📖 p.IV.418) in the exercise of their discretion.

Different interfaces for different disciplines

There is a need also to understand the different models adopted by other clinical disciplines and how these will (differently) interface with the law in a particular context. For example, the categorical approach to disorder frequently pursued by psychiatry, arising from its medical roots which emphasize disease entities, will often tend to fit better with legal thinking, which is frequently binary in its approach both to evidence and to determining verdict, than will the characteristically dimensional approach of clinical psychology. There may therefore be varying degrees of incongruity between any mental science and law depending upon the particular field of law concerned.

Cooperation not contamination

The proper role of a doctor is to aid the *effecting* of justice, through cooperation with the law, and not to *affect* justice, via contamination of their
medical role. However, the inherent bias of psychiatry towards welfare,
rather than justice (📖 p.IV.297), can result in psychiatrists deliberately or
inadvertently tailoring their opinions (📖 p.V.551) so as to achieve a result
that they see as in the patient's best interests, despite the law. Some may
even give evidence tailored towards their own view of what would be the
just outcome. This practice is ethically and legally indefensible. Yet tribunals, for example, may themselves collude with contamination of the role
of psychiatrists giving evidence, each side colluding in a discourse directed
solely at public protection, for example. This has the effect of transforming
a legal hearing from a forum for the protection of the patient's civil rights
into what some have described as 'a glorified case conference'.

Legal systems

Sources of law

What is the law covering this situation?

This question is often surprisingly difficult to answer. Where a legislative body such as a Congress or Parliament has passed a law that directly relates to the situation in question, and there is no other law to take into account, the answer may be relatively straightforward. Sometimes, however, there will be multiple laws or types of law to take into account. Moreover, some or all of these may require *interpretation* by a judge (see 'Interpretation of the law', 📖 p.IV.305) before it is accepted whether and how they apply to a given situation that they do not expressly cover.

Sources of law

The different sources of law or quasi-law, with examples relevant to forensic psychiatry, include:

- National or federal *constitutions* such as the US constitution: 'super-laws' that overrule all other laws in the country concerned. These tend to cover broad areas of principle rather than narrow situations. For example, the 8th amendment to the US constitution bans 'cruel and unusual punishment', and this has been held to prevent the execution of defendants with mental retardation (learning disability, 📖 p.II.80)

- *International treaties* such as the European Convention on Human Rights (ECHR)[*], article 5 of which on lawful detention was used to force the UK government to allow tribunals to release restricted patients (📖 p.IV.412) from hospital in the face of government resistance

- Acts of Parliament or Congress, otherwise known as *statutes*. Important examples in the UK and Ireland include the Mental Health Act 1983 (2001 in RoI), the Mental Health (Care and Treatment) (Scotland) Act 2003 and the Mental Capacity Act 2005 (see 📖 p.IV.426)

- *Common law*, which is the body of judgments in previous cases by higher courts, both courts applying the law and those applying *equity* (originally the Lord Chancellor's ability to remedy wrongs ignored by the law). Not all jurisdictions recognize common law (see 📖 p.IV.306). In E&W, for example, the common law doctrine of necessity empowered doctors to treat patients who lack capacity (📖 p.IV.440) against their expressed wishes, until the Mental Capacity Act replaced this area of law

- *Customs* or 'conventions' (in a different sense from international conventions such as the ECHR) can occasionally be given the force of law by courts. This is commonest in contract law. For example, if it were customary in a certain area to send a warning letter before taking legal action to recover a debt, and if both parties could be shown to have been aware of and to have accepted that custom when

---

[*] The convention itself is an international treaty, but many countries have incorporated it into domestic law as a statute. In the UK, through the Human Rights Act 1998. The case that forced the UK to allow tribunals to release restricted patients (*X v UK*, 📖 p.App. 3.648) was heard before the 1998 Act was passed.

contracting, an action to recover a debt would fail if no warning letter had been sent
- In limited circumstances, the *opinions of academic lawyers*, such as the so-called 'Institutional Writers' of Scotland in the 17th century
- *Guidance* and *codes of practice* can amount to quasi-laws, that is rules whose breach can be taken into account in determining whether a different law has been broken. For instance, breach of important parts of the Mental Health Act Code of Practice in E&W might be held to contribute to a finding of negligence (📖 p.V.516) by a psychiatrist.

Interpretation of the law

Frequently, a legal case before the courts (or legal advice given before the event) will turn on whether and how one or other law applies in the situation in question. For example, in a judicial review (📖 p.IV.309) of a tribunal's decision to uphold the detention of a patient with autism (📖 p.II.76) under the Mental Health Act (📖 p.IV.373), the case might turn on whether the Act applied to patients with autism, given that autism and autistic spectrum disorders are not mentioned anywhere within its text.[*]

When lawyers interpret laws, they adopt one of several approaches:
- The *literal* (or 'black-letter law') approach. Usually associated with political conservatives and writers such as Joseph Raz, this approach focuses on the straightforward meaning of the text in question, and minimizes the scope for adopting a less obvious meaning in order to reach a 'better' outcome in a situation that the legislators were unlikely to have foreseen
- The *pragmatic* approach. This seeks to interpret the law in such a way as to create the most favoured outcome for society. Liberal justices on the US Supreme Court during the 1960s adopted a strongly pragmatic approach that resulted in a huge expansion of judicial activism, most notably interpreting the constitutional right to privacy as including a right to abortion
- The *interpretive* approach. Most commonly identified with the work of Ronald Dworkin, this approach seeks to interpret the individual law in the given situation in such a way as to give the overall body of law of which it forms a part as much consistency and coherence as possible.

Psychiatrists implicitly adopt aspects of these approaches when interpreting the law for medical purposes, but they also face the additional complications brought by psychiatry's different constructs and models (📖 p.IV.296) and by the need to negotiate the interface with the law (📖 p.IV.299).

---

[*] Before the 2007 amendments to the Mental Health Act in E&W, autism was held to be a mental disorder within the meaning of the Act, and could therefore form part of the grounds for detention for assessment (📖 p.IV.383) under section 2, but it was not a mental *illness* and therefore could not justify detention for treatment (📖 p.IV.388) under section 3 under the rules then in force unless there was also evidence of mental retardation (learning disability, 📖 p.II.80).

Civil law and common law systems

Although every jurisdiction has a legal system with its own individual and distinctive features, the vast majority* can be grouped according to whether they are predominantly based on 'civil' law or 'common' law principles.

Table 14.1 shows the main differences between the two systems. Some of the entries are explained in more detail after the table.

Table 14.1 Main differences between civil and common law systems

Feature	Civil law	Common law
Codification of laws	Compiled in one 'code'	Many separate laws
Binding nature of judgments(precedent)	Only legislature can make laws (binding decisions)	Higher courts' decisions bind lower courts
Court method	Inquisitorial (judge investigates and decides verdict)	Adversarial (judge is umpire between parties)
Legal reasoning	Deductive (argue from general principles)	Inductive (principles derived from cases)
Standard of proof: • Criminal trials • Civil trials	 • 'Personal conviction' • 'Personal conviction'	 • Beyond reasonable doubt • Balance of probabilities
Rules of evidence (see 📖 p.IV.317)	Free evaluation of all evidence, no exclusions	Tightly restricted (e.g. no 'hearsay' in criminal law)
Judicial appointments	Judges form a separate profession with specific training	Judges are selected from amongst the most experienced lawyers

E&W, NI, RoI and most US states are common law jurisdictions, whereas Scotland has a hybrid system, originally civil in nature, but with many common law features being added after the union with E&W in 1707.

Codification

Laws in civil law jurisdictions were extensively rewritten throughout much of the civil law world in the 19th century to be both:

- Collected in a single document (or a small number of documents covering different areas of law) rather than a multiplicity of Acts
- Based upon a coherent set of principles† throughout the code, rather than different areas of law being based on different principles

---

* A small number of countries' legal systems are based primarily on religious law (chiefly Islamic Sharia law), but many of these have also adopted civil law principles.
† This was the goal of many 19th-century legislators across the continent, but as codes were updated in the 20th century to reflect changing social realities, their newer sections tended to embody different principles from the original parts, weakening the overall coherence of the code.

Precedent

The principle of *stare decisis* ('let the decision stand') found in common law systems means that each decision of the higher courts sets a precedent for other courts: lower courts must reach the same decision in future cases unless they can distinguish the case from the precedent (i.e. show that its facts are different in some important way). Even decisions of lower courts have persuasive authority: that is, courts can decide differently in subsequent cases, but must explain why they are doing so. In contrast, courts in civil law jurisdictions are free to reach their own decision on their own interpretation of the legal principles involved.

Inquisitorial and adversarial methods

As a general rule, civil law judges are investigators: they actively seek to establish facts by questioning witnesses, and in some jurisdictions oversee police investigations from the start. The judge's high degree of control over the process means that detailed rules governing the conduct of the parties, particularly rules of evidence (📖 p.IV.317), are not required.

Common law systems are generally adversarial: that is, each of the parties seeks to demonstrate the truth of its own version of events (and interpretation of the law), and the judge acts as an impartial umpire, ensuring that each party sticks to the rules and does not gain unfair advantage over the others. At the end of the process, the court decides which party's case is proved.

Deductive and inductive reasoning

Civil law systems, especially those with fully codified bodies of law, are characterized by overarching principles, expressed in a constitution (📖 p.IV.304) or in introductory sections of their legal codes. Courts typically reason by starting with these principles and deducing from them what the outcome should be in the situation presented by the current case.

Conversely, the starting point of analysis in common law courts is the facts of the case. Courts make pragmatic decisions, typically by considering how similar cases have been decided in the past (i.e. by considering the precedents set by earlier decisions, particularly of higher courts). Courts rarely state overarching principles explicitly; instead, these are inferred by legal commentators from the verdicts reached.

The origins of civil law and common law

Civil law was originally the law of the cives, the citizens of Rome. Roman law was largely forgotten during late antiquity after the fall of the Roman Empire, but it was rediscovered in the 12th century, and its principles and many of its laws were used to create new legal systems across Europe.

The main exception was England, which by this time was already subordinating its patchwork of local customs to a coherent body of national law formed by the judgments of the network of royal courts with peripatetic judges established by Henry II in 1166. The influence of rediscovered Roman law was therefore much weaker: Latin terminology and Roman methods of reasoning were imported, but Anglo-Norman procedures and substantive law continued to exist.

Courts and tribunals of UK & Ireland

There are three distinct legal systems in the UK, plus a separate system in RoI. Their intermixed legal history is in part explained by English rule of Wales from 1283; of Scotland from the 1707 Act of Union;[*] and of Ireland from the 1801 Act of Union until the independence of the southern three provinces in 1922. Wales and England now share a common legal system, and form one jurisdiction; NI is a separate jurisdiction with some independent legal structures, but very heavily influenced by English law; and Scotland has a hybrid legal system, combining earlier Roman and other civil law (📖 p.IV.306) influences with later English concepts and legal structures. 📖 pp.IV.319–IV.325 describe the details of the legal systems in each of the four jurisdictions.

The following is an overview of the types of legal courts found in almost all jurisdictions.

A Supreme Court

- The highest level of domestic[†] legal court
- The final court of appeal for all civil and criminal cases—usually only on points of law (as opposed to review of the facts)
- In jurisdictions that permit judicial review (📖 p.IV.309) on the ground of constitutionality, the final arbiter of whether a law is constitutional
- Hearings usually involve five or more judges (so that where there are legitimate differences of view on questions of interpretation a majority may prevail).

Appeals Court(s)

- Primarily hear appeals on points of law—that is, claims by a party to a trial that the trial court mistook or misinterpreted the law
- Review the facts of the case only where the decision of the lower court was unreasonable (📖 p.IV.310) or if there is substantial new evidence, in which case a retrial by the lower court will usually be ordered
- Hearings usually consist of three judges.

Trial courts

- Also known as courts of first instance as they are the first court to hear the substance of the issues in question

---

[*] There is scope for great disagreement over (and this handbook takes no position on) whether Wales, Scotland and NI are still subject to 'English rule', whether the devolution after the 1997 referenda and the 1998 Good Friday Agreement made a material difference; or whether by the 20th century there was more mutual 'British rule' across all four countries.

[†] States may, by ratifying international treaties (📖 p.IV.304), give international courts (such as the International Court of Justice in the Hague in relation to, say, disputes over international borders, or the European Court of Human Rights in relation to the ECHR, 📖 p.IV.420) and supranational courts (most notably those of the European Union, 📖 p.IV.326) supremacy over their domestic courts in relation to issues covered by those treaties.

- They are usually divided into courts for criminal matters and courts for civil matters, with further subdivision of the latter into (for example) family, administrative, general law, and equity* courts
- There are often different levels of trial court depending on the seriousness of the matter in question, with the higher-level trial courts sometimes also acting as appeals courts for points of law from the lower-level courts
- Trial courts rule on the issues before them and make a ruling on guilt and (if guilty) sentence in criminal matters; and on what 'relief' (e.g. damages, or an injunction) to grant any party in civil matters.

Tribunals

- Tribunals are similar in function to trial courts for civil matters, but are less formal, act more quickly and at lower cost to the parties
- Each tribunal (or division of a tribunal) covers a narrow field of law, such as employment law, immigration law or mental health law
- They are formed of several members with specialized training and functions (including a legally trained chair), rather than general legal & judicial training
- For example, Mental Health Tribunals† operate to review patients' detention under the MHA and consist of a legal member, a medical member and a lay member
- Appeals from tribunals on points of law (📖 p.IV.309, 'Judicial review') go to a senior tribunal in some cases (such as the Upper Tribunal (📖 p.IV.320) in E&W), or (by way of judicial review, 📖 p.309) to a civil court such as the High Court in others.

Judicial review

The general premise of judicial review within the UK jurisdictions is that a higher court may cancel the decisions of a body carrying out public functions. In Ireland and other jurisdictions, judicial review is a wider concept,

---

*In common law systems, courts of equity (📖 p.IV.304) consider matters that were previously ignored by the law and settled by the Lord Chancellor, most notably issues concerning trusts (not NHS Trusts), where one party holds property on behalf of another and has to use it for their benefit.
†We have used the term Mental Health Tribunal (MHT) throughout the handbook. In E&W, Tribunals were formerly known as Mental Health Review Tribunals, and are now technically the First Tier Tribunal (Mental Health). In Scotland, their formal title is the Mental Health Tribunal for Scotland; in NI, the Mental Health Review Tribunal for Northern Ireland; and in RoI, simply the Mental Health Tribunal.

and extends to reviewing the actions of the legislature and to striking down laws* because they conflict with the constitution (📖 p.IV.304).

Judicial review is not an appeal: the correctness of the decision is not examined, merely its legality and reasonableness (or, in Ireland, its constitutionality), and the procedure by which it was reached. In this context, a decision is only 'unreasonable' if it is 'so outrageous in its defiance of logic or of accepted moral standards that no sensible person who had applied his mind to the question could have arrived at it'.†

The range of public bodies subject to judicial review is very wide, and includes all NHS and HSE organizations (including General Practices) carrying out functions on behalf of the government.

Relevance to forensic psychiatry

There may be judicial review in a number of areas in forensic psychiatry:

• Decisions made by individual practitioners representing a public body such as an NHS Trust or Health Board: e.g. a decision to refuse leave
• Actions taken by non-NHS bodies that affect patients: for instance, a decision by the Crown Prosecution Service to prosecute (or not to prosecute) a patient
• Decisions made by Mental Health Tribunals (outside E&W).

England & Wales and Northern Ireland

In E&W and NI, permission for Judicial Review must first be sought from the Administrative Division of the High Court (📖 p.IV.321). The complaint must be about a public or quasi-public body. Time limits apply to the application. There are three grounds for review:

• Illegality, particularly acting outside the powers granted to the body
• Unreasonableness
• Reaching a decision without following the proper procedure (e.g. a Tribunal reaching a decision to discharge before hearing evidence; although, since 2007, the Upper Tribunal (📖 p.IV.320) in E&W has heard appeals on such grounds, removing the possibility of judicial review).

Scotland

The substance of the Scottish law on judicial review is essentially the same as English law, although the procedure is different (for example, there are no time limits, and applications are heard by the Court of Session rather than a special Administrative Court). Judicial review can apply to any body, public or private, carrying out a public function.

Republic of Ireland

The High Court and Supreme Court in Ireland can invalidate any legislation that conflicts with the constitution, and can issue injunctions against any public or private body or any individual citizen to prevent them acting unconstitutionally. In addition, some areas of specific concern, such as town planning and immigration, are subject to special statutory judicial

---

* In the UK, the Human Rights Act 1998 (like the European Convention on Human Rights Act 2003 in RoI) allows higher courts to declare laws incompatible with the ECHR; but the doctrine of Parliamentary supremacy prevents any wider judicial review of the actions of Parliament, and means that incompatible laws remain in effect unless amended by Parliament.
† The principles are from *Wednesbury* (📖 p.App. 3.647), the famous phrase from Lord Diplock.

review procedures, which can involve consideration of the merits of a decision as well as its legality, constitutionality, and procedural propriety. Applications must be made within a maximum 6-month period.

Remedies after judicial review

Courts exercising powers of judicial review can, if they rule against the decision or action of the body in question:

- Quash the decision concerned (in RoI, this includes invalidating legislation)
- Order the body (by injunction) to take, or refrain from, certain actions
- Award damages to anyone who suffered from the original decision or action of the body.

Judicial Review in action: R (Ashworth Hospital) v MHRT (see 📖 p.App. 3.629 for full details)

Facts

H was detained at a high secure hospital. There was clear evidence of risk of harm to others and of previous failed discharges. The Tribunal discharged him, despite the lack of aftercare (📖 p.IV.398) arrangements.

Grounds for review

- The Tribunal gave inadequate reasons for its decision (procedural impropriety)
- The Tribunal acted unreasonably by discharging the patient in the absence of aftercare arrangements, when it could have adjourned to allow time for arrangements to be put in place.

Decision

The Court of Appeal held that the Tribunal had decided unreasonably, and that its lack of adequate reasons for its decision was improper, and therefore quashed the decision to discharge H.

Roles in court

Court personnel have distinctive roles, many of which are established by law and/or long tradition. The following is a summary of those roles, as found in the UK jurisdictions and RoI. Not all personnel will be found in all courts.

Court personnel

- Judge—presides over a court; responsible for ensuring court procedure (📖 p.IV.314) is correctly followed, the law is correctly interpreted and applied, and ultimately that justice is done and seen to be done
- Jury—a body of 12 (15 in Scotland) ordinary people (peers of the defendant or litigant) who hear evidence and deliver a verdict, guided by the judge as to matters of law
- Court Clerk—responsible for maintaining records, and for giving legal advice to lay magistrates in E&W (who are not legally qualified, unlike District Judges); he or she normally sits at a table in front of the judge/sheriff, facing into the courtroom
- Usher, Court Officer, Macer (Scottish High Court) List Caller—introduces each case by calling parties to the court and telling the court who is representing whom; responsible for making sure that the comings and goings in the court operate smoothly, and often for arranging the order of cases efficiently, and for maintaining order
- Stenographer –records the proceedings verbatim
- Solicitors—lawyers who deal with most legal matters but usually only conduct trials (litigate) in lower courts
- Barristers, Counsel*, Solicitor advocates (Scotland), Advocates* (Scotland)—lawyers who conduct trials in higher courts.

The defendant and witnesses are the other parties present in court. The court may also have reporters and the public present, but they are only observers.

The Judiciary

Heads of judiciary
- Lord Chief Justice—head of the judiciary for E&W
- The Lord President of the Court of Session—head of the judiciary for Scotland
- The Lord Chief Justice of Northern Ireland—head of the judiciary in Northern Ireland
- The Chief Justice of Ireland—head of the judiciary in Ireland.

Other judiciary (criminal courts only)
See Table 14.2.

---

*Senior barristers and advocates in the UK may be appointed as 'Queen's Counsel' (QC) by letters patent issued by the Queen.

Table 14.2 Other judiciary (criminal courts only)

Court	England & Wales and Northern Ireland	Scotland	Republic of Ireland
Supreme Court	Justices of the Supreme Court	(Same as E&W, but see 📖 p.IV.322)	Justices of the Supreme Court
Appeals Courts	Lords Justices of Appeal[*]	Lords of Council and Session[†]	Judges of the Court of Criminal Appeal
	High Court Judges, Masters & Registrars	Lords Commissioners of Justiciary	Judges of the High Court
Higher criminal trial courts	Circuit Judges or Recorders[‡]	Sheriff Principal / Sheriff	Judges of the Circuit Court
Lower criminal trial courts	District Judges or Magistrates[§]	Justice of the Peace	District Judges

Tribunal and other roles

- Tribunal Presidents—responsible for the administration of their tribunal
- Tribunal Chairmen and Tribunal Judges—appointment based on qualifications for the particular tribunal
- Tribunal Panel members—vary according to the particular tribunal
- Notaries Public (Scotland)—solicitors who record certain transactions and sign specific legal documents.

Other terms

- The Prosecution—the legal party who presents the case against an individual in a criminal trial, in the name of the Crown in the UK and of the People in RoI
- The Defence—the legal party who represents the defendant
- Claimant[**]/Complainant/Pursuer—the person who initiates a legal action seeking a legal remedy in civil matters
- Defendant/Defender—the person or body answering a complaint (in civil courts) or the person charged with a criminal offence.

---

[*] These include the Lord Chief Justice, the Master of the Rolls, and from the High Court, the President of the Queen's Bench Division, the President of the Family Division, and the Chancellor (head of the Chancery Division), though not all sit in criminal appeals.
[†] Including the Lord President and Lord Justice Clerk. The same people are often both Lords of Council and Session and Lords Commissioners of Justiciary in the High Court.
[‡] A fully-qualified solicitor or barrister sitting as a judge.
[§] Magistrates and Justices of the Peace are lay people with basic training (but no legal qualifications) sitting with a legal advisor or clerk.
[**] Formerly known as 'plaintiff'.

Court procedures

Court procedures vary depending on the type of court and the jurisdiction. Many aspects will be irrelevant to psychiatrists but it is useful to have some understanding of basic procedures of the criminal justice process as a whole (📖 p.IV.330), those procedures relating directly to expert witnesses (📖 p.V.534), and a more detailed knowledge of the legal rules (📖 p.V.536) and codes of practice (📖 p.V.538) for expert witnesses.

Criminal courts

See also giving evidence in criminal courts (📖 p.V.590).

- Generally, at the beginning of the case, the charges will be read and the defendant will be asked to make a plea. If a guilty plea is made the magistrates or judge will hand down a sentence. If a not guilty plea is made, the case will be heard in full
- The defendant is not obliged to give evidence, however if they do give evidence they will be subject to cross-examination (📖 p.V.588) by the prosecution[*]
- Judges in an adversarial system (📖 p.IV.307) like those in the UK and RoI must be impartial and ensure fair play and due process; they decide what evidence (📖 p.IV.317) may be admitted, and other procedural issues
- In the lower criminal courts (Magistrates' Court, in E&W and NI, 📖 p.IV.320, District Court, in Scotland 📖 p.IV.322 & RoI 📖 p.IV.324), the hearing can take place in a court room, with a gallery for the general public, or in a private room (although people connected to the case such as solicitors and witnesses may be invited to attend). The judge will usually give their verdict immediately at the end of the trial
- In the higher criminal courts (Crown Court in E&W, 📖 p.IV.320, Sheriff Court in Scotland, 📖 p.IV.322, County Criminal Court in NI, 📖 p.IV.320, Circuit Court in RoI, 📖 p.IV.324), there may also be a gallery for members of the public and the press. The defendant is expected to take a seat on the dock (a raised platform) and to stand when requested. The average trial lasts for a day or so but may extend into weeks and months if the evidence is complex. At the end of the trial the jury will retire to a private room to discuss the case and decide on the verdict. The jury debate is confidential. Once a decision has been made the foreman juror will pass the verdict to the judge before reading it to the court
- Procedures differ in youth courts (📖 p.IV.320), whether they are wholly separate courts or (for example) part of a magistrates' court. This is also the case when serious youth trials are held in (adult) higher courts. The case is still heard in full but there may be more frequent breaks, and the defendant is given explanations of legal arguments in terms that they can understand. Media coverage and public access is heavily controlled to protect the identity of the defendant

[*] If they do not, the judge (at least in E&W) may make an *adverse inference direction* entitling the jury to make inferences from the defendant's silence (such as that they wish to avoid incriminating themselves under cross-examination)—unless there is psychiatric evidence that it would be 'undesirable' for the defendant to give evidence.

- Following the trial, if the defendant is found not guilty (acquitted), they are free to leave the court[*]
- If the defendant is convicted, they will sometimes be sentenced (📖 p.IV.361) immediately; more commonly, the case will be adjourned for pre-sentence reports (📖 p.IV.362) to be compiled, particularly if the defendant appears to be mentally disordered.

Civil courts

See also giving evidence in civil courts (📖 p.V.595).

- The duty of any participant in a civil case is to comply with the Civil Procedure Rules (📖 p.V.538) in E&W, or equivalents elsewhere
- In most trials the case is heard by a judge alone; juries are very rare (e.g. in some defamation trials)
- Cases are usually slow to pass through the system (taking months or years), and the vast majority of cases are settled out of court
- Although the defendant is required to give a statement, this statement is not subject to cross-examination by the prosecutor and is not given under oath. However, the statement is likely to be questioned by the judge
- In Scotland and NI all witnesses are required to give evidence orally, whether or not they have submitted a report
- At the end of the trial the Sheriff or judge will usually retire to consider their judgement and will deliver this in writing later.

Tribunals

See also giving evidence to tribunals (📖 p.V.592).

- Tribunals cover many areas of special jurisdiction including mental health and employment law (📖 p.V.523)
- Tribunals are usually conducted in private, although the parties may apply for a public hearing (even with mental health tribunals)
- Participants must follow the relevant set of Tribunal Procedure Rules
- As a witness in a tribunal, you will not be required to take an oath
- In RoI public inquiries are also often referred to as 'tribunals'.

---

[*] Unless, in Scotland, the court makes an order for their urgent detention (📖 p.IV.408) on mental health grounds; or they have been found not guilty by reason of insanity (📖 p.V.489).

The burden and standards of proof

In any legal proceeding, parties are required to *prove* facts that they wish to rely on. The standard to which they must prove a fact depends on the type of case, and which party is trying to prove it.

The standard of proof in civil courts and tribunals

In all non-criminal court hearings, facts are required to be proved *on the balance of probabilities**, meaning that it is more likely than not to be true, or 'more probable than not'. This is also the standard of proof used in Mental Health Tribunals (📖 p.IV.309), when facts are contested.

This is the case in the UK jurisdictions and RoI, although in civil law (📖 p.IV.306) countries such as France and Germany, the standard of proof in civil matters is the same as in criminal trials, and therefore much higher.

In the US, the 'balance of probabilities' is usually referred to as the 'preponderance of evidence', but the meaning is the same.

The standard of proof in criminal courts

The general rule in the UK and Ireland is that, in order for the court to convict the defendant, the prosecution must prove that they committed the offence *beyond reasonable doubt*. In cases held before a jury (📖 p.IV.312), the judge should explain that this means that the jury should only return a guilty verdict if they are '*sure*† that the defendant is guilty'.

However, in criminal cases, when it is the defence that is required to prove something—such as the existence of a specific defence (📖 p.IV.342)—it usually only has to do so on the balance of probabilities.

Most jurisdictions use the beyond reasonable doubt standard for criminal matters, although it may be phrased differently (for example, in France as 'a personal conviction' on the part of the judge). However, there are exceptions. For example, in the US in some circumstances facts are proven if there is 'clear and convincing evidence', which has been interpreted as just 'substantially more likely than not to be true'.

The standard of 'proof' before trial

In making decisions before trial, a lower standard of 'proof' is required: the police officer or prosecutor is not expected to convince themselves that something is the case, merely that it is sufficiently likely in order to proceed with the investigation or prosecution. Some relevant standards are:

- *Reasonable grounds for suspecting*—the lowest standard, enough to justify a police search of a person or a car for stolen property
- *Reasonable grounds for believing*—a more demanding standard, enough to justify a police officer entering a private dwelling to look for a specific individual

---

* A different phrase may be used: for example, in cases under the Children Act 1989, that the court is 'satisfied' of something. This is still taken to mean that it is more likely than not.
† This means that the word 'sure' can have particular weight in evidence: an expert witness (📖 p.V.534) stating they are not sure about a key point can be enough to result in acquittal.

- *Probable cause*—the US term corresponding to the previous point, used to justify police searches and arrests (and indictments by grand juries) when there is 'a fair probability' of finding evidence, or of conviction
- *Reasonable prospect of conviction*, meaning at least 50% probability of conviction—the standard used by prosecution agencies in the UK[*] and RoI to decide whether to prosecute, along with the public interest test (📖 p.III.289)

The burden of proof

A related issue is which party is required to prove certain matters. In civil matters, whichever party wishes to rely on a fact must prove it. The general rule in criminal cases, as stated earlier, is that the prosecution must prove all the elements of the offence, otherwise the defendant is acquitted. However, there are exceptions, including the following:

- Where the defendant puts forward certain defences, they must prove the relevant facts (on the balance of probabilities)
- If the defendant claims that they are unfit to plead (📖 p.V.474), they must prove it (again, on the balance of probabilities)
- In a prosecution for possession of an offensive weapon in a public place, if it has been proved that the defendant was in possession in a public place, they must prove (on the balance of probabilities) that they had a lawful authorization or reasonable excuse for this.

There are two different burdens of proof. The first is the *legal burden*, which is what has been described so far: the requirement to prove that something is the case. The other is the *evidential burden*, which means only that a party is required to adduce evidence that something might be the case, which the other party may then have a legal burden to disprove. Examples of evidential burdens include:

- The legal justifications (📖 p.IV.340) and the defence of duress (📖 p.IV.343), where the defendant has an evidential burden (e.g. to show that they were threatened), whereupon the prosecution has the legal burden of disproving that (say) the threats were sufficiently serious, or that the defendant had no alternative course of action
- In a prosecution for handling stolen goods, if it has been proved that the defendant was in possession of stolen goods, they then have the evidential burden of showing that they had a reasonable excuse for doing so, whereupon the prosecution must prove beyond reasonable doubt that their explanation is false.

Rules of evidence

Rules of evidence govern whether information in a case may be presented, when it is presented, and in what form. The rules of evidence

---

[*] Except Scotland, where the equivalent test is whether there is sufficient (i.e. corroborated) admissible, reliable, credible evidence.

vary between legal contexts.[*] They are very tightly drawn within the criminal law, less so within the civil courts, and even less so within the family courts. There are subtle variations between jurisdictions relating to the specific issues discussed here but the concepts are universal.

What is evidence?

Evidence is information (📖 p.III.297) that may be presented to a court to prove or rebut a civil or criminal case. The aim of the trial is to test the evidence from either side; a criminal trial will not proceed unless there is a realistic prospect of conviction (📖 p.III.317). Quasi-judicial bodies such as Mental Health Tribunals do not apply rules of evidence per se. There is therefore great latitude in what evidence can be presented and when.

Evidence can be in the form of:
- Testimony—oral statements
- Documentary—any paper records
- Real—physical objects.

Fact, inference, and opinion

There is a distinction drawn between fact and inference derived from fact. Opinion evidence amounts to inference drawn from particular facts. Witnesses who are not expert witnesses may only give evidence of fact, and not inference or opinion. Expert witnesses (📖 p.V.534) may give evidence of fact, including fact derived through practice of their own professional skills, and also evidence of opinion, drawing inferences from both expertly derived and ordinary facts. Facts may be relevant or collateral, i.e. going directly to the legal issue or merely being associated with it.

Relevance and admissibility

Relevant evidence will go some way to showing whether a fact did or did not exist. However, relevant evidence may be inadmissible, e.g. because of perceived unfairness in the way it was collected or presented, or because it is more prejudicial than probative. That is, it does little to prove one side's case, while tending to make a party appear bad or immoral.

Within a criminal trial a jury, or magistrates, must come to their conclusion on whether guilt is proven solely on the facts presented within the case. If they were to use information not presented within the trial then that information would not be open to challenge.

The law governing what evidence may be excluded makes up much of the law relating to evidence[†]. These rules cover not only what might logically help answer the question but also what it would be fair to include. For example, from the perspective of risk assessment (📖 p.II.127), a defendant's past behaviour would be a strong predictor of having committed the current alleged offence; but it might be unfair to allow a jury to hear such evidence because it might influence their evaluation of the evidence relating to the current alleged offence, and therefore information on past behaviour is admitted only in limited circumstances.

---

[*] And even more so between jurisdictions: countries following the civil law tradition (📖 p.IV.306) have few or no rules on admissibility of evidence, allowing investigative magistrates 'free evaluation' of all the evidence

[†] This area of law tends to be detailed and prescriptive in E&W and NI, whereas much is left to judges' discretion in Scotland and RoI. See, for example, the admissibility of confessions, 📖 p.V.479.

Use of evidence

The weight attached to a piece of evidence may be a matter of common sense; once it has been considered admissible the decision as to what weight is attached to it depends on ordinary factors such as:

- Support (corroboration) or contradiction by other evidence
- The status, demeanour or credibility of the witness
- The inherent credibility of the evidence.

Non-expert witnesses are not permitted to hear the evidence of other witnesses. Expert witnesses are usually encouraged to do so, as the other evidence may affect their expert opinion.

Hearsay

There are rules relating to facts described by a witness arising not directly from their own experience but from what they have heard from others.

- X gives evidence that Y told him something
- X gives evidence that Y told him something that Z said or did.

Generally this kind of evidence is excluded in criminal proceedings. The rationale for this is that the judge or jury cannot properly consider the weight of this evidence if it is not subject to any test of reliability by cross-examination. The strictness of the hearsay rule is greater within criminal compared to civil proceedings, where hearsay evidence is generally admissible. In civil proceedings the focus is on weight of evidence more than admissibility per se.

The *voir dire*

Prior to a criminal trial commencing there may be an application to exclude particular evidence, on the basis that it was unlawfully obtained, or that it would be unfair to include it. Within a *voir dire*[*] the trial judge will hear arguments as to why the evidence should or should not be admitted, and sometimes may hear the evidence himself. If the evidence is admitted, the same arguments may also be presented during the trial, asking for less weight to be given to the evidence.

The court system in England, Wales & Northern Ireland

The court systems in E&W and NI are separate (apart from sharing the Supreme Court) but identical (see Fig. 14.1).

---

[*] Literally, 'let us see what you are going to say [in the trial]'.

Supreme Court

- Is the highest appeal court in almost all cases in E&W
- Its role was previously held by the House of Lords
- It sits as the Judicial Committee of the Privy Council for appeals from Commonwealth countries.

Senior Courts of E&W and NI

- The Court of Appeal deals with appeals from other courts or tribunals. The Civil Division hears appeals from the High Court and the County Court, as well as some superior tribunals; the Criminal Division hears appeals from the Crown Court connected with a trial on indictment. Its decisions are binding on all lower courts
- The High Court of Justice comprises the Queen's Bench, the Chancery Division, and the Family Division. This court functions as a civil court of first instance (for more serious claims); the Queen's Bench Division also hears appeals from magistrates' courts, and the Family Division hears appeals from the Court of Protection (📖 p.IV.435)
- The Crown Court is a criminal court. It is the only court that has the jurisdiction to try cases on indictment (i.e. more serious crimes). In Northern Ireland it is known as the County Criminal Court
- In Northern Ireland, there can be a rehearing of a county court case in the High Court and an appeal from there to the Court of Appeal.

Subordinate courts

- County courts: local courts, each one having an area over which certain kinds of civil jurisdiction are exercised, including claims for debt repayment, personal injury, breach of contract, and housing disputes
- Magistrates' courts: these are presided over by a bench of lay magistrates (justices of the peace), or (in larger towns in E&W) a legally trained district judge. They hear minor criminal cases
- Family Proceedings court (part of the Magistrates' court): these hear family law cases, including child care cases, and they have power to make adoption orders
- Youth courts (part of the Magistrates' court) deal with almost all cases involving children. The court is served by youth panel magistrates and District Judges. Youth courts are less formal than magistrates' courts, are more open and engage more with the young person appearing in court and their family. Youth courts are essentially private places and members of the public are not admitted.

Tribunals

There are statutory tribunals for specialist areas: employment, immigration, social security, pensions, child welfare, and mental health. Appeals are either to appeal tribunals (known in most cases as the Upper Tribunal) or certain courts, depending on the statute.

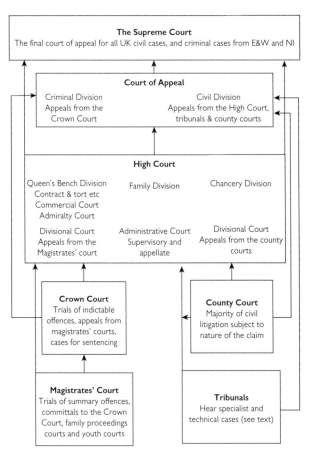

Fig. 14.1 Summary diagram of the court system in England, Wales, & Northern Ireland.

The court system in Scotland

Scotland has its own distinct courts system, which has developed separately (📖 p.IV.308) from that elsewhere in the UK or RoI. The civil courts deal with cases involving disputes between individuals and or organizations, and the criminal courts deal with criminal cases (Fig. 14.2). Notably, criminal courts in Scotland require all evidence to be corroborated by other evidence; this is no longer the case for civil courts.

UK Supreme Court
- In Scotland the Supreme Court only hears civil cases and devolution matters (disagreements about whether the Scottish authorities have the power to make certain decisions).

Court of Session
- The highest civil court in Scotland
- Divided into Inner and Outer Houses:
  - Inner House is in essence the appeal court
  - Outer House deals with a wide range of civil matters
- Judges are termed 'Senators of the College of Justice' or 'Lords of Council and Session'.

High Court of Justiciary
Court of criminal appeal
- Cases are heard by three or more judges
- There is no appeal to the Supreme Court.

Criminal trials
- Hears serious cases, such as murder or rape
- Consists of a judge and jury (15 adults)
- Has unlimited sentencing powers.

Sheriff Court
- Scotland consists of 6 sheriffdoms, each headed by Sheriff Principal
- There are sheriff courts in most districts in Scotland
- Both civil and criminal cases can be heard in this type of court
- Summary case are heard in front of the sheriff alone—maximum sentence is 3 months
- Solemn cases are heard in front of a sheriff and jury—maximum sentence is 5 years or an unlimited fine.

District Courts
- Justices of peace (JP) hear minor cases
- Can impose a maximum 60 day sentence and smaller fines.

The Mental Health Tribunal for Scotland
- This hears applications for and appeals against Compulsory Treatment Orders and other mental health orders (📖 p.IV.373)
- Other tribunals exist, covering diverse areas.

Children's Hearings

- This is a specialist system that handles the majority of cases involving allegations of criminal conduct by young people under 16 years old
- They have wide ranging powers to issue supervision orders for young people referred to them by the Scottish Children's Reporter Administration
- The children's panel is a group of people from the community who are carefully selected and trained. The panel members sit on hearings on a rotational basis. The three panel members decide on whether compulsory measures of supervision are needed for the child and, if so, what they should be
- Serious crimes are still dealt with in the usual criminal courts, at the direction of the Procurator Fiscal.

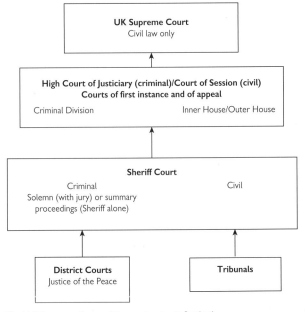

Fig. 14.2 Summary diagram of the court system in Scotland.

The court system in the Irish Republic

RoI established its own independent court system after independence from the UK in 1922 (Fig. 14.3); the principal legislation is now the Courts (Establishment and Constitution) Act 1961. The system is managed by the Courts Service of Ireland.

Superior courts
- These consist of the Supreme Court and the High Courts
- Established by the Constitution.

Supreme Court
- Defined as the Court of Final Appeal
- Main activity is hearing appeals from decisions in the High Court
- Also hears appeals from circuit courts and Court of Criminal Appeal.

Court of Criminal Appeal
- Hears appeals from the Circuit or Central Criminal Court.

High Court
- Has authority to interpret the Constitution
- Tries the most serious criminal and civil cases
- Hears appeals from the Circuit Court in civil matters
- Can review the decisions of certain tribunals
- Deals with questions of law arising from District Courts
- Termed the *Central Criminal Court* when sitting as a criminal court, when it sits with a jury. Hears mainly murder and rape trials but also tries other serious charges.

Special Criminal Court
- A court in which serious crimes may be tried in the absence of a jury
- It may be used to try defendants accused of being members of paramilitary organizations such as the Continuity IRA, or of committing organized crime.

Subordinate courts
- Circuit Court: deals with civil, criminal and family law, criminal matters that must be tried before a jury, and some appeals from the District Courts
- District Courts: deal with criminal matters (predominantly summary matters), lower value civil claims, and many family law matters
- All juvenile cases are referred centrally to the National Juvenile Office, which decides what action should be taken against them.

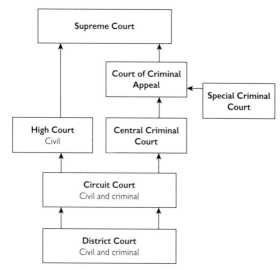

Fig. 14.3 Summary diagram of the court system in the Irish Republic.

Court systems in the EU and elsewhere

The European Union (EU)
The EU is based on a series of treaties, which set broad policy goals and establish institutions with the legal powers to implement those goals.

Supranational EU courts
- *Court of Justice of the European Union* consists of three courts: the Court of Justice, the General Court, and the European Union Civil Service Tribunal. They interpret and apply the treaties and law of the EU
- *The General Court* (previously known as the Court of First Instance) is attached to the Court of Justice. It hears and determines at first instance all direct actions brought by individuals and Member States, with the exception of those assigned to a 'judicial panel' and those reserved for the Court of Justice.

Pan-European courts not related to the EU itself
- *The European Court of Human Rights* in Strasbourg provides legal recourse of last resort for individuals who assert that their human rights have been violated by a contracting party to the Convention (one of the countries signed up to the convention). It applies the European Convention on Human Rights (📖 p.IV.420)
- *The International Court of Justice (ICJ)* is the primary judicial body of the United Nations, based in The Hague. Its main functions are to settle legal disputes and to provide advisory opinions on legal questions that have been submitted by international organizations, UN agencies and the UN General Assembly.

The United States of America and Canada
The judicial system in the US is made up of two different systems:
- The *federal court system* consists of 'article III' courts, which include: US District Courts, US Circuit Courts of Appeal, and the US Supreme Court; and two special courts; the US Court of Claims and the US Court of International Trade. With the exception of the special courts, the courts can hear almost any case and judges are appointed by the President of the United States. The second type of federal court is established by congress and includes magistrate's courts, bankruptcy courts, the US Court of Military Appeals, the US Tax Court and the US Court of Veterans' Appeals
- The *state court system*—no two state court systems are exactly the same. However most are made up of two sets of trial courts (trial courts of limited jurisdiction and of general jurisdiction), intermediate appellate courts and the highest state courts. Unlike federal courts, most state judges are not appointed for life but are either elected or appointed for a certain number of years.

The two systems are not completely independent of each other and they interact, although they are each responsible for hearing certain types of cases. The federal court system deals with issues of law relating to those powers expressly or implicitly granted to it by the US Constitution.

In Canada, the court system is a four-level hierarchy from the highest to lowest in terms of legal authority. Each court is bound by the rulings of the courts above them. At the top is the Supreme Court of Canada, then the appellate courts of the provinces and territories, the superior-level courts of the provinces and territories, and finally the provincial and territorial ('inferior') courts. There are also courts at the federal level.

Australia and the Commonwealth

The legal systems in Australia and the Commonwealth are modelled substantially on the system in E&W and so are common law jurisdictions. However, many have evolved so they no longer closely resemble the British systems. Australia now has both a state legal system and an overarching federal system with corresponding courts.

Judicial Committee of the Privy Council

The Judicial Committee of the Privy Council, comprised of judges of the UK Supreme Court, considers appeals for a number of overseas jurisdictions. It is of relevance to forensic psychiatrists because it often hears final appeals against the use of the death penalty. The extent of the jurisdiction of this committee continues to reduce as former British states establish their own courts of final appeal.

Appeal is to 'Her Majesty in Council' from the following independent nations and other territories:

- The Crown Dependencies of Jersey, Guernsey, Alderney, Sark, and the Isle of Man
- The Commonwealth realms of Antigua & Barbuda, the Bahamas, Grenada, Jamaica, St Kitts and Nevis, St Lucia, St Vincent & the Grenadines and Tuvalu
- The New Zealand associated states of the Cook Islands and Niue (though not New Zealand itself)
- The British overseas territories of Anguilla, Bermuda, British Virgin Islands, Cayman Islands, Falkland Islands, Gibraltar, Montserrat, St Helena, Ascension & Tristan da Cunha, Turks & Caicos Islands, and Pitcairn Islands
- The UK Sovereign Base Areas of Akrotiri and Dhekelia in Cyprus.

Appeal is directly to the Committee from the following countries:
- The Commonwealth republics of Dominica, Mauritius, Trinidad & Tobago and Kiribati.

Appeal is to the Head of State (i.e. The Queen) for the Commonwealth member Brunei.

Criminal law

The criminal justice process

Criminal procedure

The main elements of the process of detecting and responding to crime are shown in the flowchart in Fig. 15.1 (the specific agencies concerned, such as the police and the prosecution service, are summarized on 🕮 p.IV.448.) For simplicity, a number of details and alternative possibilities are not shown in the diagram. For example:

- Suspects do not need to have been arrested in order to be questioned: they may choose to 'help the police with their enquiries' on a voluntary basis. Arrests can be authorized by a warrant issued by a court, or under powers to arrest for 'arrestable' offences or for the investigation or prevention an offence or breach of the peace (🕮 p.IV.353)
- Often, especially in E&W, the decision to charge will be made by or in consultation with the prosecutor, rather than by the police alone. The prosecutor will not proceed unless there is a reasonable prospect of conviction (🕮 p.IV.317), usually with at least 50% probability
- The purposes of the initial appearance before the lower criminal court (Magistrates' Court, in E&W and NI, 🕮 p.IV.320, District Court in Scotland 🕮 p.IV.322 & RoI 🕮 p.IV.324) are to ensure there is sufficient evidence to justify a trial, to give the defendant an opportunity to plead guilty, to set the timetable for the trial and to consider remand
- Less serious offences can be tried summarily by the lower criminal court; more serious ones are committed to the higher criminal court (Crown Court in E&W, 🕮 p.IV.320, Sheriff Court in Scotland, 🕮 p.IV.322, County Criminal Court in NI, 🕮 p.IV.320, Circuit Court in RoI, 🕮 p.IV.324) where the trial process is more complex, guilt is usually determined by a jury, and the maximum sentences available are much greater. In a few intermediate cases the defendant may have a choice of court
- In Scotland, there is a third verdict in addition to guilty and not guilty: 'not proven', which like not guilty leads to acquittal, but which is taken to mean that there was strong suspicion that the defendant was guilty
- Suspects and offenders can be diverted (🕮 p.II.216) into mental health services from the point of arrest to that of sentencing. This might include bail or remand to hospital (🕮 p.IV.403), for example. The police, prosecutor or court may stop criminal proceedings, suspend them until the patient has recovered, or allow them to continue in parallel.

Detention, bail, and remand

During the process of investigation, the police may *detain* the suspect for a limited period of time (e.g. in E&W up to 24 hours, with the possibility of a short extension by a senior officer and then up to a total of 96 hours by a court, or longer for terrorist suspects)—or, alternatively, give them *police bail* allowing them to leave but requiring them to report back and to meet certain conditions (such as surrendering their passport, or residing at a specific place). After charging, the court can similarly bail the defendant; or *remand* them in custody, usually in a remand prison (🕮 p.V.456), but also in hospital.

Simplified criminal justice process

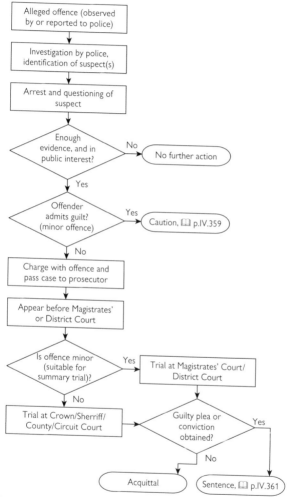

Fig. 15.1 Flowchart of the process of detecting and responding to crime.

Elements of a crime

What is a crime?

A crime is any behaviour that Parliament[*] or the courts have determined should be a crime, on the ground that the behaviour should be morally censured and the person responsible should be punished by the state. This contrasts with torts or 'wrongs' under the civil law (📖 p.V.509), such as libel, product liability, or negligence (📖 p.V.512), which attract less moral disapproval, and where the court's action is intended to restore the wronged party to the position they would have been in had there been no tort, not (usually) to punish the person responsible.

What amounts to criminal behaviour changes over time, as public attitudes change and are reflected in Parliamentary and judicial law-making (📖 p.IV.307). In recent years there has been a massive expansion of the ambit of criminal law in E&W in particular, and to a lesser extent in Scotland, NI and RoI, with the creation of large numbers of new offences.

The range of criminal offences is wide; the major categories are shown in Box 15.1. Forensic psychiatry most commonly deals with crimes against the person, both violent and sexual, and against property.

Box 15.1 Main categories of crime

- Offences against the person, e.g. assault (📖 p.IV.346), murder (📖 p.IV.345)
- Sexual offences, e.g. rape, indecent exposure (📖 p.IV.348)
- Public order offences, e.g. affray (📖 p.IV.352)
- Possession offences, e.g. of offensive weapons in public, or of drugs
- Property offences, e.g. criminal damage, arson (📖 p.IV.350)
- Offences of dishonesty, e.g. theft, fraud, deception (📖 p.IV.354)
- Offence against the state, e.g. treason, terrorism (📖 p.IV.357)
- Regulatory offences, e.g. breach of bail conditions, driving offences
- Inchoate offences (📖 p.IV.339): e.g. attempt to rob, conspiracy to rob.

The elements of a crime

Most crimes require that the prosecution prove both of the following elements beyond reasonable doubt (📖 p.IV.316):

- The actus reus ('wrongful act'): the *conduct* relevant to the offence, for example penetrating the victim's mouth, anus or vagina with the penis in the case of rape, plus the *relevant circumstances*,[†] meaning in this example the absence of the victim's consent; and in some cases, the *consequences* caused, such as death in the case of murder. The conduct can be an omission to act, such as in manslaughter (📖 p.IV.345).
- The mens rea ('guilty mind'), also known as the 'fault element': that the defendant was capable of forming, and did form, a relevant *state of mind* (see 📖 p.IV.334) at the time of the actus reus. This includes failing to consider something they should have considered (negligence).

[*] Dáil in RoI.
[†] These include the status of the defendant: for example, children under the age of criminal responsibility (📖 p.IV.338) cannot be prosecuted for conduct that would otherwise be wrongful.

However, despite proof of actus reus and mens rea, the defendant will be acquitted if they prove on the balance of probabilities* (📖 p.IV.316):

- An excuse or *justification* for their conduct, such as self-defence or the prevention of crime (see 📖 p.IV.340), or
- A *defence* to their prosecution for their conduct, such as duress or necessity (📖 p.V.502), insanity (📖 p.V.489) or automatism† (📖 p.V.483).

Vignette: making out the offence of theft

Mr B demands money for drugs from Mr C, threatening to assault him very seriously if he does not give it to him. Mr C, being penniless, steals money from the till at a shop while the shop-owner's attention is elsewhere. He is arrested, and prosecuted for theft. To obtain a conviction, the prosecution must prove:

Actus reus

That Mr C appropriated property belonging to another. The money (notes and coins) is property; it belonged to the shop-owner; and Mr C took it into his own possession (appropriated it).

Mens rea

That Mr C did so dishonestly, and with the intention of permanently depriving the other of it. Mr C was dishonest in this context: he knew the money was the shop-owner's and that he had no right to it. He also intended to give the money to Mr B, permanently depriving the shop-owner of it.

However, Mr C may be able to prove a *defence*:

Mr B forced Mr C to act by threatening him with serious injury. This could amount to the defence of duress by threats (📖 p.V.502). If the court accepts this, Mr C will be acquitted.

---

* Or, in some cases, if they raise evidence of the defence and the prosecution fails to disprove it beyond reasonable doubt, as with duress.
† Strictly speaking, these latter 'defences' (insanity and automatism) are actually proof of incapacity to form the necessary state of mind—see mens rea here and on 📖 p.IV.334.

The mental element of crime

The mental element of a crime, its *mens rea* ('guilty mind'), is the state of mind necessary for wrongful conduct to amount to a criminal offence. It is also known as the 'fault element' of the crime, by contrast with the 'conduct element', the actus reus (📖 p.IV.332). Fault is not required for some crimes of strict liability (📖 p.IV.337), where mere commission of the actus reus is all that is required for a finding of guilt.

Some crimes have forms of greater or lesser severity depending on the associated mens rea. For example, arson with *intent* to endanger life is more serious (and carries a greater maximum sentence, 📖 p.IV.361) than arson being *reckless* (📖 p.IV.336) as to whether life is endangered, which is in turn more serious than simple arson.

There may be more than one fault element within a defined crime, relating to different aspects of the actus reus. For example, the general offence of fraud (📖 p.IV.355) requires, amongst other things, knowledge (📖 p.IV.336) that a statement is false, plus an intention to gain personally from making the false statement.

Intention

To a philosopher, 'intention' refers to what a person wishes to bring about, i.e. the purpose of their actions. However, the law refers to this concept as *motive*, and for most offences this is in theory irrelevant, except as a mitigating or aggravating factor in sentencing (📖 p.IV.361).

Put simply[*], someone is said to intend something that they decide to do[†], whatever their reason for doing it. For example, imagine A wishes to save B from choking, and slaps him on the back; whereas C wishes to express his anger at D, and similarly slaps him on the back. Despite their different motives, the law views both A and C has having intended to slap B and D, and both could in principle be prosecuted for battery (📖 p.IV.347).[‡]

Intent is central to the inchoate offences (📖 p.IV.339) such as attempt, conspiracy and aiding and abetting, in which the defendant does not themselves cause the harm in question (and in that sense the offence is incomplete or 'inchoate'). Instead, the essence of their crime is their intent to bring that harm about by, for instance, trying but failing to do so themselves (e.g. attempted murder), or persuading someone else to do so (e.g. counselling to cause an explosion).

Oblique intent

Often there is no direct evidence that the defendant intended a particular harm. Deciding whether they had the intention for the crime charged may involve inference from other evidence (e.g. witnesses' descriptions of their behaviour) of their intentions, purposes, or motives. A particular

---

[*] What follows is, from the legal perspective, an oversimplification. The legal use of the word 'intention' defies robust definition, because courts continue to use the word slightly differently from one offence to another, to reflect policy considerations about who should be liable to conviction for that offence.

[†] As courts cannot know exactly what someone decided (not having direct access to their mind), judges infer that someone intended something when they 'acted so as to bring it about'.

[‡] For conviction for battery (unlawful touching), there would also need to be evidence that B and D did not consent to being slapped on the back.

instance of this is so-called 'oblique intent', which applies where the harm is a virtually certain (or 'natural and probable') consequence of the defendant's actions: e.g. where B would be virtually certain to die in consequence of A setting fire to her house when she was inside. In such cases, English law[*] allows courts to infer from other evidence (if it is sufficient) that the defendant intended the harm.

Basic and specific intent

The general sense of intending that which you decide to do is known as *basic intent*. However, certain crimes require not only that the defendant intended to act as they did, but also that they intended certain consequences. For example, GBH with intent (🕮 p.IV.346) requires a *specific intent* to cause serious injury. Imagine that A and B both deliberately push C over a wall, and she fractures her pelvis; but that whereas A intends C to be seriously injured, B is only play-fighting. Both A and B could be convicted of GBH, but only A could be convicted of the more serious offence of GBH with intent.

Crimes of specific intent include possession of a drug with intent to supply; arson with intent to endanger life (🕮 p.IV.350); burglary (🕮 p.IV.354, e.g. trespassing with intent to steal); and indecent exposure (🕮 p.IV.349, which requires an intention that another see the exposed genitals).

It is not always clear in advance which crimes involve a specific intent with respect to certain consequences, and which only basic intent: the distinction is not a coherent one, and the courts have not developed a robust rule for applying it. However, it is important to forensic psychiatrists, because psychiatric evidence of incapacity to form intent (🕮 p.V.481) is treated as negating specific intent, but is usually disregarded in crimes of basic intent, at least in E&W.[†] It is also relevant to the complex rules on how intoxication (🕮 p.V.485) affects criminal responsibility.

---

[*] A common law rule, slightly weakened by s8 Criminal Justice Act 1967. The common law rule does not apply automatically in Scotland, NI or RoI, where 'intention' is less strictly defined, and can be taken to include or exclude oblique intent as necessary.
[†] For example, consider a person with severe depression who begins reading a book in a bookshop, leaves the shop, having been distracted and forgetting that they have not paid for it, and then drops it in a puddle outside the shop, ruining it. Psychiatric evidence that their pervasive nihilistic ruminations meant that they did not have the capacity to form intent would, if accepted, prevent conviction for theft (an offence requiring specific intent to deprive the owner of the item permanently), but would not prevent conviction for simple criminal damage to the book (an offence of basic intent).

Recklessness

Where a consequence of any action is virtually certain, the law allows the inference that the defendant intended that consequence of what they did (oblique intent, 📖 p.IV.334). Recklessness is relevant when the harmful consequence is merely foreseeable: when the defendant does not intend the harm, but considers[*] that it is possible and decides to go ahead nevertheless. For example, deliberately running the risk of causing an explosion (inexpertly fixing a gas pipe, say), which then occurs and causes injury, is an offence despite the lack of intent to cause the explosion, or the injury.

In general, if the defendant themselves does not foresee the harm, there is no offence, even if the harm appears obvious. For example, in *R v Stephenson* (📖 p.App. 3.645), a schizophrenic defendant slept in a haystack and made a small fire in order to keep warm, causing the haystack to catch fire. Medical evidence suggested that because of his disorder he could not have foreseen the risk of fire, and he was therefore acquitted.

Reckless knowledge and reckless belief

In these cases, the decision to act is reckless because of what the defendant knows or believes. For example, a person who takes part in a petrol station robbery, knowing their accomplice to have a gun, may be liable under the law of joint enterprise (📖 p.IV.340) if their accomplice shoots the attendant, because of their reckless knowledge that they were armed.

Negligence

Negligence is analogous to recklessness, in that it refers to situations in which the harm is foreseeable. However, whereas recklessness is usually subjective, requiring the defendant to have foreseen the harm, negligence is objective, requiring only that a 'reasonable person' would have foreseen it. There are degrees of negligence: manslaughter (📖 p.IV.345) requires 'gross negligence', dangerous driving a standard 'far below' that of a competent and careful driver; and careless driving ordinary negligence.

Knowledge and belief

Some offences require that the prosecution prove that the defendant knew of circumstances relevant to the actus reus. For example, the offence of fraud (📖 p.IV.355) committed by making a false statement requires that the defendant knew that the statement was (or might be) false. For other offences, such as handling stolen goods, the defendant need only believe the goods to be stolen, meaning that they can be convicted even if by chance the goods are legally in their possession.

Mistaken belief

Some offences allow a mistaken belief to negate an element of the offence, such as criminal damage, in which a defendant's mistaken belief that the damaged property is theirs will prevent conviction. In other cases an objective standard is applied, and only reasonable knowledge or belief suffices. For instance, non-consensual penetrative sex is not rape (📖 p.IV.348) if

---

[*] In Scottish law, it is often sufficient that a reasonable person would have considered the risk 'serious and obvious': see the discussion on subjective and objective approaches.

the defendant believed the victim consented, provided that belief was reasonable in the circumstances.[*] See also 'Mistake', 📖 p.IV.343.

Lesser degrees of knowledge

In *wilful blindness*, also called 'connivance', the defendant realizes that the relevant circumstances might exist and deliberately avoids finding out (i.e. is reckless as to whether they exist); it has been held to be sufficient for offences such as driving an uninsured or dangerously loaded vehicle. *Constructive knowledge*, on the other hand, refers to the situation where the defendant did not contemplate the existence of the circumstances, but had reasonable cause to believe they might exist (i.e. the defendant was negligent), as in the unauthorized disclosure of information protected by the Official Secrets Acts.

Subjective and objective approaches

A conviction often hinges on whether the law applies a subjective test (e.g. recklessness, mistaken belief) or objective test (e.g. negligence, constructive knowledge) in a case. There is no coherent general principle as to when one or the other is used. A further complication is the variation between jurisdictions, the most notable being that in Scotland defendants are sometimes held to an objective standard for offences of recklessness, making them effectively indistinguishable from offences of negligence.[†]

Objective tests favour victims and public welfare at the expense of individual autonomy (📖 p.III.275); they disadvantage mentally disordered defendants in particular. Some argue that the 'reasonable person' in objective tests should be a reasonable person with the same mental capacities as the defendant, but others argue that this would introduce a slippery slope allowing (for example) criminals of low IQ to escape conviction.

Strict liability

Many 'regulatory' offences, and a small number of others, have no requirement of mens rea, and are known collectively as offences of strict liability. Examples include unlawful parking; fishing (or watching TV) without a licence; and outraging public decency (📖 p.IV.349). For the defendant to be convicted, they only need to be shown to have done the acts or omissions concerned, such as watching their unlicensed television.

---

[*] In E&W, an earlier case (*DPP v Morgan*, 📖 p.App. 3.635) had held that the mistaken belief that the victim had consented prevented conviction for rape. The requirement for belief in consent to be reasonable was introduced by the Sexual Offences Act 2003.

[†] This was also the case in E&W from 1982, after *Caldwell* (📖 p.App. 3.633), until 2004, when that authority was overturned by the House of Lords in *R v G* (📖 p.App. 3.636).

Capacity and criminal responsibility

Incapacity due to youth

Children under the *age of criminal responsibility* are deemed to lack the capacity to commit crime, as they may be insufficiently capable of moral reasoning (though they will often still be held responsible, and punished, by their parents, teachers and others). From a purely utilitarian perspective, an age of criminal responsibility of up to 12 accords with evidence (📖 p.II.30) that children do not commit behaviours amounting to criminal offences against society[*] in significant numbers until age 11–12. However, a general age of criminal responsibility ignores the fact that children develop at different rates, and that some under the age will be capable of being held criminally responsible, whereas some over the age will not.

In E&W and NI, the age of criminal responsibility is 10; in RoI it is 12 (but with the possibility of trying 10- and 11-year-olds for serious offences including murder and rape), and in Scotland 12[†] (although younger children can still be dealt with through the children's hearings system, 📖 p.IV.323). In other countries it ranges from 6 in some US states, to 18 in Belgium and Argentina.

The European Commissioner on Human Rights has recommended that the UK adopt an age of criminal responsibility in line with the European norm, on the grounds that children of 10, 11, and 12 cannot have sufficient consciousness of the nature and consequences of their actions to be held criminally responsible, as their cognitive abilities and self control may not be sufficiently developed,[‡] and they may be particularly susceptible to peer pressure.

Protections for child defendants

E&W (📖 p.IV.320), Scotland (📖 p.IV.322), NI (📖 p.IV.320), and RoI (📖 p.IV.324) all have their own youth justice systems, which attempt to balance the youth and inexperience of the defendant against the interests of their victims and of society. These systems tend to be more informal and less frightening in style; to allow relatives and friends to support the young defendant; make less use of remand procedures (📖 p.IV.330); detain young offenders in smaller institutions such as secure children's homes (📖 p.V.458) with access to schooling; and tend to employ less punitive sentences (📖 p.IV.361) with a stronger emphasis on promoting healthy, pro-social development.

An additional rule known as *doli incapax*, means that children aged under 14 cannot be convicted of a crime unless the prosecution has shown that they knew that what they were doing was wrong. This rule was abolished for E&W and NI in 1998, but continues to apply in RoI. (It has never applied in Scotland.)

---

[*] As opposed to hitting (assaulting) each other and taking toys and other items (stealing) from each other, which is rife amongst toddlers and other children.

[†] In addition, children under 16 can only be prosecuted in Scotland (as opposed to being dealt with under the Children's Hearing system) with the consent of the Lord Advocate.

[‡] However, the British government is not currently minded to accept this, as evidenced by its refusal to follow the Law Commission recommendation for E&W of including developmental immaturity as a ground for diminished responsibility (📖 p.V.491).

Incapacity due to mental disorder

As with other forms of mental capacity (📖 p.V.424), adults and children over the age of criminal responsibility are presumed capable of committing crime, and therefore of being prosecuted for it. However, some will in fact be incapable (in the loosest sense) in one way or another because of some form of mental disorder, and this is recognized by the law in different ways:

- Mental disorder *at the time of legal proceedings* may render a defendant unfit to plead and stand trial (📖 p.V.474). For example, a person with severe Alzheimer's dementia might be unable to concentrate on or comprehend the proceedings
- Mental disorder *at the time of the alleged offence* may:
  - Prevent the defendant forming the necessary state of mind or mens rea (📖 p.IV.334) for the offence, particularly intent (📖 p.V.481), or
  - Give rise to a defence (📖 p.IV.342) such as insanity (📖 p.V.489), automatism (📖 p.V.483) or the partial defence of diminished responsibility (📖 p.V.491).

Incapacity due to intoxication

Intoxication with alcohol or drugs can alter one's criminal responsibility for one's acts and omissions. However, the law on whether and how intoxication affects liability in a given case is highly complex. A broad principle is that unintended intoxication (for example, your drink being spiked) is a defence, whereas voluntary intoxication is not. This is discussed in detail on 📖 p.V.485.

Who is a party to the offence?

Usually, there is no confusion over who should be charged with an offence: if A hits B, A can be charged with assault; if A dishonestly takes B's money, A can be charged with theft. However, what if C is also involved, but without hitting B or taking B's money? There are two main ways in which C can be charged with an offence relating to A's crime.

Inchoate offences

These are 'incomplete' offences, in which C does not cause the relevant harm themselves, but is involved in one of the following ways:

- *Attempting* to commit the offence (e.g. attempted robbery: threatening the victim with a weapon, say, but not obtaining anything from them)
- *Aiding and abetting* (e.g. aiding and abetting murder: providing A with a club, knowing they will later beat B to death with it; or knowingly providing A with information that enables them to commit the offence)
- *Inciting*, also known as encouraging or assisting in E&W, and as counselling or procuring (e.g. inciting terrorism: training A to become a terrorist, and suggesting they cause an explosion, which then kills B)
- *Conspiring* (e.g. conspiracy to defraud: agreeing with A to defraud B, which is an offence even if B is not in the end defrauded).

The mental element (📖 p.IV.334) of inchoate offences is often different from that for the main offence: e.g. subjective recklessness as to causing injury suffices for murder, but only intent to kill suffices for attempted murder.

Defences such as duress (📖 p.V.502) apply in the usual way (e.g. if a violent husband coerces his wife into assisting the offence, she may have a defence).

Joint criminal enterprise or joint venture

This law governs situations in which C takes part in a crime or crimes (a 'criminal enterprise') along with A. Broadly speaking, C and A are both responsible for each others' actions in carrying out the criminal enterprise. Joint enterprise goes further than conspiracy in that it covers not only actions that are agreed or jointly planned in advance, but also any other action that C foresees A might take. It is a complex area of law that aims to make all members of criminal gangs responsible for the acts of each gang member.

The law of joint enterprise is most often relevant where A and C are jointly committing an offence such as burglary or robbery, with the intention that nobody will be hurt; but where during the offence A kills or seriously injures B. If C foresaw[*] the killing or injury (i.e. if C had reckless knowledge (📖 p.IV.336) that A had a knife, or the reckless belief (📖 p.IV.336) that A had a gun when A in fact had a knife), then C can be convicted of murder or GBH along with A;[†] but if C had no such knowledge or belief—if, in other words, A's act is 'fundamentally different' to anything foreseen by C—then C must be acquitted.

Entitlement to control

The common law has sometimes held C liable for A's actions in the absence of an inchoate offence or joint enterprise, where C was found to be 'entitled to control the actions' of A and failed to do so. For example, in one case a passenger was liable for the driver's dangerous driving because they could have stopped the driver; in another, a publican was liable for customers' illegal drinking outside licensed hours because he could have prevented them drinking; and in a third, a company was liable for failing to stop its drivers falsifying their tachograph records.

However, the rule on 'entitlement to control' represents a breach of the general principle that people are not responsible for what they do not do, and its extent is unclear. It could in principle be applied to a party host who walks in on a guest raping another guest and does nothing; or, applying it even more widely, to a homeowner who looks out into their front garden and sees one stranger assaulting another there but who fails to intervene. However, these possibilities have not been tested in the courts.

Self-defence & other justifications

Legal justifications, when present, excuse conduct (📖 p.IV.332) that would otherwise be unlawful—in contrast to defences (📖 p.IV.342), which allow the defendant to escape conviction (or receive a lesser conviction, in the

---

[*] Psychiatric evidence may be relevant on this point, to determine whether C was capable of fore-seeing what A went on to do (by analogy to capacity to form intent, 📖 p.V.481).
[†] As famously (and controversially) occurred in R v Bentley (📖 p.App. 3.630).

case of partial defences) for unlawful conduct. Five justifications are recognized by the law[*]:

- Defending oneself against attack (self-defence or 'legitimate defence')
- Defending another person against attack (public defence)
- Preventing the commission of an offence
- Apprehending an offender, and
- Preventing serious damage to property.

The justifications apply to all offences, not merely assaults and homicide offences; for example, apprehending an offender has been held to justify what would otherwise amount to the offence of dangerous driving.

Necessity

For any justification to apply, the conduct concerned must have been necessary:[†] that is, the aim of defending oneself or apprehending an offender etc. could not reasonably have been achieved in an otherwise lawful manner (such as by running away in the case of self-defence).

Reasonable force and proportionality

With each justification, the degree of force used[‡] must have been reasonable in the circumstances,[§] which includes that it must have been proportionate to the harm that could have resulted if such force had not been used to prevent it. For instance, considerable force, possibly resulting in the death of the attacker, may be justified in defending oneself or one's children against a potentially fatal attack, but little or no force would be justified in preventing someone damaging property by daubing graffiti on a wall.

Objective and subjective tests

The test of whether the force used was reasonable is objective: would a reasonable person have used that type and amount of force in those circumstances, bearing in mind the difficulty of making such a judgement in the heat of the moment? However, the circumstances are addressed subjectively: they are the circumstances that the defendant believed (reasonably or otherwise) to exist.[**]

---

[*] There are different mixtures of common law and statute in each jurisdiction;, the rules are similar, but there are minor differences (such as that in RoI, public defence applies only to family members in certain cases; and that the common law duty to retreat or escape if possible before using force in self-defence still applies in RoI & Scotland but has been abolished in E&W and NI).
[†] The necessity and proportionality requirements are particularly important in homicide cases, where they balance the victim's right to life (📖 p.V.418) against that of the self-defending attacker.
[‡] Or by analogy, the dangerousness of the driving etc.
[§] s3(1) Criminal Law Act 1967 for E&W, s3(1) Criminal Law (NI) Act 1967, and common law for Scotland and RoI. In E&W, s76 Criminal Justice & Immigration Act 2008 defines 'reasonable force'.
[**] Unless that belief resulted solely from voluntarily induced intoxication (📖 p.V.486). At least in E&W, a genuinely-held mistaken belief is sufficient for self-defence, whether or not it is 'reasonable': s76 Criminal Justice and Immigration Act 2008.

Relevant circumstances include whether the defendant was committing an offence (such as burglary) at the time, or whether they initially provoked their attacker, or struck the first blow, or sought revenge, all of which make it more difficult (but not impossible) for them to claim a justification. The location of the attack is also relevant: it is easier to claim self-defence, for example, if one is attacked in one's own home.

Burden of proof

Once the defendant has put forward enough evidence to raise the issue of one or more of the justifications, the burden of proof (📖 p.IV.317) is on the prosecution to prove beyond reasonable doubt that the justification does not apply (e.g. that the force used was not reasonable in the circumstances).

Relevance of mental disorder

The role of psychiatric or psychological evidence in support of a justification such as self defence is limited to assistance in understanding how mental disorder might have affected what the defendant might have believed the circumstances to be. The courts have repeatedly refused to allow evidence of mental disorder to be taken into account within the objective test of whether the force used was reasonable and proportionate*.

For example, in *R v Martin (Anthony)* (📖 p.App. 3.641), the court held that the defendant's misperception of risk due to his paranoid personality disorder (📖 p.II.64) and depression was not relevant to the objective test. Even in a case involving a floridly psychotic patient (*R v Jason Cann*, 📖 p.App. 3.639), the defendant's mental disorder was held not to be relevant to the objective test.

Defences and partial defences

The term 'defence' is often used in a broad sense, to refer to anything that a person may argue to rebut a charge, including alibis and other evidence that disproves one or other elements of the actus reus (📖 p.IV.332) or mens rea (📖 p.IV.334), or that shows their actions were justified (📖 p.IV.340).

In contrast, the legal term 'defence' has a more narrow meaning, referring specifically to facts that, if proven, reduce the defendant's liability for their crime. Full defences result in acquittal, whereas partial defences result in a lesser conviction (for manslaughter or culpable homicide).

Psychiatric testimony is highly relevant to many of the defences, and these are therefore described in detail in the section Legal tests relevant to psychiatry (📖 p.V.473).

Full defences

- The essence of the *insanity* defence is that the defendant's mental disorder was so severe that they were incapable of bearing criminal responsibility for their own behaviour, because they did not understand the true nature of what they were doing. See 📖 p.V.489.

---

*In contrast to the partial defences of provocation (📖 p.V.498) and diminished responsibility (📖 p.V.491), which allow mental disorder to be considered to a limited extent.

- *Automatism* is a state in which the defendant acts without exercising conscious control, as for example when they are in a hypoglycaemic state, or when someone else moves their body or part of it. Many of the causes involve a psychiatric or medical condition. See 📖 p.V.483.
- *Duress*, also known as *coercion* or necessity in Scotland, is concerned with the situation in which the defendant commits the crime but only because another person threatens to harm them or someone else if they do not (duress by threats), or because of the situation they find themselves in (duress of circumstances). See 📖 p.V.502.

Partial defences

Each of the following applies only to murder (📖 p.IV.345), and if successfully pleaded, reduces the offence to manslaughter or culpable homicide (📖 p.IV.345).[*]

- *Diminished responsibility* is similar in principle to insanity, in that the defendant is excused from criminal responsibility because of mental disorder present at the time of the offence. However, the required degree of mental disorder is much less, and the reduction in liability to punishment correspondingly smaller. See 📖 p.V.491.
- The essence of the partial defence of *provocation* (now known as loss of control in E&W and NI) is that the defendant was provoked into killing by something that another person did or said. See 📖 p.V.498.
- Deliberately killing a person who wishes to die would normally be murder. However, killing in pursuance of a *suicide pact* (where the defendant intended to kill themselves after killing the other person, but was not successful in doing so), if proved, reduces the conviction to manslaughter in E&W and NI[†]. Unlike other partial defences, the defendant bears the full burden of proof (📖 p.IV.317) of demonstrating the existence of the pact.

Mistake

A mistake by the defendant does not, of itself, give rise to a defence. However, it may have a similar effect if it negates an element of the offence (e.g. where a defendant mistakenly believes (📖 p.IV.336) the victim

---

[*] The partial defences, which are anomalous in that they only apply to murder, exist only because of the strict definition of murder (📖 p.IV.345) and because of the desire to avoid passing the mandatory life sentence (📖 p.IV.365) on more 'deserving' defendants. Infanticide (📖 p.IV.345) is also a partial defence as well as an offence in E&W, NI and RoI.

[†] In RoI & Scotland, the defendant can in theory be charged with (and convicted of) murder but is more likely to be charged with manslaughter (culpable homicide in Scotland) or assisting suicide.

to have consented to assault or indecent exposure[*]); or if it amounts to a belief in facts which would, if true, give rise to a defence or justification ([book] p.IV.340; for example, where a defendant assaults someone, mistakenly believing that they are defending themselves[†]). This is particularly relevant to psychiatrists where the mistaken belief is the result of a delusion.

Potential defences

- A few judicial decisions in E&W have hinted at a general defence of *necessity*,[‡] broader than the defence of duress of circumstances, in that it does not require a realistic fear of death or serious bodily harm. However, such a broad defence has never been firmly established.
- In E&W, the Law Commission is considering recommending a defence or partial defence of *mercy killing*, which would probably subsume the partial defence of killing in pursuance of a suicide pact. Mercy killing would cover cases where the defendant killed someone else in order to end their pain and suffering.
- There have also been proposals in E&W and RoI for a partial defence to murder of excessive *force in self-defence* (i.e. where the defendant believed they were using reasonable force, but objectively it was unreasonable, and the justification ([book] p.IV.340) of self-defence therefore fails). In such cases, where the result is merely injury, a lesser sentence can be given, but if death results the current outcome is a mandatory life sentence.

Homicide offences

Homicide is the killing of another human being. It is not necessarily an offence.

In most jurisdictions, there are at least two homicide offences: one indicating intentional, culpable killing (murder), and another indicating less intentional or culpable killing (manslaughter). Manslaughter may be voluntary (as a result of successfully pleading a partial defence to murder) or involuntary (as a result of recklessness or criminal negligence).

---

[*] e.g. *Kimber* ([book] p.App. 3.639). The same principle was applied to rape in *DPP v Morgan* ([book] p.App. 3.635); in E&W the Sexual Offences Act 2003 introduced the requirement that the mistaken belief be reasonable.
[†] This is arguably the same point as that about negating the offence, as a person who believes they are acting in self-defence does not intend to commit assault (i.e. to hit someone unlawfully).
[‡] The Scottish courts recognize a general defence called 'necessity', but only where there is imminent danger of death or great bodily harm—i.e. equivalent to duress of circumstances.

Definitions

Murder

In E&W, NI & RoI, to kill a person unlawfully with the intention (📖 p.IV.334) of killing them or doing them serious harm*; in Scotland, to kill a person unlawfully with 'wicked recklessness (📖 p.IV.336) or intent'. 'Unlawfully' in this context refers to the absence of a justification (📖 p.IV.340) such as self-defence, or being an active soldier in a legally-declared war.

Manslaughter

In E&W, NI and RoI, to kill a person recklessly or grossly negligently (📖 p.IV.336) or through an otherwise unlawful and dangerous act. In Scotland, the equivalent offence of culpable homicide is to kill a person with intent only to assault them non-fatally, or through a grossly negligent act. Grossly negligent medical care resulting in the death of a patient has resulted in doctors concerned being convicted of manslaughter.

Infanticide

Many cultures treat the intentional killing by the mother of a child aged up to 12 months, i.e. infanticide, differently from other homicide offences. In E&W, NI, & RoI, infanticide is both a specific offence, and a partial defence to a murder charge; the same penalties are available as for manslaughter. The court must be satisfied that the balance of the mother's mind was disturbed by the childbirth or lactation. In Scotland, the same mother would be convicted of culpable homicide by reason of diminished responsibility, with the same effect.

There are also a number of other specific homicide offences in some of the jurisdictions, including causing death by dangerous driving, child destruction (to which being a registered medical practitioner performing an authorized abortion is a defence), and assisting suicide.

Defences specific to murder

The partial defences (📖 p.IV.343) are only available on a charge of murder. If a partial defence to murder is accepted by the prosecution or the court, the defendant will be convicted instead of voluntary manslaughter (in Scotland, voluntary culpable homicide). The current† partial defences in all four jurisdictions (although the detailed criteria vary between them) are:
- Diminished responsibility (📖 p.V.491), which is of great relevance to psychiatrists
- Loss of control or provocation (📖 p.V.498)
- Infanticide
- Killing in pursuance of a suicide pact (📖 p.IV.343).

---

* The Law Commission for E&W has proposed new offences of first- and second-degree murder, with the mandatory life sentence and the partial defences applying only to first-degree murder. Second-degree murder would cover the more serious forms of manslaughter. If adopted, these proposals would radically alter the homicide offences in E&W.
† In E&W, the Law Commission has proposed that duress (📖 p.V.502) be added to these, as it applies to most other offences. In Scotland, it is possible that the equivalent defence of coercion (📖 p.V.502) already applies to murder, but this point has not been settled by the High Court.

Sentencing guidelines for murder

Because murder carries a mandatory life sentence (📖 p.IV.365) in all four jurisdictions, special sentencing guidelines (📖 p.IV.362) have been developed to take into account the seriousness of the killing. A minimum term or tariff (📖 p.IV.365) is set by the trial judge (from 12 years for a child defendant with no aggravating factors, to whole-life for exceptionally serious murders); it is open to appeal. A hospital disposal (📖 p.IV.405) is not a sentencing option after conviction for murder but it may still be possible to arrange for the prisoner to be transferred to hospital (📖 p.IV.410) after sentencing.

Attempted murder

In E&W, NI and RoI, this consists of doing an act which is more than merely preparatory to an unlawful killing, with intent to kill. In Scotland, there is no specific offence of attempted murder; instead, the charge would be assault to the danger of life (📖 p.IV.347), with the severity of the nature of the crime taken into account at sentencing. In both cases, the maximum penalty is a life sentence.

The partial defences do not apply to attempted murder, which can give rise to the anomalous situation that a defendant may be in a more advantageous position, in terms of pleading a partial defence, if the victim dies than if they survive.

Assault and other violent offences

Assault is a non-fatal violent crime committed against another person. Other violent crimes include homicide offences and attempted murder (📖 p.IV.346), robbery (📖 p.IV.355), and sexual offences (📖 p.IV.348), considered elsewhere. In E&W and NI there are many separate offences, classified by method or severity of injury and intention; in Scotland, there is only really one offence, that of assault, with an extraordinarily wide range of sentences.

Assault offences in E&W and NI*

In order of severity from most to least severe, the main offences are:

- *Wounding with intent* to cause GBH (grievous, i.e. 'really serious', bodily harm), and *causing GBH with intent*. These two related offences are sometimes referred to as 'section 18 GBH' or 'GBH with intent'. Defined as intentionally or recklessly wounding (causing an injury that breaks the skin) or causing GBH, with specific intent (📖 p.IV.335) to cause someone (not necessarily the victim) GBH or to resist or prevent arrest or detention.† Maximum sentence life imprisonment
- *Unlawful wounding* and *inflicting GBH*. Sometimes referred to as 'section 20 GBH' or just 'GBH'. Intentionally or recklessly (📖 p.IV.336) wounding or inflicting GBH. Maximum 7 years' imprisonment (5 in E&W)

---

* Mostly offences under the Offences Against the Person Act 1861. There are also a number of rarely-used specific offences such as poisoning, or causing bodily injury by gunpowder. More commonly used are a series of specific offences of assaulting police, prison officers etc.
† The commonest relevance of mental disorder to a charge of section 18 GBH is where it is pleaded as evidence that the defendant was not capable of forming the specific intent (📖 p.IV.335).

- Assault causing *actual bodily harm* (ABH). Any hurt or injury calculated to interfere with the health or comfort of the victim, which is not transient or trifling. Maximum 5 years' imprisonment
- *Battery* Charged as 'assault by beating'. Intentionally or recklessly touching or applying unlawful force (e.g. pushing) to another person. Maximum 6 months' imprisonment
- *Common assault* Causing a person to fear an immediate touching or application of unlawful force, or actually doing so. Maximum six months' imprisonment (2 years in NI)
- *Aggravated assaults* These are a group of specific offences where an aggravating factor (📖 p.V.506) is present and the maximum sentence is therefore greater. They include assault with intent to rob, racially aggravated assault, and religiously aggravated assault

Assault offences in RoI[*]

- *Causing serious harm* Intentionally or recklessly causing another person, not necessarily by assaulting them, a substantial risk of death, serious disfigurement or substantial loss or impairment of mobility or function. Maximum life imprisonment
- *Assault causing harm* Intentionally or recklessly assaulting another person, causing harm to body or mind (including pain and unconsciousness). Maximum 5 years' imprisonment
- *Assault* Intentionally or recklessly directly or indirectly applying force or impact to another person, or causing them reasonably to fear immediate force or impact. Maximum 6 months' imprisonment.

The offence of assault in Scotland

Scotland has one general offence[†] of *assault* under common law, although charges often use additional words to indicate the nature or severity of the assault, such as 'serious assault', 'assault to injury' or 'assault to the danger of life'. It has been defined as intentionally or recklessly directing an attack to take effect physically on the person of another, whether or not actual injury is inflicted. It includes threats of attack.

Assault is usually charged as 'serious assault' if the victim's injuries require inpatient treatment in hospital, or involve fractures, internal injuries, severe concussion, loss of consciousness, or lacerations requiring sutures which may lead to impairment or disfigurement.

The maximum penalty for assault in Scotland is life imprisonment.

---

[*] Under the Non-Fatal Offences Against the Person Act 1997. There are also, as in E&W and NI, a number of more specific offences.
[†] And one specific statutory offence, that of assaulting a police officer contrary to s41(1) of the Police (Scotland) Act 1967.

Sexual offences

Different jurisdictions define and classify sexual offences differently, based in part on social attitudes towards sexual behaviour (📖 p.l.25). Sexual offences are often separated into contact and non-contact offences; some apparently non-sexual offences may have a sexual motive or component. Table 15.1 summarizes the definitions, mostly statutory, of the more common sexual offences in the UK and RoI.

Table 15.1 Definitions of sexual offences

	E&W and NI	Scotland	RoI
Primary legislation	Sexual Offences Act 2003; Sexual Offences (NI) Order 2008	Sexual Offences (Scotland) Act 2009	Criminal Law (Rape) Act 1981; Criminal Law (Rape) (Amendment) Act 1990
Rape	A penetrates B's vagina, anus or mouth with penis; B does not consent; A does not reasonably believe that B consents (Note that B can be male or female in UK jurisdictions)	Without B consenting Without reasonable belief that B consents A penetrates B to any extent, either intending to do so or reckless as to whether there is penetration with penis	A has unlawful sexual intercourse (penile penetration of mouth or anus, or penetration by any object of vagina) with a woman who does not consent, knowing she does not consent or being reckless as to whether she consents
Sexual assault (Indecent assault)	*Assault by penetration* A intentionally penetrates the vagina or anus of B with part of his body or anything else; the penetration is sexual; B does not consent; A does not reasonably believe that B consents *Sexual assault* A intentionally touches B; the touching is sexual; B does not consent to the touching; A does not reasonably believe that B consents	Without B consenting Without reasonable belief that B consents: *Sexual assault by penetration* . . . A penetrates B to any extent, either intending to do so or reckless as to whether there is penetration with body or anything else *Sexual assault* . . . A intentionally or recklessly: sexually penetrates B; or touches B sexually; or has any other form of sexual activity; or ejaculates semen onto B; or sexually emits urine or saliva onto B	*Sexual assault* Any indecent assault (defined by courts as 'conduct that right-thinking people would consider an affront to the sexual modesty of a woman') *Aggravated sexual assault* A sexual assault that involves serious violence or the threat of serious violence or is such as to cause injury, humiliation or degradation of a grave nature to the person assaulted

Table 15.1 (*Contd.*)

	E&W and NI	Scotland	RoI
Indecent exposure	A intentionally exposes his genitals, and intends that someone will see them and be caused alarm or distress	A exposes their genitals in a sexual manner to B with the intention that B will see them; obtaining sexual gratification thereby; and humiliating, distressing or alarming B.	Offending against recognized standards of propriety by virtue of a lewd, obscene or disgusting act in public.
Sexual offences against society	*Outraging public decency* A public act of such a lewd, obscene or disgusting nature as to amount to an outrage to public decency, whether or not it tends to deprave and corrupt those who see it	*Public (shameless) indecency* A lewd act in public that offends a witness to it *Lewd, indecent or libidinous practices* As for shameless indecency, but without the requirement of a witness being offended	*Public indecency* Any act to offend modesty or cause scandal or injure the morals of the community *Offensive conduct* Any unreasonable behaviour which, having regard to all the circumstances, is likely to cause serious offence or serious annoyance
Child offences	Unlawful sexual intercourse and other offences against a child under 13 (most serious) Similar offences against a child over 13 Offences of inciting or arranging sexual activity involving children	Unlawful sexual intercourse and other offences against a 'young' child Similar offences against an 'older' child Intercourse of person in position of trust with child under 16	Defilement (sexual intercourse, buggery or aggravated assault) of child under 15 Defilement of child under 17 Child trafficking & sexual exploitation

Other offences

Other sexual offences, often with definitions that differ in detail between jurisdictions, include incest and related offences; abuse of trust offences against children or vulnerable adults; offences related to prostitution and trafficking; and offences related to the production and possession of pornographic images, especially of children.

Historic offences

The offences listed in Table 15.1 for the UK jurisdictions are all relatively new law, only applying to recently-committed offences. Sexual offences, particularly against children, are often prosecuted many years after they occur. Offences committed before the new Acts came into effect are still tried under the law in effect at the time.

Arson and criminal damage

These are offences that relate to a person destroying or damaging property. The damage may be caused wilfully or as a result of recklessness. Arson or fire-raising involves causing damage by setting fires (setting a fire that causes no damage might not be an offence, but might still be a behaviour of clinical interest: see 📖 p.II.38). The act may be further classified as to whether there was an intention to endanger life.

Arson causes up to 90 deaths per year in the UK. The estimated annual cost of arson is over £2.1 billion. There appears to be an upward trend in rates of arson over the last 20 years (see Table 2.3).

Most judges routinely request an expert psychiatric report in cases of arson, because of the association with mental disorder.

Typology of arson and criminal damage

The act of arson has been classified into four broad categories, which apply also to non-fire related criminal damage:

- Youth disorder: young children (accidental); vandalism
- Malicious: using fire as a weapon/malicious damage
- Psychological: communication of frustration, pain, or hostility
- Criminal: covering up evidence of other crime; fire for financial gain.

The offences

In E&W, NI and RoI, the relevant statutes* are broadly the same:

- *Criminal damage:* a person who without lawful excuse destroys or damages any property belonging to another intending to destroy or damage any such property shall be guilty of an offence
- *Arson:* destroying or damaging property by fire is charged as arson
- The mental element (see 📖 p.IV.334): *intending* to destroy or damage any property *or being reckless* as to whether any property would be destroyed or damaged
- Aggravating factors (📖 p.V.506): intending by the destruction or damage to *endanger the life of another* or being reckless as to whether the life of another would be thereby endangered.

---

*The Criminal Damage Act 1971, Criminal Damage (Northern Ireland) Order 1977, and Criminal Damage Act 1991 respectively.

The effect of the aggravating factors is to create three arson offences: arson with intent (to endanger life); reckless arson; and simple arson. The specific intent (📖 p.IV.335) can be difficult to prove, meaning that defendants charged with arson with intent are often convicted of reckless arson.

In Scotland, vandalism is defined by statute, but excludes fire-raising, which remains a common law offence as follows:

- *Vandalism:* without reasonable excuse, wilfully or recklessly destroying or damaging any property belonging to another
- *Fire-raising:* the raising of fire, without any lawful object . . .
- The mental element:
  - Wilful fire-raising requires the *deliberate intention* of destroying certain premises or things
  - Wicked, culpable and reckless fire-raising requires only *recklessness* as to the risk of destruction.

Public order offences

Public order offences are intended to penalise the use of intimidation or violence by groups or individuals, particularly if it could pose a threat to the State. These offences can generally be committed in private as well as public places. They can be controversial because of the scope for misuse in order to suppress legitimate political protest. See Table 15.2.

Table 15.2 Definitions of public order offences

	E&W	NI	RoI
Primary legislation	Public Order Act 1986; Common law	Public Order (NI) Order 1987; Common law	Criminal Justice (Public Order) Act 1994
Riot	Using unlawful violence as part of a group of 12 or more using or threatening unlawful violence for a common purpose, where the group's conduct would cause a person of reasonable firmness present* to fear for their personal safety	Where three or more persons assist each other in carrying out acts of violence, which alarms or terrifies at least one person	Using unlawful violence as part of a group of 12 or more, using or threatening unlawful violence for a common purpose, where the group's conduct would cause a person of reasonable firmness present to fear for their or another's safety
Violent disorder (Riotous & disorderly behaviour in NI)	Where three or more people together use or threaten unlawful violence and their conduct would cause a person of reasonable firmness present to fear for their personal safety	Where a person in any public place uses disorderly behaviour or behaviour whereby a breach of the peace is likely to be occasioned	Where three or more people together use or threaten unlawful violence and their conduct would cause a person of reasonable firmness present to fear for their or another's safety
Affray	Where a person uses or threatens unlawful violence towards another and their individual conduct would cause a person of reasonable firmness present to fear for their personal safety	Affray involves the fighting of two of more persons, which terrifies at least one person	Using or threatening unlawful violence to another person (who uses or threatens violence) where the joint conduct would cause a person of reasonable firmness present to fear for their or another's safety

Table 15.2 (Contd.)

	E&W	NI	RoI
Threatening abusive or insulting words or behaviour, or displaying signs	Using or threatening such words, signs or behaviour: (1) with intent to cause fear of immediate violence; or (2) with intent to cause (or (3), unintentionally causing) harassment, alarm or distress	Using such words, signs or behaviour in a public place or at a public meeting or procession, with intent to cause a breach of the peace, or by which a breach of the peace is likely	Using or engaging in any such words, signs or behaviour in a public place with intent to provoke a breach of the peace, or being reckless as to breaching the peace
Disorderly conduct or intoxication in a public place	Behaving in a disorderly fashion while drunk in a highway or other public place	Where a person in any public place uses disorderly behaviour or behaviour whereby a breach of the peace is likely to be occasioned	Engaging in any unreasonable behaviour in public at night likely to cause serious offence or annoyance; or being intoxicated in public to such an extent as would give rise to a reasonable fear endangering oneself or others nearby.

* In all the E&W and RoI offences, no person of reasonable firmness need actually be present.

Breach of the peace

This common-law concept, which applies across the UK and in RoI, is not strictly defined; it is usually taken to mean a situation in which violence is used or threatened and/or disorder occurs. A person may be arrested or removed to prevent a breach of the peace (📖 p.IV.441). It is not an offence as such, but those arrested may be 'bound over' for a period, meaning that they must pay the court money that they lose if they later offend.

Scotland

In contrast to the range of specific offences in other jurisdictions, there are only two common law public order offences in Scotland.
- *Mobbing and rioting*, where a group convenes for an illegal purpose, or to carry out a legal purpose by illegal means, e.g. violence or intimidation
- *Breach of the peace* is also an ordinary offence in Scotland, with penalties as severe as imprisonment. It covers conduct that is 'genuinely alarming and disturbing' to any reasonable person.

Additional public order matters

- All jurisdictions have laws relating to public processions and meetings. These are particularly clearly defined in NI legislation. Most of these laws relate to the risk of stirring up hatred or arousing fear.
- Wilful obstruction of people or vehicles, especially those of emergency services, can be a public order offence.

Acquisitive offences

Acquisitive crime refers to offences where the offender derives material gain from the crime, by obtaining something that is of direct benefit to them, or that can be used to obtain what they want (such as illicit drugs).

In E&W, NI and RoI these offences are almost entirely defined in statute, with the precise wording shown or summarized in Table 15.3. In Scotland, most of the offences exist only in common law (p.IV.306) and do not have a precise wording.

Table 15.3 Definitions of acquisitive offences

	E&W and NI	Scotland	RoI
Primary legislation	Theft Act 1968; Theft Act (NI) 1969 Fraud Act 2006	Common law; Civic Government (Scotland) Act 1982	Criminal Justice (Theft and Fraud Offences) Act 2001; Criminal Justice (Public Order) Act 1994
Theft	Dishonestly appropriating property belonging to another with the intention of permanently depriving the other of it	The taking and appropriating of property without the consent of its rightful owner or other lawful authority	Dishonestly appropriating property without the consent of its owner and with the intention of depriving the owner of it
Burglary (Theft by housebreaking in Scotland)	Entering a building as a trespasser with intent to steal, or by stealing after entering a building as a trespasser No distinction in definition between burglary of dwellings or other premises but there is distinction in sentencing Other forms of burglary exist, e.g. with intent to commit criminal damage or GBH	Theft by Housebreaking occurs whenever the security of a 'house' is overcome and an article is abstracted or removed for the purpose of being carried off Housebreaking with Intent to Steal—person breaks into 'house' with the intention of stealing property	Entering a building or part of a building as a trespasser and with intent to commit an arrestable offence Or Having entered a building or part of a building as a trespasser, commits or attempts to commit any such offence therein

Table 15.3 (Contd.)

	E&W and NI	Scotland	RoI
Robbery	When stealing, and immediately before or at the time of doing so, and in order to do so, using force on any person or putting or seeking to put any person in fear of being then and there subjected to force	The felonious appropriation of property by means of violence or threats of violence	When stealing, and immediately before or at the time of doing so, and in order to do so, using force on any person or putting or seeking to put any person in fear of being then and there subjected to force
Blackmail/ Extortion	Blackmail—the making of an unwarranted demand, reinforced by menaces, with a view to making gain or inflicting loss	Extortion— obtaining money or any other advantage by threat	Blackmail—the making of an unwarranted demand, reinforced by menaces, with a view to making gain or inflicting loss
Handling stolen goods (including those obtained by fraud etc.)	Dishonestly receiving or arranging to receive stolen property, or undertaking, assisting or arranging to retain, remove, dispose of or realize it, knowing or believing it to be stolen	With intent to deprive the owner, to receive and keep property knowing that it has been appropriated by theft, robbery, embezzlement or fraud (known as 'reset' in Scottish law)	Dishonestly receiving or arranging to receive stolen property, or undertaking, assisting or arranging to retain, remove, dispose of or realize it, knowing or believing it to be stolen
Other related offences	Fraud by false representation Fraud by failing to disclose information Fraud by abuse of position Obtaining services dishonestly Making off without payment	Falsehood—false representations by words, writing or conduct Fraud—intention to deceive or defraud Wilful imposition—the cheat designed has been successful to extent of gaining benefit or advantage or of prejudicing or tending to prejudice the interests of another	Making gain or causing loss by deception Obtaining services by deception Making off without payment Unlawful use of a computer False accounting

Juvenile offences

Rates of offending are high (p.II.30) during adolescence. The peak age of offending for males is 18 and for females is 15, and a significant proportion of crime is committed by young people. Although official statistics can only provide a crude estimate, they suggest that around a quarter of all crime is committed by 10–17-year-olds, and over two-fifths is committed by those under 21. A study by the Home Office indicated that one-third of females and over half of males aged 14–25 admitted to committing one or more criminal offences at some point; in this age range, females account for 21% of proven offences.

Type of offences

A distinction can be made between status offences and index (or notifiable) offences.

- *Status offences* refer to acts that would not usually be illegal if committed by an adult. They are relatively trivial e.g. truancy, drinking alcohol, and driving a motor vehicle under age, and rarely result in conviction
- *Index offences* refer to all other offences (such as murder, rape and sexual assault, burglary, arson, and robbery) where the age of the offender is irrelevant to determining the crime.

The number of status offences committed each year by juveniles greatly exceeds the number of index offences committed. Violent offences account for 20% of proven offences; and are equally likely to be committed by girls and boys under 21.

Police decision-making in relation to young offenders is discretionary; and structured by the cautionary guidelines and local arrangements for dealing with young defendants. There are crimes for which a person under 18 would not be prosecuted whereas a person over 18 would be. For example, an adult may be charged with ABH following an assault on a peer where as a 10-year-old would not.

Other offences relevant to psychiatry

Offences involving the care of children

Where there are concerns about the care of children, proceedings may be brought against parents/carers in the family court (in care proceedings) alongside criminal charges. Typically, the social services authority will bring care proceedings against a parent/carer, and the police will bring criminal charges (e.g. neglect or cruelty to a child). Psychiatrists who are asked to give expert opinion need to be very clear what proceedings they are being asked to provide testimony for, and that a report in one context may be used in the other.* Ordinary psychiatric defences (🕮 p.IV.342) may be raised to criminal charges of violence against a child.

Offences involving the care of psychiatric patients

It is an offence for care staff to assault, or to have sexual contact with a detained patient. Conviction can result in imprisonment, as well as professional sanctions such as being struck off the professional register.

Offences of cruelty to animals

This may (rarely) arise in the context of antisocial personality disorder, or conduct disorder in young people.

Terrorism and treason

Both are crimes with a political aim, using means that harm others. Terrorist offences are varied, but commonly include causing (or credibly threatening to cause) widespread death and destruction, such as through an explosion; or making preparations for or assisting such an act. Treason is more specific, covering harm to the head of state or a small number other key political figures, such as killing the monarch or raping a senior member of the royal family. It is an offence to fail to give information to the police about acts of terrorism, past or future, or about possible treason. Governments often limit or even break human rights laws (🕮 p.IV.418) when combating terrorism and treason, and the impact on suspects of measures such as indefinite detention without trial† can result in mental disorder. Forensic psychiatrists may also find themselves involved in the care of alleged terrorists who are said to be mentally ill; and who may be detained under mental health law.‡

Making threats to kill

The making of a threat to kill is an offence where the defendant intends the victim to fear that it will be carried out. It does not matter whether it is premeditated or said in anger. Although the normal maximum sentence is 10 years in E&W and NI, offenders thought to present a 'significant risk' of 'serious harm' to the public can receive a life sentence (🕮 p.IV.364). The corresponding offence in RoI includes threats to cause serious harm. Making threats to kill is notoriously difficult to prove, as there is rarely clear evidence that the defendant intended the victim to believe the threat would be carried out.

* e.g. a diagnosis of personality disorder made in a psychiatric report for criminal sentencing purposes might be used by a social services authority in family court proceedings in support of a case that that parent poses a continuing risk of harm to the child.
† In the UK, for example, the Anti-Terrorism, Crime & Security Act 2001 allowed such detention without trial of certain suspected terrorists until after it was ruled incompatible (🕮 p.IV.310) by the House of Lords in 2004. Similarly, the UK government had a policy of detention without trial ('internment') of suspected IRA terrorists in Northern Ireland during the 1970s.
‡ They have also in the past been involved, along with psychologists, in claims that indefinite detention, detention without trial, or repeated retrials (all of which have occurred in terrorist cases in the UK) are disproportionate under human rights law (🕮 p.IV.418) in part because of their effect on the alleged terrorists' mental health.

Stalking and harassment

These are the terms used in Scotland and elsewhere respectively for the crime of deliberately and repeatedly acting in such a way as to cause a victim significant fear, alarm or distress—for example, through multiple unwanted communications or intrusive approaches. Psychiatric evidence may be relevant both in assessing the harm caused to the victim, and in assessing the offender (mental disorder is common in stalkers, 📖 p.II.40). In addition to punishing the offender, courts also often issue injunctions (📖 p.IV.372) and restraining orders (📖 p.IV.371) preventing them from repeating the stalking behaviours. In some cases, injunctions may be available by application to a civil court, with a lesser burden of proof (📖 p.IV.316).

False imprisonment

This is the restraint of a person in a bounded area without justification or consent. Criminally, a person convicted of false imprisonment can be punished by probation, heavy fines or imprisonment. Civilly, they can be liable for punitive damages related to pain and suffering.

Poisoning

Criminal poisoning occurs when an individual, or a group of individuals, deliberately attempt to inflict harm on others by using a toxin. Historically, poisoning cases have proved difficult to diagnose, investigate and prosecute, even if death results (in which case the more common charge is murder). The methods of delivery may be highly sophisticated and subtle. Poisoners are often hard to detect.[*]

Contempt of court

This occurs when an individual disobeys a court order or is disrespectful of the court's authority, such as by showing disrespect for the judge, by disrupting the proceedings through poor behaviour, or by publication of material deemed likely to jeopardize a fair trial. This may result in a fine or imprisonment. Mental disorder is an obvious possible cause of such behaviour.

Crimes under international law

Criminal law is usually thought of as peculiar to each individual country, and based upon that country's custom and the kind of behaviour it wishes to control, albeit with great similarity between countries with similar cultures. However, since World War II a body of international jurisprudence has arisen[†] which criminalizes certain very serious behaviours.

---

[*] An example of a high profile case is that of the medical serial killer Dr Harold Shipman of Hyde near Manchester, who killed over 200 of his patients in the 1980s and 1990s through poisoning them with overdoses of morphine and other drugs before he was caught.
[†] The Hague Conventions of 1899 and 1907 (after the Boer War) and the Geneva Conventions (which were revised & expanded after World War I and then World War II), all setting out war crimes; and the Charters setting up the Nuremburg Tribunal 1945, tribunals in Tokyo 1945, Yugoslavia 1993 and Rwanda 1994, and that of the International Criminal Court 2002, which developed international human rights law.

Cases involving such war crimes and 'crimes against humanity' are very rare. However, the highly contested nature of the latter in particular means that psychiatrists may be called to examine defendants and give evidence in such cases. Cases may be brought at the International Criminal Court in The Hague, or in national courts of countries such as the UK that recognize universal jurisdiction for such crimes.

Crimes against humanity

These are committed when an individual, as part of a 'widespread or systematic attack directed against any civilian population, with knowledge of the attack', commits any of the following, amongst others:

- Murder
- Extermination (mass killing, directly or through, say, starvation)
- Enslavement
- Deportation, or forcible transfer of population
- Illegal imprisonment or 'disappearance' (secret abduction)
- Torture
- Rape, sexual slavery, enforced prostitution, and related offences.

War crimes

War crimes are crimes committed by agents of an aggressor state against individuals (including that state's own citizens), and include using unlawful weapons such as poison gas; mistreating civilians, the sick & wounded, and prisoners of war; and causing destruction not warranted by military or civilian necessity.

Cautions, reprimands, and warnings

Where there is evidence of guilt and the offender is prepared to admit it, but the offence is relatively minor, in E&W, NI, and RoI a senior police officer and/or the prosecutor[*] may give a *caution* or equivalent, instead of charging them (Table 15.4). This speeds the administration of justice, can be used as a mechanism for reducing a backlog of trials, and avoids the expense and distress of a trial when the likely sentence on conviction would be minor (e.g. a conditional discharge, 📖 p.IV.369).

Requirements for a caution

- Sufficient evidence of guilt, such as a reasonable suspicion that the individual is guilty, coupled with reasonable grounds to believe that further investigation will reveal evidence sufficient for a reasonable prospect of conviction
- An offence and consequences that are sufficiently minor: for example, in E&W a caution is not permitted for indictable-only offences (📖 p.IV.330)
- A clear and reliable admission of guilt by the suspect
- No overriding public interest in prosecution

---

[*] i.e. the solicitor acting for the Crown Prosecution Service in E&W, for the Public Prosecution Service of Northern Ireland, or for the Director of Public Prosecutions in RoI.

- Reason to believe that the caution will be effective: for example, it will usually be inappropriate to caution someone for an offence for which they have been cautioned in the past
- The offender's consent to the caution.

Effects of a caution

Cautions are not convictions, and therefore appear separately (or not at all) on criminal records. However, the admission of guilt may be taken into account in sentencing for any future offences, as evidence of 'bad character'; and some jobs involving work with vulnerable individuals may require applicants' cautions to be disclosed.

Cautions are recorded as a 'result' and as a successful detection of an offence for the purposes of police statistics, giving police and prosecutors an incentive to use cautions where possible. See Table 15.4.

Reprimands and (final) warnings

In E&W, young offenders are ineligible for cautions. Instead, for a first offence they can receive a *reprimand* from the police, which is essentially identical to a caution. The requirements are the same as for a caution, except that an appropriate adult must be present—and, controversially, that the young offender or their parent/guardian does not need to consent to the reprimand (or warning).[*]

For subsequent offences, they can receive a *warning* (originally called a 'final warning', although now it is possible to receive a second warning before prosecution). Unlike a reprimand or caution, a warning usually involves referral to the Youth Offending Team (YOT, 📖 p.IV.463). If the young offender fails to cooperate with the YOT, there are no immediate consequences, but their non-cooperation may be taken into account in any subsequent prosecution. See Table 15.4.

Table 15.4 Approximate frequencies of reprimands and warnings, and cautions

Age group	Males	Females
12–14	67%	80%
15–17	45%	67%
Adults	20%	33%

[*]These rates and the averages presented in Table 15.5 are not directly comparable, because they cover slightly different geographical areas and different time periods.

Fixed penalties

For certain specific offences, police officers and others such as traffic wardens have discretion to give a fixed penalty notice to an offender as an alternative to prosecution. Relevant offences vary from one jurisdiction

---

[*] This appears to be a breach of the ECHR (📖 p.IV.420), and might be ruled incompatible (📖 p.IV.310) by the Supreme Court (📖 p.IV.308) in future.

to another, but often include road traffic and cycling offences, public disorder, theft, and minor environmental offences such as littering.

Conditional cautions

In E&W (and possibly soon in NI, where there are proposals for its introduction), the prosecutor has discretion to give adult and child offenders a caution with conditions that, if breached, result in the original prosecution resuming. The conditions may include paying a financial penalty, attending particular places, or conditions aimed at rehabilitation or reparation.

Scotland

No cautioning system exists in Scotland: the police must either refer the offender to the Procurator Fiscal for prosecution, or take no further action. However, the Procurator Fiscal has several options for pre-trial diversion that are wider in range than, but similar in intent to, cautions and conditional cautions. These include offering the offender, as an alternative to trial, the opportunity to accept a formal warning; to pay a fixed penalty (a 'Fiscal Fine') of up to £300; to pay compensation; to do unpaid work; or to receive counselling or psychiatric treatment.

Principles of sentencing

Sentences are passed by courts after conviction—that is, after the individual's criminal responsibility has been established. Sentencing has been described as 'the authoritative statement by the criminal justice system of its response[*] to the offence'.

Purposes of sentencing

Sentences may attempt to serve a number of incompatible purposes:
- Incapacitating the offender (protecting the public from them)
- Punishing the offender (giving them their 'just deserts', 📖 p.IV.297)
- Deterring the offender and others from future offending
- Treating them (e.g. for drug use) in the interest of their welfare (📖 p.IV.297)
- Rehabilitating them (e.g. by teaching new skills)
- Reforming them (e.g. through changing their attitudes and moral views)
- Making reparation to the victim and/or society (e.g. through compensation or community service: the 'restorative justice' approach), and
- Obtaining retribution on behalf of the victim and/or society at large.

Sentences in the UK and RoI focus on different purposes depending on the legislature's view of the nature of the offence. For example, sentences of imprisonment (📖 p.IV.364) focus on incapacitation, retribution, punishment

---

[*] Although using discretion not to arrest, not to charge or not to prosecute (📖 p.IV.330)—or to divert (📖 p.II.216)—the alleged offender are alternative responses.

and deterrence*; fines (📖 p.IV.369) focus on retribution and reparation; community orders with a drug testing requirement (📖 p.IV.368) focus on reform; and hospital orders (📖 p.IV.405) focus on treatment.

Process of sentencing

In deciding the appropriate sentence, judges take the following steps:[†]

- Applying statutory mandatory or automatic[‡] sentences (such as the mandatory life sentence (📖 p.IV.365) for murder) if they apply; otherwise:
  - Determining the seriousness of the offence (the harm caused, and the offender's degree of responsibility for that harm)
  - Taking into account aggravating factors (📖 p.V.506) such as committing the offence whilst on bail; being motivated by racial or religious hatred, or hatred of a sexual orientation or disability; or certain past convictions
  - Taking into account mitigating factors (📖 p.V.507) such as having been provoked, offending because of a genuine misunderstanding, having mental disorder, showing remorse after committing the offence, admitting the offence to police, or making an early guilty plea (📖 p.IV.330), and
  - Considering orders ancillary to the sentence (📖 p.IV.370), such as a compensation order or binding over to keep the peace.

Pre-sentence reports

Judges frequently request reports from probation officers before making a decision on sentence, and may[§] also request them from others including psychiatrists, psychologists, schools and social work departments where relevant. Psychiatric reports on disposal (📖 p.V.569) usually address whether a mental health disposal is recommended (such as admission to hospital, or compulsory outpatient treatment), but may also be used in mitigation; a psychiatric risk assessment (📖 p.II.127) may also be taken by a court as evidence of dangerousness (📖 p.V.547) giving grounds for an increased or indeterminate (📖 p.IV.364) sentence, which can pose ethical problems (📖 p.II.261) for the assessing psychiatrist.

Sentencing guidelines

In E&W, criminal courts are required to consider prescriptive guidelines issued by the Sentencing Advisory Council, as well as directions issued by the Court of Appeal (📖 p.IV.320) and the Lord Chief Justice (📖 p.IV.312). Offences are mostly defined by statute, with maximum sentences and some rules on the purposes of sentencing.

In RoI and NI, the superior courts have produced a substantial body of case law that establishes general principles of sentencing, the most notable

---

* Many prisons (e.g. 'training' prisons in the UK) also have facilities that attempt to rehabilitate and reform the offender.
† These steps are taken from the Sentencing Council Guidelines that Magistrates' Courts (📖 p.IV.320) are required to follow in E&W. Higher courts follow a similar procedure. Sentencing steps are not laid down in NI, Scotland or RoI, but judges may follow a similar process in more informal fashion.
‡ The distinction is that there are no exceptions to mandatory sentences, but automatic sentences (e.g. imprisonment for a third burglary) can be overridden in exceptional circumstances.
§ In some cases, the law requires them to do so (e.g. in E&W, after conviction for arson, 📖 p.IV.350).

in RoI being that the sentence must be proportionate to the gravity of the offence and the circumstances of the offender. Offences are mostly defined by statute, with maximum sentences, and in NI some rules on the purposes of sentencing.

In *Scotland* the judge's sentencing discretion is almost entirely unfettered. Offences are mostly defined only in case law, with few or no maximum sentences. The High Court has made only a few decisions on sentencing principles, and there are almost no statutory sentences except for a mandatory life sentence for murder. However, a new Scottish Sentencing Council was established in 2010 to begin creating guidelines.

Sentencing vulnerable offenders

The same general process is followed when sentencing mentally disordered offenders, although the fact of the mental disorder may make treatment the primary purpose of the sentence. This is discussed further on 📖 p.V.547.

There are special rules on sentencing children: see 📖 p.IV.363.

Sentencing children and adolescents

The sentences applicable to convicted children and adolescents, and in some cases also young adults (aged 18–21), differ in many cases from those applicable to adults. For example, they cannot be sentenced to life imprisonment (📖 p.IV.364), but receive an alternative form of indeterminate sentence; instead of ordinary imprisonment, they are subject to detention (📖 p.IV.365) with a substantial educational or training element, usually in a special institution such as a secure children's home or Young Offender Institution (📖 p.IV.458) instead of a prison; and their community sentences (📖 p.IV.368) are usually more focused on rehabilitation than on other aims of sentencing (📖 p.IV.361), such as punishment.

Principles of sentencing young people

Whereas society is usually content to regard adults as having had a choice whether to offend or not, and to be able to weigh up the alternatives in a rational fashion, it tends to regard children as less able to do so because of their youth. As a result, the first purpose of sentencing children is, in general, not to punish but to prevent offending; in E&W, this 'principal aim' is enshrined in law.[*]

In E&W, NI, and RoI, if it appears to the court that a first- or second-time young offender charged with a minor offence can be better dealt with informally rather than by sentencing them, it may offer them a referral order (E&W, 📖 p.IV.372) or diversionary youth conference (📖 p.IV.372). The law in E&W requires judges in the Youth Court to give all first-time offenders who plead guilty a referral order (the only exception is if the charge is very serious and the Youth Court commits the defendant for trial in the Crown Court as an adult).

---

[*] In s37 of the Crime and Disorder Act 1998, which states that the principal aim of the youth justice system is the prevention of offending, and in s142A of the Criminal Justice Act 2003, which adds that the second consideration is children's welfare, followed by the usual purposes of sentencing.

The system in Scotland goes considerably further, and its de facto principal aim is to rehabilitate and reform children in the interests of their welfare. This is done most notably by diverting the vast majority of child offenders out of the criminal justice system and into the Children's Hearings system (📖 p.IV.323), but even within the Scottish youth justice system the culture opposes punitive sentences for children.

The use of custody

There is a presumption against the use of custody for children, both on remand and as a sentence. Although detention, even for long or indefinite periods, is possible in the UK and RoI, it is used much less frequently than for adults, as shown for E&W by the figures for 2010 in Table 15.5.

Table 15.5 The use of custody in E&W in 2010

Sentence type	Adults		Children	
Total	1,435,330	100%	165,101	100%
Cautions etc.	151,596	11%	91,235	55%
First-tier sentences*	1,044,865	73%	21,901	13%
Community sentences	141,575	10%	47,846	29%
Custodial sentences	97,294	7%	4,219	3%

*Conditional and absolute discharges, fines, bind-overs and other orders, plus for children, referral orders.

Life and indeterminate sentences

Sentences of imprisonment come in two basic forms: determinate sentences (📖 p.IV.366), of a fixed maximum length, and indeterminate sentences such as 'life' sentences, which involve a minimum term after which the offender must show they are fit for release. Indeterminate sentences form a small proportion of all sentences of imprisonment—see Table 15.6.

Table 15.6 Numbers of people sentenced to immediate custody* in E&W in 2010

Total prison sentences	101,513	100%
Determinate sentences	100,110	98.6%
Life sentence	384	0.4%
Other indeterminate (i.e. IPP)	1019	1.0%

* i.e. excluding suspended sentences of imprisonment

Life sentences

In the UK and RoI, there are two[*] types of life sentence for adults:

- The *mandatory* life sentence applies to murder (📖 p.IV.345) and in RoI to treason, rape by penetration and certain serious sexual and violent assaults; the judge has no discretion to pass any alternative sentence
- *Discretionary* life sentences are available for serious offences ranging from manslaughter to aggravated burglary.

Minimum terms (tariffs)

Before being considered for release, life sentence prisoners must serve a minimum term, known as a 'tariff' in NI (and formerly in E&W also), and as the 'punishment part' of the sentence in Scotland. The minimum term is set by the trial judge[†] but can be modified on appeal. In the most serious cases, the minimum term can be the whole of the offender's life.

Release on licence

After serving the minimum term, offenders can apply to the Parole Board (📖 p.V.459) to be released from prison. If their application is granted, however, they remain on licence, and are liable to recall to prison to serve the rest of their sentence, if they breach the conditions of that licence or reoffend. Like other offenders on licence, they must report regularly to their probation officer (📖 p.V.462).

Indeterminate sentences for Public Protection (IPPs)

Whereas offenders sentenced to life remain in prison or on licence until their death, other indeterminate sentences can in principle end. IPPs in E&W and NI and Orders for Lifelong Restriction (OLR) in Scotland apply to convictions for serious sexual and violent offences where the maximum sentence is over 10 years, and the court deems the offender dangerous (📖 p.V.547), in Scotland under a risk assessment order (📖 p.IV.408).

IPPs comprise a minimum term of imprisonment and a period of licence of at least 10 years. After 10 years, offenders can apply to the Parole Board once per year for their licence to be revoked.

Corresponding sentences for children and young adults

The life and indeterminate sentences described for adults cannot be imposed on children (and, in some cases, young adults). Instead, there are a variety of specific alternatives, as shown in Table 15.7. Only small numbers of children receive such sentences, even in E&W: around 25 under 21s each year are detained at Her Majesty's Pleasure, and around 50 receive DPPs.

---

[*] In E&W, between 1998 and 2004 there were also 'automatic' life sentences for certain serious offences (as opposed to mandatory, because judges had a limited discretion not to impose them). They were replaced by IPPs when the Criminal Justice Act 2003 came into force. In Scotland, there is a presumption in favour of passing a discretionary life sentence for such offences.
[†] The Home Secretary (in RoI, Minister for Justice) set the tariff, often in response to political considerations in high-profile cases, until in 2002 this was found to breach the ECHR (📖 p.V.420).

Table 15.7 Indeterminate sentences for under 21-year-olds

Age group & sentence	E&W	Scotland	NI	RoI
Under 18 Life	Detention during Her Majesty's Pleasure	Detention without limit of time	Detention during the Secretary of State's pleasure	None unless tried as adult*
18–20 Life	Custody for life†	Detention for life	Life imprisonment as for adults over 21	Life imprisonment as for adults over 21
Under 18 IPP	Detention for public protection	Order for Lifelong Restriction	Detention for public protection	N/A
18–20 IPP	IPP as for adults over 21	Order for Lifelong Restriction	IPPs as for adults over 21	N/A

*In RoI, children as young as 10 (i.e. below the usual age of criminal responsibility) can be tried in adult court for very serious offences such as murder and rape, and receive adult sentences.
†Custody for life was abolished and replaced with life imprisonment as for adults by the Criminal Justice and Court Services Act 2000, but this provision has never been brought into force.

Determinate prison sentences

'Determinate' prison sentences run for a fixed maximum period, unlike life sentences and IPPs (📖 p.IV.364). See Table 15.8.

Table 15.8 Numbers of people sentenced to immediate custody* in E&W in 2010

Total prison sentences	101,513	100%
Up to 3 months	38,316	38%
3 months to 1 year	27,233	27%
1 to 5 years	31,251	31%
Over 5 years	3310	3%
Life sentences & IPPs	1403	1%

* i.e. excluding suspended sentences of imprisonment.

Ordinary determinate sentences

The length of an ordinary determinate sentence is intended to be proportionate to the seriousness of the offence, and to reflect the culpability of the offender in terms of the current offence and any past offending.

Short sentences, particularly those of three months or less, provide little or no opportunity for training, rehabilitation or reform, whilst still interfering with offenders' employment and family responsibilities, and are discouraged by law in Scotland and in sentencing guidelines in E&W.

Parole and release on licence

Prisoners can often apply for release before the end of their sentence, or may be released automatically. The rules vary between jurisdictions, and the details have changed repeatedly over time. In general, those in E&W and NI, and those in RoI on sentences of up to eight years, are released automatically on licence at the PED, whereas those on longer sentences in RoI may apply to the Parole Board (📖 p.V.459) for release from their PED, and if unsuccessful are released automatically on their NPD.

In Scotland, the trial judge sets a 'custody part' of half to three-quarters of the sentence, after which the prisoner is automatically released.

- PED: Parole Eligibility Date (halfway through sentence)
- EDR: Expected Date of Release (varies depending on parole decisions)
- NPD: Non-Parole release Date (two-thirds point; automatic release)
- LED: Licence Expiry Date (three-quarter point; older sentences only)
- SED: Sentence Expiry Date (and licence expiry for most sentences).

Extended sentences for Public Protection (EPPs)

In E&W, Scotland and NI, those convicted of serious sexual or violent offences who are regarded as dangerous (📖 p.V.547) by the court may receive an extended sentence licence period, up to an extra 5 years (8 for serious sexual offences; 10 years in both cases in Scotland), provided this does not exceed the maximum sentence for the offence.

Furthermore, in Scotland the release of any determinate sentence prisoner after the custody part of their sentence can be refused by the Scottish Ministers if they deem them likely to cause serious harm to the public, in which case the prisoner can appeal to the Parole Board, but if unsuccessful are not released until their SED.

Corresponding sentences for children and young adults

The sentences described previously cannot be imposed on children and young adults. The corresponding sentences are shown in Table 15.9.

Table 15.9 Determinate sentences for under 21-year-olds

Age group & sentence	E&W	Scotland	NI	RoI
Under 21 Ordinary	Detention and training order (DTO)[*]	Detention in YOI	Juvenile Justice Centre Order	Children detention order[†]
Under 21 EPP	Extended DTO	Extended detention in YOI	Extended detention in YOI	N/A

[*]DTOs last up to 2 years; however, children convicted of certain very serious offences such as manslaughter and rape where the adult maximum sentence would be 14 years or more may be sentenced to detention up to the adult maximum. These are known as 'section 91' sentences.

[†]Children Detention Orders last for up to 3 years; however, children convicted of very serious offences may be sentenced as adults.

Other forms of imprisonment

Several variations are found in some or all of the jurisdictions:

- Ordinary determinate sentences (e.g. sentences of 12 months or less in E&W) can be *suspended*, meaning that the offender does not have to serve the sentence unless they reoffend within a specified period
- In *intermittent custody*, currently being piloted in E&W, the offender spends (for example) the weekend in prison but can continue their employment on licence during the week
- *Custody plus* combines prison and a community sentence (📖 p.IV.368)
- Eligible prisoners may be released up to 135 days early on *home detention curfew* in E&W and NI, during which period they are tagged and monitored by the probation service.

Community sentences

Community sentences restrict an offender's liberty less severely than imprisonment, imposing a variety of requirements on them rather than totally depriving them of liberty.

The details of community sentences vary between jurisdictions, and between the adult and youth justice systems: for example, in E&W there is a single community order to which can be added a variety of requirements, whereas in Scotland there are a variety of different orders. Moreover, some orders/requirements are available in some jurisdictions but not in others. The arrangements across the UK & RoI, and examples of different requirements, are listed here and in Box 15.2.

- In *E&W*, there is a single order for adults, the Community Order, and one for children and young people, the Youth Rehabilitation Order. Unless the relevant law specifically provides for an adult Community Order, one can only be made if the offence carries a potential sentence of imprisonment
- *Scotland* has individual probation, community service, community reparation and restriction of liberty orders applicable to both adults and children that together allow for most of the requirements in Box 15.2
- In *NI*, there is a similar range of orders covering similar requirements (reparation, community responsibility, community service, probation, drug treatment and testing, combination, youth conference, attendance centre and juvenile justice orders)
- There is more reliance on short custodial sentences in *RoI*, and less use of community sentences. Probation and community service orders are available for adults, and in addition for children there are youth conferences, mentoring, day centre and restriction orders.

At least in E&W, roughly twice as many community sentences are imposed than are sentences of imprisonment (189,321 as compared to 101,513 in 2010, approximately 12% as opposed to approximately 6% of all sentences).

Box 15.2 Examples of community order requirements

- Unpaid work
- Activity (e.g. helping at an old persons' home)
- Programme (e.g. probation-run offending behaviour group)
- Prohibited activity (e.g. not carrying an otherwise legal firearm, or not associating with a particular person)
- Curfew
- Exclusion (e.g. not to enter certain streets or areas)
- Residence
- Mental health treatment
- Drug rehabilitation (including drug testing)
- Alcohol treatment
- Supervision (e.g. attending appointments with probation officer)
- Attendance centre (e.g. attending the centre during football matches)
- Reparation (e.g. having to meet, talk to and apologize to the victim)
- Education
- Electronic monitoring (e.g. with a 'tag')
- Intensive supervision and surveillance (ISSP)
- Fostering.

Fines and other sentences

Fines

A fine is a payment to the court ordered as part (or the whole) of the offender's punishment. Failure to pay can result in bailiffs seizing the offender's property, or in imprisonment for contempt of court (📖 p.IV.358). Parents are responsible in the event of non-payment of children's fines. See Table 15.10 for rates of fines and other 'first-tier' sentences.

Conditional discharge and binding over

A *conditional discharge* imposes no immediate punishment on the offender. However, if they reoffend within the period specified in the order they will not only be sentenced for the new offence, but also resentenced for the previous offence. Conditional discharges can last from 6 months up to 3 years.

Binding over is a related order that applies where the court believes that there is a risk of the offender being violent in the future—i.e. of them 'breaching the [Queen's] Peace', in the original common law (📖 p.IV.306) terminology. It requires them to refrain from certain acts specified in the order (e.g. visiting the home of an ex-partner whom they have assaulted) for a certain period, and to make a recognisance (i.e. pay a sum of money) which they lose if they breach the order. Where the offender is a child, the parents or guardians may also be bound over.

Absolute discharge and admonition

An order for *absolute discharge* means that the offender receives no punishment, although the conviction will remain on their criminal record.

In Scotland, the offender may also be dismissed with an *admonition*, a reprimand from the judge.

Mental health disposals

Convicted offenders whom the court accepts are suffering from a mental disorder may, instead of being punished, be:

- Sent to hospital (e.g. for treatment under a hospital order, 📖 p.IV.405)
- Required to accept outpatient treatment (e.g. under a compulsion order, 📖 p.IV.405, or a community order with a mental health treatment requirement, 📖 p.IV.368), or an intervention order (📖 p.IV.434)
- Given an order combining the possibility of imprisonment with hospital treatment (e.g. a hybrid order, 📖 p.IV.408).

Table 15.10 Offenders sentenced in 2010 in E&W

Total sentences	1,600,431	100%
Fines	886,321	55%
Conditional or absolute discharge	99,245	6%
Mental health & other	33,082	2%
Cautions	242,381	15%
Community sentences	189,321	12%
Suspended sentence	48,118	3%
Imprisonment	101,513	6%

Ancillary orders

Courts in the UK and RoI may combine many of the sentences in the previous topics with additional orders, often intended to fulfil different sentencing purposes (📖 p.IV.361) to the sentence itself. These ancillary orders are listed here; some are unavailable in some jurisdictions.

Compensation order This requires the offender to pay money to the victim to compensate them for the loss the offender has caused them (e.g. to pay for the replacement of property that has been damaged).

Drinking **banning orders**, and football banning orders, prevent offenders convicted of relevant offences (e.g. affray while under the influence of alcohol, or assault on other football spectators) from visiting specified premises where alcohol is served, or attending specified football matches. In the case of overseas football matches, offenders may be required to surrender their passports. Breach of the order may result in a fine, or in the case of football banning orders, a short sentence of imprisonment (📖 p.IV.366).

An order for **confiscation, deprivation**, or **forfeiture** allows the state to remove the means and the proceeds of crime from the offender, by seizing specific assets (forfeiture,[*] particularly of weapons or drugs), by depriving them of the use of specific items (e.g. a car), or by seizing property of a certain value (confiscation). £153m was seized under these orders in E&W and NI in 2009–10.

Offenders convicted of driving-related offences can be **disqualified** from driving for a specified period (or have 'points' added to their licence, which cumulatively can lead to disqualification). Likewise, directors of companies can be disqualified from holding such directorships in the future if they commit fraud (📖 p.IV.355) or other related offences.

Parenting orders require the parents or carers of a young offender to attend counselling or guidance sessions or a parenting course for up to three months, and may include conditions lasting for up to a year, such as that the parents must attend meetings at school, or must ensure their child is at home at certain times or is not left unsupervised in certain places. Failure to comply can result in prosecution.

Orders for **restitution** require an offender convicted of theft (📖 p.IV.354) or related offences to restore specified property, or assets of equivalent value, to the person lawfully entitled to it.

Restraining orders, Sexual Offences Prevention Orders (SOPOs) and **Violent Offender Orders** are all civil injunctions (📖 p.IV.372) that courts can impose, usually on those convicted of serious violent or sexual offences. The injunction typically prevents offenders from entering certain places at specified times, or from being in contact with certain people, especially former victims.

Sex offenders can be placed on a **register** that requires them to inform police of their address at all times, and to be monitored by police under the MAPPA (📖 p.V.468). Registration can be for a fixed period, or for life.

Lastly, all courts can make **costs orders** requiring one party to pay not only their own costs, but some or all of the other party or parties' costs.

---

[*] Forfeiture originally referred to the automatic loss of property in cases of treason or murder, and especially to rules preventing those who had killed from inheriting property from their victim. Weaker versions of these forfeiture rules still exist in various forms in the UK and RoI, in addition to the forfeiture orders described in this topic.

Civil orders and quasi-punishments

Referral orders and diversionary youth conferences

In E&W, referral orders, and in NI & RoI, diversionary youth conferences,[*] allow the court and/or the prosecutor to refer children accused of offences to community panels instead of proceeding with a trial. The victim is often invited to panel meetings as well as the accused child and their parents. If the panel can agree an alternative to prosecution that is agreed by the child and acceptable to the court, the case can be suspended. If the child breaks the agreement with the panel, the prosecution can resume.

Non-criminal measures for antisocial behaviour

An *Acceptable Behaviour Contract* (ABC) is an agreement between a young person, their parents, the police, and a Youth Offending Team (📖 p.V.463). It involves a signed written promise by the young person not to engage in certain minor antisocial behaviour. It is not a sentence, and breaking the contract does not directly give rise to criminal penalties, but the breach can be used in evidence in future criminal proceedings.

Anti-Social Behaviour Orders (ASBOs) are civil orders taken out by local authorities against young people or adults because of their past antisocial behaviour, if that behaviour caused or was likely to cause harassment, alarm or distress. The order requires the person to do or not do certain things, such as not to enter a certain area. As a civil order, the antisocial behaviour need only be proved on the balance of probabilities (📖 p.IV.316), but breaching the order can result in imprisonment. ASBOs are therefore, in effect, suspended criminal punishments imposed without the safeguards of a criminal trial (such as the exclusion of hearsay evidence, 📖 p.IV.317, or the requirement of proof beyond reasonable doubt, 📖 p.IV.316), which has given rise to considerable controversy.

Other non-criminal measures

In E&W, *Child Curfews* allow young people under 16 to be banned from entering public places during prescribed hours unless they are with a responsible adult. As a civil order, it includes children under 10.

A *Child Safety Order* applies to children under 10 who have acted in a way that could have resulted in conviction had they been over the age of criminal responsibility (📖 p.IV.338). It allows the child to be supervised for a set period by a social worker or an officer of the Youth Offending Team. Child Safety Orders only exist in E&W, but in Scotland Children's Hearings (📖 p.IV.323) can make similar orders for children's protection under broader social welfare legislation.

Lastly, most courts have a general equitable (📖 p.IV.304) power to issue orders, known in most cases as *injunctions*, to individuals and organizations. Many such injunctions are now regulated by statute (such as the SOPO and Violent Offender Order, 📖 p.IV.371). Injunctions requiring a party to do a specific thing are sometimes still referred to as 'mandamus', and those requiring a party to refrain from doing a specific thing as 'certiorari'.

---

[*] the Children's Hearings (📖 p.IV.323) system in Scotland is a non-criminal procedure that allows for a similar outcome.

Mental health and mental capacity law[*]

[*] The intention of this chapter is not to offer a comprehensive and definitive rehearsal of all mental health law across the UK and RoI, but to show in broad terms how the law operates, and its relationships with other branches of law that affect those with mental disorder.

Historical development

For a considerable period after the recognition of mental disorder as an entity in its own right, there was no specific mental health law: mentally disordered people were treated informally, with or without their consent[*] (especially if they were rich enough to have a personal physician, 📖 p.l.11), or were dealt with under general laws for the poor and destitute.

In the UK & Ireland, this amounted to the Poor Laws and the Vagrancy Acts, under which mentally disordered people unable to support themselves would be placed in an almshouse, those able to work would do so in a workhouse, and those deemed idle would be confined in a House of Correction or prison; from the 17th century onwards, they could also be confined in the new private 'madhouses'. If detained unwillingly (on the order of a magistrate or relative, or under a medical certificate), inmates could only force their release under the law of *habeas corpus*,[†] if their detention was illegal (e.g. because the madhouse was not registered).

The Lunacy Acts

The first specific mental health law[‡] in the UK was the Criminal Lunatics Act 1800 (📖 p.ll.216); this diverted mentally disordered offenders into lunatic asylums, but did not affect the vast majority of mentally disordered patients. They had to wait for the Lunacy Act 1845 and associated legislation, which established a network of county asylums across E&W (and later Scotland and Ireland) and instituted a system of inspection of institutions by Commissioners who could order minimum standards of treatment and the release of patients. The right of appeal to the courts was removed, however. The Act was the product of the therapeutic optimism of the period, the belief that patients could recover if given 'asylum' from harsh social conditions, and the advent of the railways, which made a national supervisory regime possible. At the same time, public fear of 'dangerous lunatics' such as Daniel McNaughten (📖 p.V.489) made it politically possible to pay for a new generation of asylums.

There was eventually an outcry against the abuses that arose because any person purporting to be a doctor could commit someone to an asylum or madhouse, and because there was no legal mechanism for challenging the truth of statements made in the doctor's certificate. A series of amendments culminating in the Lunacy Acts 1890 & 1891 required specialist magistrates to authorize all admissions, allowed for leave, permitted 'boarding out' with friends and relatives, and effectively restricted admission to patients with serious forms of mental disorder.

---

[*] Informal treatment without consent usually meant being forced into treatment by your family.
[†] *Habeas corpus* was a writ requiring any person detaining any other (e.g. in prison) to bring the detainee before the courts and to show that they had the legal power to detain them. In practice, it was only available to the wealthy who could afford solicitors.
[‡] Discounting feudal laws that gave the King custody of the land and property of lunatics and idiots, and 18th century Acts regulating private madhouses.

The Mental Deficiency and Mental Treatment Acts

Until the 20th century, so-called idiots and mental defectives (broadly speaking, people with learning disability, 📖 p.II.80) were cared for by relatives, or were placed in workhouses or lunatic asylums. However, at the turn of the century there was public fear of being 'overrun' by people with learning disability, who were perceived to have many children, and the Mental Deficiency Act 1913[*] set up specific institutions for their care and control, with a Board of Control to inspect them, modelled on the Lunacy Commission. The system then expanded to take in the many victims of the encephalitis lethargica epidemic of 1915–26. At first, it was seen as progressive despite its origins, but concern grew in the 1940s at prevalent abuses, including using patients as a cheap source of labour.

The Mental Treatment Act 1930[†] began a gradual process of liberalization and de-institutionalization. Patients could be admitted and treated voluntarily, i.e. without compulsory powers, all institutions were renamed Mental Hospitals, and outpatient and aftercare (📖 p.IV.398) services were developed. At the same time, the first genuinely effective (though still poor, and over-used) treatments for mental disorder, including ECT and psychosurgery (📖 p.II.158) allowed many more patients to be discharged.

The Mental Health Acts

The first Mental Health Acts[‡] marked a decisive break with the legalism of the Lunacy Acts and continued the processes of liberalization and medicalization. Doctors were given the leading role in making decisions on compulsory as well as voluntary treatment, and courts were replaced by less formal Tribunals (📖 p.IV.414). However, such trust was placed in this benignly paternal system that the Lunacy Commission and other independent inspectorates were abolished; a fresh round of public scandals led to their re-creation under new names in the 1960s.

Divergence in mental health law

Mental health law in the UK and RoI remains true to many of the principles of the first Mental Health Acts, particularly medical dominance within the legal process. However, the details have diverged in the four jurisdictions, and the current laws reflect each nation's different emphasis on individual freedom, paternalism, legalism, and public protection: see 📖 p.IV.377.

---

[*] The Mental Deficiency and Lunacy (Scotland) Act 1913 brought in similar provisions for Scotland, but there was no special system for people with learning disability in Ireland, partly because the debate over its autonomy ('Home Rule') overshadowed any other legislative developments.
[†] In NI, The Mental Treatment Act (NI) 1932; there was no corresponding Act in Scotland. By this time RoI was an independent country, and later passed the Mental Treatment Act 1945, which went much further and abolished the need for judicial orders for any patients.
[‡] The Mental Health Act 1959 for E&W, the Mental Health (Scotland) Act 1960, the Mental Health (NI) Act 1961, and the Mental Treatment Act 1961 in RoI.

Relationship to other areas of law

Mental health law should not be viewed in isolation from the values and principles (📖 p.IV.377) of the society it serves, or from the areas of law with which it coexists. In these different areas of law, mental disorder is constructed in a variety of different ways, because of the different social aims or goals of each area of law, and therefore the effect of a given type of mental disorder on the outcome of a case will vary considerably depending on the field of law concerned.

Mental capacity law

Whereas mental health law governs the compulsory treatment of people with mental disorder for that disorder, mental capacity law (📖 p.IV.424) provides rules for determining who lacks the capacity (because of mental disorder, or from other causes such as brain injury) to perform a variety of acts with legal consequences, such as buying, selling and willing property, marrying, voting, and accepting or refusing medical treatment (where mental health law does not apply).

Medical treatment in the absence of consent is possible under both laws, but on very different grounds, reflecting very different ethical principles. Hence, some authors have argued for unification of the two areas of law within in a single mental capacity law applicable to treatment for both mental and physical disorder.

Family and social care law

Both mental health law and mental capacity law are specific examples of a broader field of public law that aims to protect the rights and interests of potentially vulnerable members of society. This includes laws on child protection (📖 p.V.510) and protection of vulnerable adults, laws prohibiting discrimination on the grounds of disability and other characteristics, health and safety law, social security laws (the successors to the Poor Laws, 📖 p.IV.374), and social welfare law (📖 p.IV.440).

Criminal law

Criminal law (📖 p.IV.329) is concerned with the regulation of behaviour, through punishing and/or reforming individuals who behave in socially unacceptable ways. Unlike mental health law, which is paternalist in approach, criminal law assumes that individuals are able to make rational choices about how to behave, and that they are therefore responsible for those choices. It overlaps with mental health law in that it recognizes several exceptions to the rule of personal responsibility based upon mental disorder (for example, insanity, 📖 p.V.489, and unfitness to plead, 📖 p.V.474), and it allows for mentally disordered offenders to receive psychiatric treatment either as part of or instead of a penal sentence (📖 p.IV.361). It also takes mental disorder into account as a factor indicating risk of harm to others that may justify an indeterminate sentence (📖 p.IV.364) for public protection.

Which branch of law should do what?

The relationship of the purposes of mental health law to the purposes of other fields of law raises the following questions, amongst others:

- Should there be similar principles or separate law dealing with treatment for mental and physical disorders?
- What rights to treatment or to other benefits, if any, should be granted specifically within mental health legislation, by comparison with other law?
- Should mental health law allow preventive detention directed towards public protection, as an alternative, or in addition to use of the criminal law?
- Where, and how should the 'boundary' between criminal and mental health law be drawn?

Should we have mental *health* legislation, directed at individual mental health and welfare, or mental *disorder* legislation, directed to a greater degree at the control of mentally disordered individuals for the public good?

Principles of mental health laws

Ethical principles underlying law

The law regulates relationships between individuals and the State (public law); and also between individuals or groups in different types of relationship (private law). Laws embody society's views on questions such as:

- What should society do about a 'dangerous' individual?
- Should we help a citizen who doesn't want to be helped in that way?
- When should we allow one group of citizens to use force against another, and in what circumstances?
- When is it right to detain or treat someone against their will, if ever?

Mental health laws provide specific answers to these questions in relation to mentally disordered individuals, and set out who has the power to detain or force treatment on them, and in what circumstances.

Intention, capacity, and paternalism

Criminal law (📖 p.IV.376) and much of the civil law (📖 p.V.509) assume that, generally, individuals have the capacity to make rational, voluntary decisions about actions and their consequences; and for this reason, the primary basis of criminal liability is an individual's intention (📖 p.IV.334) to commit crime. However, mental health laws recognize that mental disorder may impair the capacity to avoid crime or to seek treatment. From this perspective, mental health laws are based on one of two principles:[*]

- Protection of those who lack the capacity to desist from crime or seek treatment (mental health law as an extension of capacity law, 📖 p.IV.424)

---

[*] There is also a third principle, ignored in this debate, of mental health law assisting those who are capable of seeking treatment, but actively unwilling to do so (against their own best interests).

- Protection of others from those deemed 'objectively' to need treatment, and/or to pose an unacceptable risk of harm (📖 p.II.127) to themselves or others.

In E&W, the MHA, as emphasized by its 1995 and 2007 amendments, ignores capacity in determining whether a person can be detained (although capacity is relevant to treatment, 📖 p.IV.390), and focuses heavily on *protection of the public* and the individual. In Scotland, by contrast, the MHCTA requires evidence of impaired capacity before allowing civil detention, even in an emergency (📖 p.IV.386).

The laws in NI and RoI fall between these two extremes. Both the MHNIO and the MHA in RoI allow detention without reference to capacity,* but in more restrictive circumstances than in E&W: for example, in both jurisdictions detention cannot be for treatment of PD alone, and the risk of harm to the patient or others must be serious and imminent; and in RoI, there must be evidence that the proposed treatment is likely to benefit the patient's condition to a material extent.

The dichotomy between physical health and mental health

Throughout the UK and RoI, there is a legal distinction between compulsory treatment for physical ill-health, and for mental disorder. The former can only be given to patients who lack capacity, in their best interests; or (in very limited circumstances) where there is a risk to public health (📖 p.IV.440). However, even Scotland's capacity-based mental health law is distinct from its general capacity law, with a less stringent test of incapacity ('significant impairment' of capacity).†

Rights of the individual

Both under the Lunacy Acts (📖 p.IV.374) and the mid-20th-century Mental Health Acts, there were very few protections for the patient against abuse (📖 p.IV.422) by those detaining and treating them, and public scandals arose frequently. Modern mental health laws have been repeatedly amended, partly in response to human rights law (📖 p.IV.418), and now include:

- Legal definitions (📖 p.IV.381) of key concepts, to limit discretion
- Procedures (📖 p.IV.381) requiring two or more professionals from different disciplines to agree on the need for compulsory treatment
- Built-in reviews of detention and treatment at various stages
- Rights to appeal (📖 p.IV.414) to independent tribunals or courts
- Restrictions on long-term or irreversible treatments (📖 p.IV.390).

---

* This is the case in NI at the time of writing. However, the NI Executive proposes to introduce the Mental Capacity (Health, Welfare and Finance) Bill (📖 p.App. 2.624) in summer 2011, which as currently drafted would replace the MHNIO with a system based on mental capacity.
† The Richardson committee's first draft of a new Mental Health Act for E&W in 1999 was capacity-based, but this was rejected by the government.

As much ethics as law

Mental health law represents a significant intrusion by the State into an individual citizen's private life. It allows for people to lose their liberty and have their movements controlled without having been convicted of a crime —known as *administrative* (i.e. non-criminal) *detention*. It allows people to be forced to do things, and have things done to them, against their will. It places great power in the hands of those who are approved by the State to utilize these laws. These intrusions are ethically justified by the future benefits that people are expected to perceive when they are restored to health; and the benefits to society of caring for the vulnerable; and public protection.

However, the wide discretion allowed to clinicians under these laws create the possibility for abuse (📖 p.IV.422) and require ethical decision-making (📖 p.II.229). For those who use these laws, it is important to ask oneself, 'If I, or someone I love, became mentally unwell, would I be comfortable with the use of these laws on me or them?'.

Roles of professionals and relatives

A variety of individuals have legally-defined roles under mental health law. The following is a glossary of those roles across the UK and RoI.

Medical or clinical roles

Appointed doctor (NI) A doctor appointed by the Secretary of State either to issue medical recommendations for compulsory admission (like an AMP or S12 doctor), or to give second opinions on treatment (like a SOAD or DMP).

Approved Clinician (AC, E&W) A mental health professional approved by the Secretary of State to exercise powers under the MHA associated with being in overall charge of a patient's care.

Approved Medical Practitioner (AMP, Scotland) A doctor with appropriate training and experience who has been approved by a Health Board under s22 of the MHCTA.

Clinical Director (CD, RoI) A doctor in charge of an Approved Centre.

Designated Medical Practitioner (DMP, Scotland) A doctor appointed by the MWC to give second opinions under the treatment (📖 p.IV.390) provisions of the MHA, and who is independent of the hospital concerned.

Responsible Clinician (RC, E&W) The AC with overall responsibility for the patient's case. (Before 2008, the doctor in overall charge of the patient's case was known as the Responsible Medical Officer, RMO.)

Responsible Medical Officer (RMO, Scotland & NI) The doctor with overall responsibility for the patient's case.

Section 12 approved doctor (S12 doctor, E&W) A doctor, usually a GP or a psychiatrist, approved by the Secretary of State as having special expertise in the assessment or treatment of mental disorder.

Second Opinion Approved Doctor (SOAD, E&W) A doctor appointed by the Secretary of State to give second opinions on treatment under the MHA, and who is independent of the hospital concerned.

Social work and related roles

Approved Mental Health Professional (AMHP, E&W) A mental health practitioner (other than a psychiatrist) who has undergone special training in working with mentally disordered patients and their relatives. (In the past, only social workers could fulfil this role, and were known as Approved Social Workers or ASWs.)

Approved Social Worker (ASW, NI) or *Mental Health Officer* (MHO, Scotland) A social worker with appropriate training and experience who has been approved under s32 of the MHCTA or under the MHNIO.

Relatives' and others' roles

Independent Mental Health Advocate (IMHA, E&W) A person trained in advocacy appointed to support and advise detained patients.

Named person (Scotland) A person nominated by a patient (or their carer or nearest relative) under s250 MHCTA to support them and protect their interests, and in certain circumstances to receive information and make decisions on their behalf.

Nearest relative (E&W, Scotland & NI) The relative deemed to be closest or most significant to the patient, and able in limited circumstances to apply for their detention or for their discharge (or in Scotland, the default named person); the first of the people listed in Box 16.1, but with preference given to those who live with or care for the patient.

Box 16.1 Potential nearest relatives, in order of priority

The nearest relative is usually the first of those in this list who is adult, alive, and resident in the UK. Where two or more people are of equal priority, the nearest relative is usually the oldest of them:
- Husband or wife or civil partner, or person lived with as a spouse for at least 6 months
- Son or daughter (including step-children)
- Father or mother
- Brother or sister (full siblings before half-siblings)
- Grandparent
- Grandchild
- Uncle or aunt
- Nephew or niece.

Organizational roles

Approved Centre (RoI) A mental hospital approved and registered with the MHC for the detention and treatment of patients under the MHA.

Care Quality Commission (CQC, England) A healthcare inspectorate one of whose duties is the inspection of mental health facilities to ensure that they and their staff comply with their duties under the MHA. (Previously a separate organization known as the Mental Health Act Commission (MHAC) carried out this role.)

First-Tier Tribunal (Mental Health) (FTTMH, E&W) A special Tribunal (📖 p.IV.308) to which patients (and in some instances their nearest relatives) can appeal or be referred (📖 p.IV.414) for release from detention in hospital. (Before 2008, known as the Mental Health Review Tribunal, MHRT.)

Mental Health Review Tribunal (MHRT, NI & RoI) An appeals tribunal analogous to the FTTMH in E&W.

Mental Health Tribunal (MHT, Scotland) A tribunal similar to the FTTMH in E&W, but with broader powers to make and renew Compulsory Treatment Orders in the first instance, as well as to hear appeals.

Mental Health Commission (MHC, NI & RoI) and ***Mental Welfare Commission*** (MWC, Scotland) Bodies with wide-ranging powers to ensure compliance with mental health law and to supervise its operation.

Procedures for using civil powers

The procedures for the use of compulsory civil powers to detain and treat patients comprise the same main elements throughout the UK and RoI: an application* is made, supported by one or more medical recommendations, which must meet a definition of mental disorder, and a risk criterion. In some cases, there are also urgency or necessity criteria, capacity tests, and treatability tests.

The application

The process of compulsory detention begins with a person who knows the patient, or a suitable professional, recognising that they appear to be mentally unwell and in need of treatment that they are thought likely to refuse. In E&W, NI and RoI certain relatives can apply, but in Scotland only doctors can do so, although they need the consent of a specially-trained social worker.

The recommendations

Except in emergency (📖 p.IV.386), the application must come with a recommendation from one or more doctors (often specially approved), certifying that the requirements that follow are met.

Definition of mental disorder

The law defines what can amount to a mental disorder, to limit discretion and reduce opportunities for abuse (📖 p.IV.422) of the law, such as by detaining those one dislikes, or political opponents. However, the definitions are very broad and reflect social views on when forced treatment is appropriate: for example, in NI and RoI a diagnosis of personality disorder

---

* In the case of patients before the criminal courts, the 'application' is in fact a court order.

alone is never sufficient, and in all jurisdictions alcohol or drug addiction and sexual deviation* alone are likewise insufficient.

In E&W, the broad definition of mental disorder ('any disorder or disability of the mind') is qualified by the requirement that in the case of learning disability it must be associated with 'abnormally aggressive or seriously irresponsible conduct' in order to justify compulsory treatment (📖 p.IV.388) after an initial assessment period. A requirement for such conduct is also incorporated in the definition of 'significant intellectual disability' in RoI and of 'severe mental impairment' in NI.

The mental disorder must also cross a threshold to qualify in E&W and NI: it must be of a nature (the type and past history of the disorder) and/or of a degree (the current severity of the disorder) sufficient to warrant the use of the particular compulsory power in question.

Risk criterion

Suffering from mental disorder is not enough to justify compulsory detention and/or treatment; there must also be grounds for believing that, without treatment, harm would result. This usually means harm to the patient's health, or to their welfare or personal safety; or harm to other people's personal safety.

In Scotland and RoI, where there is no threshold for mental disorder, there is instead a threshold for the risk criterion, e.g. that the harm to the patient's health or safety must be 'significant'.

Urgency and necessity criteria

In order to use the simplified procedures available in emergency situations or with patients already in hospital (📖 p.IV.386), there must usually be some reason why the situation is urgent and the usual, longer procedure cannot be employed. By extension, for longer-term treatment beyond an initial assessment period to be authorized, there must be some reason why the use of compulsory powers are necessary (e.g. because the patient continues to refuse to agree to the treatment).

Capacity test

The basis of mental health law (📖 p.IV.377) is not, in general, whether or not the patient lacks capacity. However, in RoI 'impaired judgement' is a basis for detention as an alternative to risk of harm; in Scotland 'significantly impaired ability' is a general criterion for the use of compulsory powers; and in all jurisdictions capacity after admission is relevant to the patient's consent justifying certain treatments (📖 p.IV.390).

Whether the capacity tests in RoI and Scotland rule out compulsory admission of all patients with capacity, or whether some patients who met the test for capacity under mental capacity law (📖 p.IV.424) could nevertheless be deemed to have 'impaired judgement' or 'significantly impaired decision-making ability', has not been tested in court.

---

*In E&W, the specific exclusion for sexual deviancy was removed with effect from 2008, although that for alcohol and drug dependence remains. If the sexual deviancy amounts to a diagnosable mental disorder, then it alone can now be the basis for detention and compulsory treatment.

Treatability test[*]

Concerns about the risk of administrative detention (📖 p.IV.379) of people who have committed no crime but who may be at high risk of harming others, yet for whom there might be no effective treatment, have led to various forms of 'treatability' test before compulsory treatment beyond an initial assessment period can be authorized. These range from a requirement that treatment is likely to benefit or alleviate the condition to a material extent in RoI, to a much vaguer requirement that 'appropriate' treatment is available in E&W. There is no treatability test at all in NI.

Civil admission for assessment

Relevant legislation

- E&W: MHA s2: admission for assessment
- Scotland: MHCTA part 6 s44: short-term detention order. The short-term detention order may be for treatment as well as assessment, unlike the corresponding orders in E&W, NI and RoI
- NI: MHNIO art.4: application for assessment
- RoI: MHA s9: application for involuntary admission.

In E&W, the second recommendation must be either from a registered medical practitioner who knows the patient (e.g. their GP), or from a second approved doctor.

See Table 16.1 for the grounds, and Table 16.2 for the process, of civil admission for assessment in each jurisdiction.

---

[*] This term can be confusing to those used to the test for the categories of psychopathic disorder and mental retardation under the pre-2008 Mental Health Act in E&W, which was explicitly known as the 'treatability test'. In this section of the handbook, we use this term much more broadly, to cover any test considering the appropriateness or otherwise of treatment.

Table 16.1 Grounds for admission for assessment

	E&W	Scotland	NI	RoI
Mental disorder	Any disorder or disability of the mind, of sufficient nature or degree	Any mental illness, personality disorder or learning disability, however caused or manifested	Mental illness, mental handicap or any other disorder or disability of mind, of sufficient nature or degree	Mental illness, severe dementia or significant intellectual impairment (i.e. not personality disorder alone)
Risk criterion	In the interest of the patient's own health or safety or for the protection of others	Significant risk to the patient's health, safety or welfare, or to the safety of others	Substantial likelihood of serious physical harm to himself or to other persons	Serious likelihood of the patient causing immediate and serious harm to themselves or others
Purpose	Assessment, or assessment followed by treatment	Determining what medical treatment should be given to the patient, or giving medical treatment	Assessment, or assessment followed by treatment	Assessment for an admission order
Capacity test	None	Significantly impaired ability to make decisions about medical treatment	None	(as an *alternative* to the risk criterion) Judgement so impaired that without compulsory treatment a serious deterioration would be likely

Table 16.2 Process of admission for assessment

	E&W	Scotland	NI	RoI
Recommendations	Two medical recommendations, one of which must be by a doctor approved under s12	One approved medical practitioner (AMP)	One recommendation from an appointed doctor followed by report to responsible authority on admission by a second doctor	Doctor not working at the approved centre where the patient is to be admitted
Applicant	Approved Mental Health Professional or nearest relative	No application as such, but the doctor must obtain the consent of a Mental Health Officer to the order, who must interview the patient if practicable	Nearest relative or Approved Social Worker, who must consult the nearest relative if practicable. (If they object, the ASW must consult another ASW before proceeding.)	Spouse or relative, an authorized officer (of the Health Board), a Gard (police officer) or any other adult with no conflict of interest
Maximum duration	28 days	28 days	7 days (48 hours if the second doctor was not the RMO or an approved doctor)	The recommendation lasts for 7 days, but detention is authorized for only 24 hours to allow assessment for an admission order
Renewal	Cannot be renewed	Cannot be renewed, but can be extended for 3 days to allow an application for a compulsory treatment order to be made, plus a further 5 days once the application has been made	One further occasion of 7 days, on the order of the RMO	Cannot be renewed

Emergency civil procedures

These comprise simpler, more rapid emergency assessment procedures (not required in NI and RoI, where the main procedure is itself simple and quick), and procedures for patients already in hospital voluntarily.

Relevant legislation
- E&W: MHA s4: emergency admission, s5: inpatient application
- Scotland: MHCTA s36: emergency detention order, s299: nurse's holding power
- NI: MHNIO art.7: application in respect of inpatient
- RoI: MHA s23: power to prevent patient leaving approved centre.

See Table 16.3 for the grounds, and Table 16.4 for the procedures, for emergency assessments.

Table 16.3 Grounds for emergency admission for assessment

	E&W	Scotland	NI	RoI
Mental disorder	Any disorder or disability of the mind, of sufficient nature or degree	Any mental illness, personality disorder or learning disability, however caused or manifested	Mental illness, mental handicap or any other disorder or disability of mind	Mental illness, severe dementia or significant intellectual impairment (i.e. *not* personality disorder alone)
Risk criterion	In the interest of the patient's own health or safety or for the protection of others	Significant risk to the patient's health, safety or welfare, or to the safety of others	Substantial likelihood of serious physical harm to himself or to other persons	Serious likelihood of the patient causing immediate and serious harm to themselves or others
Urgency criterion	For s4, urgent necessity, and s2 would involve undesirable delay; for ss5(2), 5(4), immediately necessary to stop patient leaving hospital	Urgent necessity, and s44 would involve undesirable delay; for s299, immediately necessary to stop patient leaving hospital	For art7(3), not practicable to secure the immediate attendance of a doctor	None—merely that the patient indicates they wish to leave
Capacity test	None	For s36 only, significantly impaired ability to make decisions about medical treatment;	None	(as an *alternative* to the risk criterion) Judgement so impaired that without compulsory treatment a serious deterioration would be likely

Table 16.4 Process of emergency admission for assessment

	E&W	Scotland	NI	RoI
Recommendations	For s4, one medical recommendation, by a doctor who knows the patient or by a s12-approved doctor	For s36, one medical practitioner	None	None
Applicant	For s4, an approved Mental Health Professional or nearest relative; for s5(2) the doctor or AC in charge of treatment or their nominee; for s5(4) a mental health nurse	For s36, no application as such, but the doctor should if practicable obtain the consent of a Mental Health Officer to the order; for s299, a mental health nurse	For art7(2), a doctor on the staff of the hospital; for art7(3), a mental health nurse	Consultant psychiatrist, doctor or registered nurse on the staff of the hospital
Maximum duration	72 hours, or 6 hours in the case of s5(4)	72 hours, or 2 hours in the case of s299	48 hours, or 6 hours in the case of art7(3)	24 hours
Renewal or extension	S4 cannot be renewed, but when converted to s2 will then last for a total of 28 days if a second doctor completes a recommendation; s5 cannot be renewed or extended	Cannot be renewed or extended	Cannot be renewed or extended	Cannot be renewed or extended, but can be converted into an admission order (🔲 p.IV.388) if a second consultant psychiatrist makes a recommendation

Civil admission for treatment

Relevant legislation
- E&W: MHA s3: admission for treatment
- Scotland: MHCTA part 7, s57: compulsory treatment order. A mental health officer has a *duty* to apply for a CTO if the conditions apply
- NI: MHNIO art12: detention for treatment. Only applies to patients already detained under article 4 (🕮 p.IV.383) or article 7 (🕮 p.IV.386)
- RoI: MHA s15: admission order. Only applies to patients detained under s10 (🕮 p.IV.383), s12 (🕮 p.IV.400) or s23 (🕮 p.IV.386).

See Table 16.5 for the grounds, and Table 16.6 for the procedure, of civil admission for treatment in each jurisdiction.

Table 16.5 Grounds for admission for treatment

	E&W	Scotland	NI	RoI
Mental disorder	Any disorder or disability of the mind, of sufficient nature or degree	Any mental illness, personality disorder or learning disability, however caused or manifested	Mental illness or severe mental handicap (i.e. *not* mild LD or PD alone), of sufficient nature or degree	Mental illness, severe dementia or significant intellectual impairment (i.e. *not* personality disorder alone)
Risk criterion	In the interest of the patient's own health or safety or for the protection of others	Significant risk to the patient's health, safety or welfare, or to the safety of others	Substantial likelihood of serious physical harm to himself or to other persons	Serious likelihood of the patient causing immediate and serious harm to themselves or others
Treatability test	Appropriate medical treatment is available	Available treatment likely to prevent disorder worsening or to alleviate its symptoms or effects	None	Likely to benefit or alleviate the condition of that person to a material extent
Capacity test	None	Significantly impaired ability to make decisions about medical treatment	None	(as an *alternative* to the risk criterion) Judgement so impaired that without compulsory treatment a serious deterioration would be likely
Necessity test	Cannot be treated without section	Making of CTO is necessary	Other methods are not appropriate	None

Table 16.6 Process of admission for treatment

	E&W	Scotland	NI	RoI
Recommendations*	Two medical recommendations (one must be approved under s12)	Two medical recommendations (one must be approved under s22)	One recommendation from an appointed doctor	Consultant psychiatrist
Applicant	Approved Mental Health Professional or nearest relative	Mental Health Officer, who applies with a proposed care plan to the Tribunal, which decides whether or not to grant a CTO (or interim CTO)	N/A. Original application for assessment made by ASW or nearest relative	N/A. See ☐ p.IV.383 for details of the initial application and recommendation process
Maximum duration	6 months	6 months, or 28 days in the case of interim CTO	6 months	21 days
Renewal	6 months then annually	6 months then annually (or for further periods of 28 days, but not longer than 56 days in total, for interim CTOs)	6 months then annually	3 months then 6 months then annually
Additional Information		CTOs can authorize community treatment (☐ p.IV.394) as well as inpatient treatment	Article 12 detention for treatment is only after assessment under art. 4 or 7	Consultant must inform the Commission on making or renewing order, for a Tribunal to be arranged

*In E&W and Scotland, the second recommendation must be either from a registered medical practitioner who knows the patient (e.g. their GP), or from a second approved doctor.

Consent to treatment

The patient's consent (see also 📖 p.III.275) is required for all medical treatment except where that treatment is given under a specific legal power to treat without consent. Powers to detain a patient for treatment include power to give treatment, but only certain kinds of treatment, and subject to certain safeguards, as described in this section. There are very different rules for treatment without consent under mental capacity law (📖 p.IV.424).

The detained patient

Although the treatment of people detained under mental health law involves consideration of the patient's capacity to decide, most mental health legislation ultimately allows for the over-riding of a patient's refusal even when they retain the capacity to refuse (except in Scotland, where compulsory treatment under the MHCTA only applies to patients with 'significantly impaired' decision-making ability, which may exclude patients with capacity). There are safeguards in the different laws for the use of such compulsory treatment, for example, that an independent doctor agrees that the treatment should be given, but it still raises important philosophical (📖 p.IV.371) and ethical (📖 pp.III.235, III.275–III.280) issues.

What counts as treatment?

In all cases, the proposed treatment must be for mental disorder, or for its consequences (for example, refeeding is accepted as a treatment for severe anorexia: psychological treatment alone will be ineffective, partly because of the depressive cognitions and rigidity of thought caused by starvation). Treatment of physical illness is not covered.

In E&W, treatment had been defined by the courts (as it still is in NI) as 'treatment, care habilitation or rehabilitation'; the MHA 2007 has substituted 'medical treatment [including nursing care, psychological intervention and specialist mental health habilitation, rehabilitation and care] the purpose of which is to alleviate, or prevent a worsening of, the disorder or one or more of its symptoms or manifestations', a definition arguably broad enough to encompass some forms of administrative detention (📖 p.IV.379) despite the ethical objections.

In Scotland, the MHCTA defines treatment as 'nursing, care, psychological intervention, habilitation or rehabilitation'. In RoI, the MHA 2001 states that treatment includes (but is therefore not limited to) 'the administration of physical, psychological and other remedies . . . intended for the purposes of ameliorating a mental disorder.'

The ethics of these various definitions are discussed on 📖 p.III.282.

Mental health laws and consent to treatment

Table 16.7 shows the legal position in each jurisdiction. Accompanying codes of practice provide guidance on consent. In all cases, consent can only be a valid basis for treatment if the patient has capacity to consent.

Table 16.7 Consent to treatment provisions

	E&W	Scotland	NI	RoI
Relevant law	MHA part IV, IVA (ss56–64K)	MHCTA part 16 (ss233–249)	MHNIO part IV (arts 62–69)	MHA part 4 (ss56–61)
Treatment covered	For mental disorder only	For mental disorder only	For mental disorder only	Intended to ameliorate mental disorder
Default position	Inpatient treatment may be authorized by AC without consent. Under CTO, need capacity & consent; if lacks capacity, need authorization under MCA or passive assent	Treatment may be authorized by RMO without consent	Treatment may be authorized by RMO without consent	Treatment only with consent unless patient lacks capacity and treatment necessary to save life, restore health, alleviate condition or relieve suffering
Restricted treatments	Psychosurgery (need consent and a second opinion)	Psychosurgery (need consent and two second opinions)	Psychosurgery (need consent and a second opinion)	Psychosurgery (need consent and tribunal authorization)
	ECT[†], or medication after three months (need consent or a second opinion)	ECT or long-term treatment (need consent unless treatment is urgent)	ECT, or medication after three months (need consent or a second opinion)	ECT, or medication after three months (need consent or a second opinion)
Exceptions to restrictions (and to CTO requirements)	Treatment immediately necessary to save life, or non-irreversible, non-hazardous treatment immediately necessary to prevent serious deterioration, serious suffering, or violence	Urgent treatment to save life, or non-irreversible, non-hazardous urgent treatment to prevent serious deterioration, serious suffering, or violence	Treatment immediately necessary to save life, or non-irreversible, non-hazardous treatment immediately necessary to prevent serious deterioration, serious suffering, or violence	None

[†] In E&W ECT, unlike medication after three months, can only be given to an adult patient lacking capacity if this does not conflict with a valid applicable advance directive (p.IV.430) or decision of a donee (p.IV.432) or deputy (p.IV.434); also, ECT can only be given to competently consenting children (p.IV.430) if the second opinion certifies this is appropriate.

Leave from hospital

For the vast majority of patients in secure care (📖 p.II.209), periods of thera-peutic leave (📖 p.II.154) outside the secure environment are a cornerstone of the rehabilitation (📖 p.II.213) phase of the care plan. However, for patients detained under mental health law,* and particularly for patients subject to special restrictions (📖 p.IV.412), there are legal procedures that must be complied with before such leave may be taken, as shown in Table 16.8.†

Leave versus suspension

Whereas the laws in E&W, NI, and RoI use the concept of leave from hospital, Scottish law employs an alternative concept, that of the tempo-rary suspension of measures. The latter is considerably more flexible, as it not only allows the leave of absence from a place of detention subject to certain conditions, but also allows for other aspects of an order—such as requirements to accept a particular treatment, or to reside in a certain place—to be lifted temporarily.

Leave for restricted patients

Leave outside the hospital or unit to which a patient is admitted or trans-ferred from court or prison can only be granted to patients subject to restriction orders or restriction directions (📖 p.IV.412) with the consent of the relevant government department (such as the Ministry of Justice in E&W). In such situations, it is important to consider what the court or department has defined as the 'hospital' or 'unit' in the order or warrant authorizing the patient's admission. For example, if the order specifies a single ward, then the patient cannot go outside the ward without a leave application being approved. Conversely, if the order specifies an entire hospital, then the patient may be permitted into the grounds of that hos-pital at the discretion of the treating team—although if the grounds of the hospital are not within a secure perimeter, and the patient would be in prison if not in hospital, it may be unwise for the treating team to authorize this, particularly if the patient is unescorted.

---

* The arrangements for leave under other laws, notably mental capacity law (📖 p.IV.436) are very much simpler.
† If they are not complied with, the leave is legally unauthorized (📖 p.II.139).

Table 16.8 Leave and suspension provisions

	E&W	Scotland	NI	RoI
Relevant law	MHA s17	MHCTA ss41, 53, 127, 179, 221, 224	MHNIO art15	MHA s26
Leave authorized by	Responsible Clinician (RC)	Responsible Medical Officer (RMO)	Responsible Medical Officer (RMO)	Consultant Psychiatrist responsible for the patient's care
Nature of leave	Indefinite, or on specified occasions or for any specified period	A period (not exceeding 6/9 months); the duration of an event or series of events, plus associated travel	On specified occasions or for any specified period	For any period less than the unexpired period of the admission order
Criteria	Leave for more than 7 days can only be authorized if a community treatment order (🕮 p.IV,394) considered first	Leave for more than 28 days must be notified to the mental health officer, GP and others first, and to the MWC within 14 days	Leave for more than 28 days must be notified to the Mental Health Commission within 14 days	None
Escort	Patient may be kept in the custody of any named person during the leave	Patient may be in the charge of any authorized person	Patient may be in the custody of any named person during the leave	No specific provision, but could be made a condition
Leave conditions	Any necessary in the interests of the patient or for the protection of others	Any necessary in the interests of the patient or for the protection of others	Any necessary in the interests of the patient or for the protection of others	Any the consultant psychiatrist considers appropriate
Revocation	At any time by the RC provided the patient is still liable to detention*	At any time by the RMO	At any time by RMO provided the patient is still liable to detention*	At any time by the consultant psychiatrist

*i.e. provided the period of detention specified by the original section or article (e.g. s2, s3, art4, art12) has not yet expired.

Civil community treatment

Relevant legislation

- E&W: MHA s17A: community treatment order, s7: guardianship
- Scotland: MHCTA part 7, s57: compulsory treatment order. This covers community as well as inpatient treatment
- NI: MHNIO art18: guardianship
- RoI: No powers to enforce treatment in the community.

Any second medical recommendation must be either from a registered medical practitioner who knows the patient (e.g. their GP), or from a second approved doctor.

See Table 16.9 for the grounds, and Table 16.10 for the process, of civil community treatment.

Table 16.9 Grounds for compulsory community treatment

	E&W CTO	E&W Guardianship	Scotland	NI
Mental disorder	Any disorder or disability of the mind, of sufficient nature or degree	Any disorder or disability of mind, of sufficient nature or degree	Any mental illness, personality disorder or learning disability, however caused or manifested	Mental illness or severe mental handicap (i.e. not mild LD or PD alone), of sufficient nature or degree
Risk criterion	In the interest of the patient's own health or safety or for the protection of others	In the interests of the patient's welfare or for the protection of others	Significant risk to the patient's health, safety or welfare, or to the safety of others	In the interests of the welfare of the patient
Treatability test	Appropriate treatment can be provided without continuing detention in hospital	None	Available treatment likely to prevent disorder worsening or to alleviate its symptoms or effects	None
Capacity test	None	None	Significantly impaired ability to make decisions about medical treatment	None
Necessity test	The power of recall is necessary (particularly taking into account the risk of relapse)	Guardianship is necessary	Making of CTO is necessary	Guardianship is necessary

Table 16.10 Process of enforcing community treatment

	E&W CTO	E&W Guardianship	Scotland	NI
Recommendations	Supporting statement from an Approved Mental Health Professional	Two medical recommendations (one must be approved under s12)	Two medical recommendations (one must be approved under s22)	Two medical (one by an appointed doctor) plus one by an ASW
Applicant	Responsible Clinician	Approved Mental Health Professional or nearest relative	Mental Health Officer, who applies with a care plan to the Tribunal	Nearest relative or Approved Social Worker (ASW)
Maximum duration	6 months	6 months	6 months, or 28 days in the case of interim CTO	6 months
Powers available	Attendance for examination, and any condition necessary or appropriate for ensuring treatment, for health or safety or for protection of others	Residence; attendance at appointments for medical treatment, education, occupation or training; access for visits	Giving treatment; attendance to receive treatment or community care services; residence; access for visits	Residence; attendance at appointments for medical treatment, education, occupation or training; access for visits
Enforcement provision	Recall to hospital for 72 hours if conditions breached, then revocation of order (meaning detention under s3 or s37) if they require treatment and the risk criterion is met	Reasonable force can be used to ensure compliance	Reasonable force to ensure compliance and/or 72 hours' detention in hospital in the event of non-compliance	Reasonable force can be used to ensure compliance

Renewal	6 months then annually	6 months then annually	6 months then annually	6 months then annually
Additional Information	Patient must be under section 3 (📖 p.IV.388) or section 37 (📖 p.IV.405) for the order to be made	The guardian may be the local social services authority, or with its agreement, any other person	CTOs can authorize inpatient treatment (📖 p.IV.388) as well as community treatment	The guardian may be the responsible social services authority, or with its agreement, any other person

Aftercare

Historically, mental healthcare was provided solely in institutions such as the asylum (📖 p.IV.374) and the madhouse; when inmates left such institutions, they were expected to be ready to cope with the outside world. However, from the late 19th century it became clear that many people released from mental institutions needed support to adjust to life in the community, and in the UK charities such as the Mental After-Care Association were formed to provide it. Eventually the UK government recognized a duty to ensure that patients who needed it received aftercare.*

Table 16.11 summarizes the aftercare provisions across the different jurisdictions.

Aftercare should not be confused with the Care Programme Approach (CPA) in the UK. For example, all patients detained for treatment in E&W are entitled to aftercare,† but only those with greater needs are treated under the CPA.

The Republic of Ireland

Chiefly because of its separate historical development, the mental health system in RoI has never had a duty to provide aftercare, although many public and private hospitals provide community and aftercare services on a discretionary basis. There is a currently debate about whether there should be a duty to provide aftercare to children leaving state care services at the age of 18, including mental health aftercare, but there are no proposals for a general duty to provide mental health aftercare.

---

* There is no clear conceptual distinction between 'after care' provided on discharge from hospital, and treatment provided in the community without any hospital admission, but the concept of aftercare persists because of the specific legal duties to provide it.
† Even those that do not fall within s117 (e.g. because they were only detained for assessment under section 2) still have a right for assessment of their needs under other legislation such as s47 of the NHS and Community Care Act 1990, but they do not have the automatic right to free provision of services to meet those needs that they would have under s117.

Table 16.11 Aftercare provisions

	E&W	Scotland	NI
Relevant law	MHA s117	MH(CT)A ss25–27	MH(NI)O arts 112, 113
Application	Patients detained under s3 (admission for treatment, ☐ p.IV.388), ss37, 37/41, 45A (court-ordered admission for treatment, ☐ p.IV.405) or ss47, 48 (transfer from prison, ☐ p.IV.410)	All persons not in hospital who have or have had a mental disorder	Patients in general (there is no specific duty to provide specific services to individual patients)
Responsible bodies	Primary Care Trusts/Local Health Boards, and local social services authorities	Local Authorities, in cooperation with health bodies and voluntary organizations	Health and Social Services Boards, and Health and Social Services Trusts
Nature of the duty	To provide, in cooperation with voluntary organizations, after care services	To provide care and support services, and services to promote well-being and social development; and associated travel assistance	To make arrangements to promote mental health, prevent mental disorder, and promote the treatment, welfare and care of people with mental disorder
Specific powers (not associated with a duty)	N/A	To provide residential accommodation; social, cultural and recreational activities; training; employment support; to provide similar services to inpatients	To pay inpatients personal expenses; financial assistance to those on leave (☐ p.IV.392) if needed for treatment or resettlement; to contribute to maintenance of those on guardianship (☐ p.IV.394); to provide training and occupation for all patients
Extent of the duty	Until satisfied the person is no longer in need (and has been discharged from any CTO ☐ p.IV.394)	Indefinite; To minimize the effect of mental disorder and promote living a normal life	Indefinite
Notes	Charges may not be made (in contrast to identical services provided otherwise than under s117)	Charges may be made for some services	All subject to the approval of the Department of Health and Social Services

Police powers under mental health law

Frequently, the first professionals to have contact with mentally disordered people are the police. In other situations, a person may be known to be suffering from a mental disorder and to need immediate assistance, but be on private property where staff do not have permission to enter to assess them. Mental health law provides the police with powers to assist in these situations.

See Table 16.12 for police powers in public places, and Table 16.13 for powers in private property.

Table 16.12 Powers available in public places

	E&W	Scotland	NI	RoI
Relevant law	MHA s136	MHCTA s297	MHNIO art. 130	MHA s12
Power held by	Police constable	Police constable	Police constable	Gard (police officer)
Criteria for removal	Appears to be suffering from mental disorder and to be in immediate need of care or control	Reasonable suspicion that they have a mental disorder and are in immediate need of care or treatment	Appears to be suffering from mental disorder and to be in immediate need of care or control	Reasonable grounds for believing they suffer from mental disorder
Risk criterion	In the interests of that person or for the protection of others	In the interests of that person or for the protection of others	In the interests of that person or for the protection of others	Serious likelihood of the patient causing immediate and serious harm to themselves or others
Removal to	Place of safety (can include police station)	Place of safety (can only include police station if nowhere else available)	Place of safety (can include police station)	Into custody
Detention period	72 hours	24 hours	48 hours	No maximum
Purpose of detention	Assessment by AMHP and doctor and making arrangements for treatment or care	Assessment by doctor and making arrangements for treatment or care	Assessment by ASW and doctor and making arrangements for treatment or care	Assessment by a doctor in order to make (or refuse) a recommendation for an admission order (📖 p.IV.388)

Table 16.13 Powers available in private premises

	E&W	Scotland	NI	RoI
Relevant law	MHA ss135(1)*	MHCTA s293*	MHNIO art 129*	MHA s12
Power held by	Justice of the Peace (magistrate)	Sheriff or (in urgent cases) a Justice of the Peace	Justice of the Peace (magistrate)	Gard (police officer)
Applicant	AMHP	Mental Health Officer	Health staff, or constable	N/A
Criteria for forcible entry and removal	Reasonable cause to suspect that a person believed to be suffering from mental disorder has been or is being ill-treated, neglected or not kept under proper control, or lives alone and is unable to care for themselves	Satisfied that a person over 16 has a mental disorder, is suffering or at risk of ill-treatment, neglect etc., loss of or damage to property, or lives alone and is unable to care for themselves; and likely to suffer serious harm if not removed	Reasonable cause to suspect that a person believed to be suffering from mental disorder has been or is being ill-treated, neglected or not kept under proper control, or lives alone and is unable to care for themselves	Reasonable grounds for believing they suffer from mental disorder and are to be found in the premises concerned; and serious likelihood of the patient causing immediate and serious harm to themselves or others
Conditions on forcible entry and removal	Constable must have warrant and be accompanied by an AMHP and a doctor	Constable must have warrant and be accompanied by MHO and doctor	Constable must have warrant and be accompanied by a doctor	None
Removal to	Place of safety (can include police station)	Place of safety (can not include police station)	Place of safety (can include police station)	Into custody
Detention period	Up to 72 hours	Up to 7 days	Up to 48 hours	No maximum

*s135(2) in E&W, s292 in Scotland and art129(2) in NI provide a similar power when a constable or other person authorized to take or retake a patient to hospital etc. applies to a magistrate stating that they believe the patient to be on certain private premises and that permission to enter has been or would be refused. No AMHP or doctor is involved in this case.

Court-ordered pre-sentence assessment

Relevant legislation

- E&W: MHA ss35,36: remands to hospital
- Scotland: CPSA ss52A-52U: assessment and treatment orders, s200: pre-sentence report (sentences of imprisonment only)
- NI: MHNIO arts42,43: remands to hospital
- RoI: CLIA ss4(6), 5(3): committal for examination. Note the dramatically narrower legal grounds for such orders compared to the UK.

See Table 16.14 for the grounds, and Table 16.15 for the process, of court-ordered pre-sentence assessment.

Table 16.14 Grounds for pre-sentence admission

	E&W	Scotland	NI	RoI
Mental disorder	For s35, reason to suspect any disorder or disability of the mind; for s36, any such disorder of sufficient nature or degree	Any mental illness, PD or LD, however caused or manifested; for assessment order and s200, reasonable grounds for believing such disorder is present	For art42, reason to suspect mental illness or severe mental impairment; for art43, such illness/ impairment of sufficient nature or degree	No specific requirement, but presumably the court must suspect that a doctor might diagnose mental disorder
Risk criterion	None	Significant risk to the patient's health, safety or welfare, or others' safety (not s200)	None	None
Necessity test	Impractical to obtain medical report on bail	Detention necessary for assessment; or for treatment order, that available treatment likely to prevent deterioration or alleviate symptoms	Impractical to obtain medical report on bail	None
Purpose	For s35, a report on mental condition; for s36, treatment	Assessment and treatment; for s200, inquiry into mental condition required to decide sentence	For art42, a report on mental condition; for art43, treatment	For examination by an approved medical officer, for the court to decide whether to make order for treatment (📖 p.IV.405)

Table 16.15 Process of pre-sentence admission

	E&W	Scotland	NI	RoI
Stage of legal proceedings required for order to be considered	Charged with offence punishable with imprisonment; and for s36, be in Crown Court*	Be in Sheriff Court*	Charged with offence punishable with imprisonment; and for art43, be in Crown Court	For s4(6), meets criteria for unfitness to plead (🕮 p.V.474); for s5(3), meets criteria for insanity (🕮 p.V.489)
Evidence (medical recommendation)	Written or oral evidence of a S12 doctor (and a second doctor for s36), plus evidence of a hospital representative that a bed will be available within 7 days	For assessment order and s200, written or oral evidence of a doctor; for a treatment order, one approved and one other doctor; in all cases, evidence that a bed will be available within 7 days	Written or oral evidence of an appointed doctor (and a second doctor for art43)	None
Applicant	N/A	Prosecutor or Scottish Ministers (not s200)	N/A	N/A
Maximum duration	Up to 28 days	Assessment order, 28 days; s200, 3 weeks; treatment order, until disposal	Up to 28 days	Up to 14 days
Renewal	Can be renewed by request of the AC/RC up to a maximum of 12 weeks	Cannot be renewed, but assessment order can be extended once for 7 days, s200 once for 3 weeks	Can be renewed by request of the RMO up to a maximum of 12 weeks	S4(6) (unfitness to be tried) cannot be renewed; s5(3) (insanity) can be renewed up to 6 months

*For the magistrates' court in E&W or NI to remand a person under s35, it must have convicted them, or have satisfied itself that they did the act or omission charged (i.e. the actus reus, 🕮 p.IV.332); or they must consent to the remand.

†However, s52A allows District Courts to remit the case to Sheriff Court if they are charged with a offence punishable by imprisonment and appear to have a mental disorder.

Court-ordered sentence of treatment

Relevant legislation
- E&W: MHA s37: hospital order, s38: interim hospital order
- Scotland: CPSA ss53,57A: (interim) compulsion order
- NI: MHNIO art44: hospital, order, art45: interim hospital order
- RoI: CLIA ss4(3),(5), 5(2): committal for treatment. Note the dramatically narrower legal grounds for such orders compared to the UK.

See Table 16.16 for the grounds, and Table 16.17 for the process, of court-ordered sentences of treatment.

Table 16.16 Grounds for court-ordered sentence of treatment

	E&W	Scotland	NI	RoI
Mental disorder	Any disorder or disability of the mind, of sufficient nature or degree (and if LD, abnormally aggressive or seriously irresponsible)	Any mental illness, PD or LD, however caused or manifested	Mental illness or severe mental impairment, of sufficient nature or degree (severe mental handicap for guardianship)	Mental illness, severe dementia, or significant intellectual impairment; or for outpatient treatment if unfit to plead, any disease of the mind
Risk criterion	None	Significant risk to the patient's health, safety or welfare, or to the safety of others	None	For inpatient treatment, serious likelihood of the patient causing immediate and serious harm
Treatability test	For hospital order, appropriate treatment is available	Available treatment likely to prevent disorder worsening or to alleviate its symptoms or effects; for interim order, reasonable grounds for believing this	None	For inpatient treatment, likely to benefit or alleviate the condition of that person to a material extent
Necessity test (capacity test in the case of RoI)	For interim order, a hospital order might be appropriate	Medical treatment can only be given if detained in hospital (unless the compulsion order is only for community treatment)	For interim order, a hospital order might be warranted	For inpatient treatment (as *alternative* to the risk criterion) Judgement so impaired that without compulsory treatment a serious deterioration likely

Table 16.17 Process of court-ordered sentence of treatment

	E&W	Scotland	NI	RoI
Stage of legal proceedings required for order to be considered	Convicted (or, in magistrates' court, found to have done the act or omission) of offence punishable with imprisonment	Convicted of offence punishable with imprisonment	Convicted (or, in magistrates' court, found to have done the act or omission) of offence punishable with imprisonment	For s4, meets criteria for unfitness to plead (☐ p.V.474); for s5, meets criteria for insanity (☐ p.V.489)
Evidence (medical recommendation)	Written or oral evidence of a S12 doctor, and a second doctor, plus evidence of a hospital representative that a bed will be available within 28 days	Written or oral evidence of one approved doctor and a second doctor, plus evidence that a bed will be available within 7 days, plus report from a mental health officer	Oral evidence of an appointed doctor, and written or oral evidence of a second doctor, plus an ASW for guardianship	None
Maximum duration	6 months (12 weeks for interim order)	6 months (12 weeks for interim order)	6 months (12 weeks for interim order)	Indefinite
Renewal	For 6 months and then a year at a time; for interim order, 28 days at a time up to a year	For 6 months and then a year at a time; for interim order, up to 12 weeks at a time up to a year	For 6 months and then a year at a time; for interim order, 28 days at a time up to a year	No necessity for renewal as such, but the order must be reviewed by the Review Board at least every 6 months
Additional information	S37 also authorizes guardianship	Compulsion order; like compulsory treatment order (☐ p.IV.388), can compel community treatment. An order for lifelong restriction (☐ p.IV.365) is automatically available as an alternative sentence	Art44 also authorizes guardianship	Review Board can terminate order, and also restart legal proceedings

Other court orders

Urgent detention of acquitted persons

In general, if a court acquits a person it has no further power to deal with them. Even if it has evidence from an earlier stage of the proceedings that they may require treatment, it can only hope that either the patient will be willing to accept treatment voluntarily, or that the relevant professionals will consider a civil admission for assessment (p.IV.383) or treatment (p.IV.388).

However, if this situation arises in Scotland (meaning that the court has before it the written or oral evidence of two doctors that the defendant is suffering from a mental disorder of a type required for a compulsion order (p.V.405), and that the risk criterion and treatability test for that order are met), then if it satisfied that it is not immediately practicable for a doctor to examine them with a view to making a short-term detention order (p.IV.383) or emergency detention order (p.IV.386), it can order them to be taken to a place of safety and detained there for up to six hours in order to enable such an examination to take place.

Risk assessment order

All three UK jurisdictions have a system for extended (p.IV.367) or indefinite (p.IV.365) detention of people convicted of serious violent or sexual offences who are thought by the court to be dangerous (p.V.549). Whereas in E&W and NI the court may make its assessment of dangerousness based on whatever conviction and other information is before it, in Scotland the court must usually make a risk assessment order, requiring the Risk Management Authority (p.V.469) to compile a risk assessment report on the offender.

Hybrid order and hospital direction

In the UK, successive governments have been concerned about the possibility of offenders with personality disorder alone being transferred to hospital but then proving untreatable and having to be released, possibly many years earlier than they would have been released from prison. The *hospital and limitation direction* in E&W (usually known as a hybrid order) and the hospital direction in Scotland were therefore added to the MHA and CPSA in 1997, in effect allowing a patient with personality disorder to be given both a prison sentence and a hospital order or compulsion order with restrictions (p.IV.412) simultaneously: should treatment then prove unsuccessful, they would be remitted to prison to serve the remainder of their prison sentence. The orders were unpopular with clinicians, however, and only a handful have ever been made.[*] They remain in the Acts, and are currently available for offenders with any mental disorder who meet the criteria for a hospital order or compulsion order (p.IV.405).

---

[*] An average of 6 hybrid orders have been made each year since 2005 in E&W, as compared with an average of 837 hospital orders per year.

Supervision and treatment order

This order is available throughout the UK (though known as a supervision order in E&W), and applies only to those found not guilty by reason of insanity (📖 p.V.489) or unfit to plead (📖 p.V.474), where neither admission to hospital nor an absolute discharge (nor, in Scotland and NI, guardianship) would be appropriate. It makes the defendant subject to the supervision of a social worker or (in E&W and NI) probation officer* for up to two years (three years in Scotland), during which time they must submit to any pre-scribed medical treatment for mental disorder, under medical supervision. There is no appeal to a Tribunal (📖 p.IV.414) against a supervision order or supervision and treatment order; appeals must be made to the relevant court.

Guardianship orders and intervention orders

Guardianship is available in E&W and NI as an order for mentally disor-dered persons, both as civil guardianship (📖 p.IV.394), and as a variant on a hospital order (📖 p.IV.405). However, in Scotland, court-ordered guard-ianship (📖 p.IV.434) and the associated intervention order (📖 p.IV.434) are available only for defendants who lack capacity (📖 p.IV.424).

Restriction orders and restriction directions

These are covered on 📖 p.IV.412.

Courts-martial

Military courts trying a member of the armed forces have limited powers to order treatment for mental disorder.

In the UK, defendants who have been found unfit to plead (📖 p.V.474) or not guilty by reason of insanity (📖 p.IV.489) can be given an *admission order* authorizing detention and treatment in hospital, a *supervision and treatment order* equivalent to the order described earlier in this section, or a *guardianship* order. In each case, the defendant is then treated as if a local criminal court had made the order.

In RoI, if a court-martial finds a member of the defence forces unfit to plead or insane at the time of the offence, the defendant is transferred to a designated centre for treatment as if they had been committed for treatment (📖 p.IV.405) under the CLIA.

---

* In practice, Home Office guidance states that it should be an approved social worker (i.e. now an AMHP in E&W).

Transfer from prison for treatment

These are not court orders, but directions issued by the government department that runs the prison service (🕮 p.V.456) in each jurisdiction.

Relevant legislation

- E&W: MHA s47: transfer of prisoner, s48: urgent transfer
- Scotland: MHCTA s136: transfer for treatment direction
- NI: MHNIO arts53, 54: removal of prisoners
- RoI: CLIA s15: transfer of prisoner.

See Table 16.18 for the grounds, and Table 16.19 for the process, of transfer from prison.

Table 16.18 Grounds for transfer from prison

	E&W	Scotland	NI	RoI
Mental disorder	Any disorder or disability of the mind, of sufficient nature or degree	Any mental illness, personality disorder or learning disability, however caused or manifested	Mental illness or severe mental impairment, of sufficient nature or degree	Mental illness, mental disability, dementia or any disease of the mind
Risk criterion	None	Significant risk to the patient's health, safety or welfare, or to the safety of others	None	None
Treatability test	Appropriate treatment is available	Available treatment likely to prevent disorder worsening or to alleviate its symptoms or effects	None	None
Necessity test	In the public interest, and expedient in all the circumstances; and for s48, in urgent need of treatment	The transfer for treatment direction is necessary	In the public interest, and expedient in all the circumstances; and for art54, in urgent need of treatment	Cannot be afforded appropriate care or treatment in the prison in which they are detained

Table 16.19 Process of transfer from prison

	E&W	Scotland	NI	RoI
Stage of legal proceedings required for order to be considered	Convicted, serving sentence of imprisonment (or for s48, detained pending civil or criminal trial or deportation)	Convicted, serving sentence of imprisonment	Convicted, serving sentence of imprisonment (or for art54, detained pending civil or criminal trial or deportation)	At any stage
Evidence (medical recommendation)	Reports by a s12 doctor, and by a second doctor	Reports by one approved doctor and a second doctor, plus evidence that a bed will be available within 7 days	Reports by an appointed doctor, and by a second doctor	Report by two doctors, or one doctor with consent of patient
Maximum duration	Until EDR (🕮 p.IV.367), after which detention continues under 'notional' unrestricted hospital order (🕮 p.IV.405)	Until end of custody part (🕮 p.IV.367) of sentence	Until EDR (🕮 p.IV.367), after which detention continues under 'notional' unrestricted hospital order (🕮 p.IV.405)	Until they cease to be a prisoner, at which point further detention only possible if an admission order (🕮 p.IV.388) made
Return to prison	At any time, if RC or Tribunal states that treatment no longer needed or no further effective treatment available	At any time (or at annual reviews), if RC and MHO, Scottish Ministers or Tribunal no longer think conditions met	At any time, if RMO or Tribunal states that treatment no longer needed or no further effective treatment available	If prisoner refuses treatment (unless two doctors certify they should stay in hospital nevertheless); or if Clinical Director or Review Board concludes conditions no longer met
Additional information	In practice, s49 restrictions (🕮 p.IV.412) are always applied for s47; they are mandatory for s48	Prisoners on remand can be treated under an assessment or treatment order (🕮 p.IV.403)	Art55 restrictions (🕮 p.IV.412) are mandatory for art54	Detention reviewed by Review Board at least every 6 months

Restriction orders and directions

In the UK, the philosophy underlying the court orders and transfer directions on 📖 pp.IV.403–IV.411 is that where offenders or potential offenders are assessed as suffering from treatable mental disorder, they should be diverted (📖 p.II.216) to hospital for treatment, or occasionally to the community for outpatient treatment. Where the offence is relatively minor and/or the offender's risk assessment (📖 p.II.127) suggests that they are not a danger to society (📖 p.V.549), that is usually the end of the matter. However, if they are charged with or convicted of a serious sexual or violent offence, or are deemed 'dangerous' for some other reason, they will usually be treated in secure services (📖 p.II.209), and they will be subject to restrictions that limit the treating clinicians' powers.

In RoI, there is no general power to sentence offenders to treatment, and no order under which offenders can be treated in an unrestricted fashion. All court treatment orders and transfers from prison are automatically subject to what in the UK would be regarded as restrictions.

Orders and directions to which restrictions can be applied

Orders marked with an asterisk* either require that restrictions be applied automatically, or imply restrictions by having no mechanism for the RC/RMO/CD to discharge, transfer or grant leave to the patient.

Sentences of treatment
- Hospital order (E&W, MHA s37/41; NI, MHNIO art44/47)
- Compulsion order (Scotland, CPSA ss57A/59)
- Committal for treatment (RoI, CLIA ss4, 5).*

Other court orders
- Hybrid order (E&W, MHA s45A)*
- Hospital direction (Scotland, CPSA s59A).*

Transfer directions
- Transfer/removal of prisoner (E&W, MHA s47; NI, MHNIO art53)
- Urgent transfer/removal (E&W, MHA s48; NI, MHNIO art54)*
- Transfer for treatment (Scotland, MHCTA s136)*
- Transfer of prisoner (RoI, CLIA s15).*

Criterion for making a restriction order

Where the court or the relevant Minister† has discretion over whether or not to apply restrictions, it may do so if the restrictions are *necessary for the protection of the public from serious harm,* having regard to the offence they have been convicted of, and to their past criminal record, as well as any risk assessment that may be available.

Where a court is considering making a restriction order, it can only do so if it has heard oral evidence from at least one of the doctors recommending admission to hospital.

---

† The government minister or department responsible for running the prison service: the Ministry of Justice in E&W, the Scottish Ministers, or the Secretary of State in NI. See 📖 pp.V.464, V.467.

Restrictions when in hospital

During the period that the restrictions apply, the RC/RMO/CD cannot:

- Grant leave (📖 p.IV.392) from hospital (or suspend detention in Scotland)
- Transfer the patient to another hospital or unit outside the boundaries of the hospital or unit named in the order
- Discharge the patient from hospital.

Instead, the CD, RC or RMO must apply to the relevant Minister,† who will decide whether or not to transfer the patient, or grant leave or in the case of sentences of treatment, to discharge the patient; in other cases, discharge is not usually possible but the Minister may decide to return the patient to prison.

In addition, the order cannot expire and therefore does not need renewal; it lasts until the restrictions are lifted by the relevant Minister or a Tribunal, or (in the case of transfer directions, hybrid orders and hospital directions) until the patient would have been released from prison had they not been transferred, after which it may end completely or continue as an unrestricted form of the order (see 📖 pp.IV.405–IV.411 for details).

Restrictions after discharge from hospital

Patients treated under a hospital order or compulsion order with restrictions (or committed for treatment in RoI) can be *conditionally discharged* from hospital by a Tribunal, or in E&W and NI by the relevant Minister. After a conditional discharge, the patient may leave hospital, but if they relapse or breach the conditions (and there is evidence to suggest risk of relapse), the relevant Minister can recall (📖 p.V.467) them to hospital to continue treatment under the original order.

Common conditions include a requirement to reside in a particular place, often a mental health hostel; to accept treatment; to submit to drug testing; and to attend appointments with the RC/RMO, social supervisor (📖 p.V.467) and other staff. The conditions can be varied at any time by the relevant Minister.

Where a Tribunal in E&W, Scotland or NI grants a conditional discharge, it may *defer* it taking effect until whatever arrangements it thinks necessary (such as obtaining funding for a placement) have been made.

Reporting requirements

When restrictions apply to a patient, the law requires the RMO/RC to keep the relevant Minister informed of developments in their care and treatment. This includes an update on their condition whenever the RMO/RC applies for leave, transfer or discharge, and also:

- An annual review for patients in Scotland
- An Annual Statutory Report (ASR) on inpatients in E&W and NI, and
- Quarterly reports on conditionally discharged patients in E&W and NI.

Appeal against detention & treatment

The cornerstone of the protection of patients' rights under mental health law is the role of the Tribunal,* which independently reviews the use of detention and compulsory treatment.

Civil detention and treatment

A Tribunal can review detention and treatment automatically, before the relevant order comes into effect; if the patient appeals against the order; and if the order is referred to it by hospital managers, the MHC/MWC, or the relevant Minister (p.IV.412), as shown in Table 16.20. There is no appeal against or review of emergency civil detention (p.IV.386) because the detention is so brief.

Table 16.20 Appeal against civil orders

	E&W	Scotland	NI	RoI
Review prior to order	None	CTO only made or varied if Tribunal approves application	None	None
Appeal against assessment	Within first 14 days of s2 order only	Any time under short-term detention certificate	Within 6 months of admission	None
Appeal against treatment or guardianship	Within 6 months of s3, guardianship or CTO being made, plus once in every renewal period	If RMO extends unvaried CTO (which does not need Tribunal review); or three months after making, varying or extending order	Within 6 months of admission or guardianship, plus once in every renewal period	None
Referral to Tribunal	At discretion of relevant Minister; and by hospital managers after 6 months then every three years, if no appeals	MWC also has power to revoke short-term detention, interim CTO or CTO, as well as to refer CTO to Tribunal	At discretion of relevant Minister; and by Hospital Boards every two years if no appeals	By MHC on making or renewal of admission order

Court-ordered treatment and transfer from prison

There is no appeal against or review of a court order for pre-sentence assessment (p.IV.403). Rules for appeal against other court orders are shown in Table 16.21.

* The First-Tier Tribunal (Mental Health) in E&W; the Mental Health Tribunal in Scotland; and the Mental Health Review Tribunal in NI and RoI.

Table 16.21 Appeal against court orders

	E&W	Scotland	NI	RoI
Appeal against treatment or guardianship	After 6 months of unrestricted hospital order (or within 6 months for guardianship) then once in every renewal period. NB nearest relative can also appeal	If unrestricted compulsion order, Tribunal must approve extension or variation; appeal three months after making, varying or extending order	Within 6 months of unrestricted hospital order or guardianship plus once in every renewal period	None, except to appeal court against the finding of unfitness to plead or insanity
Appeal against transfer from prison	If unrestricted s47, within 6 months plus once in every renewal period; otherwise, as for restriction order	During first 12 weeks, then after 6 months, then once in every 12 months	If unrestricted art53, within 6 months plus once in every renewal period; otherwise, as for restriction order	None
Restriction orders (including hybrid orders etc.; see also 🔲 p.IV.408)	After six months, and then once in every 12 months	After six months, and then once in every 12 months; plus within 28 days of recall	Within 6 months of order, then between 6 and 12 months, then once in every 12 months	None
Appeal against conditions of discharge	After 12 months, and then once in every 2 years	Once in every 12 months, plus within 28 days of variation of conditions	Within 12 months of discharge, then once every year	None
Referral to Tribunal	At discretion of relevant Minister; and by the Minister every three years if no appeals, plus within a month of recall	At discretion of relevant Minister; and by the Minister every 2 years if no appeals	At discretion of relevant Minister; and by the Minister every 2 years if no appeals, plus within a month of recall	Automatic review by Review Board at least every 6 months, plus at discretion of relevant Minister or Board

The review process

Review by a Tribunal (or the Review Board for offenders in RoI) involves the following stages:

- An examination of the patient by the RMO/RC and a care co-ordinator, social worker or social supervisor; and, if requested by the patient or their solicitor, an independent psychiatrist or other appropriate professional; each of whom must submit a report (📖 p.V.567) to the Tribunal
- In E&W, an examination of the patient by the medical member of the Tribunal
- The representation of the patient by a publicly-funded solicitor
- An oral hearing, usually in private, before the Tribunal panel[*]
- The giving of evidence (📖 p.V.592) and cross-examination of each party
- The giving by the Tribunal of written reasons for its decision, and
- The opportunity for the patient to appeal against the decision,[†] but in the UK only by judicial review (📖 p.IV.309) or on equivalent grounds.

Powers of tribunals

Tribunals must, most notably, immediately discharge unrestricted patients absolutely from detention and treatment if the criteria for the order under which they are detained and/or treated are no longer met, and have an additional discretionary power to discharge for all unrestricted patients. However, if this is not thought appropriate or is not possible for the order concerned[‡], there is no power for Tribunals to discharge *unrestricted* patients subject to conditions. Tribunals in the UK (but not RoI, except in the case of conditional discharge) can also:

Unrestricted patients[§]

- Order a *delayed discharge* in E&W or NI, that is, a discharge that is to take effect on a specified future date
- In E&W or NI, make a *recommendation* to the RMO/RC that the patient be granted leave, be transferred to another hospital, or be placed under guardianship or (in E&W) a CTO, and reconvene if the recommendation is not followed
- In Scotland, uphold the CTO or unrestricted compulsion order but *vary the measures* authorized by it.

---

[*] Comprising an independent consultant psychiatrist, a lay member (often a retired ASW or AMHP in E&W and NI), and a legally-qualified President (a high court judge or equivalent for restricted patients in E&W).

[†] In E&W, to the Upper Tribunal (📖 p.IV.320); in Scotland, to the Sheriff Principal or Court of Session (📖 p.IV.322); in NI, the Court of Appeal (📖 p.IV.320); and in RoI, to the Circuit Court (📖 p.IV.324).

[‡] i.e. prison transfers; hybrid orders, in E&W; or hospital directions in Scotland.

[§] Except patients subject to short-term detention certificates in Scotland.

Patients sentenced to treatment with restrictions
- Discharge the patient *conditionally** (including in RoI; see 📖 p.IV.413)
- Direct that the patient be conditionally discharged, but *defer* this taking effect until necessary arrangements have been made (as opposed to delaying it until a future date), and reconvene if they are not made
- Uphold the restriction order in Scotland, while *varying* the measures authorized by the associated compulsion order
- In Scotland, *revoke* the restriction order, but uphold the (now unrestricted) compulsion order
- For conditionally discharged patients, uphold the restriction order but *vary* the conditions of discharge, or discharge them *absolutely*.

Prison transfers, hybrid orders and hospital directions
- *Direct* the Scottish Ministers to revoke the hospital direction or transfer for treatment direction, in which case the patient will be returned to prison, or
- Make a *recommendation* in E&W or NI to the relevant Minister (📖 p.IV.412) that the patient be conditionally or absolutely discharged; the relevant Minister may then authorize the conditional or absolute discharge within 90 days, after which the patient is otherwise remitted to prison unless the Tribunal has recommended that they remain in hospital.

Relationship with Parole Boards

A small number of patients detained in hospital in the UK under hybrid orders or hospital directions or after transfer from prison will have received life sentences or other indeterminate sentences (📖 p.IV.364) and cannot be released into the community unless this is authorized by the Parole Board (📖 p.V.459).

In Scotland, if the Tribunal directs that the hospital direction or transfer for treatment direction be revoked for a patient who has received such a sentence, they return to prison and the normal procedure for consideration of their release by the Parole Board will apply.

However, in E&W and NI, if the Tribunal recommends conditional or absolute discharge, and states that the patient should remain in hospital in the meantime, and if the patient is eligible for parole (because they have passed their tariff, 📖 p.IV.365), the Parole Board may meet at the hospital and allow the patient to be discharged directly into the community.

---

*Absolute discharge of a patient sentenced to treatment with restrictions without an initial period of conditional discharge is also possible in the UK, but only if the tribunal is satisfied that liability to recall is inappropriate.

Human rights law

In both the UK and RoI, the European Convention on Human Rights (ECHR, 📖 p.IV.420) has been incorporated into domestic law. This means that courts must take the Convention (and judgments of the European Court of Human Rights) into account in reaching verdicts; that public bodies must exercise their powers in ways that conform with the Convention; and that the acts of public bodies, and domestic laws themselves, can be overturned by local courts through judicial review (📖 p.IV.309).

Articles of the ECHR can conflict with each other (for example, one person's right to freedom of speech can conflict with another person's right to a private life). Courts account for this by giving certain articles greater weight than others (e.g. absolute rights such as the prohibition of torture always outweigh qualified rights such as the right to private life). The articles are written in extremely broad terms; individual countries are allowed a 'margin of appreciation': that is, a degree of flexibility in the interpretation of an article to fit its domestic law.

Incorporation has had a significant impact on the detention and compulsory treatment of patients under mental health law. The articles of the Convention and associated case law that have had the most significant impact on practice are outlined here.

Article 2—the right to life

The death of a person in the custody of the State, such as someone detained under mental health law, may contravene article 2. The courts have held that the State has a positive duty to safeguard the lives of prisoners and other people in its custody, not merely a duty not to kill them. For example, in the UK the police were found to have breached article 2 for failing to protect a family adequately, resulting in a man's death, despite knowing of a 'real and immediate threat' to his life.

The State does not have an absolute duty to prevent death: for example, if a hospital or prison becomes aware of the risk of a patient or prisoner committing suicide, and takes reasonable and proportionate steps to safeguard them (such as putting them on observations, 📖 p.II.154), it may not be liable even if the patient goes on to kill him- or herself. Conversely, however, if reasonable and proportionate steps are not taken, the State may be liable even if death does not result, as long as there was a 'material risk' of death.

The courts have also held that States have a duty to investigate the deaths of people in their custody (or for whose safety they have some other responsibility, such as when the police engage in a high speed chase of a suspect), and to conduct that investigation in a prompt, fair, impartial and accountable manner.

Article 3—prohibition on torture and degrading treatment

Whether a certain treatment is 'inhuman' or 'degrading' depends on the circumstances of the case, the duration of the treatment, its purpose, and its cumulative effect on the specific patient. For example, holding a person with schizophrenia in overcrowded conditions without daylight or adequate lighting or ventilation, alongside people with infectious disease and with parasitic insects was held to breach article 3, as was force-feeding a patient when the alternative of parenteral nutrition was available.

The courts have held that the feelings of inferiority and powerlessness often associated with mental disorder create a need for vigilance to ensure article 3 is complied with.

Article 5—the right to personal liberty

Article 5 specifically authorizes detention of 'persons of unsound mind', and many cases have concerned the limits of this authorization: what amounts to detention, when detention is authorized, for how long, and in what circumstances. This has led to rulings that in a Tribunal (🕮 p.IV.309) the burden of proof (🕮 p.IV.317) is on the hospital to show that detention continues to be justified, not on the patient to show it is not; that tribunals, rather than Ministers, must be free to discharge restricted patients (🕮 p.IV.412) absolutely; and that long delays in holding tribunals are unacceptable. A desire to comply with article 5 was also the reason for creating the Deprivation of Liberty Safeguards (DoLS, 🕮 p.IV.436) in E&W, after the Bournewood (🕮 p.App. 3.631) case.

A possible future target for litigation under article 5 is the inability to appeal against specific conditions of a Community Treatment Order (🕮 p.IV.394) in E&W (as opposed to appealing against the existence of the entire order).

Article 8—the right to private and family life

This article has been interpreted very widely by the court, and as imposing positive obligations on States, not merely negative obligations not to interfere with people's lives. For example, an excessive delay in providing necessary medical treatment has been held to be a breach, as have unnecessarily disclosing a person's HIV status during court proceedings, and disclosing a private psychiatric report to a GP without consent. An earlier version of the E&W MHA was also found to be in breach of article 8 by restricting too greatly who could act as a patient's nearest relative (🕮 p.IV.380).

Other decisions have held that the following are all lawful under the Convention:
- Compulsory antipsychotic treatment causing unpleasant side effects
- Requiring limited disclosure of HIV status to protect prison staff
- Closing a residential home or day centre on financial grounds
- Restricting day care services to local residents
- Health authorities' decisions on which treatments to fund.

and, in a high security hospital (🕮 p.II.209):
- Randomly monitoring 10% of telephone calls
- Refusing to supply condoms
- Refusing to allow a patient to cross-dress.

European Convention on Human Rights

The main text of the key articles of the Convention for the Protection of Human Rights and Fundamental Freedoms is reproduced here, along with the articles from the first and 13th protocols that apply in the UK and RoI, and the articles of the fourth protocol that apply in RoI. The relevance of certain articles to forensic psychiatry is discussed on 📖 p.V.418.

Article 1 The High Contracting Parties shall secure to everyone within their jurisdiction the rights and freedoms [below].

Article 2 Everyone's right to life shall be protected by law. No one shall be deprived of his life intentionally . . . [except] when it results from the use of force which is no more than absolutely necessary in defence of any person from unlawful violence; in order to effect a lawful arrest or to prevent escape of a person lawfully detained; or in action lawfully taken for the purpose of quelling a riot or insurrection.

Article 3 No one shall be subjected to torture or to inhuman or degrading treatment or punishment.

Article 4 No one shall be held in slavery or servitude. No one shall be required to perform forced or compulsory labour.

Article 5 Everyone has the right to liberty and security of person. No one shall be deprived of his liberty save in the following cases and in accordance with a procedure prescribed by law:

- Lawful detention after conviction by a competent court [or for contempt of court];
- Lawful arrest or [remanding in custody before trial]; . . .
- Lawful detention for the prevention of the spreading of infectious diseases, [or] of persons of unsound mind, alcoholics or drug addicts, or vagrants;
- Lawful arrest or detention to prevent unauthorized entry into the country or with a view to deportation or extradition.

Everyone who is arrested shall be informed promptly, in a language which he understands, of the reasons for his arrest and the charge against him.

Everyone who is deprived of his liberty by arrest or detention shall be entitled to take proceedings by which the lawfulness of his detention shall be decided speedily by a court and his release ordered if the detention is not lawful.

Everyone who has been the victim of arrest or detention in contravention of the provisions of this article shall have an enforceable right to compensation.

Article 6 Everyone is entitled to a fair and public hearing within a reasonable time by an independent and impartial tribunal.

Article 7 No one shall be held guilty of any criminal offence on account of any act or omission which did not constitute a criminal offence under national or international law at the time when it was committed.

Article 8 Everyone has the right to respect for his private and family life, his home and his correspondence.

Article 9 Everyone has the right to freedom of thought, conscience and religion.

Article 10 Everyone has the right to freedom of expression.

Article 11 Everyone has the right to freedom of peaceful assembly and to freedom of association with others.

Article 12 Men and women of marriageable age have the right to marry and to found a family.

Article 13 Everyone whose rights and freedoms as set forth in this Convention are violated shall have an effective remedy before a national authority. [Directly applicable in RoI, but not in UK.]

Article 14 The enjoyment of the rights and freedoms set forth in this Convention shall be secured without discrimination on any ground such as sex, race, colour, language, religion, political or other opinion, national or social origin, association with a national minority, property, birth or other status.

Article 15 In time of war or other public emergency threatening the life of the nation any High Contracting Party may take measures derogating from its obligations under this Convention.

1st Protocol Article 1 Every natural or legal person is entitled to the peaceful enjoyment of his possessions. No one shall be deprived of his possessions except in the public interest and subject to the conditions provided by law.

1st Protocol Article 2 No person shall be denied the right to education… [which should be] in conformity with their own religious and philosophical convictions.

1st Protocol Article 3 The High Contracting Parties undertake to hold free elections at reasonable intervals by secret ballot, under conditions which will ensure the free expression of the opinion of the people in the choice of the legislature.

4th Protocol Article 1 No one shall be deprived of his liberty merely on the ground of inability to fulfil a contractual obligation [RoI only].

4th Protocol Articles 2, 3 and 4 guarantee freedom of movement and prohibit the expulsion of national citizens or the collective expulsion of foreigners [RoI only].

13th Protocol Article 1 The death penalty shall be abolished. No one shall be condemned to such penalty or executed.

Misuse of mental health law

Mental health law allows the State to detain people without having to prove that they have committed any offence, and without the need for a trial. Across the UK and RoI, tens of thousands of orders for compulsory detention and treatment are made every year, as shown in Table 16.22. The detainee may be able to appeal to a Tribunal (□ p.IV.414), but this is not available under some orders, and it may be weeks or even months before the hearing occurs. The potential for abuse is obvious, and mental health laws in all jurisdictions have gradually evolved to include progressively greater safeguards (□ p.IV.378) to protect patients' interests. Nevertheless, there continue to be occasional claims from patients, families and pressure groups that mental health law is used inappropriately.

Table 16.22 Frequency of detention under mental health law, 2010 (for RoI, 2009)

Order type	E&W	Scotland	NI	RoI
Civil assessment	18,385	3,352	No data	N/A*
Civil treatment	9,545	1,091	No data	1,434
Civil emergency	587	1,822	No data	590
Court-ordered	2,191	329	No data	0†
Total orders	30,774	6,594	1,043	2,024
Orders per 100,000 people	56	127	58	48

*There are no separate data for civil assessment orders (□ p.IV.383) for RoI, because the same order, the admission order, serves both assessment and treatment functions.

†In RoI, there is no general power for courts to make hospital disposals: only transfers from prison (□ p.IV.410) and hospital treatment for insanity (□ p.V.489), diminished responsibility (□ p.V.491) and unfitness to plead (□ p.V.474) are available.

Misuse for political purposes

The most egregious and well-known examples of using mental health law to detain political prisoners occurred in the former Soviet Union from the 1940s to the 1970s, initially haphazardly and later in organized fashion, with the creation of a network of psychiatric prisons under the control of the secret police. The Serbsky Institute in Moscow defined a form of schizophrenia unrecognized in the West, *sluggish schizophrenia*, in which the only symptoms were changes in social behaviour, most notably 'ideas about a struggle for truth and justice … formed by personalities with a paranoid structure'. Many hundreds of dissidents were incarcerated by psychiatrists on the grounds that they suffered from sluggish schizophrenia, in some cases because the psychiatrists were politically aware and consciously acting on behalf of the State (a grave breach of their professional ethics, □ p.III.241); in other cases the psychiatrists concerned naively believed they were correctly diagnosing genuine mental illness. Once detained, dissidents would be given antipsychotic medication and other unnecessary treatments or medical procedures, and sometimes subjected to torture masquerading as treatment, including electric shocks, radiation exposure, and beatings.

Similar political abuse occurred on a lesser scale in East European countries under Communist rule during the same period, and some authors claim that it continues today in Russia and China. Although such abuse is not believed to occur in the UK or RoI, some provisions of mental health law imply a recognition of the possibility, for example by requiring special procedures before Members of Parliament can be detained.

The focus on dangerousness

As discussed elsewhere (e.g. 📖 pp.III.239–III.289), there is a continual tension within forensic psychiatry between the duty to act in the patient's best interests and the need to protect the public from harm. Some authors regard it as an outright misuse of mental health law to use it with any purpose other than to act in the patient's best interests, and argue against ethical risk assessment and management (📖 p.III.265) being a legitimate possibility. Others accept 'double effect': that detention for public protection may be justifiable, but only if there is some scintilla of benefit to the patient (other than merely the avoidance of future offending and incarceration).

The antipsychiatry position

Since the 1960s, the antipsychiatry movement has argued that psychiatry, far from being a legitimate medical specialty, is nothing more than a form of social control. Szasz in particular has cited previous mainstream psychiatric views that are now discredited because social views have changed (such as regarding masturbation and homosexuality as signs of mental disorder) as proof that psychiatry is not objective science but merely reflects the views of powerful social groups. From this position,[*] any use of mental health law to detain or treat a person involuntarily is by definition a misuse of State power.

---

[*] A development of this position is Fulford's concept of the 'fact-to-value' ratio of medical diagnoses. Some, such as Alzheimer's disease, have a clear biological basis; others, such as personality disorder, are less clearly biologically defined, and more subject to the incorporation of value judgements that can lead to abuse.

Principles of mental capacity law

The legal term 'capacity'* refers to the mental ability to carry out or be subject to a variety of legally-recognized acts, such as making a will, marrying, selling property, consenting to treatment (📖 p.IV.390), or even, loosely speaking, being prosecuted (📖 p.IV.338). Exactly what constitutes the required mental ability varies from one legal situation to another as explained in the next section, and is subject to varying rules in different jurisdictions.

Historical development: the basis for incapacity

Capacity law developed from property law, for determining when the law should and should not allow individuals to decide how they managed and disposed of their property. Initially, certain categories of people, such as children, women (in some circumstances), 'lunatics' (people with mental illness), and 'idiots' (people with LD) were regarded as permanently lacking capacity for all decisions (a *status* approach).

As recognition spread after the Enlightenment that mental disorders varied in nature and degree and could change over time, status approaches to incapacity declined, except in relation to childhood. Instead, often those with mental disorder who made foolish or incomprehensible decisions were thought incapable: that is, it was the *outcome* of their decision-making process that indicated their incapacity.

Modern mental capacity law, however, takes a *functional* approach: what matters is not the decision reached, but the process by which it was reached. Only if a person lacks the functional ability to make a decision (being unable to understand relevant information, for instance) are they incapable of making such a decision. This is explained further in the following section:

General principles of capacity law

- Capacity relates to a specific decision at a specific time: a person may lack capacity for one decision on one day (e.g. selling their home), but have it for another decision on another day (e.g. making a gift)
- Everyone is presumed to have capacity unless they are shown to lack it
- Nobody lacks capacity merely because they make an unwise decision
- Nobody can be determined to lack capacity unless reasonable efforts have been made to facilitate their making the decision (e.g. calming anxiety, presenting information simply, etc.)
- Decisions for people who lack capacity must be in their best interests
- Decisions must be those that least restrict the person's freedom
- Decisions must take into account advance statements (whether binding or not) and the views of relatives and carers.

These principles are explicitly stated in the MCA; the last four are explicitly stated in the AWIA. The main purpose of these laws is to provide a legal framework for acting on behalf of those found incapable.

---

* The term 'competence' is sometimes used in medical and philosophical literature to refer to the same mental ability in a more general sense (i.e. without reference to any specific legal rules).

Definition of mental capacity

The legal definitions of mental capacity (or incapacity) are shown in Table 16.23. They comprise the following elements:

A cause of incapacity

There must be an identifiable reason for the alleged mental incapacity; under the AWIA this must be a recognized form of mental or (in the case of inability to communicate) physical disorder,[*] whereas the common law in NI and RoI, and the MCA, allow a broader range of factors affecting mental functioning.

Comprehension and appreciation

The person must be able to understand all the relevant information: not necessarily every detail, but the essence of it. This goes beyond an intellectual understanding: they must be able to apply the information to themselves and their situation (to 'appreciate' or 'assimilate' it, in the courts' terminology). For example, a young person or a person with learning disability might understand the notion of death but be unable to appreciate that their own death may be a possible outcome of a decision.

Using information

They must be able to make use of the information in coming to a decision. This includes:

- Retaining the information in memory for long enough to make the decision (this might be a short time for, say, a decision on what meal to order, but a much longer time for a complex financial transaction)
- Believing it as appropriate (for example, accepting that one has a heart condition requiring treatment, as opposed to believing in grandiose delusions that one is invulnerable), and
- Weighing up the different pieces of information 'in the balance' (i.e. within a reasoning process[†]) so as to arrive at a decision.

Communication

If a person is unable to communicate their decision to others (explicitly, by speaking or writing or sign language; or implicitly, by acting in a particular way) or to act for themselves, they are in effect incapable.

---

[*] This raises the possibility of mental incapacity unrelated to mental or physical disorder. For example, a mentally healthy young adult might be so emotionally overwhelmed by the information involved in a life-or-death decision that they are unable to comprehend, appreciate or use the information. Although not incapable according to the MCA or AWIA, it might be legal to assist them under the similar common law principles that existed prior to those Acts.

[†] Reasoning distorted by mental disorder can result in incapacity. For example, a depressed person's hopelessness may lead them to undervalue continued life. More controversially, it was held that a patient with severe PD who over-valued the pleasure of manipulating others as a factor in decision-making might be incapable because of 'distorted' *reasoning* (R v Brady, 🕮 p.App. 3.632).

Details of mental capacity law

The legal definitions of mental capacity (or incapacity) are in Table 16.23.

Table 16.23 Definitions of mental (in)capacity

	E&W	Scotland	NI	RoI
Relevant law	Mental Capacity Act 2005 (MCA)	Adults With Incapacity (Scotland) Act 2000 (AWIA)	Common law;* MHNIO	Common law;† Lunacy Regulation (Ireland) Act 1871 (LRA)
Definition: cause of incapacity	Impairment, or disturbance in the functioning of, the mind or brain	Mental disorder or physical disability	Impairment or disturbance of mental functioning	Permanent cognitive impairment, or temporary such as unconsciousness, fatigue, shock, pain, or drugs
Definition: components of capacity	Understand relevant information; retain that information; use or weigh that information as part of the decision-making process; communicate the decision	'Incapable' means incapable of acting; making decisions; communicating decisions; understanding decisions; or retaining the memory of decisions	Inability to comprehend and retain relevant information; inability to use it and to weigh it in the balance in the process of reaching a decision	Impairment of cognitive ability causing insufficient: comprehension of relevant information; belief in it; retention of it; assimilation of it; weighing of it in the balance
Age limit	Over 16	Adult (over 16)	None	None
Result of finding of incapacity	Decisions taken by others in person's best interests	Decisions taken by others in person's best interests	Medical decisions taken by doctors in patient's best interests	Person may be made a ward of court under LRA (p.IV.435)
Appeal against finding of incapacity	To CoP‡ for declaration, or by judicial review (p.IV.309) of assessor's decision	To Court of Session, by person or anyone with interest in their property	To the High Court	To the High Court

*This is the position at the time of writing, and the leading case is Re C (p.App. 2.633). However, the proposed Mental Capacity (Health, Welfare and Finance) Bill (p.App. 2.624) would, if enacted, create a new capacity-based mental health and mental capacity regime in NI; † Specifically, Fitzpatrick (p.App. 3.636); ‡ The Court of Protection—a division of the High Court.

Fluctuating capacity

A person may have capacity in relation to one decision, but not to another (which requires more complex information to be understood for longer, for example). In addition, even in relation to the same decision, a person may have capacity on one day and not on another, because of confusion, pain, anxiety, the effects of drugs or alcohol, or the variable symptoms of mental disorders such as Alzheimer's disease.

If a person with fluctuating capacity loses capacity temporarily, those acting for them may rely on consent given when they had capacity, or delay the decision if practical to do so.

Emergency situations

It is a common misconception that different rules apply in emergencies, but this is not the case. The only difference is that there may not be time to assess a person's capacity, give them relevant information or check for an advance statement (📖 p.IV.430). In this situation, urgent treatment necessary to save life or prevent a major deterioration can be given, after which capacity must be assessed in the usual way.

Advocates

In addition to receiving support from friends and relatives, people who lack capacity often benefit from the advice and support of a trained advocate who understands the issues involved. In Scotland, NI and RoI such advocates are available on an informal basis; in E&W, there is a statutory system of Independent Mental Capacity Advocates (IMCAs). Doctors in E&W are required to request and consult an IMCA for major treatment or residence decisions if no appropriate relative or friend is available.

Research

Research on subjects who lack capacity, who cannot consent (📖 p.III.286) to the risks involved, requires special permission from an ethics committee, and is only appropriate if it could not be carried out on subjects with capacity, There must be a chance of the research benefiting the subject, and the costs of participating (such as the time taken, and the risk of discomfort or pain) must be reasonable when balanced against the possibility of benefit. Alternatively, if there is no personal benefit, unintrusive research carrying a negligible risk of harm can go ahead if it is likely to increase knowledge about the subject's condition or a related condition.

Certification

To treat a person without capacity under the AWIA in Scotland, the doctor must complete a form certifying that they lack capacity in relation to the treatment decision in question, similar to completing a 'section' form in order to treat someone under mental health law (📖 p.IV.373). By contrast, under the MCA in E&W, and the common law in NI and RoI, no special forms are required; it is advisable, however, to document any capacity assessment and actions taken in the patient's medical notes.

Capacity in children and adolescents

The same general principles of capacity law (p.IV.424) apply to children as to adults, but with two significant variations:

- Children under a certain age are presumed to *lack* capacity
- In some cases, children under this age can be shown to have capacity if certain criteria are met

Table 16.24 shows how these variations apply in each jurisdiction.

Table 16.24 Capacity in children and adolescents

	E&W	Scotland	NI	RoI
Relevant law	MCA; Family Law Reform Act 1969; *Gillick* (p.App. 3.637)	Age of Legal Capacity (Scotland) Act 1991	Age of Majority (NI) Act 1969; *Gillick* (p.App. 3.637)	Non-Fatal Offences Against the Person Act 1997
Under 16s presumption	Lack capacity	Lack capacity	Lack capacity	Lack capacity
Under 16s exception	If they have sufficient understanding and intelligence to understand fully what is proposed	If they are capable of understanding the nature and possible consequences of the treatment	If they have sufficient understanding and intelligence to understand fully what is proposed	Not tested in court; guidelines suggest following the same rule as in E&W
16–17 year olds	Have capacity for medical treatment	Have capacity for all purposes	Have capacity for medical treatment	Have capacity for medical treatment
If parents and child disagree	A Gillick competent child can give consent even if parents refuse it, but parents can also give consent if child refuses it	Parents cannot override consent or refusal of consent by a competent child.	A Gillick competent child can give consent even if parents refuse it, but parents can also give consent if child refuses it	Not tested in court; parents can override competent child's refusal; unclear whether competent child can overrule parental refusal
Additional information	MCA applies to 16- & 17-year-olds. High Court can overrule both child's and parents' competent refusal of consent	All under-16s have legal capacity to make 'reasonable' transactions 'of a kind commonly entered into' by children		

As shown in Table 16.24, the legal presumption in all jurisdictions is that under-16-year-olds lack mental capacity, until they are shown to have it. However many child and adolescent services in practice assume that children between 12 and 16 do in fact have capacity, unless there is a reason to doubt it, or unless their capacity needs to be confirmed for legal purposes.

The ability of parents in E&W and NI to overrule a competent child's refusal of consent (including that of a 16- or 17-year-old child) may contravene human rights law (☐ p.IV.418), but this has not yet been tested in court.

The zone of parental control (ZPC)

The concept of the 'zone of parental control' is used in judgments of the European Court of Human Rights (☐ p.IV.326). It is helpful for thinking through when it is appropriate to facilitate parents (or others with parental responsibility, such as a Local Authority in the case of a child in care) in overriding the decision of a competent child, and vice versa. A decision is within the ZPC if it is one which:

• Parents would normally be expected to make in that society; and
• The parents appear able to make in the best interests of the child.

The E&W MHA Code of Practice suggests that, at least in relation to treatment for mental disorder, doctors should only rely on parental consent in the absence of the child or young person's consent if the decision is within the ZPC, and the child or young person lacks capacity. If these criteria are not met, doctors should consider using mental health law (☐ p.IV.373) if it applies, or applying to the High Court (Court of Protection) for a ruling.

Advance statements, powers of attorney and court powers

In general, these options for managing the affairs and personal welfare of adults who lack capacity are not available for children under 16. Instead, those with parental responsibility can decide for them, or others can be appointed to manage their affairs or welfare under child protection legislation.[*]

Criminal prosecution

The mental capacity law described here does not apply, by and large, to criminal proceedings. Instead, there is a separate age of criminal responsibility (☐ p.IV.338) and related rules of the youth justice system (☐ p.IV.294).

---

[*]Principally the Children Act 1989, Social Work (Scotland) Act 1968, Children (NI) Order 1995, and the Child Care Act 1991 in RoI. A discussion of the complex field of child welfare and child protection law is beyond the scope of this book; readers are advised to consult a textbook of child psychiatry or child & family social work.

Advance statements

Anyone can make a statement in advance about what they would like or not like to happen in a given situation in the future. In some circumstances, such advance statements can be relevant in deciding how to treat a person who has subsequently lost the capacity to decide for themselves.

Advance decisions to refuse treatment in E&W

The MCA makes advance statements that contain a decision to refuse treatment binding on doctors in certain specific circumstances.[*] Such binding 'advance decisions' can only be made by over-18-year-olds (even though the MCA as a whole applies to over-16-year-olds). To be binding, an advance decision must be both *valid* and *applicable*.

Criteria for validity and applicability of advance decisions in E&W
An advance decision is valid if, at the time of the proposed treatment:
- It has not been withdrawn while the patient still had capacity
- It has not been superseded by a relevant lasting power of attorney (📖 p.IV.432)
- The patient has not done 'anything else clearly inconsistent' with it remaining a 'fixed decision' (e.g. ordering new nightwear for a move to a nursing home, despite having previously made an advance decision to refuse such a move).

An advance decision applies if, at the time of the proposed treatment:
- The patient lacks capacity
- The proposed treatment is specified in the decision
- The current situation is envisaged by the decision
- There are no 'reasonable grounds for believing' that the patient would not have made the advance decision if they were in the situation that has now arisen.

In addition, advance decisions can only allow a refusal of life-sustaining treatment if they contain an explicit written, signed and witnessed statement that they apply to such treatments.

A valid, applicable advance decision to refuse treatment overrules a decision made by the donee of a Lasting Power of Attorney (📖 p.IV.432).

In general, even a valid and applicable advance statement is overridden by the MHA—but there is a major exception in the case of ECT (📖 p.II.158), which can be refused in advance (see 📖 p.IV.391).

---

[*] Advance directives can only bind doctors *not* to give a certain treatment; they can never require them to give a treatment.

Other advance statements in the UK and RoI

Apart from advance decisions to refuse treatment in E&W, advance statements (or 'advance directives' in Scotland and RoI) have no specific legal status and are not binding. However, a variety of provisions of mental capacity and mental health laws require doctors and others to take into account the previously-expressed wishes of patients, before they make a decision in the patient's best interests—and this obviously includes any advance statements the patient may have made.

The most notable of these is the MHCTA in Scotland, which requires psychiatrists to take into account any written, signed, and witnessed advance statement when they make decisions on treatment for mental disorder under the Act.

Moreover, some authors believe that article 8 (📖 p.IV.418) of the European Convention on Human Rights (📖 p.IV.420) makes at least some advance statements directly binding—although this has not yet been tested in court.

The following questions may help in deciding whether an advance statement (not amounting to an advance decision in E&W) should be taken into account in a given situation:

- Does the statement clearly envisage the current situation? For example, a statement refusing resuscitation in the context of terminal cancer would not apply for resuscitation after a myocardial infarction
- Is the course of action in the statement both legal and clinically justifiable? For example, an advance statement, no matter how specific and clearly drafted, could not justify a decision to give a drug in order to cause death[*], or to give amphetamines for bipolar disorder
- Has the patient since done anything to withdraw the statement, or that is inconsistent with it and suggests they have forgotten it or consider it to have been withdrawn?
- Is the statement consistent with what relatives and friends say the patient would have wanted? (If it differs, that does not necessarily invalidate it, but it may reduce the weight given to it.)

---

[*] At the time of writing, euthanasia is illegal throughout the UK and RoI, although there have been debates in E&W in particular about not prosecuting those who assist in euthanasia for terminally ill relatives.

Powers of attorney

What is an attorney?

An attorney is someone appointed to take decisions on behalf of someone else. Originally, in an age before the rapid communication made possible by the telephone and the Internet, people travelling abroad for several weeks or more might appoint a trusted attorney to take decisions on business or financial matters that could not wait until their return.

This basic form of the power of attorney can be revoked by the donor (the person who appointed the attorney[*]) at any time. The power can only apply to decisions involving financial matters or other property—not to health or personal welfare decisions. Also, because the attorney can only make a decision or exercise a power that the donor could themselves have exercised, if the donor loses capacity (and therefore cannot make such decisions themselves), the attorney's power to act also ceases.

A power of attorney puts the donee in the position of making decisions as if made by the donor. There are no rules relating to what decisions should specifically be made.

Enduring, continuing, and lasting powers of attorney

Recognizing the limitations of the original power of attorney allowed by common law, governments have legislated to create the Enduring (or Continuing) Power of Attorney (EPA/CPA), and the more extensive Welfare Power of Attorney (WPA), and Lasting Power of Attorney (LPA). Table 16.25 shows which forms apply in each jurisdiction.

Like simple powers of attorney, in all cases the donor must be over 18 (or over 16 in Scotland) and have capacity when granting the power. The donor can grant a general power, or one limited to specific decisions or types of decisions. It would almost always be inappropriate for a treating psychiatrist or other similar professional to be the donee of an LPA or WPA covering health, welfare or personal care decisions.

---

[*] Therefore; the attorney is sometimes known as the donee, i.e. the person who has been given the power. In Scotland, the donor may be called the granter, and the donee the grantee.

Table 16.25 Power of attorney in each jurisdiction

	E&W	Scotland	NI	RoI
Name of the power	Lasting Power of Attorney	Continuing or Welfare Power of Attorney	Enduring Power of Attorney	Enduring Power of Attorney
Relevant law	Mental Capacity Act 2005	Adults With Incapacity (Scotland) Act 2000	Enduring Powers of Attorney (NI) Order 1987	Powers of Attorney Act 1996
Decisions covered	Personal welfare, property and affairs	Property and financial affairs (CPA); personal welfare (WPA)	Property and affairs (after donor loses capacity)	Property, money and personal care (after donor loses capacity)
Conditions on making welfare decisions	Donee must reasonably believe donor now lacks capacity	Donee must reasonably believe donor now lacks capacity	N/A	Donee must consult family and act in accordance with what donor was likely to do
General restrictions on donee	Must act in best interests of donor	Must be satisfied act will benefit donor, and is least restrictive option	Must act as common law fiduciary (in donor's interests & for their sole benefit)	Must act in best interests of donor
Restrictions on welfare power	Cannot restrain* donor unless restraint is necessary, and proportionate to the harm prevented	Cannot authorize treatment for mental disorder against the will of the donor	N/A	Does not include healthcare decisions (but covers residence, contacts, diet, benefit etc.)
Other information	LPA must be registered with the Public Guardian before it has effect	CPA or WPA must be registered with the Public Guardian before they have effect	EPA must be registered with the High court when the donor loses capacity	EPA must be registered with the High Court when the donor loses capacity

*In this context, 'restraint' refers to using; force or the threat of force, or restricting the donor's liberty or movement.

Court powers in mental incapacity

Intervention orders

In Scotland, anyone with an interest in the personal welfare or property of a person without capacity (or that person themselves) can apply to the Sheriff Court for an intervention order. This can authorize anything that the person would have been able to do themselves, if they still had capacity. It can include appointing someone to perform specific acts or make specific decisions on their behalf.[*]

A criminal court can also make an intervention order as an alternative to another sentence (📖 p.IV.370) if the defendant lacks capacity and it believes this to be the most appropriate disposal.

Decisions, deputies, and controllers

Under the MCA in E&W and the MHNIO in NI, the High Court (but not criminal courts) can make decisions on behalf of a person lacking capacity, or appoint a deputy ('controller' in NI) to make a specific decision or class of decisions. This is analogous to the Scottish intervention order. The decisions covered can include health and welfare decisions in E&W but only decisions on property and financial affairs in NI.

Guardianship orders in Scotland

In E&W and NI, civil guardianship (📖 p.IV.394) is a form of community treatment for mental disorder under mental health law, and does not require evidence of incapacity. By contrast, in Scotland a guardianship order[†] can only be applied to a person who lacks capacity, although that incapacity need not be the result of mental disorder. As with intervention orders, a guardianship order can be made by a criminal as well as a civil court.

Anyone with an interest in the personal welfare or property of someone without capacity (or, as with an intervention order, that person themselves) can apply to the Sheriff Court for a guardianship order, on the grounds that the person's long-term incapacity means they cannot safeguard their own interests adequately. In addition, the local authority is under a duty to apply for one if it thinks these conditions are met.

A guardianship order can last for any period, the default being three years, and can be renewed by the court. The guardian can be any appropriate relative or friend, or a social worker in the case of a guardianship order on the grounds of personal welfare alone. The guardian is required to visit the patient regularly, investigate their affairs and report to the Public Guardian and/or the local authority on their actions every month.

As with a welfare power of attorney (📖 p.IV.432), a guardian appointed on the grounds of personal welfare may (if the guardianship order permits it) consent to medical treatment, but cannot consent to treatment for mental disorder against the person's will.

---

[*] The court can require the appointee to pay a deposit (to 'find caution'), which they forfeit if they act improperly or cause loss to the person. It may also require a guardian to do the same.
[†] Before the AWIA, there was a similar form of guardianship for those under 18 and (loosely) those who lacked capacity, known as curatorship; the guardian was known as the 'curator bonis'.

The Court of Protection

In E&W, there used to be a special court known as the Court of Protection (CoP) that was responsible for managing the property and financial affairs of those who lacked capacity; it exercised the king's so-called *parens patriae* ('father to the country') jurisdiction on his behalf. To reduce costs and simplify proceedings, the old Court of Protection was abolished by the MCA, and corresponding powers, revised and updated, were granted to the High Court—such as the power to appoint deputies. However, only specially-designated High Court and other judges do this work, and when doing it they are deemed to be sitting for a division of the High Court still known as the 'Court of Protection', which can sit in any region of E&W.

Wardship and receivership

In RoI, being made a ward of court is the approximate equivalent of being subject to a Scottish guardianship order, or to the jurisdiction of the High Court in E&W and NI. It is the only system for making decisions on behalf of incapacitated adults in RoI who have not made an enduring power of attorney (📖 p.IV.432) before losing capacity.[*]

However, the law governing such wardship, the Lunacy Regulation (Ireland) Act 1871, has not been updated as social views about mental disorder and incapacity have changed. It contains no definition of incapacity, implicitly equating it with mental illness (lunacy). It provides for 'all matters relating to the person and estate' of a lunatic to be managed on their behalf by a 'receiver' under the supervision of the High Court. The receiver has complete power over the affairs of the lunatic, who cannot (for example) marry, have a bank account, take part in legal proceedings or change their residence without the Court's permission.

An outline of a new Mental Capacity Bill was proposed by the Justice Minister in 2008. It would replace wardship with a system of guardianship similar to that in the UK. However, at the time of writing, a detailed draft of the Bill has not yet been published.

---

[*] The common law power to make individual treatment and other decisions on their behalf is also available, as described on 📖 p.IV.426, but this does not provide a system for managing their affairs in a comprehensive way.

Detention in mental incapacity

The European Court of Human Rights has ruled that any detention or other 'deprivation of liberty' amounts to a breach of article 5 of the Convention (📖 p.IV.419) unless it follows a legal procedure and the patient has access to a court or Tribunal to challenge it. Whereas mental health law provides a statutory procedure (📖 p.IV.381) for detention and compulsory treatment and affords patients with the opportunity to appeal to a Tribunal (📖 p.IV.414) at an early stage, general* mental capacity law (📖 p.IV.424) does not provide adequate procedural safeguards or access to a Tribunal, and therefore cannot be used to authorize detention or other forms of deprivation of liberty. This problem has been approached in different ways in different jurisdictions.

What amounts to a deprivation of liberty?

The ECtHR has not established any clear rule for determining whether measures amount to a deprivation of liberty. It has, however, said that:

- The distinction between a (lawful) *restriction* of liberty and a potentially unlawful *deprivation* of liberty is 'merely one of degree or intensity, not one of nature or substance'†
- 'Each case has to be considered on its own particular range of factors', and
- Factors suggesting deprivation include the use of restraint and control of social contacts, residence or movement for a significant time.

Deprivation of Liberty Safeguards (DoLS)

In E&W, there was a desire to avoid having to detain large numbers of people without capacity who did not object to treatment (estimated at 11,000 in 1998 during the Bournewood case, 📖 p.App. 3.631) under mental health law, in order to give them access to a Tribunal. Instead, since 2008 the MCA has contained a special regime, known as the 'deprivation of liberty safeguards'. Its main provisions are as follows:

Measures amounting to a deprivation of liberty are only permissible if:
- They are ordered by a court as part of a decision on behalf of the person lacking capacity (📖 p.IV.434), or
- They apply to someone resident in a hospital or care home and special authorization has been obtained, or
- They are necessary to give treatment to sustain life or prevent a major deterioration, while a declaration is sought from the court.

Authorization to deprive someone of their liberty in a hospital or care home may only be granted by a 'supervisory body' (PCT or Local Authority) after an independent assessor has confirmed that the deprivation of liberty is for the purpose of care or treatment; and that the person:
- Is over 18
- Has a mental disorder

---

* That is, mental capacity law excluding the special regimes to deal with detention that are described in this topic.
† *HL v UK* (📖 p.App. 3.638).

- Lacks capacity in relation to the decision to accept care or treatment
- Is not covered by any other safeguards such as under the MHA
- Does not refuse the care or treatment (including by a valid, applicable advance decision, 📖 p.IV.430, or by a decision of an attorney, 📖 p.IV.432 or deputy, 📖 p.IV.434), and that
- The deprivation of liberty is in his or her best interests, necessary to prevent harm and a proportionate response to the likelihood and severity of that harm.

All elements are necessary for the authorization to be granted. Such authorizations must be reviewed by the supervisory body on request of the person concerned or their representative. There is also a right of appeal against the deprivation of liberty to the High Court.

Deprivation of liberty in Scotland, NI and RoI

In Scotland, measures amounting to a deprivation of liberty would not normally be authorized under general capacity law, but under a specific court order: either an intervention order, or a guardianship order (📖 p.IV.434). These provide the procedural safeguards and right of appeal required under the ECHR.

As the law in NI stands at the time of writing, there is no mechanism under capacity law that would meet the ECHR requirements for authorizing care or treatment that involves a deprivation of liberty. Patients must therefore be treated under mental health law (such as guardianship, 📖 p.IV.394), or the treating institution risks a legal challenge. The proposed Mental Capacity (Health, Welfare and Finance) Bill is expected to provide a legal mechanism that would comply with the ECHR.

In RoI the legal mechanism by which care and treatment involving a deprivation of liberty can be authorized is wardship (📖 p.IV.435) under the Lunacy Regulation (Ireland) Act 1871. This would probably be found not to comply with article 5 (📖 p.IV.419) of the ECHR were it to be challenged, because it does not provide modern procedural safeguards or an effective system of appeal. The proposed new Mental Capacity Bill is expected to remedy these defects.

Mental capacity and other social roles

Marriage

There is a principle that a person must have mental capacity in order to marry, and that a decision to marry* cannot be taken on their behalf by anyone who would be able to take other decisions on their behalf, such as an attorney (📖 p.IV.432) or a deputy (📖 p.IV.434).

However, the test of capacity is not the usual general test of capacity (📖 p.IV.426). For example, in E&W a marriage can be voided by a court if it is shown that a person did not 'validly consent' because of 'unsoundness of mind'. In general, the courts have held that the standard of capacity required is very low: a basic understanding that the two people will stay together indefinitely is sufficient.

Conducting legal proceedings

A complainant or defendant in civil legal proceedings must have adequate mental capacity to conduct the proceedings, even with professional legal representation. The general test of capacity (e.g. under the MCA in E&W, 📖 p.IV.424) applies. If they are found to lack capacity, despite adjustments to the process to assist them, their interests will be represented instead by an Official Solicitor from the Office of the Public Guardian.

In criminal law, defendants currently face a quite different test of ability, known in E&W as the *Pritchard* criteria: see 📖 p.V.474.

Entering into contracts

People with mental disorder can make valid contracts. However, if a person lacks mental capacity when they make a contract, then the contract is invalid under common law if the other party knew at the time that the person lacked capacity.† In addition, a contract may be set aside by a court if they consider it sufficiently 'unconscionable' or 'improvident', which might be the case if it appeared to exploit the vulnerability of a person without capacity.

Wills and testamentary capacity

Disputes may arise over the making of a will. A psychiatrist may be requested to provide an opinion on whether the testator (maker of the will) possessed testamentary capacity, defined as follows:

- *E&W* and *NI* Ability to understand the nature of the act and its effects; to understand the extent of the property of which he is disposing; and to appreciate the claims (of others) to which he ought to give effect. They should not have mental illness that influences their decisions
- *Scotland* The person must comprehend what a will is and what would be the consequences of making one
- *RoI* They must have 'understanding and reason' and not suffer from mental conditions such as 'delusion, insane suspicion or aversion'.

---

* The same applies to decisions on other family matters such as divorce and adoption, and to a decision to consent to sexual acts.
† However, in E&W the MCA requires that even in this situation a person lacking capacity must pay 'a reasonable price' for the supply of any 'necessary' goods or services.

Voting

The law is currently unclear on whether electors must pass a test of mental capacity in order to be allowed to vote, especially in E&W. Old common law rules disenfranchising those with mental disorders have been abolished; and in the UK the rules preventing people detained in hospital or in prison from voting have been amended so that those who are on remand (📖 p.IV.330) or are detained under civil mental health law (📖 p.IV.388) may vote, if necessary using the hospital or prison as their address.* Electoral Commission guidance is therefore that people who lack capacity probably cannot be stopped from voting, but that they do need capacity if they wish to appoint a proxy to vote on their behalf.

Jury service

There are considerable restrictions on jury service for those suffering from mental disorder.† The rules often ignore mental capacity, and are based merely on diagnosis and treatment. In E&W, RoI, and Scotland, anyone who suffers from mental disorder and is still receiving treatment (or is under an order such as guardianship) cannot be a juror. In NI, anyone with a diagnosis of mental disorder is automatically excluded.

Driving

There are complex rules governing fitness to drive in the presence of various mental (and physical) disorders. In the UK, the Driver and Vehicle Licensing Agency (DVLA), and in RoI the Road Safety Authority (RSA), must be informed of any medical condition that might affect fitness to drive. In some cases, this means that doctors will be required to breach confidentiality (📖 p.III.263) and inform the DVLA or RSA if the patient refuses to do so. The DVLA's rules relating to mental disorder currently forbid the following from driving, amongst others:

- A person who is currently psychotic
- A person with bipolar disorder who has had more than three episodes in the last year, unless they have been well for 6 months
- A person with epilepsy who had daytime seizures in the last 10 years
- A person with severe LD
- A person with dementia who has poor short-term memory, disorientation, lack of insight, and judgement.

Other powers to detain or treat

Powers to remove persons in need of care

In E&W and Scotland, a vulnerable adult (📖 p.V.453) may be removed from their home by a local authority in the interests of their health or safety or that of others*. A psychiatrist may be asked for an assessment before or after the removal, depending on the circumstances.

In Scotland, in addition to removing the vulnerable adult to a hospital or other place of safety, certain people may be banned from having contact with them if they have been intimidating, exploiting or otherwise endangering them. This provides a much more extensive, and enforceable, system than is available under the non-statutory safeguarding of vulnerable adults (📖 p.II.202) procedure in E&W.

There is no equivalent system of removal in NI or RoI.

Infectious diseases

All UK and Irish jurisdictions provide† for a magistrate to order a person with a serious infectious disease to be detained and treated in hospital if they are refusing treatment or otherwise acting in a way that makes the spread of the infection likely. This might be relevant to patients with mental disorder who also have conditions such as tuberculosis (TB), who cannot be treated for their TB under mental health law (📖 p.IV.373).

Common law emergency powers‡

The UK courts have held that, separate to the specific statutory powers described here and elsewhere, there is a general common law power to 'take such steps as are reasonably necessary and proportionate to protect others from the immediate risk of significant harm'. In the leading case on this issue (*Munjaz*, 📖 p.App. 3.642), the court also made clear that the power 'applies whether or not the patient lacks capacity to make decisions for himself.' Another case (*Black v Forsey*, 📖 p.App. 3.630) added that all private individuals have a legal power to restrain or detain 'in a situation of necessity, a person of unsound mind who is a danger to himself or others'.

The former power was specifically held to include a power to seclude informal patients. By extension, it includes a power to *give treatment in prison*, or in hospital or elsewhere, if that is 'reasonably necessary and proportionate' to the 'immediate risk of significant harm'. Whether the power applies if the significant harm is only to the patient themselves and not to others has not been tested in court. An alternative possibility is that the latter power, from *Black v Forsey*, could be considered to include treatment, but the courts were clear that this power can be exercised

---

* Under s47 of the National Assistance Act 1948 in E&W, or s14 of the Adult Support and Protection (Scotland) Act 2007. Both Acts contain a variety of different safeguards, involve doctors at certain stages, and require a court order before the person may be removed from their home.

† Under s37 of the Public Health (Control of Disease) Act 1984 in E&W, s39 of the Public Health etc (Scotland) Act 2008, s3B of the Public Health Act (Northern Ireland) 1967, and s38 of the Health Act 1947 in RoI.

‡ These are mostly specific applications of the general common law doctrine of (medical) *necessity*, which also governs the treatment of those lacking capacity (📖 p.IV.424) in NI and RoI where there is no statutory framework like the MCA (📖 p.IV.426).

only by individuals, and only until detention and treatment under mental health law is possible; it cannot be operated by staff on behalf of a hospital or other institution.

It is likely that courts in RoI would recognize similar common law emergency powers, but this too has not been tested in court.

Making an arrest and preventing crime

In addition to the general common law emergency power, criminal law* provides a power to members of the public to 'use such force as is reasonable in the circumstances in the prevention of crime, or in effecting or assisting in the lawful arrest (📖 p.IV.450) of offenders or suspected offenders or of persons unlawfully at large'. This would include restraining and secluding an inpatient, whether informal or detained, if that is reasonable to prevent them committing an offence (such as assaulting another patient or member of staff); or restraining someone in the community who has absconded from detention in hospital.†

Preventing a breach of the peace

The common law also provides every citizen, not just police officers, with a power to use reasonable force to prevent a breach of the peace (📖 p.IV.353), meaning the use or threat of violence or disorder. In the leading case (*Laporte*, 📖 p.App. 3.640), the House of Lords ruled that 'every citizen enjoys the power and is subject to a duty to seek to prevent, by arrest or other action short of arrest, any breach of the peace occurring in his presence, or any breach of the peace which (having occurred) is likely to be renewed, or any breach of the peace which is about to occur'. This would enable, for example, a nurse or doctor in a hospital or a CPN or social worker in the community to restrain a person or patient whose abusive or threatening behaviour is likely to provoke imminent violence.

---

*Specifically, s3(1) of the Criminal Law Act 1967 for E&W, and s3(1) of the Criminal Law (NI) Act 1967, which are identically worded. S4(1) of the Criminal Law Act 1997 in RoI, which allows for citizen's arrests (📖 p.V.450), implies a similar power to use reasonable force. In Scotland, a similar rule applies under common law.

†This is in addition to statutory powers under mental health law to retake such patients. Technically, the power to use reasonable force in these circumstances does not apply to people who meet the legal test for insanity (📖 p.V.489), at least in E&W; but the power in *Black v Forsey* could apply in such cases.

The rights of victims of patients

Victims' rights in general

The prosecution service (p.V.448) is meant to promote the interests of victims as well as the Crown (or the People in RoI). However, there have been calls for increased recognition of victims' experience and needs, following successful campaigns by crime victims in the US. In practice, crime victims can expect assistance:

- At the time of any criminal trial where they are witnesses
- At the time of any offender's discharge where they may be affected.

Standards of support for victims

Victims' Charters are in place in E&W, NI, and RoI that indicate standards of service provision that victims of crime can expect to receive from the CJS. However, these services are not founded on a legal right of the victim; rather, the charters take a 'needs-based' approach to victim services and distinguish between those victims who are eligible for special service provision and those who are not.

The Code of Practice for Victims of Crime 2006 sets out requirements for various agencies within the CJS; these include the police (p.V.449), Probation Service (p.V.462), Prison Service (p.V.456), Witness Care Units, HM Court Service (p.IV.308) and Youth Offending Teams (YOTs, p.V.463). It represents a minimum standard of service and its aim is to ensure that victims of crime are provided timely, accurate information about their case at all stages of the criminal justice process. The victim may choose not to receive services, or request modification of the services that they receive.

In Scotland, the Executive has produced National Standards for Victims of Crime, which includes three main rights: the rights to information, support and participation. The Victim Notification Scheme was introduced to provide the victim with information about offenders sentenced to custodial sentences of more than 18 months.

Victim support services

Victims of crime in E&W, may also be supported by Victim Support, an independent charity, which offers free assistance, including advice and help for psychological and emotional needs as well as practical help. Other charity based victim groups include Support After Murder and Manslaughter (SAMM). There are similar organizations in Scotland, NI and RoI. These charitable organizations have recently turned their attention towards a 'rights-based' approach to victim's needs. The US has used this latter approach for some time and has introduced the Victim's Rights Act across different states as statutory legal requirements affording rights to a range of victims.

Victims' rights under mental health law

In the UK, victims of crime by a mentally disordered offender who has committed a serious sexual or violent offence have the right to information about their detention in (or transfer to) and release from hospital, and to make representations about those issues, whether or not the patient is subject to a restriction order (📖 p.IV.412).[*] In Scotland, however, the law only applies to offenders sentenced to 4 or more years' imprisonment, and therefore excludes those only sentenced to treatment (📖 p.IV.405).

Rights of victims of mentally disordered offenders in the UK

To make representations about:

- Whether any discharge or release should be subject to conditions or supervision requirements if applicable (e.g. under a restriction order or a licence)
- If so, what those conditions should be.

To be informed:

- When the patient is to be discharged or released from hospital
- What conditions or supervision requirements (if any) they will be subject to after discharge or release.

In NI, the law also allows victims to make representation and to receive information about leave from hospital and its conditions.

The law in E&W and NI also places a number of statutory duties on the Probation Service (and their Victim Liaison Officers) and on hospital staff, as well as Tribunals and other bodies, all of whom have a duty to consider victims' views. In inpatient facilities, the MDT social worker (📖 p.II.180) will often take on the statutory role of liaising with past or potential victims in order to assess their needs and rights.

Mental Health Tribunals have addressed cases on whether to admit victims' testimony into evidence; and to what extent information from MHTs may be shared with victims,

There is no equivalent system in RoI.

[*] The relevant laws are the Domestic Violence, Crime and Victims Act 2004 (DVCVA) for E&W and NI, and the Criminal Justice (Scotland) Act 2003. The rules under the DVCVA apply to offences committed after 1.11.07, and to offences committed after 1.7.05 in the case of offenders given restriction orders or directions.

Psychiatry within the legal system

The criminal justice system

The system

The Criminal Justice System (CJS) comprises a variety of government and private agencies and institutions that define (📖 pp.II.18, IV.332), detect, prosecute, try, and punish crime according to criminal process (📖 p.IV.330). Other organizations that have a role in crime prevention (including education, health and social services) are not usually seen as part of the CJS.

Detection and investigation

The police (📖 p.V.449) are the organization with primary responsibility for indentifying crime, by responding to reports of possible crime from victims and others (including police officers), and by investigating those reports so as to gather evidence for prosecution. Other specific bodies, some of which are part of the police service in the UK and RoI, include:

- The UK Serious Organised Crime Agency (SOCA), which focuses on major criminal gangs. During 2011 it will become the National Crime Agency, partly modelled on the US Federal Bureau of Investigation (FBI). The equivalent in RoI, the National Bureau of Criminal Investigation, has a broader remit, encompassing any serious crime with which the local force needs assistance
- The Royal Military Police and the Póil´n´ Airm, each of which is a corps responsible for policing British and Irish armed forces respectively, at home (when on duty in military facilities) and abroad
- Specialist intelligence agencies with their own powers of investigation and sometimes arrest, including MI5 (the Security Service) and MI6 (the Secret Intelligence Service) in the UK, and G2 (the Directorate of Military Intelligence) in RoI
- The UK Border Agency (UKBA) in immigration (📖 p.V.525) matters and Her Majesty's Revenue and Customs (HMRC) also have powers of investigation and arrest. In RoI, these tasks are performed by the police.

Prosecution

In E&W the Crown Prosecution Service (CPS), headed by the Director of Public Prosecution, is a non-ministerial department responsible for the public prosecution of individuals charged with a criminal offence. The same role is performed by the Public Prosecution Service in NI, the Office of the Director of Public Prosecutions in RoI, and the Crown Office and Procurator Fiscal Service in Scotland (headed by the Lord Advocate). These services are responsible for criminal cases beyond the police investigation, and involve giving advice to the police on bringing charges, and preparing and presenting cases for court.

Trial

Criminal charges are heard in criminal trial courts (📖 p.IV.308), comprising lower courts that hear less serious charges such as Magistrates' Courts (📖 p.IV.320) in E&W and NI, and higher courts for more serious charges such as Sheriff Courts (📖 p.IV.322) in Scotland and Circuit Courts (📖 p.IV.324) in RoI. These courts have their own roles at court (📖 p.IV.312), procedures (📖 p.IV.314) and rules (📖 pp.IV.312, IV.316).

Offences committed by serving members of the armed forces and by prisoners of war are tried by Courts-Martial, according to military law. Their processes and personnel are similar to those of ordinary criminal courts, but in addition to ordinary offences courts-martial try offences relating to breaches of military discipline, and can impose military penalties such as demotion to a junior rank.

Hopefully only very occasionally, miscarriages of justice may occur in which an innocent person is wrongly convicted. The Criminal Cases Review Commissions* exist in the UK to review doubtful cases if new evidence comes to light, and can refer them back to an appeal court (📖 p.IV.308).

Sentences and punishment

Sentences (📖 p.IV.361) imposed by criminal courts can be divided into three main types:

- Sentences of imprisonment (📖 pp.IV.364, IV.366), carried out by the *prison service* (📖 p.V.456)
- Community sentences (📖 p.IV.368), supervised by the *probation service* (📖 p.V.462), which also advises the court on sentencing options, and
- Fines (📖 p.IV.369) and other sentences, which are monitored by the court itself or by its agents such as bailiffs.

In addition, court-imposed mental health orders (📖 p.IV.373) are supervised by a government department if restrictions (📖 p.V.412) are added to the order. In E&W and RoI, this is the Ministry of Justice; in Scotland, the Directorate of Criminal Justice, and in NI the Department of Health, Social Security and Public Safety. Each department contains a unit that manages restricted patients (📖 p.V.466), approving decisions on leave, transfer, and discharge.

Police services

Whereas there is a single national civilian police service in RoI, the Garda Síochána na hÈireann (Guardians of the Peace of Ireland), a patchwork of different police services perform police functions in the UK:†

- Territorial police forces, such as the Metropolitan Police in London or the Yorkshire Police, which carry out the majority of policing
- Special national police forces such as the. British Transport Police, and
- Small, specific police forces created by miscellaneous laws, such as local parks police and port police forces.

---

*The CCRC covers E&W and NI. The Scottish Criminal Cases Review Commission performs the same role in Scotland. There is no equivalent in RoI.

†This is largely because of the historical British aversion to creating a single civilian organization that a tyrannical government could use to subjugate and control the population. The Gardai, by contrast, evolved from the former colonial police in Ireland: rulers in London had no compunction about controlling the Irish population, and a single force was therefore formed.

Personnel

All police officers are legally known as 'constables' in the UK, and 'guards' (Gardai) in RoI. More senior officers include sergeants, who are in charge of a team of constables or Gardai; inspectors, who are in charge of day-to-day policing on a given shift; superintendents, who are in charge of a police station; and chief superintendents ('borough commanders' in London), responsible for policing a subdivision of the police area.

Many forces in E&W, but not elsewhere, also employ civilians (i.e. staff who are not trained police officers and therefore lack police powers of arrest[*]) to patrol streets and public places and to provide information and reassurance (a community policing strategy, see 📖 'Policing strategies', p.V.451).

Throughout the UK and RoI, all police forces have a Criminal Investigation Department (CID) staffed by detectives whose role is solely to investigate reported crime and gather evidence.

Functions of the police

The original role of the earliest police forces was to maintain public order. Police roles have diversified since then, and now include:

- Maintaining public order (preventing a breach of the peace, 📖 p.IV.353)
- Protecting people (especially politicians and royalty) and property
- Detecting and recording crime
- Investigating reported crime and gathering evidence for prosecution
- Arresting and detaining (suspected) criminals for prosecution
- Recovering and restoring stolen property[†]
- Deterring crime by having a high profile.

Police powers

Most police officers can exercise most of the following powers, all of which only apply in certain circumstances (e.g. where an officer has reasonable grounds to suspect the person has committed a serious crime):

- To stop and search a person
- To arrest a person and detain them for questioning
- To search vehicles and premises and seize and retain property
- To take fingerprints and bodily samples for testing.

Citizen's arrest

All citizens, not merely police officers, have limited powers to prevent a breach of the peace (📖 p.IV.441), to detain a mentally disordered person (📖 p.IV.440) if they pose a danger to themselves or others, and most notably to make a 'citizen's arrest'. This limited power[‡] only applies if it is not reasonable or practical to wait for a police officer, and:

- If the suspect is (or the person has reasonable suspicion that the suspect is) *in the act* of committing a serious offence, or

---

[*] Although specific laws give some such support officers limited powers to detain suspects until police officers arrive, in addition to powers to issue fixed penalty notices (📖 p.IV.360), confiscate alcohol and drugs, or seize vehicles, and the power of citizen's arrest.

[†] Originally a function of the privately-employed 'thief-takers' found in 18th-century England.

[‡] Under s24A of the Police and Criminal Evidence Act 1984 in E&W, art26 of the Police and Criminal Evidence (NI) Order 1989, s4 of the Criminal Law Act 1997 in RoI, and under common law in Scotland. Serious offence means 'indictable offence' in E&W, and 'arrestable offence' in NI and RoI.

- If a serious offence *has been committed* and the suspect is (or the person has reasonable suspicion that the suspect is) guilty of it.

Policing strategies

The techniques police services use, and the functions they prioritize, have varied as technology and social expectations have developed. Some alternative strategies include:

- Reactive policing: responding rapidly to reports of crime
- Community policing: high-profile officers getting to know a local area and its inhabitants well, deterring crime and reassuring the public
- Intelligence-led policing: actively gathering information on possible crime
- Problem-oriented policing: analysing patterns of crime in order to prevent crime.

The role of the psychiatrist

A significant proportion of people who come into contact with the police have a mental disorder. Psychiatrists may be involved with assessments of suspects at various stages of police contact including:

- In response to the use of police powers (📖 p.IV.400) when a person in a public place appears to be suffering from a mental disorder
- Advising on diversion from custody and attending to medical needs
- Advising on fitness to be interviewed (📖 p.V.452)
- Advising on the need for an appropriate adult (📖 p.V.453) during interview.

In the police station

Arrest

If someone is reasonably suspected of an offence they may be arrested for questioning. They will then be taken to a police station unless the police exercise powers under mental health legislation to take them to hospital* for psychiatric assessment (📖 p.IV.383).

On arresting a suspect, the police officer must caution them about their rights. In RoI, NI and Scotland, suspects have the *right to remain silent*, but anything they say may be recorded and used in evidence against them. In E&W, the right to silence is restricted by the fact that courts are allowed to draw inferences from it[†] (such as that they are trying to avoid revealing information that could be used to convict them).

---

* Except in areas where local policies allow the assessment to take place at the police station (e.g. where it is the designated 'place of safety' under the E&W MHA).
[†] This makes the assessment of fitness to be interviewed all the more important, as someone interviewed when unfit might wrongly have such inferences drawn later from their silence.

Initial procedure

The custody officer* is independent of the investigating officers, and is responsible for:

- Ensuring that the detainee's rights are upheld
- Informing them of the reasons for arrest and the grounds for detention
- Informing them of their right to private consultation with a solicitor
- Keeping a record of detention in custody
- Deciding whether there is sufficient evidence to charge the detainee
- Calling in a healthcare professional:
  - For assessment of possible mental or physical disorder
  - For any injuries or after allegations of excessive force or assault
  - If medical examination is requested
- Requesting an appropriate adult (📖 p.IV.453) to be present during interviews for all children and vulnerable adults.

Forensic medical examiner (FME)

The FME or police surgeon may be called for any of the previously mentioned reasons and will usually be the first person to carry out a more thorough examination of mental health. There is similar provision in all jurisdictions. They may consider the following specific issues:

- The need for a formal assessment under mental health law (📖 p.IV.373)
- The fitness to be interviewed of the detainee.

Many FMEs are approved to participate in formal mental health assessments, but this is not a requirement for appointment to the role.

Other mental health professionals may be available to the police, including members of YOTs linked to mental health services.

Fitness to be interviewed

Judging whether a person is fit to be interviewed is required for two primary reasons:

- To assess whether they may be harmed by the interview
- To assess whether the interview may later be considered unreliable.

The assessment is both an assessment for the presence of mental disorder, and a functional assessment akin to a capacity assessment (📖 p.IV.424). Any mental disorder may or may not render a person unfit to be interviewed. The assessment should include an assessment of mental state and how it might affect their ability:[†]

- To understand the nature and purpose of the interview
- To comprehend the questions put to them
- To appreciate the significance of any answers given
- To make rational decisions about whether they want to say anything
- To reply in a way that is unaffected by their mental condition (without necessarily having to be fully rational and accurate)

The questions in Box 17.1 may assist in addressing these issues.

---

* In RoI, the Gardaí in charge of the station is the equivalent of the UK custody officer. These duties are less clearly set out than is the case in the UK.
† These tests are not laid down in law, but taken from the psychiatric literature.

Box 17.1 Sample questions for assessing fitness to be interviewed

- Do you understand why you have been arrested?
- What does the caution you were given mean?
- What will the police want to find out in the interview?
- What impact might it have if you said [give a relevant example of an incriminating statement]?
- What would you do if you did not want to answer a question?

Police options for dealing with vulnerable suspects

- Charge and bail (📖 p.IV.330) with or without conditions until the next court hearing
- Charge and remand into custody (📖 p.IV.330) until the next court hearing
- Give police bail to return to the police station at a later date
- Give a caution for the offence (📖 p.IV.359)
- Release and take no further action ('NFA')
- Arrange admission to psychiatric hospital (i.e. diversion, 📖 p.II.216), as an alternative to, or in conjunction with any of the other listed options.

The psychiatrist

A psychiatrist may be involved in assessments at the police station including giving an opinion on all of the issues described in this topic. The unique clinical skill in the police station is assessing fitness to be interviewed.

Vulnerable suspects

Appropriate adults

Any suspicion of mental disorder or other vulnerability with regard to understanding or replying to questions should lead to a request for an 'appropriate adult' to be present in E&W, Scotland, or NI*, whether or not they have requested a legal representative.

Who can be an appropriate adult?

- A relative or guardian
- Someone with experience of dealing with the mentally disordered or otherwise vulnerable (commonly a psychiatric social worker)
- Any person aged over 18
- *Not* a police officer
- In Scotland, the appropriate adult must have professional training.

The role of the appropriate adult

- To offer advice and assistance
- Observation that interview is being conducted properly and fairly

---

* The appropriate adult system is statutory in E&W and NI, but purely informal in Scotland. There is no official appropriate adult system in RoI.

- To facilitate communication with the interviewee (both to protect them, and to ensure that the decision whether or not to charge is not based upon misunderstanding between them and the police)
- To help avoid false or unreliable confessions by abnormally suggestible or compliant (📖 p.II.123) mentally disordered people.

Increasingly, organized groups of trained volunteers or professionals carry out the role of the appropriate adult.

The guidance relating to appropriate adults in Scotland is subtly different. The appropriate adult is not limited to assisting with detainees suspected of offences but also helps both victims and witnesses. There is greater emphasis on their training in mental disorder, and the appropriate adult may not be a friend or relative. The primary aim is to provide support and reassurance.

Children and young people

- An appropriate adult should also be appointed for anyone under the age of 18 years (in E&W, Scotland, and NI)
- In RoI there are laws that place special duties on the Gardai in dealing with child suspects. Children under the age of 12 years cannot be arrested or detained in a Garda station unless the offence is murder, manslaughter, rape, or aggravated sexual assault; otherwise the Gardai must take them to be questioned in front of a parent or guardian
- Children under 14 years old cannot be charged in RoI without the permission of the Director of Public Prosecutions.

Protections for child and vulnerable adult defendants

Once in court, the judge has discretion to adapt the proceedings in order to make it easier for a vulnerable defendant to understand what is happening and to participate appropriately. This might include providing a sign language interpreter, providing information slowly and in written form as well as orally, allowing a supporter to sit or stand with the defendant and explain proceedings to them, or taking more frequent breaks ('adjournments') than is usual.

A defendant who, even with all reasonable special arrangements in place, would still be unable to comprehend may be unfit to plead and stand trial (📖 p.V.474).

Investigative psychology

Investigative psychology is a large and rapidly expanding subdiscipline of forensic and criminal psychology. It was originally developed to provide a scientific approach to 'offender profiling', adopting the approach that any contributions that psychologists might make to police investigation or to legal process must have an empirical, systematic and scientific basis.

❧ Investigative inferences: Offender profiling

Offender profiling is the attempt to draw inferences about the mind and other characteristics of a perpetrator, from the available evidence. Other terms for this type of activity include psychological profiling, criminal profiling, and crime scene analysis.[*] There are many myths that surround offender profiling because of its portrayal in detective fiction and the media.

Profilers attempt to answer such questions as, 'What plan, intention, or fantasy might the offender have had?' and 'Why did the offender choose that specific victim, crime, or method ("modus operandi")?' From these answers hypotheses are generated about the type of person the offender might be (e.g. sex, age, occupation, geographical location, criminal history). This form of profiling has been employed most often in murder and rape cases, especially high-profile serial cases where the police investigation is not progressing well.

There are three broad methods of profiling, with some overlap between the three:

- The clinical practitioner approach: a practising clinical or forensic psychologist (or possibly psychiatrist) extrapolating from their expertise to profiling
- The criminal investigative approach: an investigative specialist utilizing psychological training or experience
- The statistical/actuarial approach: an academic or group of academics deriving patterns from analysis of a number of past similar cases.

The Behavioural Science Unit (BSU) was set up by the US FBI in the 1970s to develop methods of collating information regarding offenders, victims, and crime scenes in order to develop profiles of potential suspects. The Unit identified two distinct types of offenders—organized and disorganized. It was suggested that crime scenes should be classified according to this dichotomy and thereby provide clues to the offender's characteristics, although other researchers disputed this. More recently the FBI has adopted a more scientific approach to behavioural investigative research and this has been adopted by services in Canada, the UK, Australia, and other countries.

⚠ The evidence of the effectiveness of profiling is varied at best, with the least evidence in support of the pure clinical practitioner approach.[†]

Currently offender profiling is used to provide the police with supportive investigative advice through experience, statistics, and the sharing of information. It would appear that many police officers view profiling favourably, but nevertheless it is rarely used as a basis for an arrest, merely for further investigation.

---

[*] These should be contrasted with geographical profiling, which is uncontroversial, and involves plotting offence locations and other characteristics on a map in order to spot patterns and infer where the offender might live.

[†] Offender profiling deriving from a clinical paradigm and aimed at direct self-incrimination by a suspect can prejudice a trial. In E&W the trial of Colin Stagg for the murder of Rachel Nickell was terminated by the judge on the first day, when it was made plain that the defendant had been induced to make incriminating statements to an undercover police officer who asked leading questions based on the profiling psychologist's advice. Some years later, another man was convicted of the murder.

Investigative and legal material

Investigative psychologists examine material collected during investigations and presented in court to detect deception, identify potentially false confessions, and evaluate eyewitness testimony. The study of factors influencing the reliability of witness testimony, of facial recognition, of the evaluation of children's evidence, and of deception and whether it can be detected, have become significant areas of work for investigative psychologists, and have produced a considerable literature, possibly greater than that for offender profiling.

Researching the investigative process

Investigative psychologists research detective decision-making and investigative strategies and develop procedures for interviewing suspects.

Prison services

Prisons and jails* perform two main functions: detaining people before trial (on remand, 📖 p.IV.330), and isolating them from the rest of society as a punishment (a sentence of imprisonment, 📖 pp.IV.364, IV.366). They can be divided into the following major groups, although in practice a single institution will often perform functions from more than one group:

• Secure or 'closed' prisons
• Resettlement or 'open' prisons with minimal security
• Juvenile prisons and Young Offender Institutions (YOIs, 📖 p.V.458).

Women and men (and male and female young offenders) are detained separately, usually in separate prisons. Closed prisons provide varying levels of 'perimeter' security (physical security, 📖 p.II.152) and 'internal' security (procedural and relational security, 📖 p.II.152); in E&W, they, and their inmates, are described as category A (maximum security), category B (medium security†), and category C (low security), with open prisons being described as category D.

Prisons in E&W, NI and RoI often specialize in a single function (such as housing remand prisoners or young offenders), whereas those in Scotland more often comprise several units with different functions. Table 17.1 refers to the largest unit of each prison. Prisons have been categorized using the security categories from E&W.

---

* Also spelt gaols (the old British spelling; 'jails' is the US spelling). In the UK and RoI the two terms tend to be used interchangeably, whereas in the US a jail is a local remand institution and a prison houses convicts. The term 'training prison' is often used in E&W to indicate what in the US would be called a prison.

† These are not equivalent to the security levels of secure hospitals (📖 p.II.209). A high secure hospital corresponds roughly to category B, a medium secure unit to category C, and a low secure unit falls somewhere between categories C and D.

Table 17.1 Prison Estates in the UK & Ireland, 2010–11

Prison type	E&W	Scotland	NI	RoI
Adult category A	8	2	1	1
Adult category B	39	7	1	9
Adult category C	50	3	1	1
Adult category D (open)	9	2	0	2
Young offender institution	38	3	1	1
Total	144	17	4	14
Number of prisoners	82,991	7967	1507	3881

Prison is expensive, costing from around £20,000 per year per prisoner in an open prison to £50,000 per year in maximum security (though still far cheaper than a secure hospital). Reoffending rates (📖 p.II.18) after release are high; this may in part reflect the nature of offenders who are imprisoned (as opposed to being given other sentences), not merely the failure of prison to change their behaviour.

Areas of a prison

A typical British or Irish prison comprises the following units, although not all will be found in all prisons, depending on the prison's functions:

- A reception centre, where new inmates are assessed (including a brief assessment of mental health, suicide, and self-harm risk and drug dependency), and where searches and other checks take place
- A first night centre, where new inmates undergo an induction before moving into the main prison accommodation
- A number of wings (long open galleries of cells) or houseblocks (cells/rooms on separate enclosed floors) providing accommodation for prisoners on 'ordinary location'
- A vulnerable prisoner unit for groups of prisoners at risk of victimization by other prisoners (e.g. sex offenders, former police officers, etc.)
- A segregation unit for individual detention of prisoners who have seriously breached prison rules, or who are at extreme risk of victimization by others
- A special unit (in some prisons, a Close Supervision Centre) for prisoners at very high risk of violence and/or escape
- A healthcare centre or wing for the assessment and treatment of physically or mentally unwell prisoners, including outpatient facilities
- An education and training centre
- A workshop in which prisoners can learn practical skills, and make items that can be sold by the prison
- One or more indoor and outdoor recreation areas
- A visitors' centre where supervised visits can be held.

The Prison GP or Medical Officer

Every prison has one or more doctors, usually former or part-time GPs, who provide general medical services to the prisoners, from an outpatient clinic at the healthcare centre. Prisoners can usually refer themselves or be referred by prison officers.

Those requiring treatments that cannot be provided by a GP in an outpatient setting can be referred to local NHS secondary care services; a few services will offer specialist outpatient clinics within the prison, but in most cases (and for all urgent or inpatient treatments) prison officers will need to escort the prisoner to the hospital.

The role of the psychiatrist

The prison medical officers are supported by a number of other specialist staff, including in particular drug misuse and mental health 'inreach' (outpatient) and inpatient teams, often led clinically by a psychiatrist. Prison psychiatric services are described in more detail on 📖 p.II.217.

Youth custody services

In addition to adult prisons (📖 p.V.456), a variety of services exist to keep children and young people in the custody of the State (Table 17.2). Unlike prisons, youth custody services not only detain people on remand (📖 p.IV.330) and as a sentence (📖 p.IV.361), but also under civil child care law, when their behaviour cannot be managed in foster care or an ordinary children's home.

Young Offender Institutions (YOIs)

These are the juvenile equivalent of a prison and are run by the prison service, although the aethos is intended to be one of care, education and rehabilitation rather than one of punishment. Young men are far more likely to be held in YOIs than young women (2700 as compared with 300, for instance, in E&W in 2010).

In E&W, there are two groups of detainees in YOIs: young offenders aged 18–21, and juvenile offenders aged 15–17; units that take only the latter group are sometimes referred to as 'juvenile units' instead of YOIs. In Scotland and RoI, children in YOIs are aged 16–21. In NI, children aged 10–17 can be detained in the sole Juvenile Justice Centre; those over 18 are held in adult prisons.

Secure training centres and detention schools

STCs are purpose-built centres for young offenders up to the age of 17 years, and are found only in E&W. They are run by private operators under contracts. STCs house vulnerable young people who are sentenced to custody or remanded to secure accommodation. They differ from YOIs in that they have a higher staff to young offender ratio and are smaller in size, which means that individual's needs can be met more easily. The four STCs in E&W hold around 9% of the young people in custody at any given time.

In RoI, there are a number of similar institutions known as children detention schools, which take children under 16.

Secure children's homes

These are usually used to accommodate young offenders between the ages of 12–16 years (14 in E&W), as well as girls up to the age of 16 years and 15–16-year-old boys who are assessed as vulnerable. In RoI, children aged 11–17 may be held there. They are run by local authority social care departments and are overseen by national government health and education departments.

In E&W, around 8% of young people in the secure estate are held in secure children's homes.

Adolescent secure hospitals

There are six forensic adolescent secure psychiatric units in England (Manchester, Newcastle, Birmingham, Southampton, and two in London). These are medium secure forensic psychiatric hospitals (p.II.210) providing care for under 18s suffering from mental illness associated with difficult or offending behaviour. Four of the six units are mixed gender but the two in London only accept males. These units accept referrals from a single managed resource centre.

Table 17.2 Youth custody in the UK & Ireland, 2008–10

Institution type	E&W	Scotland	NI	RoI
Young offender institution	38	3	1	1
Secure training centre	4	–	–	4
Secure children's home	17	6	2	2
Adolescent secure hospital	6	–	–	–
Total	65	9	3	7
Number of detainees	3000	940	63	217

Parole Boards

The general role of Parole Boards in all jurisdictions is to make directions or recommendations regarding the release of prisoners serving longer sentences. Their membership includes judicial, mental health, probation criminology, and community or lay members in all jurisdictions. Hearings may be oral or paper-based, and are usually held in prisons.[*] Decisions of the Parole Boards may be challenged by way of judicial review (p.IV.309).

The Court of Appeal in E&W has emphasized (with persuasive authority in other jurisdictions) that the Parole Board should not just be independent but avoid any appearance of lack of independence.

See Table 17.3 for details of each jurisdiction's Parole Board.

[*] Hearings for prisoners transferred to hospital may occasionally be held at the hospital: see p.IV.417.

Psychiatry and the Parole Boards

There are three main roles for psychiatrists in relation to Parole Boards:

Providing reports on patients under their care, usually as a psychiatrist working in a prison but also where transferred prisoners are detained in hospital. In these circumstances the duty is as a doctor and psychiatrist and ordinary report writing advice (📖 p.V.555) should be followed. There will be a particular requirement that risks associated with release into the community are considered but this should be no different from that expected by a Mental Health Tribunal. Parole Board reports in this context should cover the areas listed on 📖 p.V.570.

Providing independent reports can be on behalf of either the prisoner or the Ministry of Justice. Here the psychiatrist will be required to read the prisoner's file and to advise on risk in the community. Only where there is a diagnosable psychiatric condition, which may then imply risk, is it ethically acceptable to assess risk and recommend a community regime, since doctors have no special expertise in assessing the risk presented by ordinary offenders. And, even then, involvement results in a very different ethical position than is usual in ordinary clinical practice.

Sitting as a parole board member is practically and ethically distinct in that the process is one of weighing up all of the available evidence in a somewhat 'judicial' fashion so as to contribute to the making of a decision, somewhat similar to sitting as the medical member of a Mental Health Tribunal (📖 p.V.592).

However, unlike Tribunals the Parole Board is concerned almost solely with protecting the public. Other factors, including the prisoner's interests, are considered but are given much less weight, and certainly less than would a psychiatrist in clinical practice. Whereas attempting to predict harms (as opposed to assessing risk of harm; see 📖 p.II.127) is discouraged in psychiatric practice, the advice of a psychiatrist member may be sought and given significant weight by the Board, particularly when considering prisoners with mental disorder. Furthermore, the contractual duty of the psychiatrist in this situation is to the Board, and this may conflict with their ethical professional duties (📖 p.III.244).

Parole Boards may also seek advice from the psychiatric member on:
- The prisoner's emotional development and personality factors
- The interpretation of psychiatric reports
- The contribution of knowledge on the science of risk assessment, prediction and outcome
- The role of drug and alcohol abuse
- Management strategies or interventions.

Table 17.3 Details of the Parole Board in each jurisdiction

	E&W	Scotland	NI	RoI
Primary function	Risk assessing prisoners to decide whether they can be safely released into the community	Ensuring those prisoners no longer regarded as presenting a risk to the community are released	Consideration of the suitability for release of prisoners who had been sentenced to life imprisonment	To advise the Minister for Justice, Equality and Law Reform in relation to the administration of long-term prison sentences
Primary relevant legislation	Criminal Justice Act 1967 Criminal Justice and Public Order Act 1994	Prisons (Scotland) Act 1989 Prisoners and Criminal Proceedings (Scotland) Act 1993	Life Sentences (Northern Ireland) Order 2001	Non-statutory
Sentences considered by the Parole Board	All life and. indeterminate sentences (IPPs) (📖 p.IV.364). All extended sentences (EPPs) and determinate sentences (📖 p.IV.366) for serious sexual or violent offences, or if recalled after release on licence	All life sentences Imprisonment >4 years	All life sentences	All life sentences

Probation services

Probation began in the US as an informal system allowing sentencing (📖 p.IV.361) to be delayed while convicted offenders submitted to the supervision of a local volunteer and 'proved' that they had reformed their behaviour; those who demonstrated moral improvement received a lighter eventual sentence. In the early 20th century, the system spread across the UK and Europe, became regulated by statute law (📖 p.IV.304), and became available as a sentence in its own right.

In the mid- to late-20th century, probation officers in the UK and RoI came to see themselves as social workers specializing in work with offenders, and probation as a form of social therapy in the interests of offenders' welfare, rather than simply as a supervised testing of the offender. However, from 1993 onwards successive UK governments recast probation as a punishment, particularly in E&W, and probation officers as 'offender supervisors' acting on behalf of the courts—against resistance from probation officers who asserted the welfare model (📖 p.IV.297).

Roles of probation services

Modern probation services perform some or all of the following roles:

- Assessing offenders before sentencing, to advise the court on the suitability of various sentencing options through a pre-sentence report (PSR)
- Monitoring the progress of offenders sentenced to imprisonment (📖 p.IV.364)
- Advising the Parole Board (📖 p.V.459) on prisoner's suitability for release
- Supervising offenders released from prison under licence (📖 pp.IV.365, IV.367), and recalling them to prison if they breach the licence terms
- Supervising offenders' compliance with community sentences (📖 p.IV.368) and reporting them to court if they breach the terms of their sentence
- Advising offenders on available services and resources in their local area, with the aim of helping them avoid reoffending
- Directly providing support, counselling or treatment to offenders, especially group psychology programmes (📖 p.II.171) such as Think First.

England and Wales

National Probation Service (NPS)—adults

Each year the NPS commences the supervision of 175,000 offenders. Its primary aims are to protect the public and reduce reoffending; although many individual probation officers believe strongly in promoting the welfare of (ex-)offenders, this is not an official priority.

- Approximately 70% of supervised offenders are on community sentences, and 30% on licence following release from prison
- The NPS's work with offenders combines assessment, including the use of risk assessment (📖 p.II.127) measures such as OASys (📖 p.II.133), and the management of risk through the provision of accredited offender behaviour programmes designed to reduce reoffending.

Youth Offending Teams—age 10–17 years

YOTs are multi-agency teams made up of staff including:

- Police officers
- Probation officers
- Social workers
- Psychologists (from CAMHS)
- Teachers and/or education welfare officers
- Substance misuse counsellors
- In some cases, housing officers and other staff from local charities.

There is a YOT in every local authority in E&W. The team identifies the needs of, and risks posed by, each young offender using a structured assessment process (ONSET and ASSET, 🕮 p.II.134) developed by the Youth Justice Board (🕮 p.IV.464), and plans suitable programmes and interventions according to the results of this assessment.

Unlike the NPS, the emphasis of YOTs is the welfare of the offender, and how they can be helped to avoid reoffending in the future. There is a strong focus on re-engaging the young offender in education and on involving parents and other family members; and in the case of restorative justice (🕮 p.IV.361) measures such as the referral order (🕮 p.IV.372), also involving victims and representatives of the local community.

Northern Ireland

The probation system is NI has a stronger focus on rehabilitation than the E&W NPS, but is otherwise similar, with a split between the Probation Board for NI, which supervises adult offenders, and the Youth Justice Agency (YJA, 🕮 p.V.465), which does the same for young offenders.

The local offices of the YJA organize diversionary youth conferences (🕮 p.IV.372), and provide a variety of community services to help young offenders re-integrate into their local community and avoid reoffending. Unlike YOTs, the YJA directly employs all its local staff, who liaise with staff from other agencies as needed.

Republic of Ireland

A single agency in RoI, the Probation Service, supervises both adult and (through its Young Persons Probation division) young offenders. Its focus is on providing assessments to the courts, and supervising offenders on licence and on community sentences. It also supports a number of practical (as opposed to psychological) training and outreach programmes.

Scotland

There is no probation service in Scotland. Instead, local authorities employ Criminal Justice Social Workers who assess and supervise over-16-year-old offenders, alongside social workers who supervise young offenders through the non-criminal Children's Hearings (🕮 p.IV.323) system.

Psychiatrists and the probation service

Psychiatrists commonly have contact with probation officers through joint management of MDOs, on community orders (🕮 p.IV.368) with a condition of treatment, or patients on licence (🕮 p.IV.365), or through contributing to the risk management (🕮 p.II.189) of a patient subject to MAPPA (🕮 p.V.468).

Offender management

From the late 20th century onwards, governments in the UK in particular have come to see sentencing less as a semi-private matter between an individual judge and an individual offender, and more as a public act of a single over-arching Criminal Justice System. The collection of courts, prisons (📖 p.V.456) and probation services (📖 p.V.462) that deal with convicted offenders came to be seen as engaged in 'offender management', and new bodies were created to oversee those agencies and to ensure that they worked to achieve the System's aims consistently and coherently.

England and Wales

National Offender Management Service & Youth Justice Board

NOMS, an agency of the Ministry of Justice, aims to join up prison and probation services, in order to facilitate the management of offenders and to strengthen and streamline commissioning so as to improve service efficiency and effectiveness. It commissions prison and probation services (such as prison offender treatment programmes, 📖 p.II.176, probation hostels and 'approved premises', and victim support services, 📖 p.II.186), including from the private sector. It also conducts research to improve its specification, benchmarking and costing of services. It advises government departments on the needs of offenders, and provides judges with information on the costs and benefits of sentencing options.

The YJB performs the same roles in relation to the Youth Justice System. Whereas adult prison and probation staff are directly employed by the Prison Service and NPS (📖 p.V.462), the staff of children's homes and YOTs (📖 p.V.463) are employed by local authorities, and the YJB therefore makes grants to local authorities for these services.

Mental Health Unit

The Ministry of Justice's Mental Health Unit (MHU) performs a more limited offender management role in relation to mentally disordered offenders subject to restriction orders and directions (📖 p.IV.412). Its 60 staff consider applications from clinicians for prisoners to be transferred to hospital (📖 p.IV.410) for treatment, and for restricted patients to have leave (📖 p.IV.392), be transferred elsewhere, be remitted to prison, or be discharged. They also write statements to Tribunals (📖 p.IV.414) considering discharge, and have the power to recall (📖 p.V.467) conditionally discharged patients and to vary their conditions or absolutely discharge them. They apply their own risk assessment criteria to clinical reports.

Scotland

Community Justice Authorities & National Advisory Board

Scotland has no single body comparable to NOMS in E&W, but has instead created regional Community Justice Authorities (CJAs) that aim to create a coherent, flexible network of services in their area, supported by a National Advisory Board that sets standards and a national strategy. CJAs are responsible for allocating resources to local authority criminal justice social work services (📖 p.V.463).

Scottish Ministers' Restricted Patients Team

This small nine-member team managers restricted patients in Scotland on behalf of the Scottish Ministers. Like the MHU in E&W, each caseworker takes responsibility for a group of patients on an alphabetical basis. The team is responsible for approving transfers between hospitals, returns to prison, cross-border transfers, suspension of detention (📖 p.IV.392), recall from conditional discharge, and variations of conditions.

Northern Ireland

Offender Management Groups & Youth Justice Agency

There is no equivalent of NOMS or the CJAs for adult offenders in NI. Instead, the 'offender management model' in the NI Prison Service aims to improve the risk assessment of prisoners, make safer decisions about release, and improve liaison with the probation service. Each prison has an Offender Management Group, responsible for oversight of the review system, supported by senior probation officers and psychologists.

The Youth Justice Agency (YJA) is responsible for dealing with offending by children and young people, through the delivery of a range of community based, court-ordered and diversionary interventions, including youth conferences (📖 p.IV.372) and custody (📖 p.V.458) where necessary.

Department of Justice Criminal Justice Policy Division

Staff in this division perform the same functions in relation to restricted patients as the MHU in E&W and the Scottish Restricted Patients Team.

Republic of Ireland

There is no overarching organization responsible for offender management in RoI, only individual prison and probation organizations. Neither is there any equivalent of the MHU: the movements of the small number of restricted patients are approved by the same unit as other prisoners.

Reoffending and the effectiveness of offender management

Studies of the effectiveness of national CJSs in reducing reoffending are plagued by methodological problems (📖 p.II.18) related to varying definitions and methods of data collection. Table 17.4 shows one 'harmonized' international comparison that attempts to overcome these problems, and a number of un-harmonized figures for individual jurisdictions.

Table 17.4 Rates of reoffending after one year

	E&W	Scotland	Holland	
Harmonized rate (2004)	45.1%	44.3%	38.0%	
Rates on different bases:	**E&W**	**Scotland**	**NI**	**RoI**
Imprisonment	51.4%	46.7%	37.7%	27.4%
Community sentences	36.8%	42.1%	24.7%	No data
Restriction orders	5.8%	No data	No data	N/A

Managing the restricted patient

The care of patients subject to restriction orders (📖 p.IV.412) must be co-ordinated* with the national mental health offender management agency (📖 p.V.464), such as the MoJ Mental Health Unit (MHU) in E&W. Clinicians therefore discuss proposed admissions, transfers (📖 p.IV.410), leave (📖 p.IV.392), and conditions of discharge (📖 p.IV.413) with the patient's allocated caseworker at the MHU or its local equivalent.

In hospital

The clinical care of restricted patients detained in hospital should not differ from that which they would have received if unrestricted. Like all other compulsorily detained patients, their care will be supervised by a Responsible Medical Officer (RMO, or RC in E&W, 📖 p.IV.379); this will usually be a consultant forensic psychiatrist, except where the MHU or equivalent has approved admission to a PICU or general psychiatric unit.

Leave

Leave (or in Scotland, suspension of detention, 📖 p.IV.392) outside the ward, unit, or hospital† specified on the court order or transfer warrant must first be approved by the MHU or equivalent, which will require a standard form to be completed detailing the patient's condition, the purposes of the leave, the risks it would involve, and the contingency plans. This process can take several weeks at busy times.

Permission is not required in advance for escorted leave to allow urgent medical treatment, but the MHU or equivalent must be informed as soon as possible. Permission is also not required for court appearances in E&W, although it is required in Scotland.

Transferred prisoners who would not be eligible for parole or release (because they have not yet reached their EDR, 📖 p.IV.367, or completed their minimum term or tariff, 📖 p.IV.365) are usually refused leave.

Incidents

Incidents involving a restricted patient that result or could have resulted in serious harm must be reported to the MHU or equivalent, including:
- Incidents causing serious injury or death, or serious property damage
- Hostage-taking (📖 p.II.195)
- Public protests (e.g. following access to a rooftop)
- Escape or absconding (📖 p.II.200), or
- Any other incident requiring a formal critical incident review.

Transfer between hospitals or wards

Restricted patients cannot be transferred between hospitals without the permission of the MHU or equivalent—even in an emergency where they are being transferred to a higher level of security (although in such cases permission will usually be given immediately by telephone, by the on-call

---

* The MHU wishes the co-ordination to be on the basis of a partnership between it and the clinician, and many clinicians accept this model. Others, however, see the relationship as one of a 'productive tension' to balance patient and public welfare.
† If the court order or transfer warrant specifies an entire hospital, leave within the hospital grounds can legally be granted without permission from the MHU or equivalent, although this may be unwise if there is no secure barrier between the grounds and the community.

manager outside working hours). Transfers between wards may be possible without permission, even if they involve a reduction in security, if the court order or warrant specifies a whole unit or hospital and both wards are within that unit or hospital. A standard form will be required, and the process may take several weeks at busy times.

After conditional discharge

The main impact of the restriction order is seen when patients are conditionally discharged. The discharge planning for a restricted patient should be thorough as for any patient in forensic services. The conditions for each patient are derived from individual risk assessments and are designed to manage relevant risk factors. They usually include:

- Residing at a particular hostel or other address
- Compliance with medication and other aspects of the care plan
- Attending appointments, or accepting visits, from supervisors
- Giving samples for drug or alcohol testing (and occasionally, refraining from drug or alcohol use entirely or only with permission[††])
- Not entering an exclusion zone (specific streets or a whole postcode near a former victim's home or place or work, for example).

The MHU accept that junior doctors and junior social workers (or other care coordinators, who can act as social supervisors with appropriate training) often manage conditionally discharged patients in practice. However, there must be a supervising RC/RMO and/or senior social supervisor who also countersigns their statutory reports (☐ p.IV.413).

The psychiatric supervisor must have contact with the patient at least once every 3 months, and ideally every month; the social supervisor must see them weekly at first, reducing to no less often than monthly. Patients must be seen at home on a regular basis.

Recall to hospital

Patients who relapse, or breach conditions in such a way that the risk of relapse is increased (e.g. drug use in a patient known to become psychotic when regularly using drugs) may be recalled from conditional discharge. The MHU and equivalents will recall patients on the advice of supervisors, or by itself if it is concerned about patients' reported behaviour, or if patients are admitted informally for more than 6 weeks. It is crucial to discuss concerns openly with the MHU or equivalent, even if you oppose recall, so that you maintain the trust of caseworkers.

[††] This condition is only really practical if the patient accepts the legitimacy of it (e.g. because they are trying to stop using drugs, but have poor self-control). Imposing this condition on a non-compliant patient will result in rapid and frequent recalls to hospital.

Public Protection Arrangements: MAPPA

In the three UK jurisdictions, the process of inter-agency cooperation for protecting the public has been formalized under the Multi-Agency Public Protection Arrangements (MAPPA) for E&W and Scotland, and the Public Protection Arrangements for Northern Ireland (PPANI) in NI. Under this statutory scheme,[*] the so-called Responsible Authorities (RA)—the police, probation, and prison services[†]—must jointly manage offenders deemed to pose a 'serious risk of harm to the public', and are entitled to cooperation from other relevant agencies, such as health, housing, education and social services.

Identification of offenders to be supervised

This is generally determined by the offender's offence and sentence, but also by assessed level of risk. There are three formal categories, as shown in Box 17.2. Note that agencies can also cooperate in the management of offenders not covered by MAPPA, under informal arrangements (see 🕮 p.II.203).

Box 17.2 MAPPA offender categories

Category 1: Sex Offenders
This includes all sex offenders on the Sex Offenders Register (🕮 p.IV.371), and also any other convicted or cautioned (🕮 p.IV.359) sex offender assessed as posing a high risk (🕮 p.II.127) to the community.

Category 2: Violent Offenders
This comprises all offenders convicted of a violent offence (one which led, or was intended or likely to lead, to death or physical injury) who are sentenced to at least 12 months' imprisonment (🕮 p.IV.366), or a hospital order (🕮 p.IV.405).

Category 3: Potentially Dangerous Offenders
Offenders who have been cautioned for or convicted of an offence that indicates they are capable of causing the public serious harm.

Only the RA can definitively allocate referred offenders to a category and thereby make them subject to MAPPA. Category 3 offenders can only be managed under MAPPA for up to 3 months, unless they can be reallocated to category 1 or 2.

---

[*] Brought in by the Criminal Justice and Courts Services Act 2000 and extended under the Criminal Justice Act 2003 for E&W; and brought in elsewhere in the UK by the Criminal Justice (Northern Ireland) Order 2008 and the Management of Offenders (Scotland) Act 2005.
[†] Except in Scotland, where the responsible authorities are the police, prison service, social services, and health boards.

On 31.3.2009, there were 32,336 offenders in category 1 in E&W and 2967 in Scotland, compared with 44,761 in categories 2 and 3 in E&W and 3145 in Scotland.

Sharing of information about offenders

MAPPA promotes information sharing between all the agencies by providing a statutory basis for such; with the intention of more effective supervision and better public protection. However, breach of confidence (📖 p.III.263) in sharing information under MAPPA is governed by the usual legal rules, including by the test in *Egdell* (📖 p.App. 3.635): that is, breach requires that there is a 'significant risk of serious harm to others'. Hence, reports given to MAPPA agencies should be fashioned for that purpose, and there should not be disclosure of clinical reports and records as a whole.

Assessment of the risks posed by offenders

MAPPA enables resources and attention to be focused on offenders who present the highest risk (most MAPPA offenders do not present a serious risk to the public). Victims' needs are represented, and additional measures are put into place to manage the risks posed to known victims.

Management of the risk posed by individual offenders

MAPPA offenders are managed at one of three levels. While the assessed risk is an important factor, it is the degree of management intervention required which determines the level.

- *Level One: involves normal agency management* by one or sometimes two agencies. Generally offenders managed at this level will be assessed as presenting a low or medium risk of serious harm to others. In 2007/08 around 75% of MAPPA offenders were managed at this level.
- *Level Two: often called local inter-agency risk management*
  Most offenders assessed as high or very high risk of harm. In 2007/08 around 23% of MAPPA offenders were managed at this level.
- *Level Three: known as Multi-Agency Public Protection Panels (or MAPPPs)*
  Appropriate for those offenders who pose the highest risk of causing serious harm or whose management is so problematic that multi-agency cooperation and oversight at a senior level is required with the authority to commit exceptional resources. In 2007/08 around 2% of MAPPA offenders were managed at this level.

The Risk Management Authority

The Risk Management Authority (RMA) is a Scottish public body that was established in 2003. It is concerned with the assessment and management of serious violent and sexual offenders who would present a risk to the public if at liberty. It has a special responsibility in respect of the small number of offenders who sentenced to an order for lifelong restriction (OLR, 📖 p.IV.365). Note that it is *not* specifically or solely concerned with mentally disordered offenders.

The RMA's functions are:
- To develop policy and carry out research into the risk assessment and management of offenders whose liberty presents a risk to the public at large
- To set standards for, and issue guidance to, those involved in the assessment and management of risk
- To accredit practitioners and risk management plans and monitor risk management plans for those offenders who receive an OLR from the High Court of Justiciary.

The role of an accredited risk assessor

An accredited risk assessor may come from a range of professional backgrounds including psychiatry, psychology, and social work. This role is similar to that of the 'forensicist' in the US, and is a step further on from the traditional role of the forensic psychiatrist who provides a medical report to the court: the risk assessment report on an offender is requested under a risk assessment order (📖 p.IV.408) solely for the purpose of determining what risk the person at liberty presents to the safety of the public at large. There is no requirement that risk be linked to mental disorder for the court to make an OLR. The risk assessment report needs to be written in accordance to the rigorous standards of the RMA using structured professional judgement techniques.

Ethics of the role of the accredited risk assessor

The role of the psychiatrist as a risk assessor extends the scope of traditional medical ethical duties, as the risk assessment is not done for the benefit of the offender but solely for public protection (📖 p.III.261). Given that it is rare for such assessments to make no finding at all, it could be argued that the offender's interests may well be harmed by the assessment. This raises the issue of their consent to risk assessment (📖 p.III.284). The individual must be informed that the risk assessment is being conducted because of a court order, that it is part of the sentencing process (📖 p.IV.361) and not part of a therapeutic treatment process, that any information provided might be used in the risk assessment report (i.e. there is no confidentiality, 📖 p.III.263), and that the outcome could be an indefinite sentence of imprisonment (📖 p.IV.364) or another restrictive sentence such as the OLR.

Mental health professionals, and especially doctors, may have ethical objections to their involvement in risk assessments for the RMA (much like they may to involvement in courts' assessments of dangerousness, 📖 p.V.549); but others such as forensic psychologists may believe that it is within their professional role. Clinicians prepared to act as accredited risk assessors must bear in mind that their clinical skills may be inapplicable where there is little or no discernible relationship between the offence or risk, and the offender's mental disorder, if any (see 📖 p.II.127).

Homicide and suicide inquiries

In 1994 the UK[*] Government directed that there be an external independent inquiry whenever a homicide or suicide was committed by someone who was in contact with mental health services during the previous 6 months. Inquiries now involve three stages, though not all three are always required in the case of suicides:
- An initial service review done in the first 72 hours
- A internal investigation by the Trust or Health Board concerned
- An external independent inquiry commissioned by the Strategic Health Authority in England, or the relevant Minister in Wales, Scotland, & NI, usually only after the conclusion of any criminal proceedings

Purposes of homicide and suicide inquiries

The stated purpose of these inquiries is to identify any system failures, and opportunities for prevention in the future. They produce lengthy reports which may, however, offer the basis for later negligence (📖 p.V.516) claims against employees or NHS bodies.

However, academic commentators have identified additional purposes:
- The allocation of responsibility, and
- An opportunity for catharsis for relatives of the victim and the public.

They have argued that pursuit of at least two of the purposes are mutually inconsistent (eg encouraging openness from clinicians, in order to improve services for the future, is inconsistent with allocating responsibility, which will encourage defensive caution in evidence giving).

Criticisms of homicide and suicide inquiries
- The terms of reference very rarely reflect legal criteria for judging clinical practice (e.g. criteria for negligence); practitioners may be heavily criticized for a negative outcome even though a responsible body of fellow practitioners would have acted in the same way
- Inquiries very rarely address causation (📖 p.V.512) in a legally coherent fashion in apportioning blame for any failures identified: clinicians may be blamed for a negative outcome not directly related to their actions
- There is no formal due process:[†] clinicians who may end up being blamed, with serious consequences for their career, may not be legally represented and have no opportunity to cross-examine other witnesses etc. (although to enable this would dramatically increase the cost and duration of inquiries)
- The mandatory nature of homicide inquiries betrays the assumption that a homicide must have resulted from a service failure (whilst there is no such assumption in relation to a suicide). There is no 'screening' process to determine which homicides should be the subject of a full external independent inquiry

[*] There is no equivalent requirement in Ireland, although ad hoc inquiries may be held into certain high-profile homicides and suicides by people with mental disorder.
[†] The only requirement is that the inquiry panel must formally notify those it considers vulnerable to criticism, by way of what is known as a 'Salmon letter'.

- Each inquiry is unique to itself, with no coordination to enable each to build on the developing knowledge gleaned from its predecessors.

Outcomes of homicide and suicide inquiries

The only major review of the outcome of homicide inquiries found that, assuming the conclusions of inquiry, whatever its method, to be valid, only about a quarter of homicides were deemed to have been 'predictable'; but two-thirds were thought to be 'preventable'. That is, many homicides would have been prevented if there had been proper earlier clinical intervention, driven by patient need, which would, coincidentally, have interrupted the chain of events leading to the homicide (see 📖 p.II.191 for a more detailed consideration of these findings).

Although rates of suicide and of homicide by the mentally ill fell in the UK between 1994 and 2008/9*, there is no evidence that inquiries were responsible.

Research

Suicides and homicides by mentally ill people, as well as sudden unexpected deaths, are researched by the 'National Confidential Inquiry'. The project aims to understand the details of such incidents so as to make recommendations to services on reducing the risk of further incidents.

As of 2009, the cumulative conclusions of the National Confidential Inquiry include the following:

- Fatal incidents following absconding from secure units are rare.
  A more common event is the suicide of the detained patient following absconding from an open ward
- Changing patterns of ligatures and ligature points continue to be found: recognized types of points, for example, are eliminated when wards are redesigned, but those designs introduce new, unrecognized, points
- Suicides preceded by non-compliance with treatment have become less common
- There has been a fall in the number and rate of suicides in both the general population and in-patient population
- The number and rate of homicides have increased amongst males in the general population, but not for women or for patients generally.

---

*ONS statistics for the UK show that suicide rates fell from 19.9 per 100,000 men in 1992 to 17.7 in 2008, and from 6.1 to 5.4 for women. Home Office statistics for E&W show that homicide resulting in a verdict of diminished responsibility (📖 p.IV.491), a rough proxy for homicide by the mentally ill, fell dramatically from 1.39 per 100,000 people in 1994 to 0.33 in 2009. More specifically, but for a more limited period, data from the National Confidential Inquiry for mental health service users show falls in suicide rates per 100,000 population from 3.83 in 1997 to 3.30 in 2006 for men and 1.9 to 1.61 for women; and a static rate of homicides by service users (0.12 per 100,000 population in 1997, 0.13 in 2005).

Legal tests relevant to psychiatry

Fitness to plead

A criminal trial can proceed only if the defendant is 'fit to plead', in terms of their mental ability to participate in the trial. Fitness to plead is legally defined and determined by the court, but with reference to expert psychiatric, and/or psychological evidence. Physical conditions may also be relevant (e.g. being deaf or mute). Fitness to plead is distinguished from fitness to attend court (📖 p.V.478).

All defendants are presumed fit until evidence is presented to suggest they are not, so that the relevant legal tests are actually of *unfitness*. Tests vary in detail between jurisdictions, but are all tests of cognitive ability, taking into account the degree to which it is affected by psychotic or other mental symptoms, neurological disorder or learning disability.

Tests of unfitness

E&W and NI R v Pritchard (📖 p.App. 3.643) The precise wording of the test has changed as it has been restated by judges in various cases. As set out most recently in *R v M* (📖 p.App. 3.641), a finding of unfitness to plead involves demonstrating, on the balance of probabilities (📖 p.IV.316) that the defendant is incapable of one or more of:

- Understanding the charge or charges
- Deciding whether to plead guilty or not
- Exercising his right to challenge jurors
- Instructing solicitors and counsel
- Following the course of proceedings, or
- Giving evidence in his own defence (📖 p.V.477).

Being unable to remember events even directly related to the alleged offence is insufficient for a finding of unfitness (*R v Podola*, 📖 p.App. 3.643).

Scotland Criminal Justice and Licensing (Scotland) Act 2010 The test is whether the defendant is incapable, by reason of a mental or physical condition, of participating effectively in a trial. As in E&W, being unable to remember the alleged offence is insufficient; the court must consider the defendant's ability to:

- Understand the nature of the charge
- Understand the requirement to tender a plea to the charge and the effect of such a plea
- Understand the purpose, and follow the course, of the trial
- Understand the evidence that may be given against them, and
- Instruct and communicate with their legal representative.

RoI Criminal Law (Insanity) Act 2006 An accused person shall be deemed unfit to be tried if he or she is unable by reason of mental disorder to understand the nature or course of proceedings so as to:

- Plead to the charge
- Instruct a legal representative
- Make a choice (where available) on trial summarily or by jury
- Make a proper defence
- Understand the evidence, or, where appropriate,
- Challenge a juror to whom he or she might wish to object.

Problems with the tests of unfitness

There has been much criticism of the definitions of unfitness, in that the tests are based solely upon cognitive disabilities, ignoring other types of mental symptoms likely to influence decision-making capacity, as well as factors such as suggestibility and compliance (📖 p.II.123), or cultural background. This very narrow approach is thought to explain why findings of unfitness to plead are very rare.[*] As a result the E&W Law Commission is currently consulting on proposals to replace the current test with a broader one based upon mental capacity, similar in terms to that within the Mental Capacity Act (📖 p.IV.424) applicable in civil law.

Other problems

- The current tests distinguish between abilities *per se* (lack of which can affect fitness to plead), and *use* of those abilities (abnormality of which cannot): for example, in *R v Robertson* (📖 p.App. 3.644), a defendant of low intelligence who had delusions relating directly to the alleged offence was held capable of meeting the *Pritchard* tests, and as merely 'failing to act in his own best interests' (because of his delusions and low IQ)
- Human rights law (📖 p.IV.418) implies that a defendant should be able to plead with understanding. Hence, if a defendant is deluded about the consequences of a particular plea (for example that, as in *R v Erskine*, 📖 p.App. 3.636, if he acknowledges his killings he will be deported to America and executed), then he cannot plead with understanding; yet he might still be held fit to plead on the current tests
- A mentally disordered defendant who has killed might meet the criteria for diminished responsibility (📖 p.IV.491), but still be fit to plead because their abnormality of mind (or, in E&W or NI, abnormality of mental functioning) does not affect those cognitive abilities required by the current tests of fitness to plead. Hence, if they lacked insight into the presence and nature of their mental disorder, they might be allowed to refuse to plead diminished responsibility, resulting in an unfair conviction for murder.[†] That is, the disorder which would lay the basis for a successful plea of diminished responsibility might well be the reason they refuse to plead it; and they may well be found fit to do so, because of narrowness of the current tests of fitness to plead
- Psychiatrists are commonly encouraged to give evidence directly about whether the defendant is fit to plead (i.e. the ultimate issue, 📖 p.V.543). This can mean that they interpret the legal test for themselves, rather than describing the relevant mental disabilities and leaving the court to determine whether they amount to unfitness. Hence, apparent disagreements between psychiatrists may not be about the defendant's medical disabilities, but about their legal interpretation.

---

[*] Numbering in the tens or hundreds in a typical year in E&W, as compared with around 12,000 in the US.

[†] The defence can only be raised by the defence, not the prosecution or the court.

Procedures

The issue of fitness to plead can be raised by the defence, the prosecution or the judge.

E&W Criminal Procedure (Insanity) Act 1964 (amended 1991, 2004)
- At least two medical practitioners must give evidence on the issue
- If raised by the prosecution, it must be proved beyond reasonable doubt; if by the defence, on the balance of probabilities (📖 p.IV.316).
- Determined by the judge in the Crown Court (📖 p.IV.320), not a jury.[*]

Scotland Criminal Procedure (Scotland) Act 1995 (amended 2010)
- Referred to as unfitness for trial (previously 'insanity in bar of trial')
- No longer any requirement for medical evidence
- The case may be adjourned so that investigation of the defendant's mental condition can occur.

NI Mental Health (Northern Ireland) Order 1986
- Referred to as the question of fitness to be tried
- At least two medical practitioners must give evidence (one oral)
- The judge determines the issue.

RoI Criminal Law (insanity) Act 2006
- Determined by the Court
- Based on evidence of an approved medical officer.

Delaying trial

Where a defendant is likely to be found unfit to plead but has a mental condition which is likely to be treatable, so as to make them fit to plead within a reasonable period of time, it is sensible to advise the court to delay trial, rather than to proceed to an unfitness hearing.

Even where a defendant is fit to plead, yet still seriously mentally unwell, if there is a prospect of improving their mental health through treatment, and that would be likely to further improve their ability to participate in their trial, then again it is sensible to advise the court of this and to suggest delay, on the basis of 'natural justice'.

Outcome following a finding of unfitness to plead

After a finding of unfitness to plead, there is a 'trial of the facts' to determine whether the defendant did the acts or omissions charged (i.e. the conduct element, 📖 p.IV.332, of the offence).[†] This is to avoid the possibility of

---

[*] There is no procedure for testing unfitness to plead in the magistrates' court. However, under s37(3) of the MHA, magistrates can make a hospital order (📖 p.IV.405) or guardianship (📖 p.IV.405) if the offence is punishable with imprisonment and they are satisfied that the defendant did the acts or made the omissions charged.
[†] In E&W, the Law Commission has proposed allowing consideration of the mental element (📖 p.IV.334), such that if there is clear evidence (unrelated to the cause of the unfitness to plead) that the defendant lacked the relevant mens rea, they can be acquitted notwithstanding their unfitness to plead.

the long-term detention of a defendant who might not have done what is alleged. The acts or omissions need only be proved on the balance of probabilities (except in RoI). If proved, the court may make one of the following orders:

E&W, NI, and Scotland

- Hospital order (compulsion order in Scotland) (📖 p.IV.405)
- Hospital/compulsion order with restrictions (📖 p.IV.412)[*]
- Interim compulsion order (Scotland only)
- Guardianship order (📖 p.IV.409) in Scotland and NI
- Supervision & treatment order (Supervision order in E&W) (📖 p.IV.409)
- Absolute discharge.

In E&W, even if there has been a definitive disposal, the patient can be retried if they become fit to plead.

RoI

- Committal for treatment (📖 p.IV.405) to a designated centre for inpatient or outpatient care or treatment.

Return to court

A finding during a trial of the facts that the defendant did the acts or omissions alleged does not amount to a conviction. If later fit to plead, therefore, the defendant might sometimes have an interest in being tried. In practice, however, subsequent trial is unusual, partly because the policy of both governments and prosecution services opposes it (for example, after the passage of time, the memories of witnesses may be dimmed, and important documents and samples may have been lost).

Fitness to give evidence

Whereas fitness to plead and fitness to stand trial (📖 p.V.474) apply only to defendants, all witnesses, not only defendants, must be fit to give evidence. Whether they are fit to do so is an issue for the judge, aided where necessary by psychiatric or psychological evidence.[†]

There is a long history of trials not being pursued, or being abandoned, because of concerns or assumptions that witnesses were unfit, or that their evidence was likely to be unreliable. This most often applies to prosecution witnesses, particularly victims (e.g. of rape, 📖 p.IV.348, where their evidence may be the sole evidence on which conviction could be based). Commonly, witnesses considered to be vulnerable are young, elderly and frail, or learning disabled, but other mental disorders may also be relevant.

---

[*] In E&W, this is mandatory if the charge was murder.

[†] It is of particular relevance to defendants in E&W, because s35 of the Criminal Justice and Public Order Act 1994 allows courts or juries to regard a defendant's 'failure' to give evidence as a factor supporting the prosecution case (the so-called '*adverse inference*' from the defendant's silence)—unless the judge accepts that they were unfit to give evidence.

The question of whether a witness is fit to give evidence must be distinguished from:

- Concerns about the reliability of their evidence (📖 p.II.120), which might lead to it being excluded (📖 p.IV.318), or admitted only with caution
- Concerns about the vulnerability of the witness (📖 p.II.119), which might lead to the court taking special measures to protect them, such as concealing their identity.

Test of fitness to give evidence

Specific tests have not evolved in each jurisdiction. One model is that provided in E&W by *R v M* (📖 p.App. 3.641), in which the judge ruled that the defendant giving evidence—and by extension, other witnesses—must be able to:

- Understand the questions that are put to them
- Apply their mind to answering them
- Convey intelligibly to the jury the answers they wish to give.

It is not necessary for fitness that a witness's answers should be plausible or believable or reliable, or seen as such by the witness, although this might give rise to separate concerns about the reliability of the evidence.

Problems with the test

The test may not allow for subtleties of disability. There is an analogy with the validity and reliability of police interviews, where suggestibility or compliance (📖 p.II.123), for example, must be taken into account. There is arguably greater protection, therefore, for vulnerable individuals being interrogated by the police than when being cross-examined in court—although it could also be argued that in court the judge is present to ensure fair questioning.

Moreover, conditions such as dysexecutive syndrome, or mild Asperger's syndrome (or, indeed, being from a very different cultural background), might not prevent a witness meeting the criteria, but might still lead to them being unable to stand up appropriately, as would an ordinary defendant, to the rapid, subtle, and pointed cross-examination by a barrister who wishes to discredit their evidence. The impact of such a defendant's relative vulnerability can sometimes be counterbalanced by allowing expert evidence to describe the nature of the defendant's mental disorder and how this may influence their answers to questions and their body language (evidence which may be allowed under current rules on expert evidence, 📖 p.V.531). However, this may not always amount to adequate counterbalancing. Again, special measures may assist, such as allowing frequent breaks for the witness to regain their composure.

Fitness to attend court

A witness who is unfit to give evidence will not be required to attend court, but a defendant may still be expected to attend. For some mentally disordered defendants, therefore, it may be necessary for a psychiatrist to consider whether they are indeed fit to attend court. This is more likely to be an issue with inpatients, where severe psychotic or other symptoms, or suicidal ideation, determine that they cannot safely be allowed to attend court, even with staff escorts.

If you consider that this applies to one of your patients, it is important to communicate this to the clerk of the court in good time, as some hearings will have to be adjourned if the defendant cannot be present, whereas others may still be able to proceed. If you report that a defendant is unfit to attend court it is very helpful to give an indication of how soon the defendant may become fit, in order to allow proceedings to be rescheduled appropriately.

Confessions

A confession is usually thought of as an admission of guilt, but can include any statement by a suspect that is in some way adverse to their legal interests. It may be admitted in evidence if it is relevant and is not excluded by the court. In E&W, NI, and RoI a defendant may be convicted on the basis of a confession alone; in Scotland, confessions, like all evidence, must be corroborated.

- A *genuine confession* is one in which the suspect confesses truthfully.
- A *retracted confession* is one in which the suspect, after having made a confession, later claims that their original confession is untrue. Retracted confessions are common in criminal proceedings.
- A *false confession* is one in which the suspect confesses to a crime they did not commit.

False confessions may lead to unjust and unsafe conviction, and failure to apprehend the actual offender, who may go on to offend again. Genuine and retracted confessions are legally problematic only if they are obtained by threats or coercion, or are otherwise legally unreliable.

False confessions
There are three types of false confessions:
- A *voluntary* false confession occurs in the absence of obvious external pressure, and may result from ulterior motives for being prosecuted (e.g. to protect the true criminal, for financial gain, or public notoriety)
- A *coerced-compliant* confession occurs in full awareness that the confession is false, but where the suspect complies (📖 p.II.124) because of coercion. It can be related to eagerness to please, to a need for self-esteem in the company of others, or to a desire to avoid conflict.
- A *coerced-internalized* confession occurs when the suspect comes to believe (wrongly) that the confession they are making is true. This is usually related to suggestibility (📖 p.II.123) affecting responses during a high-pressure interrogation.

Factors impacting on false confessions
Situational and individual factors, and the interaction between them, can lead to an interviewee making a false confession. The conditions in which the interrogation takes place can therefore be crucial to the veracity of a confession. Demonstrating the trait of being suggestible or compliant is insufficient to show a confession is false; what is also required is demonstration, through analysis of the interviews, that the such traits were operative in making the confession.

Situational factors include the effects of custody and isolation prior to interview; the process of police interrogation; coercion or pressure by the interrogator; and interrogators' prior beliefs that the suspect is guilty (which may lead to giving information about the offence, which is then taken as proof of guilt when repeated by the interviewee).

Individual factors include mental disorder; lacking mental capacity (📖 p.IV.424), e.g. because of learning disability; distress leading to confusing reality with fantasy; guilt leading to false confession as a means of absolution; a desire for publicity or notoriety; and a desire to protect the true perpetrator, out of love or fear or for personal gain.

Individual factors may be beyond the control of the police or other interviewers, but they may be mitigated by requesting an appropriate adult (📖 p.V.453), or by an effective solicitor. A degree of situational pressure may be desirable in interviews where the suspect might lie or dissemble; a balance must be struck between this and risking false confessions, and guidelines such as those under PACE* in E&W aim to assist in this.

Admissibility of confessions†

In *E&W* and *NI*, confessions must be excluded if they were obtained by 'oppression' (torture, coercion, threats etc.) or anything else likely to render them unreliable. Any evidence, including confessions, may be excluded at the court's discretion if it would have too great an adverse effect on fairness. Confessions made by 'mentally handicapped' persons may still be admitted, but the jury or magistrates must be warned that there is a 'special need for caution' before convicting on the basis of it.

In *Scotland*, there are no special rules on the admissibility of confession evidence, and fewer rules of evidence in general (📖 p.IV.317); the main protection against conviction on the basis of false confessions is the requirement of corroborating evidence.

In *RoI*, there are no special rules on the admissibility of confessions, but the jury or court must be warned about any absence of corroboration before convicting.

Assessment of false confession for court reports

An expert psychologist might be required to carry out an assessment of an individual when there concerns about the reliability of a confession. Often a psychiatrist will also be required if there is evidence of mental disorder. In addition to following the usual principles of assessment (📖 p.II.90) and rules for criminal court reports (📖 p.V.569), experts should:

• Ask for copies of the police transcripts and interview tapes—when reviewing or listening to these there should be attention paid to leading or closed questions, undue pressure by the interrogator, and to the possible effects of the absence of an appropriate adult or solicitor

---

* The Police and Criminal Evidence Act 1984 and its associated Codes of Practice. Code C, and Code H in relation to suspected terrorists, are particular relevant to interview procedure.
† SS76–78 PACE in E&W, arts 74–76 PACE(NI)O1989, and s10 Criminal Procedure Act 1993 in RoI.

- Assess individual characteristics that may make the suspect more vulnerable to confessing, using where appropriate psychometric tests (📖 p.II.101) of intelligence, memory, suggestibility and compliance, and assessing mental disorder, especially psychosis or personality disorder.

Capacity to form intent

Psychiatrists and psychologists are often called upon to assess whether the defendant would have been capable of forming the relevant mental element (📖 p.IV.334) of the alleged crime (📖 p.IV.332) at the relevant time. Most often, this involves determining whether they could have formed a particular intent (📖 p.IV.334) at that time.

The legal test

What legal test will be applied will depend on:
- The mens rea (📖 p.IV.334) for the offence, usually specific intent[*] (📖 p.IV.335) or recklessness (📖 p.IV.336), and
- The jurisdiction (broadly speaking, E&W has very detailed, precise definitions of the different mental elements in case law, and Scotland leaves great discretion to the judge, with NI and RoI in between).

Some examples are shown in Box 18.1. Exactly what legal test will apply in a given case should be specified in the written instructions (📖 p.V.558) you receive from your solicitor; if not, ask them to do so.

> ### Box 18.1 Examples of questions on capacity to form the mental element
>
> Did the defendant have the capacity to . . .
> - Intend to kill or cause serious injury? (Murder, E&W, NI or RoI)
> - Kill with wicked recklessness or intent? (Murder, Scotland)
> - Foresee the risk of death a reasonable person would have foreseen? (Manslaughter or culpable homicide)
> - Foresee what a co-defendant might do? (Joint enterprise)
> - Intend the bodily contact that they made? (Battery, ABH, etc.)
> - Reasonably believe the victim consents? (Defence to rape, E&W)
> - Intend life to be endangered? (Arson with intent, E&W or NI)
> - Intend permanently to deprive the owner of property? (Theft).

The role of the psychiatrist

As with all expert evidence, it is important for the psychiatrist only to answer questions within their professional expertise (📖 p.V.533), and not to attempt to answer broader ultimate questions (📖 p.V.543) that are for the court. In this context, a valid question is, would the defendant's mental

---

[*] There is a rule of law, at least in E&W, that psychiatric evidence of incapacity to form intent is usually inadmissible (📖 p.IV.318) in crimes of basic intent (📖 p.IV.335) alone—but this is a concern for your instructing solicitor, not you.

condition at the time have been likely to prevent them forming the relevant mental element?[*]

Symptoms and conditions that might prevent formation of a particular mental element include:

- Specific delusions relating to the knowledge in question, or some other relevant aspect
- An abnormal mood state (severe depression or severe mania) or associated psychomotor agitation or retardation, or impaired concentration that prevents consideration of risks or facts a reasonable person would have considered
- Severe cognitive impairment, e.g. in dementia or chronic schizophrenia.

Notably, changes in mental state brought about solely by voluntary intoxication (📖 p.V.486) are not relevant[†] to the capacity to form a mental element: the doctrine of *prior fault* states that the defendant should have foreseen the increased likelihood of criminal behaviour while intoxicated.

> Mrs Smith suffers from agitated depression. She goes shopping at the local supermarket, but walks out without paying, distracted by ruminations on her sense of guilt and worthlessness. She is charged with shoplifting, but acquitted when the court accepts psychiatric evidence that she was at that moment incapable of intending permanently to deprive the supermarket of their property because of her depressive ruminations. (If she had not been distracted but, in fact, intended to take the items in order to be punished, then she would be guilty, even though her motivation was pathologically determined.)
>
> Mr Richards has schizoaffective disorder and forms a delusion that his body is covered by beautiful, iridescent fish scales. He therefore goes outside without needing to wear clothes, and is arrested for indecent exposure. He is acquitted when the court accepts psychiatric evidence that at that moment he could not have intended that others see his naked body, because of his delusion.

Incapacity and public policy

Evidence of incapacity to form a mental element is most usually sought in relatively minor offences. This is because the result is an outright acquittal, which legislatures see as unacceptable in the case of people with mental disorders who cause serious harm to others; legal mechanisms are therefore provided in many cases to allow their detention in prison or in hospital. Examples include the partial defence to murder of diminished responsibility (📖 p.IV.391), the insanity (📖 p.IV.389) defence, and the Scottish order for the urgent detention of acquitted persons (📖 p.IV.408).

---

[*] The key question is whether a psychiatric condition would have prevented the defendant forming the mental element Evidence that they actually did so is in theory irrelevant, although clear evidence should be taken into account (and will probably be raised in cross-examination).
[†] There are two main exceptions to this rule: specific intent (📖 p.IV.335) and mistaken belief (📖 p.IV.343), as explained on 📖 p.V.487.

Automatism

An action which the mind of the defendant did not will is an automatism: the body is said to have moved involuntarily. Automatism is a full defence (📖 p.IV.342) to any offence, provided there is a total lack of control: partial control rules it out (*A-G's Reference*, 📖 p.App. 3.629). Automatism can be caused by physical or mental disorder, but not voluntary intoxication (📖 p.V.486).

Insane versus non-insane automatisms

Automatisms are *insane*, resulting in a finding of not guilty by reason of insanity (📖 p.V.489)[*], or *non-insane*, resulting in acquittal.[†] The distinction is a legal, not a medical one, based upon whether the cause of the automatism is a 'disease of the mind'. The cause is a disease of the mind if:

- The cause was 'intrinsic' to the defendant's mind (*R v Quick*, 📖 p.App. 3.644); i.e. where there was no 'external blow', either physical or mental, or
- the cause of the automatism resulted in violence and is prone to recur (*Bratty v A-G NI*, 📖 p.App. 3.632)

Medico-legal incongruence

The distinction between intrinsic and extrinsic causes is incoherent from a medical point of view. For example, consider a man with BPD (📖 p.II.61) who, hoping to manipulate others, deliberately takes an excess of insulin and becomes hypoglycaemic, in which state he assaults his victim. Does the insulin make the automatism non-insane, or the PD make it insane?

Likewise, is an epileptic fit triggered by a drug such as cardiazol insane because of the fit, or non-insane because of the drug? Or is hypoglycaemia caused by Zollinger–Ellison syndrome (an insulin-secreting pancreatic tumour) insane because the source is intrinsic to the body, or non-insane because it is extrinsic to the brain?

Epilepsy Most doctors would not classify epilepsy as a disease of the mind, or as 'insanity', and it is not a ground for detention under mental health law (📖 p.IV.373). Someone with epilepsy who kills during an insane automatism might not be detainable, and the alternative supervision order (📖 p.IV.409) might not be adequate to protect the public.

Dissociation As Box 18.2 shows, dissociation can be an insane automatism, or if it is triggered by a severe external blow, a non-insane automatism. Moreover, if the defendant has drunk alcohol and this contributed to the dissociation then the automatism defence might still be available even though voluntary intoxication is usually no defence.

Scotland and RoI

Scottish law does not recognize insane automatism as such; defendants must raise the defence of insanity instead. In Scottish law, the defence of (non-insane) automatism requires:

- An external factor causing loss of reason that must not be self-induced and could not be foreseen, and

---

[*] This raises the question, what is the legal difference between an insane automatism and insanity? The legal rules for insanity (e.g. the McNaughten rules) apply in both cases: but only those cases of insanity in which the defendant's actions are involuntary will also be cases of (insane) automatism.
[†] Provided, if non-insane, it has a 'feature of novelty or accident' (*R v Hennessy*, 📖 p.App. 3.638).

Box 18.2 Insane versus non-insane automatisms

Insane automatisms	Non-insane automatisms
An epileptic fit (R v Sullivan, 🕮 p.App. 3.646)	Concussion after head injury
Arteriosclerosis causing transient ischaemia (R v Kemp, 🕮 p.App. 3.639)	Hypoglycaemia after taking insulin without food (R v Quick, 🕮 p.App. 3.644)
Parasomnias (🕮 p.II.83) such as sleep walking (R v Burgess, 🕮 p.App. 3.632)	
Dissociation caused by 'ordinary stresses and disappointments' (R v Rabey, 🕮 p.App. 3.644)	Dissociation that is precipitated by an unusual external stressor such as rape (R v T, 🕮 p.App. 3.646)

- A resulting 'total alienation of reason' amounting to a complete loss of self-control, demonstrated by expert medical evidence.

Courts in RoI have recognized the distinction but have also, as in Scotland, often only accepted non-insane conditions as automatisms.

Resolving contentious issues

Issues such as those discussed may give rise to confusion at the medico-legal interface (🕮 p.IV.299). However, any confusion is for the court to unravel and not the expert, who should always remain within the limits of psychiatric opinion. Describe the medical condition and its precipitation (if any) and leave the court to determine whether the automatism was insane or not, or not an automatism at all, as illustrated in the example that follows.

B suffered a head injury in a car accident and developed organic PD. He now experiences dissociation triggered by being in a car. Whilst driving one day, he dissociates, and is charged with dangerous driving.

Psychiatric issues
- What is the diagnosis, including the sequelae of head injury?
- How does the diagnosis relate to the alleged behaviour?

Legal issues (for the court, not the psychiatrist, to determine)
- Was there a total loss of control, resulting in automatism?
- If so, do the head injury and its consequences make it an *insane* automatism?
- Or, if the accident was very recent, could the external trigger of getting into a car make it a *non-insane* automatism?
- Does the voluntary act of getting into the car remove the defence, in that he should have known that he was at risk of dissociation?

Involuntary intoxication

Intoxication with drugs or alcohol alters a person's mental state, and may well have an impact on their decision to commit an unlawful act. However, being intoxicated is not straightforwardly a legal defence (☐ p.IV.342): under the *prior fault* rule, people who voluntarily ingest substances are usually held responsible for their behaviour while intoxicated, whilst those who become intoxicated involuntarily are usually not.

When is intoxication 'involuntary'?

Intoxication is presumed to be voluntary (that is, intentional or reckless) unless there is clear evidence that the defendant was unaware of the risk of becoming intoxicated. Examples of involuntary intoxication include:

- Someone else putting alcohol into a soft drink unbeknownst to the defendant
- A would-be rapist drugging the defendant's drink with flunitrazepam (Rohypnol®)
- Taking a drug prescribed by a medical practitioner (even though the drug is taken voluntarily, the law treats it as involuntary because the drug is taken on the professional advice of the prescribing doctor)
- Using a substance that is not dangerous* and does not normally cause intoxication, unless the use was itself reckless for some reason
- Using a substance on which one is dependent (☐ p.II.56), if there is an 'irresistible impulse' to take it (*R v Tandy*, ☐ p.App. 3.646).

However, simply because an alcoholic drink was much stronger than expected, or by extension cannabis was more potent than expected, does not make the intoxication involuntary. The prior fault was it taking the substance at all.

---

* A 'dangerous' drug is one where it is 'common knowledge' that the person using them 'may become aggressive or do dangerous or unpredictable things' or become incapable of appreciating risks; amphetamines and LSD have been held to be 'dangerous drugs'. Diazepam has been held to be 'non-dangerous' (*R v Hardie*, ☐ p.App. 3.637).

When is involuntary intoxication a defence?

If the degree of intoxication is sufficient to make it clear that the defendant was not in the state of mind (📖 p.IV.334) required for the crime, and the intoxication was involuntary, then the defendant will be acquitted.[*]

Evidence of involuntary intoxication may be taken as evidence that the necessary state of mind was absent, but it does not prove it to be so; the fact of the intoxication must be weighed alongside the other available evidence, which might show that the defendant did, on balance, have the necessary mens rea (as, for example, in *R v Kingston*, 📖 p.App. 3.640, where despite it being accepted that the defendant was involuntarily intoxicated, he was convicted on the basis of photographic and audio evidence that the jury held showed he did in fact intend to commit indecent assault).

Where involuntary intoxication is insufficient for acquittal it may sometimes still be a mitigating factor (📖 p.V.506) sufficient to reduce the sentence.

Voluntary intoxication

The underlying principle is that the courts hold defendants responsible for their behaviour while intoxicated, unless they can show that their intoxication was involuntary (📖 p.V.485) and therefore not their fault.

However, it is not simply a matter of ignoring the voluntary intoxication as legally irrelevant. In many cases it will not be straightforward, or perhaps even possible, to determine the state of mind of the defendant while they are intoxicated and while they are committing the actus reus (📖 p.IV.332) of the offence. The courts have therefore devised a set of somewhat arbitrary rules governing such situations. These are followed strictly in E&W and often in NI; similar principles are observed in Scotland and RoI, but much more flexibly, so as to enable the court to reach whatever result it deems just.

Mens rea and 'Dutch courage'

As a general rule, the mental element of the offence (📖 p.IV.334) must still be proved; if it cannot be shown that the defendant possessed the relevant mens rea, then they cannot be convicted. However, the courts have established two major exceptions to this rule:

- If there is evidence that the defendant formed the mens rea for the offence beforehand, then deliberately became intoxicated in order to overcome their inhibitions and went on to commit the offence, they can be convicted on the basis of their earlier mens rea.[†] This was famously described as seeking 'Dutch courage' by Lord Denning
- If the criminal behaviour can be seen as a 'natural and probable' consequence of becoming voluntarily intoxicated, the defendant can be presumed to have intended or foreseen (i.e. been reckless, 📖 p.IV.336, as to) that behaviour, as happened in *DPP v Majewski* (📖 p.App. 3.641)

---

[*] For this purpose (and in contrast to the rules on voluntary intoxication, 📖 p.V.486) it is irrelevant whether the offence is one of specific or of basic intent (📖 p.IV.335).

[†] This is also an exception to the usual rule that the defendant must be shown to have the relevant mens rea at the time of the relevant acts or omissions (the actus reus, 📖 p.IV.332).

when the defendant drank heavily and then assaulted police officers, and in *R v Hardie* (📖 p.App. 3.637).

Mistake and specific intent

If *and only if* neither of the exceptions just mentioned applies, then a lack of evidence of the required mens rea leads to acquittal, even if it is clear that the lack was due to voluntary intoxication. This means, for example, that:

- If voluntary intoxication causes the defendant to form a mistaken belief (📖 p.IV.343) that negates an element of the offence, they will be acquitted. For example, a person who genuinely believes (because of the influence of drink or drugs) that they own the property they are smashing cannot be convicted of criminal damage (📖 p.IV.350).
- If the offence is one of specific intent (📖 p.IV.335) and there is evidence that the defendant was not capable of forming that intent (📖 p.V.481) because they were intoxicated, they will be acquitted. For example, a grossly drunk man who clearly cannot control his behaviour and who drops a lit cigarette into a pool of brandy he spilt earlier, causing a major fire, would be acquitted of arson with intent (📖 p.IV.350), although he might still be convicted of simple arson.

In very few cases, however, will voluntary intoxication be accepted as a defence to a crime of specific intent: a very high degree of intoxication is required. The courts have held that:

- The degree of intoxication required is not defined by any particular blood alcohol level (because tolerance can vary between individuals due to varying metabolic rates and varying cerebral susceptibility).
- Ordinary evidence showing the defendant exercised a degree of control over their actions will neutralize the defence.

Expert evidence

In cases involving voluntary intoxication, you should comment upon capacity to form intent (📖 p.V.481), not on whether the defendant actually formed a specific intent, which is for the court to determine. There may, for example, be ordinary evidence showing that intention was formed, which goes against expert evidence that he lacked the capacity to do so.

Scotland and RoI

These rules are often interpreted leniently in RoI and Scotland, where for example even recklessly voluntarily intoxicated defendants have been convicted of lesser offences (e.g. manslaughter instead of murder) where this was thought just in the circumstances.

Intoxication and specific defences

Intoxication has to be distinguished from mental disorder per se precipitated by substances (such as substance dependence, or a drug-induced psychotic episode), and from the effects of chronic brain damage resultant from chronic substance (usually alcohol) abuse. The general rule, in relation to specific defences (📖 p.IV.342), is that such mental disorder or brain damage is relevant to the defences, but the intoxication itself is not, even, in some cases, if it was involuntary (📖 p.V.485).[*]

Diminished responsibility

Mental disorder resulting from intoxication

Intoxication-related mental disorder or chronic brain damage can amount to an 'abnormality of mental functioning' (E&W, NI), and is obviously a mental disorder for the purposes of diminished responsibility (📖 p.V.491) in RoI. If the conditions of the defence are otherwise met (e.g. because of schizophrenia), the fact that the defendant is also intoxicated does not negate the defence (R v Dietschmann, 📖 p.App. 3.634).

In Scotland, any disorder arising solely from intoxication is specifically excluded from the defence.

Intoxication as a recognized medical condition

In Scotland, the position is clear: the definition of the partial defence excludes intoxication. However, the definitions in NI and E&W[†] are based on the concept of a 'recognized medical condition', and in RoI on 'mental disorder'. This raises the possibility that a plea of diminished responsibility might succeed if experts were prepared to state that acute intoxication was a mental disorder or a recognized medical condition, based perhaps on its presence in both ICD10 and DSM-IV (📖 p.App. 1.601).

On a strict literal interpretation of the wording of the statute in each case, acute intoxication could perhaps be accepted as a foundation for diminished responsibility; but it seems far more likely that the Court of Appeal would rule that Parliament[‡] could not have intended such a major change to a well-established rule without stating this explicitly, and that therefore the legal interpretation of 'recognized medical condition' excludes acute intoxication.

Automatism

If the automatism (📖 p.V.483) is induced solely by involuntary intoxication, it is a non-insane automatism, and the defendant will therefore be acquitted (assuming the criteria for automatism are met, i.e. there is evidence that the defendant totally lacked any control over their behaviour). If, however, the automatism was induced solely by voluntary intoxication, the automatism is no defence, and the defendant may be convicted.

An automatism induced by intoxication-related mental disorder or chronic brain damage will be an insane automatism (📖 p.V.483).

Insanity

Intoxication, no matter how severe, cannot cause insanity (📖 p.V.489) on its own because it is not legally a 'disease of the mind' (R v Quick, 📖 p.App. 3.644). However, intoxication-related mental disorder or brain damage may form the basis of a defence of insanity.

---

[*] However, involuntary intoxication (📖 p.V.485) may act as a general defence in the same case, if it negates an element of mens rea (📖 p.IV.334).
[†] That is, the new tests in E&W and NI are defined thus. Cases or appeals heard under the old test (📖 p.V.491) would not succeed on the basis of acute intoxication, as that is not a condition of arrested or retarded development of mind, an inherent cause, or induced by disease or injury.
[‡] Or in RoI, that the Court of Criminal Appeal would rule that the Dáil could not have intended this in relation to 'mental disorder'.

Unlawful killing while voluntarily intoxicated (NI)

This statutory provision[*], which only applies in NI, concerns people who at the time of a killing are temporarily insane as a result of voluntary intoxication.—that is, they are 'labouring under such a defect of reason . . . as not to know the nature and quality of [their] act [or, that it] was wrong' because of voluntary intoxication. If before becoming intoxicated they had the intention of killing or causing serious harm, they will be convicted of murder (this is equivalent to the Dutch courage rule, 📖 p.V.486), otherwise they will be convicted of manslaughter. In other jurisdictions, such defendants could still be convicted of murder.

Insanity

Insanity is a legal concept expressing a highly cognitive test. The threshold is also high, such that so that it very limited in its application even to severely psychotic defendants. Since automatism and insanity are the only mental condition defences (📖 p.IV.342) to offences other than murder there is potentially a gap in justice, reflected in the many convictions of severely mentally disordered defendants.

The McNaughten rules

The McNaughten rules have long been a standard test for criminal liability in relation to mentally disordered defendants in common law jurisdictions, with some minor adjustments, and continue to apply in E&W and NI. When satisfied, the accused is found not guilty by reason of insanity.

> *McNaughten rules, 1843*
> At the time of the committing of the act, the party accused was labouring under such a *defect of reason*, from *disease of the mind*, as not *to know the nature and quality of the act* he was doing, or, if he did know it, that he did not know what he was doing *was wrong*.

Defect of reason excludes all aspects of mental functioning other than reasoning and unlike in diminished responsibility (📖 p.V.491) is not 'the mind in all its aspects' (*R v Byrne*, 📖 p.App. 3.632). Uncontrollable urges do not amount to a defect of reason.

Disease of the mind includes diseases of both the mind and brain:
- Arteriosclerosis of the brain (*R v Kemp*, 📖 p.App. 3.639)
- Epilepsy (*R v Sullivan*, 📖 p.App. 3.646)
- Hyperglycaemia in untreated diabetes (*R v Hennessy*, 📖 p.App. 3.638)
- Sleepwalking (*R v Burgess*; 📖 p.App. 3.632, cf. automatism, 📖 p.IV.483), but
- *Not* external factors, eg insulin-induced hypoglycaemia (*Quick*, 📖 p.App. 3.644).

Not knowing the nature of quality of the act suggests, for example, being deluded about the act itself or the object of the act.

[*] Criminal Justice Act (Northern Ireland) 1966, s6.

Wrong means legally, not morally wrong (*R v Windle,* 📖 p.App. 3.648).

- If the delusions do not prevent the defendant from having mens rea there will be no defence, Psychosis may explain the behaviour but not prevent the defendant knowing that their actions were legally wrong
- Evidence of stopping when the police arrive would also suggest knowing that the act was illegal.

The meaning of *knowing*, narrowly interpreted, is straightforward. However, it is open to question whether someone driven to offend by powerful delusions or other psychotic symptoms appreciates or is paying attention to his knowledge that the act is unlawful.

Other forms of the insanity defence

Scotland Criminal Justice and Licensing (Scotland) Act 2010
Scotland has adopted a statutory test equivalent to insanity referred to as the 'special defence', and has abolished insanity as a legal term. The definition is accompanied by specific exclusion from this defence of personality disorder that is characterized solely or principally by abnormally aggressive or seriously irresponsible conduct.

> **Section 51A CJLSA**
> A person is not criminally responsible for conduct constituting an offence, and is to be acquitted of the offence, if the person was at the time of the conduct unable by reason of mental disorder to appreciate the nature or wrongfulness of the conduct.

RoI Criminal law (Insanity) Act 2006
- The accused was suffering at the time from a mental disorder, and
- The mental disorder was such that the accused ought not to be held responsible for the act alleged by reason of the fact that he or she—
  - Did not know the nature and quality of the act, or
  - Did not know that what he or she was doing was wrong, or
  - Was unable to refrain from committing the act.

Procedures

E&W Criminal Procedure (Insanity) Act 1964 (as amended)
- Raised by defence, prosecution or judge
- Jury may disagree with unanimous medical evidence if justified
- Burden of proof on the defence once the issue is raised

Scotland Criminal Procedure (Scotland) Act 1995
- Written/oral evidence of two or more registered medical practitioners
- Jury decision.

NI Mental Health (Northern Ireland) Order 1986
- Oral evidence of one and written/oral evidence of another doctor
- Jury decision.

RoI Criminal law (insanity) Act (2006)
- Oral evidence of one consultant psychiatrist
- Jury decision.

Outcome following a finding of insanity

E&W, NI, and Scotland
- Hospital order (compulsion order in Scotland)
- Hospital/compulsion order with restrictions (in E&W these are mandatory if the charge was murder and a hospital order is appropriate)
- Interim hospital or compulsion order
- Guardianship
- Supervision order (supervision and treatment order in Scotland)
- Absolute discharge.

RoI
- Initial committal to a designated centre for not more than 14 days for inpatient or outpatient care or treatment.

Diminished responsibility

Diminished responsibility is a partial defence (☐ p.IV.343) to murder (☐ p.IV.345)—and to no other offence. If pleaded successfully, the defendant is instead convicted of manslaughter (culpable homicide in Scotland), and therefore avoids a mandatory life sentence (☐ p.IV.365).

The partial defence can only be raised by the defence, not the prosecution[*] or the judge; the defence will succeed if it can be shown on the balance of probabilities (☐ p.IV.316) that the defendant meets the criteria shown as follows (which vary by jurisdiction). As only the defence can raise the issue, and given the possibility that the defendant who lacks insight may refuse to plead 'diminished' despite supportive psychiatric reports, it is always important to assess their fitness to plead (☐ p.V.474).

Tests of diminished responsibility

E&W and NI S52,53 Coroners and Justice Act 2009
This new test (☐ p.V.494) applies to offences committed from 4.10.10 in E&W; and 1.6.11 in NI.

A defendant, D, is not to be convicted of murder (but only manslaughter) if D was suffering from an *abnormality of mental functioning* which:
- Arose from a *recognized medical condition*
- *Substantially impaired* D's *ability* to understand the nature of D's conduct; to form a rational judgement; or to exercise self-control, and
- Provides an *explanation* for D's acts and omissions in doing or being a party to the killing (meaning that it caused, or was a significant contributory factor in causing, D to carry out that conduct).

E&W and NI S2 Homicide Act 1957; S5 Criminal Justice Act (NI) 1966
This test applies to offences committed in E&W before 4.10.10 and in NI before 1.6.11 (and therefore to appeals for some years to come).

---

[*] Except in a case in E&W in which the defendant pleads insanity alone, when s6 of the Criminal Procedure (Insanity) Act 1964 allows the prosecution to raise diminished responsibility as an alternative.

A defendant shall not be convicted of murder if:
- He was suffering from such *abnormality of mind**
- (whether arising from a condition of arrested or retarded development of mind or any inherent cause or induced by disease or injury)
- As *substantially impaired* his *mental responsibility* for his acts and omissions in doing or being a party to the killing.

Scotland *Galbraith v HM Advocate* (📖 p.App. 3.637)
Diminished responsibility requires:
- An *abnormality of mind*, other than one caused solely by the consumption of drink or drugs, or by psychopathic personality disorder (📖 p.II.66)
- Which need not 'border on insanity', and
- Which has the effect that the accused's *ability to determine or control* his actions was *substantially impaired*.

RoI *S6 Criminal Law (Insanity) Act 2006*
If the jury or court finds that a defendant charged with murder:
- Did the act alleged
- Was at the time suffering from a *mental disorder*, and
- That disorder did not amount to insanity (📖 p.V.489), but
- It *diminished substantially* his or her *responsibility* for the act,

the jury or court, shall find them not guilty of murder, but guilty of manslaughter on the ground of diminished responsibility.

Which mental disorders qualify?

'Abnormality of mind' has been defined as 'a state of mind so different from that of ordinary human beings that the reasonable man would term it abnormal', and as covering 'the mind in all its aspects': *R v Byrne* (📖 p.App. 3.632). This is not therefore a medical test, but requires medical evidence in support of it (*R v Dix*, 📖 p.App. 3.634). It includes abnormalities of consciousness, perception, cognition, mood and volition. It has been interpreted loosely, such that the courts have allowed the following examples to qualify in the UK:
- Schizophrenia and paranoid psychosis (*R v Sanderson*, 📖 p.App. 3.645)
- Paranoid personality disorder (*R v Martin (Anthony)*, 📖 p.App. 3.641)
- Pre-menstrual stress and post-natal depression (*R v Reynolds*, 📖 p.App. 3.644)
- Battered woman syndrome (*R v Ahluwalia*, 📖 p.App. 3.629)
- Chronic alcoholism causing brain damage (*R v Tandy*, 📖 p.App. 3.646)
- Irresistible perverted sexual desires (*R v Byrne*, 📖 p.App. 3.632).

Intoxication, whether voluntary (📖 p.V.486) or involuntary (📖 p.V.485), is insufficient, but mental disorder or brain damage arising from substance misuse may qualify in E&W, NI, and RoI.

In RoI, there was no defence of diminished responsibility at common law; there is therefore very little case law to date on what mental disorders are accepted. It is also uncertain which disorders will qualify

---

* In NI, the phrase 'mental abnormality' is used, and is not limited to the list of causes in the next bullet point.

under the reformed test (📖 p.V.494) in E&W and NI, or how the defence will be interpreted in other ways.

Who decides?

There is much case law which emphasizes that, even in the presence of unanimous medical evidence supporting diminished responsibility, it is a decision for the jury to take (most recently, *R v Khan*, 📖 p.App. 3.639). This is at least partly because the jury may reject evidence suggesting symptoms upon which the doctors rely, or because they see the abnormality as less severe than do the doctors, or because they balance other explanations for the killing (such as evidence of longstanding enmity) against the mental abnormality. Whether this ruling still applies, or applies as comprehensively, to the reformed defence (📖 p.V.494) is not yet clear.

Effect of the plea of diminished responsibility

The prosecution may accept the plea if the weight of medical evidence is sufficient, in which case the court will proceed directly to sentencing.* If the prosecution does not accept the plea, the jury will decide the issue.

The sentencing options range from absolute discharge to discretionary life imprisonment, or treatment in hospital (📖 p.IV.405). It is not uncommon for a plea of diminished responsibility to be accepted and for the defendant still be to sentenced to imprisonment—for instance, because the mental condition was a temporary one, or because the defendant does not satisfy mental health legislation criteria for detention (which are very different from definitions of 'diminished responsibility').

Controversies in Scotland and RoI

The defence has generally been used very flexibly in these jurisdictions, with much responsibility resting on juries to follow, or reject even unanimous medical evidence as they see fit. Unlike in E&W, where there was a significant amount of case law concerning the old test, and where there is likely to be substantial argument over interpretation of the reformed test (📖 p.V.494), there has been far less legal debate in Scotland and RoI.

- In Scotland, there has been some limited debate over the exclusion of psychopathy (or effectively ASPD more widely)
- In RoI, there has been some disquiet over sentencing after a finding of diminished responsibility: there is no option to send the defendant to hospital (although they may be transferred from prison, 📖 p.IV.410), and sentencing guidelines do not take the mental element of the crime into account in determining the length of imprisonment.

---

* Providing that the judge also accepts the plea. Very occasionally the judge refuses to do so, most famously in the case of Peter Sutcliffe (the 'Yorkshire Ripper'). There was therefore a trial within which the Crown attacked the opinion of both the defence and prosecution experts, whose evidence they had earlier indicated that they accepted. Sutcliffe was convicted of 13 murders and 7 attempted murders and given multiple sentences of life imprisonment. It is unclear whether the judge has a general power to refuse to accept the plea, or whether the Sutcliffe case was wrongly decided, as some lawyers allege.

Frequency of the finding

The number of cases successfully pleaded in E&W, either with the agreement of the Crown or at trial, has steadily diminished in recent decades (under the old test). There is no clear explanation for this. However, it may relate to changing social attitudes, and a reduced willingness for juries to accept what appear to be excuses for killing. Another may be the increased tendency of the CPS to see its performance as reflected in 'targets', as with other public services, with the achievement of convictions for murder being valued within such targets more highly than 'accepted diminished responsibility'. It remains to be seen whether the reformed test will lead to a resurgence in the numbers of successful pleas, or further decline. Which occurs may be determined in part by interpretation of the new defence by the Court of Appeal.

Reform of diminished responsibility

The background to reform in E&W and NI

The Law Commission recommended modernizing diminished responsibility in the light of developing medical and psychological knowledge. The essence of the reform is the removal of 'impaired mental responsibility' from the test, in favour of 'impaired mental capacities'. The reformed defence:

- Invokes the dynamic notion of abnormality of *mental functioning* (as opposed to the status of having an 'abnormality of mind')
- Requires the abnormality to arise from a *recognized medical condition*
- Limits the defence to *substantial impairment of the* ability to understand conduct or form a rational judgement (in cognitive terms akin to the insanity defence, 📖 p.V.489), or to exercise self-control, and
- Requires that the abnormality of mental functioning provides an explanation for the killing (i.e. *caused* it or was a substantial contributory factor in causing it).

The new defence (📖 p.V.491) is 'medical' rather than 'moral', more complex than the old test, and will require considerable interpretation by the Court of Appeal. It is unclear how it will operate in practice, and whether it will be interpreted more or less narrowly than the old test.

Controversial changes to the defence

Flexibility and the moral element

The old test[*] allowed a jury to strike a balance between medical and non-medical explanations of a killing, in pursuit of natural justice. The medical specificity of the new test may reduce its flexibility, and, depending how it is interpreted, may also reduce the scope for such balancing.

---

[*] '. . . suffering from such abnormality of mind (whether arising from a condition of arrested or retarded development of mind or any inherent causes or induced by disease or injury) as substantially impaired his mental responsibility . . .'

A man with psychopathy (📖 p.II.66) has killed his wife and children by dousing them with petrol and setting them alight, after finding out that his wife was having an affair.

Under the old test, a jury could accept that he had an abnormality of mind, but decide that it did not sufficiently impair his mental responsibility for the offence, taking a moral stance on psychopathy. Under the new test, the jury may be limited to considering whether psychopathy substantially impaired his ability to understand his conduct, form a rational judgement or exercise self-control, and, if they accept evidence that psychopathy causes violence, have little choice but to accept the plea of diminished responsibility.

A similar situation could arise with, say, a defendant with depression. Previously a jury could accept the diagnosis and its effects, but balance that evidence against evidence of an ordinary motivation to kill (e.g. for reasons of jealousy or financial gain); under the new test, such balancing may not be possible, so that the jury has to find in favour of the defence on the basis that the depressive illness was 'a substantial contributory factor', even though there were other factors. The removal of the moral element in favour of an 'incapacity' test may therefore have the effect of expanding the role of expert evidence.

Reliability
The loss of flexibility in the defence is likely to reduce the variability in outcomes between similar defendants, making the defence more reliable. However, this may be achieved at the expense of restricting the scope of the defence to a narrower range of qualifying mental conditions and incapacities, limiting the number of defendants to whom it is available. This will prove less, or not the case if the word 'substantial' is interpreted in similar terms to its interpretation in the old defence, that is 'less than total but more than trivial' (*R v Lloyd*, 📖 p.App. 3.640).

Developmental immaturity
Contrary to the Law Commission's recommendations, the new test does not allow a plea of diminished responsibility based on normal developmental immaturity (i.e. not amounting to a recognized medical condition). This means that a 10-year-old boy who, when emotionally overwhelmed, was substantially impaired in his ability to exercise self-control will not be able to plead the defence, whereas an adult psychopath might be able to do so. The inequity of this is emphasized by the fact that both the boy and the adult may each satisfy all the other elements of the defence and yet only the adult psychopath be able to benefit from it.

Particular areas of uncertainty

In addition to areas of uncertainty already described on the previous page, the interpretation of the legal elements in Box 18.3, and therefore the scope and operation of the defence, will remain unclear until cases are heard by the Court of Appeal.

> **Box 18.3 Aspects of the new test likely to require judicial interpretation**
>
> - What will be the threshold for mental functioning to be deemed abnormal? Would merely statistical deviation from the norm suffice, so long as there was a 'recognized medical condition', or will it have to be qualitatively abnormal in some way, and how abnormal?
> - Will 'substantially' impaired continue to mean 'less than total but more than trivial' (*R v Lloyd*, 📖 p.App. 3.640), or will its meaning change in the context of the new test?
> - Will diagnoses which have a literature and had been accepted under the old test (for instance, 'battered woman syndrome') be excluded from recognized medical conditions because they are not (perhaps yet) included in diagnostic classifications such as the ICD or DSM?
> - What does it mean to 'understand' one's own conduct? Will an intellectual understanding suffice, or will an appreciation (perhaps a moral appreciation) be required?
> - What is the relationship between 'provides an explanation' and 'caused (or was a significant contributory factor in causing)'? Does the former infer determining the 'predominant' cause, allowing the jury still to balance medical against other causes? Or will a threshold approach (because it is required only that the recognized medical condition was a contributory factor) be adopted?
> - Will 'causes' be interpreted in scientific terms? (In which case will causation ever be capable of proof?) Or will it be interpreted as in psychiatry, in terms of a narrative of the offence incorporating the abnormality of mental functioning? Or will causation (📖 p.V.513) be interpreted in the sense developed in negligence law and elsewhere?

Expert evidence in diminished responsibility

Diminished responsibility rests (perhaps more so within the reformed defence in E&W and NI), upon well-informed psychiatric expert evidence (📖 p.V.534). If you are instructed to prepare a psychiatric report in relation to a plea of diminished responsibility, we recommend that you follow these guidelines.

Who interviews when?

The simple rule is, whether you are instructed by prosecution or defence, you should interview the defendant at the earliest opportunity, and ideally without reading a report of another expert instructed.

It is common for psychiatrists instructed by the Crown to wait until they have received a report from a psychiatrist instructed by the defence before assessing the defendant, reflecting the legal process of the defence raising the defence and the Crown potentially then rebutting it. However, this practice invites an approach driven by the question of whether there is a basis upon which to counter the defence report—rather than producing an unbiased, independent opinion uninfluenced by the opinion of any other expert.

It is best practice, therefore, to asses independent of the opinion of any other expert, even when instructed by the Crown after a defence report has been submitted. If you are instructed by the defence and the Crown expert insists on seeing the report of the defence expert before carrying out their own assessment then you may wish initially to submit only a brief interim report summarizing your opinion but without including any data. This puts the Crown on notice of the opinion, and you can then submit the full report in parallel with that of the other psychiatrist.

Evidence about what?

Under the previous diminished responsibility defence it was important to avoid addressing the ultimate issue (📖 p.V.543)—that is, giving an opinion on whether the defendant met the criteria for diminished responsibility. Good practice was to limit expert evidence to describing the abnormality of mind, plus any narrative of the offence to which that abnormality appeared relevant, leaving the jury to draw its own conclusion as to whether or not this amounted to diminished responsibility, balancing the medical evidence against other explanations for the defendant's conduct[*] and translating a medical narrative into a moral conclusion.

The reformed defence has abolished the distinction between these two 'limbs' of the defence (the quasi-medical and the moral) by removing the moral element (other than in the title of the defence). Psychiatrists are free therefore, because of 'medicalizing' of the defence, to address all of the elements.

---

[*] This does not mean that, if the defendant denies the killing, it is not feasible to describe or interpret any evidence that may bear on diminished responsibility (as some experts refuse to do). By giving this evidence, you do not presume that they did kill the victim; you only explain to the court that *if* it finds that they did the killing, there is evidence that their responsibility for having done so might have been (or might not have been) substantially impaired.

Discussing the alleged offence

Experts sometimes worry about whether it is appropriate to ask the defendant about the alleged offence, in case it prejudices the case in some way, or in case they breach the *Turner* rule (📖 p.V.536): giving expert evidence on a matter within the ordinary experience and knowledge of the jury. However, it is appropriate to ask about the offence, first because the defendant's account of the alleged offence may itself reveal symptoms of mental disorder at the time (e.g. apparent delusional beliefs, or hallucinations, or misperceptions); second, because it will be necessary to develop an understanding (including through the defendant's own description) of what may be the relationship (under the new defence, the causal relationship) between the mental abnormality and the killing. Inferences drawn by an expert from such information will not breach the *Turner* rule, as they are not within the ordinary experience and knowledge of the jury. Neither does rehearsing such information in front of the jury contravene the hearsay rule (since the account is given not as being 'true' but as part of the basis upon which the expert has formed his opinion).

Causation in E&W and NI

The reformed test (📖 p.V.494) of diminished responsibility in E&W and NI explicitly requires experts to consider causation (i.e. whether the abnormality of mental functioning 'provides an explanation' for, or 'caused or was a contributory factor in causing' the killing). However, causation is a legal, not a medical concept (📖 p.IV.296). A psychiatric expert may only be able to express an opinion in terms of a narrative of the offence which incorporates the abnormality of mental functioning.

Considering disposal

Instructions from solicitors in a murder trial will typically focus on the question of diminished responsibility rather than on sentencing. However, if an expert's findings are supportive of diminished responsibility it may seem natural then also to offer an opinion on disposal (📖 p.V.555) in the event that defence were to be successful. However, if then recommendation is not for hospital admission (📖 p.IV.405), this may prejudice the defence by giving the false impression that the defendant was not truly, or seriously mentally disordered at the time at the time of the killing. It is therefore wise to exclude such a recommendation from the report unless there has been a specific request from instructing solicitors to do otherwise. It will always be possible to provide a separate sentencing report after conviction.

Loss of self-control & provocation

The common law developed the concept of provocation in the 17th century, when murder carried the death penalty; as a 'concession to human frailty' it partly excused 'loss of mastery over the mind in response to things said or done', and resulted in a manslaughter (📖 p.IV.345) conviction.[*] Over time, the defence became viewed first as too restrictive,[†] and then as too subjective,[‡] such that it was heavily criticized on various policy grounds.[§] It has been modified by statute in E&W and NI,[**] although it.has evolved more gradually in Scotland and RoI.

Tests of provocation

Scotland Robertson v HM Advocate (📖 p.App. 3.644)

- Provocation requires a *loss of self-control*, and . . .
- A reasonably *proportionate* (i.e. not grossly disproportionate) *relationship* between the provocation and the reaction to it.
- There is no requirement to show that an ordinary person might have acted in the same way (*Gillon* 📖 p.App. 3.637)
- It is unclear whether a long period of domestic violence can amount to provocation, as it can in E&W and NI but cannot in RoI
- A successful plea of provocation usually results in a conviction for culpable homicide, but could sometimes still be for murder (*Drury*, 📖 p.App. 3.635).

---

[*] In other jurisdictions, including some US and Australian states, provocation can be a defence to any offence against the person (📖 p.IV.346). In Scotland and elsewhere, the term is also used to refer to circumstances that mitigate (📖 p.V.506) offence seriousness, and therefore can reduce the sentence.

[†] For example, the old common law categories of provocation: a grossly insulting assault; witnessing an attack on a relative, or an Englishman being unlawfully deprived of liberty; a husband finding his wife in the act of adultery; and a father discovering someone committing sodomy on his son.

[‡] The peak of subjectivity within the test was represented by the decision in *Morgan Smith* (📖 p.App. 3.642), in which the defendant's depression was taken into account in deciding not just his sensitivity to things said or done, but whether his violent response to the provocation was reasonable.

[§] For example, uncertainty about the extent to which the reasonable person can be defined properly to share the defendant's characteristics (including mental disorder and personality traits)—i.e. the extent to which the defendant's response to the provocation should be partly subjective or wholly objective.

[**] The most important modifications were the Homicide Act 1957 in E&W and the equivalent Criminal Justice (NI) Act 1966, which until 2010 provided for a defence of provocation, the essence of which was a loss of mastery over the mind, where a reasonable person would have reacted similarly. The loss of mastery had to be sudden (*R v Duffy*, 📖 p.App. 3.635; *R v Ahluwalia*, 📖 p.App. 3.629).

E&W and NI *S54 Coroners and Justice Act 2009*

A defendant, D, is not to be convicted of murder (but only manslaughter) if:

- D's act's and omissions resulted from D's *loss of self-control* (which need not be sudden)
- The loss of self-control had a *qualifying trigger* (fear of serious violence and/or acts or words that constitute circumstances of an extremely grave character and give a justifiable sense of being seriously wronged[*])
- A person of D's sex and age, with a *normal degree of tolerance and self-restraint*, and *in the circumstances of D*, might have reacted in the same or a similar way to D; and
- D did not act in a considered desire for revenge.

Sexual infidelity is explicitly excluded as a ground for feeling seriously wronged.

RoI *R v Duffy* (📖 p.App. 3.635)

- Provocation is one or more acts by the victim which cause a *sudden* and *temporary loss of self-control*, and which
- Would cause such loss of self control in any *reasonable person*
- 'Temporary' means that the defendant must act before having an opportunity to regain composure (*Masciantonio v The Queen*[†]).

Once enough evidence has been adduced for a jury reasonably to conclude that provocation (or loss of control) might apply, the burden of proof (📖 p.IV.317) is then on the prosecution to prove beyond reasonable doubt that it does not.

Problems with the reasonable person test

This test, which is inherent to the defence, has caused problems in many jurisdictions, through dispute about the extent to which the reasonable person can properly be imbued with the specific characteristics, including mental characteristics, of the defendant (ranging from youthfulness to learning disability to particular personality traits).[‡] The new rules in E&W and NI are an awkward compromise between a purely objective and an excessively subjective test; how subjective the new rule is will depend on how broadly judges interpret 'in the circumstances of D', and how narrowly they interpret 'a normal degree of tolerance and self-restraint'. However, it seems that 'circumstances' is broader than the narrowed rule in *Holley* (📖 p.App. 3.638), and can include anything relevant in the defendant or his history, or 'woundability' to things said or done by the victim that are 'qualifying triggers' (though not characteristics which go to his 'reaction').

Scotland avoids these difficulties, with its simpler proportionality rule.

---

[*] The feared violence must be from the victim, to the defendant or another person. Feared violence does not count insofar as it was caused by anything D 'incited to be done or said for the purpose of providing an excuse to use violence'. Similarly, a sense of being seriously wronged is not justifiable if it was caused by something D incited for the purpose of such an excuse.

[†] Like the English case *R v Duffy*, this Australian case does not bind courts in RoI, but there is no recent local case law, and both cases have been explicitly approved by the RoI Law Commission in its report on the current law of provocation in Ireland.

[‡] The courts have adopted varying views: see *Camplin* (📖 p.App. 3.633), *Morgan Smith* (📖 p.App. 3.642) and *Holley* (📖 p.App. 3.638). This is the same tension as is found between subjective and objective approaches to intention (📖 p.IV.334).

Controversies

- Men typically react immediately to provocation, often in response to sexual infidelity or relationship loss, whereas many women react after delay, after what has been called 'slow burn'[*]. This is particularly the case in 'battered woman syndrome (a concept related to PTSD, 📖 p.II.70). The common law provocation defence was thought to discriminate against women, because of the requirement of 'suddenness' of response; the 'loss of control defence' is intended to remedy this[†]
- The rules on the qualifying trigger in E&W and NI may greatly restrict the scope of the defence, as may the policy-driven exclusion of sexual infidelity. The latter is also likely to appear counter-intuitive to juries, as well as being likely difficult to define
- The notion of 'loss of self control' that 'need not be sudden' is, on its face, mutually contradictory; whereas 'loss of mastery over the mind' was a broader notion, made problematic only by the additional requirement that it be 'sudden'
- Many authors believe that provocation should either be available as a general defence, or be abolished altogether (alongside abolition of the mandatory life sentence for murder, so that provoked killers could potentially be given a more lenient sentence)

Role of psychiatric evidence

Psychiatric evidence may be relevant where a mental disorder or characteristics might have affected a defendant's 'woundability' in response to 'qualifying triggers' in the defence. For example, evidence of a mental characteristic such as depressed mood, or a depressive illness, might make the defendant more 'woundable' by taunts (e.g. about inadequacy).

- A history of childhood sexual abuse might be relevant to a sexual assault in adulthood acting as provocation
- Chronic spousal abuse might cause PTSD or, falling short of that, otherwise affect the abused victim mentally such that they are the more easily 'wounded' by things said or done, for example further taunts or violence, by their abuser.

Relationship with diminished responsibility

Pleading defences in tandem

It is possible to plead both self defence (E&W, NI) or provocation (other jurisdictions) and diminished responsibility simultaneously, in which case the jury considers diminished responsibility first, and only considers provocation if the plea of diminished responsibility fails.

---

[*] *R v Ahluwalia* (📖 p.App. 3.629).

[†] However, the requirement of 'loss of self-control' (as opposed to 'loss of mastery over the mind') might actually disadvantage abused women, who typically kill in a very considered fashion, often having developed learned helplessness. Only if the non-sudden loss of control is interpreted to include distorted and restricted reasoning on a defendant's options will the defence afford itself to most abused women who kill.

Legal polarizing of a psychological spectrum
The partial defences of provocation (or loss of control) and diminished responsibility (💭 p.V.491) represent two poles of a psychological spectrum: in the purest form of the latter, the ground for killing is entirely internal (i.e. solely the product of mental disorder, as in *Clunis*, 💭 p.App. 3.633), whereas in 'pure' provocation, the cause is entirely external. In between lie varieties of mixed causation, such as where the other's words, actions or identities play upon an abnormality of mental functioning (e.g. in delusional misidentification or severe depression), or where the provocation is slight and, although someone else might not be particularly woundable by such provocation and retaliate, someone with the characteristics (provocation defence), or 'in the circumstances' of the defendant ('self control' defence) might do so. However, the spectrum is defined legally discontinuously, so as to have a large gap in its middle, where neither defence is available. The new provisions for 'diminished responsibility' and 'loss of control' in E&W and NI have altered, perhaps widened, the gap.

Duress, coercion, and necessity

Duress is a defence to a defendant having acted in a way that would otherwise be unlawful as a result of specific *threats* or *circumstances*. It is a complete defence. In Scotland, duress by threats is known as coercion; duress of circumstances is known as necessity* in Scotland and RoI.

Duress by threats (coercion)

The basis of the defence is that another person's threats overwhelmed the defendant's will (a subjective test) and would have overwhelmed the will of a person of ordinary courage or fortitude (an objective test).

E&W and NI R v Hasan (💭 p.App. 3.638) Threats can amount to duress[†] if:
- They concern serious bodily harm or death to the defendant, their immediate family, or someone else close to them

---

* Not to be confused with the potential general defence of necessity in English law (see 💭 p.IV.343).
[†] In addition, the courts may still recognize a related defence of marital coercion, where a married woman commits an offence with her husband present, whose coercion has overborne her will.

- A reasonable person of their age and background[*] would have been forced to act in the same way
- The threats directly caused the criminal conduct
- The criminal conduct could not have been avoided without incurring the threatened harm
- The defendant did not voluntarily run the risk of such threats (including by associating with the threatener, e.g. a fellow gang member).

Scotland Thomson v HM Advocate

'It is only where, following *threats*, there is an *immediate danger* of *violence* . . . that the defence of coercion can be entertained, and even then only if there is an *inability to resist or avoid* that immediate danger . . . It is the danger which has to be 'immediate', not just the threat.'

RoI A-G v Whelan (📖 p.App. 3.629) Duress requires the following:

- 'Threats of immediate death or personal violence . . .
- so great as to overbear the ordinary power of human resistance'
- The defendant's will must actually have been overborne
- The duress must be operating when the offence is committed
- There must be no opportunity for the defendant to escape.

Once evidence suggesting duress has been raised, the burden of proof (📖 p.IV.317) is on the prosecution to show that the defendant did not act under duress.

The defence does not apply to murder, attempted murder or treason, on the ground that the law must protect the 'sanctity of life'.

Duress of circumstances (necessity)

This defence concerns situations in which the defendant commits an offence in order to avert death or serious physical injury. It applies if:

E&W, NI and RoI R v Martin (📖 p.App. 3.641)

- The defendant had good cause to fear death or serious injury . . .
- and was therefore impelled to commit the offence to avert this . . .
- because of what they reasonably believed to be the situation
- They acted reasonably and proportionately to the danger
- A sober person of reasonable firmness, sharing their characteristics, would have responded to the situation in the same way
- The danger was not brought about by the defendant themselves.

Scotland Moss v Howdle (📖 p.App. 3.642)

- The defendant acted under an immediate danger of death or great bodily harm to themselves or another person
- The criminal conduct was an endeavour to escape the danger
- There was no reasonable alternative course of action.

The burden of proof, and the exclusion for murder, attempted murder, and treason are the same as for duress by threats.

---

[*] This can include pregnancy and serious physical disability or mental disorder, but none of their other special characteristics or 'woundability', such as timidity or emotional instability (R v Bowen, 📖 p.App. 3.631). Unlike in provocation or loss of control (📖 p.V.498), 'characteristics' are insufficient to modify 'reasonable fortitude'. There must have been a diagnosable mental disorder.

In addition, the common law doctrine of medical necessity (📖 p.IV.440) provides a defence to offences such as battery (📖 p.IV.346) which would otherwise have been committed by giving treatment.

Duress and undue influence in civil law

Duress also applies if force or violence is used to compel a person to enter into (or discharge) a contract. If the defence succeeds, the contract is invalidated and may be rescinded. There are two broad categories:

- Physical duress (the use or threat of physical force or violence), and
- Economic duress (the use or threat of financial inducements or penalties, such as threatening to withhold a person's salary or bonus).

There is a related civil law equitable doctrine (📖 p.IV.304) of *undue influence* in making a contract or will. It occurs if the plaintiff and defendant have a 'special relationship', so that the contract is made on unfairly advantageous terms, or the bequest is over generous. If the relationship is a recognized one (e.g. parent and child, or doctor and patient), there need be no proof of actually placing special trust in the defendant.

Relevance of psychiatric evidence

Psychiatric evidence may be relevant in criminal proceedings where the defendant had a recognized mental disorder[*] which can be held to have reduced the defendant's fortitude to below 'reasonable fortitude' (see 📖 p.V.502). For example, an abused woman with PTSD whose children are threatened with harm if she does not smuggle drugs may not have the 'reasonable fortitude' to resist the threats.

Amnesia

Amnesia for an alleged offence is potentially relevant within criminal proceedings because:

- It *can* be suggestive of an abnormal state of mind at the time of the offence
- The defence may wish to call expert evidence to validate the defendant's claimed amnesia, so as to rebut lack of credibility
- An amnestic syndrome, or other generalized memory disorder, can be relevant to fitness to plead, fitness to be interviewed, and the reliability of interviews, either for a defendant or witness.

Law

Amnesia for events surrounding an alleged offence cannot itself be a defence or render a defendant unfit to plead (*R v Podola*, 📖 p.App. 3.643). This is justified on the basis that, even if the defendant validly cannot recall the relevant events, they can respond to the evidence presented in the trial; and because it would be too easy to claim 'I can't remember' in order to avoid trial. The rule may put a defendant at a disadvantage, however, if only they and the victim were present and the issue is whether the victim is telling the truth; or if the victim is dead. However, if the amnesia is due to a generalized memory disorder or other cognitive impairment, that disorder or impairment can be relevant to fitness to plead (📖 p.V.474).

---

[*] i.e. a diagnosable condition, not merely a 'characteristic' (as in provocation, 📖 p.V.498).

If amnesia for an offence is genuine, this can clearly bear upon the reliability of a defendant or witness (📖 p.II.119), especially if they attempt to 'do their best' to remember ('I must have done . . .' rather than 'I remember . . .). A more generalized memory disorder will also be relevant to reliability, most obviously where there is amnestic syndrome and the likelihood of confabulation.

Questions put to experts

- Is the defendant's amnesia for relevant events genuine?
- Does the amnesia suggest an underlying condition which could be a basis for a mental condition defence (📖 p.IV.342)?
- Does the amnesia suggest the defendant lacked the capacity to form the requisite mens rea (📖 p.IV.334) for the alleged offence?
- Does the defendant have a generalized memory disorder relevant to fitness to plead (📖 p.V.474), or to reliability (📖 p.II.124) in police interviews?

Clinical assessment

Assessment (see also 📖 p.II.89) must include reading all medical records, plus reviewing legal papers for evidence of the consistency or otherwise of the claimed amnesia or its extent. Police interviews and witness statements should be read with care: it is embarrassing to argue for amnesia at the time of the alleged offence and then to be directed in cross-examination to evidence which clearly suggests relevant memories.

Specific clinical issues relevant to amnesia include whether there have been multiple episodes of amnesia, and whether the amnesia is solely for events surrounding the offence, with no other episodes. If the latter, it is very unlikely to represent an underlying chronic disorder, and is most likely to arise either from a disorder of consciousness at the relevant time (organically or psychologically determined, with events not laid down in memory) or from 'psychogenic amnesia' (dissociation from memories that were laid down).

Dissociative disorders and dissociative amnesia

Clinically it is difficult to distinguish between *dissociative* (or psychogenic) *amnesia* (not necessarily representing anything abnormal about the mental state at the time of the offence but only of retrieval[*]) and the effects on memory formation of a *dissociative state* at the time of the offence.

Dissociative amnesia has a number of characteristics: it is often patchy; it is associated with events of emotional significance (e.g. related to the offence); and it can be either dense or patchy for the offence itself but can gradually resolve. Further evidence is required to demonstrate that there was dissociation at the time of the offence, such as:

- Depersonalization and/or derealization recalled as occurring prior to the time of the offence
- A period of dense amnesia for the offence, with clear previous and next memories
- Pursuance of acts out of character with apparently purposeful behaviours despite lack of memory

---

[*] Some authors, confusingly, also use the term 'dissociative amnesia' to include amnesia resulting from dissociation at the time when memory would otherwise have been formed.

- Observed confusion after the offence
- Presence of other factors predisposing to dissociation e.g. head injury/traumatic brain injury, previous episodes of dissociation, depersonalization or derealization
- Precipitation by a psychologically significant event e.g. being sexually assaulted when there is a personal history of sexual abuse.

Dissociative amnesia is the most likely explanation of amnesia for an offence; amnesia resulting from dissociation at the time of the offence is uncommon. There is often suspicion that such amnesia may be at least partly deliberate, and cross-examination is therefore often robust.

Alcohol-induced amnesia
Alcohol-induced amnesia can occur in the context of chronic alcohol abuse and is likely to reflect alcohol blackout syndrome, in which the individual wakes with no recollection of the events of the previous day/evening. Since violent offending is also often associated with intoxication the two commonly occur together.

Other organic causes
Head injury occurring at the time of the offence can cause a transient organic amnesia. A history of any neurological condition that might explain amnesia for the offence, requires thorough assessment and investigation, especially if there are no records of previous diagnosis.

Aggravating and mitigating factors

Aggravating and mitigating factors are taken into account by judges when sentencing (p.IV.361) convicted offenders. In some jurisdictions, most notably E&W, judges are constrained to a degree by strict sentencing guidelines (p.IV.362) as to what can amount to such factors, how they can affect the sentence, and how this should be explained to the defendant; in others, most notably Scotland, judges have wide discretion to take factors into account, and explain their reasoning (or not), as they see fit.

What are aggravating factors?
These are features of an offence that indicate either that particularly grave harm was caused, and/or that the offender bears particularly great responsibility for the harm caused (i.e. a greater degree of culpability). Examples of factors indicating greater degree of harm include:
- Victimizing someone particularly vulnerable
- Offending against someone serving the public (e.g. police officer, nurse)
- Harming multiple victims
- Causing particularly serious injury, mental trauma or other harm
- Committing the offence against or in the presence of children.

Examples of greater culpability include:
- Offending while on bail awaiting trial for another offence
- Being motivated by hatred for the victim's religion, sexuality, race, etc.
- Planning the offence in advance, or being a 'professional' criminal
- Committing the offence while using drugs or alcohol
- Using a weapon
- Abusing a position of power or trust (e.g. MP, teacher, doctor).

What are mitigating factors?

Some factors may indicate that an offender's culpability is low, or that the harm caused by an offence is less serious than usual. Examples include:
- Being provoked (📖 p.V.498) into committing an offence other than murder
- Suffering from a relevant disability or mental disorder
- Being young or otherwise vulnerable or immature
- Playing only a very limited role in the offence
- Showing remorse or otherwise trying to make amends
- Reporting oneself to the police, or pleading guilty at the first opportunity.

Weighing up the two

Even within the prescriptive guidelines of E&W, there is no formula to decide what weight should be given to one or other factor, although there are suggested thresholds above which community or custodial sentences may be appropriate. Beyond this, the weighing up of aggravating and mitigating factors remains an issue for the judge.

Relevance of psychiatric evidence

A psychiatrist may be instructed to prepare a report on a defendant's mental disorder for the purpose of sentencing (📖 p.V.547), the contents of which may be used in mitigation (but also for determining dangerousness, 📖 p.V.549, in some cases, which may pose an ethical dilemma, 📖 p.III.261). Expert reports may inadvertently raise or imply other aggravating or mitigating factors even though written for other purposes:
- Psychological or psychiatric formulations may suggest a motivation for offending, including arising out of mental pathology
- A psychiatric history may contain information to indicate that aggravating or mitigating factors (such as being abused, or hating people from a certain minority group) are present
- There may be comments recounted of the defendant's attitudes towards or remorse for an offence, and
- Some diagnoses may themselves be seen as aggravating factors, especially certain personality disorders such as narcissistic (📖 p.II.63) or antisocial (📖 p.II.60) personality disorder.

Example from E&W sentencing guidelines for magistrates

Sentencing and mitigation in *common assault*
- The starting point is a fine
- If one aggravating factor indicating greater culpability is present, the threshold for a community sentence is normally passed
- If two such factors are present, the threshold for a custodial sentence is normally passed.

Common aggravating factors indicating *greater culpability*
- Use of a weapon
- Planned or sustained offence
- Head-butting, kicking, biting, or attempted strangulation
- Motivated by sexual orientation or disability
- Motivated by hostility towards a minority group
- Abuse of position of trust
- Offence as part of a group.

Common aggravating factors indicating *greater harm*
- Serious injury
- Victim was providing a public service, or was highly vulnerable
- Additional degradation of victim
- Offence committed in the presence of a child
- Forced entry into victim's home
- Offender prevented victim seeking or obtaining help
- Previous threats or violence to the same victim.

Common *mitigating factors* for common assault
- Provocation
- Single push, shove, or blow.

Civil legal issues

Family law

Family law encompasses divorce, adoption, wardship (the court supervising a child's care), residence of and contact with children, parental responsibility, and care proceedings. It covers both private and public law.[*]

- **E&W and NI** Hearings may take place in County Courts; in Family Proceedings courts (Magistrates Courts in E&W and NI), where they are bound by Family Procedure Rules; or in the Family Division of the High Court
- **Scotland** The vast majority of hearings take place in the Sheriff Courts
- **RoI** Hearings take place in the District or Circuit Court.

Legislation

Family law is complex and much of it is not relevant to a psychiatric expert, although knowledge of it can be relevant to understanding patients' situation in relation to their children. The following is a non-exhaustive list of relevant legislation:

- **E&W** Family Law Act 1996, Children Acts 1989 & 2004
- **Scotland** Family Law (Scotland) Act 2006, Children (Scotland) Act 1995
- **NI** Children (Northern Ireland) Order 1995
- **RoI** Family Law Act 1995, Children Acts 1997 & 2001.

Principles

Family law upholds the principle that the welfare (📖 p.IV.297) of the child is paramount; and the law operates to protect the interests of vulnerable children (and by extension, those who care for them). Other aims, such as doing justice (📖 p.IV.294) to the parents and other parties, are secondary.

Role of psychiatric evidence

Divorce

Most divorce cases do not have to address issues of parental contact, or residence because these are settled amicably between the parties. The court will only be involved where there is disagreement (about 30% of cases). Psychiatric evidence may be called where one party claims to have been abused by the other, usually in cases of domestic violence, and in other cases where one parent seeks to restrict access to the children by the other parent. There may be misguided attempts to 'prove' that domestic violence has taken place because one parent suffers from post-traumatic stress disorder (📖 p.II.70).

Annulment

Rarely, psychiatric evidence may be introduced to support the annulment of a marriage on the grounds that one or other party lacked the mental capacity to marry (📖 p.IV.438) at the time; but this is unusual.[†]

---

[*] Private law concerns the rights and duties of individuals towards each other (e.g. marriage, divorce); public law concerns the rights and duties of the State (e.g. taking a child into local authority care).
[†] This may be more relevant to Catholic couples who cannot remarry in church if they divorce, and therefore seek annulment instead.

Parenting and child protection

Child psychiatrists, general psychiatrists and forensic psychiatrists may all be asked to provide the family courts with expert reports (📖 p.V.555) and testimony (📖 p.V.585). Experts are usually agreed by all parties in advance.

The questions before the courts that require psychiatric advice include:

• Does this parent have a mental disorder that impacts on their capacity to parent, i.e. to care safely for their child?
• Does this parent pose a risk of harm to their child because of mental disorder? (It is important not to attempt to advise on risk of harm arising from causes other than mental disorder.)
• Can any mental disorder be treated, and if so what is the time scale?
• Does this child have a mental disorder?
• If so, to what extent is it caused or exacerbated by the home environment or by the actions of one or other parent?
• What attachment relationship is there between parent and child?

This list is not exhaustive. The family courts use this testimony to make decisions about where a child will live; and whether they will have access to their parents.

A note of caution

It will be obvious that these are complex questions with far-reaching consequences. There is no established evidence base for many of the questions (for example: does having schizophrenia impact on parenting capacity? This has not been studied in detail). Often formulation is more helpful than simple diagnosis, and a forensic psychotherapy (📖 p.II.163) consultation may assist with this.

Where there is a role for forensic psychiatrists and psychotherapists in assessing an individual parent it should not trespass into the domain of child and family psychiatry, within which experts directly assess children and parenting. Forensic psychiatrists can only ever give evidence about parenting by way of inference from diagnosis or formulation of a parent's mental disorder, and this no substitute for direct observation. Forensic assessment should therefore always only be an addendum to a family psychiatry assessment, offering a secondary perspective on the same question.

Tort law and negligence

Tort is the branch of civil law that deals with civil wrongs: that is, breaches of general duties owed to other individuals,[*] as opposed to breaches of duties owed to society (crimes, 📖 p.IV.332) or of a duty taken on by agreement with a specific individual (breach of contract).

The aim of tort law is to restore the victim (claimant or pursuer) to the position they would have been in had the wrong not occurred, by the payment of damages (financial compensation) by the defendant. In a few cases, other equitable remedies (📖 p.IV.304) such as specific performance will be applied (e.g. requiring the return of an item of sentimental value[†], as no alternative object purchased with damage payments will be of equal value); very occasionally there will be punitive damages.

Box 19.1 lists the main torts. Only negligence is of real relevance to forensic psychiatrists, though rarely they may give evidence in intentional torts (e.g. on the mental state of the defendant at the time and its relevance to capacity).

Box 19.1 Major categories of torts

- Negligence
- Nuisance (e.g. noise or pollution)
- Libel and slander
- Intentional torts[‡] (e.g. battery, false imprisonment, trespass, conversion)
- Economic torts (misrepresentation, restraint of trade)
- Statutory torts (competition law, product liability, etc.).

Negligence

The law of negligence is built upon the principle of *neighbourship*: that we each have a legal duty to pay regard to the welfare of those near whom we live. Where there is failure to be a good neighbour, and where that failure causes harm to another, the law requires the bad neighbour to pay damages equivalent to the harm. Key questions therefore are:

- Who is my neighbour? (To whom do I owe a *duty of care*?)
- What is the standard of being a good neighbour in this case? (What amounts to *breach* of that duty?)
- What harm (*damage*) did my neighbour suffer?
- Did my being a bad neighbour *cause* the harm to my neighbour?
- How will the amount (*quantum*) of damages be calculated?

Duty of care: who is my neighbour?

In simple terms your neighbour is anyone you ought to have in mind when you do something. Examples include:

- Individuals who occupy adjacent property: neighbours in a literal sense

---

[*] 'Individuals' can include corporations (companies and other organizations with a legal identity).
[†] This example would be a claim for the tort of conversion, in which the defendant (the 'tortfeasor', the person who has done wrong) has used the victim's property as if it were their own.
[‡] Many intentional torts are similar to crimes. In tort, however, the victim sues for damages for the harm suffered, whereas the State prosecutes crimes and inflicts punishment.

- The user of a product or service[*] (*Donoghue v Stevenson*, 📖 p.App. 3.634)
- The client of someone claiming to have special expertise or knowledge, e.g. the patient of a doctor (see 📖 p.V.516).

For a person to be regarded as owing a duty to another, they must be 'so closely and directly affected' by the person's acts that it is reasonable to expect them to take them into account (there must be 'proximity'). For a duty to arise, a particular harm must also be *reasonably foreseeable*; and it must be *fair, just, and reasonable* for a duty to exist.[†]

What amounts to breach of duty?

- Someone who knowingly exposes their neighbour to a substantial risk of harm is in breach of their duty to their neighbour (this is analogous to recklessness in the criminal law, 📖 p.IV.329)
- Someone who fails to realize that they are exposing their neighbour to a substantial risk of harm is in breach of duty if a *reasonable person* would have foreseen the potential harm.[‡]

Causation: did my actions cause the harm?

This underlying principle is simple: would the harm[§] have resulted if the defendant had not acted as they did? It is often complex in practice:

- If a *third party* or event intervenes before harm occurs, and this was not reasonably foreseeable, the defendant has not legally caused the harm.
- If the harm was too *remote* from the defendant's actions, they have not legally caused it (this is similar to saying the harm must be reasonably foreseeable). For example, depression caused to bystanders witnessing an accident is too remote for compensation (📖 p.V.514).

Quantum: how much must I pay in damages?

The aim is to restore the claimant to the position they would have been in had the breach not occurred. In practice, it is often difficult, even arbitrary, to assign monetary values to non-monetary harms, such as pain, the loss of a limb, or psychological trauma.

If there are several defendants, the quantum will be shared between them. If the claimant is deemed to have *contributed* to the negligence by their own carelessness, the quantum will be reduced.

---

[*] Not merely the person who buys it, who is owed a duty in contract law.
[†] This is the 'threefold test' laid down by the House of Lords in *Caparo v Dickman* (📖 p.App. 3.633).
[‡] If the defendant holds themselves out as having special knowledge or experience, the test involves a reasonable member of that profession: e.g. the Bolam test (📖 p.App. 3.631).
[§] However, the claimant does not need to prove that the defendant's breach was the sole cause of harm, merely that it 'materially increased the risk of harm'.

Compensation after injury

So-called 'personal injury claims', based upon claims that someone was negligent in allowing an injury to occur, make up a multi-billion pound industry. Psychiatric injury is often the harm on which a claim is based.

Basis for a claim for compensation for psychiatric injury

Compensation for psychiatric injury requires that:
- A recognizable psychiatric illness is present (not just 'mental distress')
- The disorder was caused or aggravated by the acts or omissions of a negligent defendant (see 📖 p.V.512 for how negligence is proved).

Specific legal issues in psychiatric injury cases

- Both *primary* and *secondary victims* may be entitled to compensation but the distinction can be complex. 'Innocent bystanders' are not entitled to compensation as harm to them is too remote (📖 p.V.513).
  - A primary victim is someone who suffers psychiatric illness as a result of being directly (physically) injured or put in fear of injury[*]
  - A secondary victim is someone who suffers psychiatric illness as a result of being in a 'close tie of love and affection' with a primary victim, being present at and directly perceiving an incident that caused them direct injury (or its immediate aftermath)
- A situation can only be considered dangerous in terms of compensation if it was *reasonably foreseeably* so: a harm that no person could reasonably have foreseen will not attract compensation. Conversely, if danger could reasonably have been foreseen, and the fear of this danger caused psychiatric illness, there need not be proof of actual danger
- People who act as *rescuers* (either private individuals or professionals such as police and fire officers) may claim compensation for psychiatric injury on the ground that it is reasonably foreseeable that people will attempt to rescue victims of a dangerous situation
- People who are *involuntary participants*[†] in the creation of a dangerous situation that results (or could reasonably foreseeably have resulted) in injury may be entitled to compensation if they suffer psychiatric illness
- Psychiatric illness caused by *workplace stress* can be a ground for compensation, if the psychiatric illness was reasonably foreseeable
- Ill-treatment by prison officers, and insensitively breaking bad news, have both also been held to be grounds for compensation when reasonably foreseeable psychiatric illness has resulted.

---

[*] According to the House of Lords, the primary victim must be 'directly involved in the accident . . . and well within the range of foreseeable physical injury': *Page v Smith* (📖 p.App. 3.643). The E&W Law Commission has proposed reforming these rules, and abolishing the shock requirement.
[†] For example, the crane driver in *Dooley v Cammell Laird* (📖 p.App. 3.635) was an involuntary participant in feared injury caused by his employer's negligence.

The shock requirement for secondary victims[*]

The psychiatric illness must have been induced by a shock: a 'sudden assault on the nervous system', as the courts have put it. For example, the courts have ruled that psychiatric illness resulting from years spent caring for a negligently injured spouse, or dealing with a negligently brain-damaged child's challenging behaviour, did not warrant compensation because there was no shock; nor, for the same reason, did viewing a disaster involving loved ones on live television.

The shock requirement is deliberately restrictive: the courts fear opening the 'floodgates' to a large number of claims, which might lead to general increases in insurance premiums.

What is a recognizable psychiatric illness?

The mental disorder most clearly related to injury or trauma is PTSD (📖 p.II.70). Depression (📖 p.II.69), anxiety disorders, and adjustment disorders (📖 p.II.72) are also common bases of claims. Other conditions that the courts have accepted as 'recognizable psychiatric illness' include hysterical (histrionic) personality disorder (📖 p.II.58), pathological grief (📖 p.II.72), and chronic fatigue syndrome (📖 p.II.74).

The 'eggshell' rule

There is a general legal rule that you take your victim as you find them: any unknown vulnerability they may have (meaning that they suffer more serious injury than you could have foreseen, or suffer injury when another person would not have done) does not reduce your liability either in criminal law (📖 p.IV.329) or in tort law (📖 p.IV.312), provided in the latter case that *some* degree of injury was reasonably foreseeable.

This is known as the 'eggshell skull' rule in the context of head injury: if you are negligent (or act criminally), the fact that the victim suffered serious brain injury instead of mere bruising only because they have an abnormally thin cranium does not reduce your liability for the actual damage they have suffered. This has been generalized to mental states, to vulnerable or 'eggshell' personalities, and to previously-traumatized individuals who are more likely to be traumatized by subsequent events.

Compensation under other arrangements

Victims of injury, including psychiatric illness, that resulted from a *violent criminal offence* can also claim for compensation under statutory schemes.[†] Close relatives who are *bereaved* may also sue those who caused the death, particularly if they were financially dependent on the person who was killed.

---

[*] The term 'nervous shock' is sometimes used by the courts to refer to the psychiatric illness caused, but in the case of the primary victim there is no shock requirement, despite the term.
[†] From the Criminal Injuries Compensation Authority in E&W and Scotland; the Compensation Agency in Ni; and the Criminal Injuries Compensation Tribunal in RoI.

Clinical negligence

The same general legal rules apply to clinical or medical negligence cases as to any other negligence (📖 p.V.512) case where a party is seeking compensation (📖 p.V.514) for harm they have suffered. A number of cases have laid down how these rules apply specifically in clinical negligence cases.

Grounds for clinical negligence

Claims can arise from any aspect of a doctor's professional interaction with a patient: not merely technical procedures (e.g. ECT, 📖 p.II.158), but, for example, for not giving all required or relevant information in seeking consent, or for unreasonably failing to recommend detention under mental health law (📖 p.IV.373) in order to prevent harm to self or others.

The elements of a claim for clinical negligence are the same as for any other negligence claim (see 📖 p.V.512): the doctor must owe the claimant a *duty of care*; they must be shown to have *breached* that duty; and that breach must have *caused the harm* the claimant suffered. Only then will the court assess the *quantum* of damages that apply.

When doctors owe a duty of care

Doctors owe duties of care to the following:
- A patient they have treated personally
- A potential patient to whom they have offered their services
- A patient reasonably referred to them whom they failed to assess or treat
- A patient treated by someone for whom the doctor is responsible (e.g. a trainee working for a consultant).

What amounts to a breach of duty

The leading case on breach of duty in clinical negligence is *Bolam* (📖 p.App. 3.631), which adopts a 'peer review' approach: would the allegedly negligent practice be accepted as proper by a responsible body of doctors,[*] and does it have a logical basis (*Bolitho*, 📖 p.App. 3.631)? Evidence of following the logical practice of a responsible minority of doctors is a valid defence, even if the majority of practitioners would have behaved differently.

Trainees

The law holds all doctors, including trainees, to the same standard of care. Those who are not yet experts in a particular field (because they are in training, or perhaps because they normally practice in another field) are expected to know their own limitations and to seek expert advice when they need it.

---

[*] In the language of the judgment, did the defendant act 'in accordance with a practice accepted as proper by a responsible body of medical men skilled in that particular art'?

Causation in medical negligence

The complexities of establishing the 'chain of causation' (📖 p.V.513) in medical negligence cases is often greater than in other cases, because:

- It may be unclear what harm would have resulted from the underlying medical condition with non-negligent treatment
- In many cases, there may be a separate negligence claim for the underlying medical condition (e.g. a workplace or road traffic accident, or an industrial disease such as pneumoconiosis from coal mining)
- There may have been many different practitioners from several different professions involved in the care provided in a modern hospital, and disentangling the effects of breaches of duty by one or a small number of them may be very difficult.

Doctors as employees and as private practitioners

Doctors who practise privately are wholly liable for any negligence claims against them. However, those who are employees will share liability for negligence with their employer: the employer, in other words, is *vicariously liable* for the employed doctor's actions.

In the NHS, this brings both advantages and disadvantages from the doctor's point of view:

- Cases will usually be managed, and damages will usually be paid by, the NHS Litigation Authority* (this is called NHS indemnity); and
- The doctor will benefit from Crown immunity† for certain actions; however,
- The interests of the employing NHS body may be different from those of the doctor (e.g. the NHS may want to settle a claim out of court, while the doctor might want to defend it in order to preserve their reputation); and
- If the claim relates to any work the doctor does which is outside their contract of employment, the doctor will not be covered by NHS indemnity and will be personally liable for the proceedings and any damages.

For these reasons, you are strongly advised to have personal medical defence cover, so that you can be independently legally represented if necessary, and can continue proceedings in your own name if the NHS wishes to settle its part of the claim. Cover should also apply in situations where the employer takes action against you, e.g. under employment law, at inquests (📖 p.V.527) or in professional conduct proceedings (📖 p.V.521).

---

* The Authority runs the NHS Clinical Negligence Scheme, which helps NHS employers learn from past negligence cases and avoid acting (or having employees who act) in ways that may be negligent. For example, it produces advice on safe record-keeping and good communication, failures in which are two of the most common reasons for being unable to defend a negligence claim successfully.

† The Crown (i.e. the Queen, or the State) is often exempted from laws allowing other bodies or individuals to be prosecuted or sued for various wrongs.

Professional liability in practice

A number of potential pitfalls account for a large proportion of all cases of clinical negligence (📖 p.V.516) claims against psychiatrists, and of disciplinary or professional proceedings (📖 p.V.521). The largest of these is one form or other of boundary violation, which is discussed on 📖 p.V.519.

Multiple liability

Proceedings in relation to professional activity can involve both civil and criminal actions; and may run in parallel with personal legal liability and a complaint to the GMC. For example, a doctor who drinks heavily at work and is later apprehended driving home may be subject to:

- An action for clinical negligence by any patient harmed by professional decisions they took whilst intoxicated
- Personal criminal charges in relation to driving whilst intoxicated
- Disciplinary action by their employer, and
- Professional conduct proceedings by the General Medical Council or in RoI the Medical Council.

Common scenarios

Psychiatric situations that most often result in liability, according to medical defence organizations, include:

- Poor quality clinical care, e.g. prescribing and failing to change an antipsychotic (📖 p.II.159) that then produces severe tardive dyskinesia
- Missing a diagnosis, particularly organic conditions (📖 p.II.85) with psychiatric presentations, and incidental comorbid conditions
- Breaches of confidentiality (for example, through inappropriate disclosure, 📖 p.III.263,* at a MAPPA meeting, 📖 p.V.468)
- Sexual boundary violations (📖 p.V.520)
- Inadequate risk assessment (📖 p.II.127) or management (📖 p.II.189) leading to suicide (📖 p.II.199), escape (📖 p.II.200), assault or killing (📖 p.II.191)

Issues for expert witnesses

If you are instructed to produce a report on an issue in such a scenario, you should consider the following issues:

- Which type of proceedings are these, and therefore which legal or other questions do you need to address? (For example, in disciplinary proceedings you might need to consider whether the subject's practice was grossly inappropriate [gross misconduct], whereas in a negligence (📖 p.V.512) case, the standard is whether the treatment given would be supported by a responsible body of opinion, and was logically sustainable.)
- How can the actions of the subject of the report be separated out from those of other team members? For example, a nurse on observations fails to notice a suicidal patient on an open ward leaving through the unlocked main door. Is whether this is unacceptable practice affected by a junior doctor's decision to set the observation frequency at once every 15 minutes, despite the evidence of increased risk?

---

*See in particular the case of *W v Egdell* (📖 p.App. 3.635) discussed on 📖 p.III.263.

- What would have happened if no inappropriate action had been taken, or if (in a different case) the patient had received optimal care? A negative outcome might have been inevitable in either case, and unrelated to inappropriate or inadequate care. For instance, a patient with an undiagnosed glioma might have died even if the correct diagnosis had been made in time; this does not excuse the failure to make the diagnosis, but might affect whether the negligent doctor is held fully liable for the negative outcome, as the wrong diagnosis did not affect the outcome. This issue is often relevant to alleged negligent care of patients with chronic or relapsing and remitting psychiatric conditions, where the ultimate prognosis, beyond the litigated event, is poor.

Professional liability for the actions of patients

Persons under your control The UK courts have held that there is a duty of care towards those who might reasonably foreseeably be harmed by the actions of those under your control, if you fail to exercise proper control (*Home Office v Dorset Yacht Co*, 📖 p.App. 3.638). Whilst this could not be applied to patients treated in the community, it is possible that a court could hold a doctor or hospital liable for harm caused by detained inpatients over whom it negligently failed to exercise proper control. This might even extend to a duty to prevent them acting violently (📖 p.III.242).

Duty to warn or to protect In the US, the courts have stated that psychiatrists and therapists have a legal duty to protect identifiable third parties who are at risk from patients under their care, by warning them, notifying the police, or taking other reasonable steps to protect them (*Tarasoff*, 📖 p.App. 3.646). Courts in the UK, however, have not laid down such a duty, avoiding doing so in cases where they might have done this (e.g. *Palmer v Tees* 📖 p.App. 3.643; *Surrey v McManus* 📖 p.App. 3.646; *K v Home Office*, 📖 p.App. 3.639)—although the reasoning of these judgments leaves open the possibility that they might impose a duty to protect a specific victim who could be identified in advance. No similar cases have been litigated in RoI.

Duty to the patient themselves Doctors and hospitals owe a duty of care to their patients to diagnose and treat them adequately, and in certain cases will be liable for consequent harm if they fail to do so (e.g. for the pain and suffering caused by a missed diagnosis). However, they are not liable to the patient for failing to prevent them offending: the courts have held that a patient cannot base a claim for negligence on their own offending behaviour (*Clunis*, 📖 p.App. 3.633), even if they were found not guilty by reason of insanity (📖 p.IV.489).

Professional boundary violations

Boundary violations refer to those lapses in medical care in which the doctor (or other professional) has 'lost' or abandoned their professional identity in the workplace; and may have placed their personal needs above the needs of the patient, their employer, their colleagues, or others. Depending on the nature of the boundary violation, this may represent a breach of professional codes of ethics (📖 pp.III.241, App. 3.649), and also infer professional liability (📖 p.V.518).

By putting their personal interests first, the doctor runs the risk of harming the patient: by failing to provide an adequate standard of care, and by potentially exploiting the patient's vulnerability. Most regulators also take the view that doctors who breach professional boundaries do harm by bringing the profession into disrepute; and so reducing trust.

Professional boundary violations may be categorized according to whether they involve physical touching, and whether they concern the patient or others. It is also possible to see boundary violations as more or less severe in terms the degree of harm caused (e.g. psychological injury).

Non-physical boundary violations

These most commonly involve the inappropriate disclosure or use of information:

- Inappropriate self-disclosure (this rarely results in disciplinary proceedings or other action, but may be the first sign of a loss of professional identity, and is likely to be raised in any future hearings if the clinician's behaviour deteriorates)
- Disclosure of confidential information (📖 p.III.263) without consent or lawful excuse (these can and do result in disciplinary hearings, professional proceedings or even negligence claims)
- Using patient information for personal gain (for example, in funded research without consent, or for paid market research)
- Having a dual relationship with a patient (e.g. using the services of a professional tax advisor who is your patient, or accepting your cleaner as a patient).

Physical boundary violations

The most serious (and relatively common) such violations are sexual relationships with patients, which often involve a vulnerable patient unable to protect themselves from a predatory doctor (patients in such relationships may believe they wanted, and even that they started, the relationship until after it has finished and they are able to re-evaluate it free of the doctor's influence). They include:

- Having a sexual or otherwise improper personal relationship with a patient or former patient[*]
- Inappropriate touching (especially sexual touching) of patients, such as during a physical examination.

Psychiatrists are over-represented at the GMC amongst doctors who are accused of boundary violations. These concerns about boundary violations would suggest a 'no-touch' policy is safest for psychiatrists, especially for those who are doing individual psychotherapeutic work—although many psychiatrists would argue for limited exceptions, such as briefly touching a distressed patient in an appropriate place, such as on the arm or shoulder, to indicate their support and concern.

---

[*]One with a former patient where there has been no contact for many years may be acceptable, as long as they no longer have mental disorder or other vulnerability.

Boundary violations not involving the patient

These are more commonly the subject of disciplinary proceedings (☐ p.V.521), and may be viewed less seriously, but are unacceptable boundary violations none the less.

- Theft of the employer's property
- Use of the employer's assets for personal gain without permission (ranging from sending a fax relating to a private medicolegal report, to paying for a holiday on a company credit card)
- Deliberately giving a false or biased opinion (e.g. providing 'expert' advice or testimony as a 'hired gun': that is, giving the opinion wanted by those who pay you, as opposed to a genuine professional opinion)
- Allowing your practice to undergo 'baseline drift' over time (through bias in your methods or interpretation of data, your opinions tending to favour a particular side in a case, e.g. prosecution or defence)
- Misusing professional knowledge and status for personal gain (e.g. involving oneself in a case without instructions to do so, particularly if this involves something outside one's area of expertise[*])
- Acting in an unprofessional manner (by, for example, publicly personally derogating other clinicians or experts who disagree with your views).

Disciplinary & professional proceedings

Regulatory bodies and their responsibilities

Members of professions are generally regulated by a professional body for that profession, or for a group of related professions (e.g. the Health Professions Council in the UK oversees the regulation of many health-related professions other than medicine, such as psychologists, dietitians and radiographers). Doctors in the UK are regulated by the General Medical Council (GMC), and in RoI by the Medical Council.

---

[*] For example, Professor David Southall was banned from child protection work for 3 years, after an incident in which he telephoned the police and suggested that a couple might have murdered their child, after watching a television documentary about her death. He was struck off in 2007 after a second such incident (he was reinstated by the High Court on a technicality in 2010, and at the time of writing his case is currently being reheard by the GMC).

Professional fitness to practise proceedings

There are five grounds for fitness to practise proceedings by the GMC:
- Misconduct
- Poor professional performance
- A criminal conviction
- Physical or mental ill-health
- A decision by a regulatory body elsewhere that fitness to practice is impaired.

The Medical Council in RoI adopts the same grounds, plus failure to comply with a condition of registration, a requirement of a previous inquiry, or a requirement of the Medical Practitioners Act 2007.

A complaint that appears to show grounds for impaired fitness to practise will result in a preliminary information-gathering investigation. This can result in a warning, an undertaking by the doctor to change their practice or behaviour, mediation between doctor and employer, or a referral for a formal inquiry by the Fitness to Practise Panel (Committee in RoI).

The formal inquiry will be chiefly concerned with the protection of patients and with public confidence in the profession. For example, the GMC states that cases in which there is proof of sexual assault or indecency, violence, an improper sexual or emotional relationship with a patient or someone close to them, or dishonesty, are likely to lead to suspension or erasure from the register.

Controversially, the GMC and the Medical Council apply the civil standard of proof (📖 p.IV.316) of the balance of probabilities; until 2007, the GMC applied a higher standard of proof analogous to the criminal standard of beyond reasonable doubt. This means that doctors' careers can be limited or even terminated while substantial doubt remains about the truth of the allegations against them.

It is possible to appeal to the High Court against a decision of the GMC or the Medical Council.

Disciplinary proceedings

These are conducted by the employer and relate solely to the doctor's contract of employment, although they may run in parallel with professional or negligence proceedings. The grounds for dismissal in the NHS consultant's contract are shown in Box 19.2; those in trainee doctors' contracts are very similar, though those in the private sector may be significantly less generous.

Box 19.2 Grounds for termination of employment in the NHS consultants' contract

- Conduct
- Capability
- Redundancy
- Failure to maintain registration with the GMC etc.
- In order to comply with a relevant statute
- Any other 'substantial reason in a particular case'.

The role of psychiatric evidence

There may be scope for a forensic psychiatric opinion in professional or disciplinary proceedings in the following situations:

- If there is evidence of mental disorder which might provide some explanation, for example, of inappropriate conduct in the workplace (e.g. hypomania causing sexual disinhibition). In such circumstances, the employer or regulatory body might agree to withhold or suspend disciplinary sanctions to allow treatment of mental disorder
- Where proceedings relate to alleged clinical malpractice or incapability on the part of a fellow forensic psychiatrist.

Before accepting instructions in either of these cases, the expert should ensure they are aware what legal standard of proof (📖 p.IV.316) applies within the proceedings, and what definitions of key concepts (such as 'breach of duty of care') are adopted within the relevant employment contract or professional guidelines (📖 p.III.240).

Employment & equality law

Employment law is relevant to forensic psychiatrists instructed to prepare reports on people with mental disorder who are involved in employment-related legal proceedings. Alleged workplace harassment, and therefore requests for expert reports on its psychiatric effects, are on the increase. Issues of negligence (📖 p.V.512) including compensation after workplace injury (📖 p.V.514) may also arise.

Equality law is concerned with eliminating unlawful discrimination. It places responsibilities on employers and others* to prevent or avoid discrimination. Most employees with mental disorder are eligible for the protection offered by the legislation described in the following section; psychiatrists may be involved in demonstrating how the disorder places the claimant in a protected group, or how alleged discrimination might have affected them.

Specific legislation

Equality Act 2010 (UK), 2004 (RoI)

These almost identical Acts implement EU law (📖 p.IV.326). The UK Act replaced the Disability Discrimination Acts, and consolidated others such as the Race Relations Act and Sex Discrimination Act.

In broad terms the relevance to people with mental disorder is that the Act protects anyone who has, or has had, a disability (along with seven other 'protected characteristics': age, gender reassignment, marriage or civil partnership, race, religion or belief, sex, and sexual orientation). Disability includes people who have *any substantial mental impairment*, if it has a substantial and long-term adverse effect on their ability to perform normal day-to-day activities. The prohibited forms of discrimination are

---

* Such as those running businesses or providing services to the public.

shown in Box 19.3. The third form, discrimination because of a consequence of the characteristic, only applies to disability.[*]

Box 19.3 Prohibited forms of discrimination

Direct discrimination
Refusing to serve a person in a shop because they are black.

Indirect discrimination
Requiring all prospective employees to be at least a certain height, as this will prevent many more women obtaining a job than men.

Discrimination arising from disability
Evicting a tenant with schizophrenia who has sublet their property in breach of the tenancy agreement, if the symptoms of schizophrenia made it harder for them to control their behaviour and adhere to the rule prohibiting subletting.

Health & Safety Acts[†]

These Acts place duties on employers to their employees including people with mental disorder, to ensure a safe workplace and safe working practices. There is also a duty to protect the mental health of employees.

Tort law

Separately, the common law provides remedies for damage to mental health caused by employers' negligence:

- If psychiatric harm has occurred then whether this kind of harm to the individual concerned was reasonably foreseeable (p.V.513) is a key issue. Foreseeing harm relates to the nature of the job and any known individual vulnerabilities
- Employers must take reasonable preventive action if harm is foreseen.

Tribunals

- Employment tribunals are independent judicial bodies that determine disputes between employers and employees. They consist of three members including a legally qualified chair. The Employment Appeal Tribunals is the higher tribunal
- In RoI an employee can present a complaint to the Rights Commissioner Service with referral on to the Employment Appeals Tribunal. Complaints under equality legislation are heard by an Equality Tribunal.

---

[*] This disability-specific third form was added in order to reverse the decision of the House of Lords in *Lewisham v Malcolm*, (p.App. 3.640), which was thought too unfavourable to disabled persons.
[†] Health & Safety at Work Act 1974 in the UK; Health & Welfare at Work Act 2005 in RoI.

Legal issues encountered by psychiatric experts

- *Work related stress* This issue may arise with respect to the link between work, stress and mental disorder, particularly conditions such as depression (📖 p.II.69), adjustment disorder (📖 p.II.72) and PTSD (📖 p.II.70)
- *Fitness to work* in relation to psychiatric disorder may have many implications for employee and employer. Psychiatric opinion is unlikely to be sought unless there is a complex or highly contentious issue. General practitioners and occupational health departments are more likely to involved in writing reports in this area
- *Unfair or wrongful dismissal* If the employee contends that they were unfairly or wrongfully dismissed[*] because of their mental disorder or its consequences (which might also amount to a breach of equality law), a psychiatrist may be instructed to give an opinion on the nature and symptoms of the mental disorder, its cause, its impact on work, and the patient's response to work.

Immigration and extradition law

Immigration law deals with the rights of non-citizens to enter and stay in the UK and RoI. In both countries, European Union citizens may usually enter and stay freely, whereas there are many restrictions on those from outside the EU. Particularly relevant to psychiatric practice are:

- Asylum seekers—those who have lodged an application for asylum
- Refugees—those who have been found to be at risk of persecution and have had their asylum claim accepted
- Mentally disordered offenders with no right to remain in the country.

People may have no right to remain because of illegal entry, overstaying or breaching conditions of immigration (for example, engaging in paid employment without permission). Unless the matter is dealt with as a criminal offence, the usual outcome of breaches of immigration law is deportation to the country of origin. Direct appeals to immigration appeals tribunals, and further appeals to courts under human rights law (📖 p.IV.418) are available, and these often take many months or years to complete. Psychiatric evidence may be relevant to some appeals.

Access to mental healthcare

Those who are not citizens[†] of the UK or RoI are, in general, not entitled to the benefits of citizenship, such as free healthcare from the NHS or HSE,

---

[*] Wrongful dismissal is any kind of sacking that is in breach of the contract of employment (for example, because the required notice period was not given, or because there was no adequate reason for it). Unfair dismissal is a subcategory of wrongful dismissal, where the dismissal did not follow a procedure required by statute, or was for a prohibited reason (such as because a female employee has become pregnant).

[†] Technically, not only citizens, but also those with certain immigration statuses such as 'indefinite leave to remain' are entitled to healthcare and other benefits of citizenship. Moreover, citizenship of certain other countries, especially former countries of the British Empire, may confer some benefits of UK citizenship when that person is in the UK.

or social care from local authorities, or benefit payments. However, a major exception is compulsory treatment provided under mental health law (📖 p.IV.373), which no person can be charged for. In E&W and Scotland this also means that non-citizens can be provided with free aftercare (📖 p.IV.398) health services, although this does not extend to social care services (such as accommodation that does not count as 'continuing healthcare').

Detention of mentally disordered people

- Detention of those suffering from *serious medical conditions* or *mental illness* will be avoided pending deportation if possible (but this does not apply to people with personality disorder)
- Mental healthcare in detention centres is limited and has been heavily criticized in inspection reports
- Transfer to hospital (📖 p.IV.410) using mental health legislation can be carried out if necessary.

Deportation of mentally disordered people

- The deportation of mentally disordered people is permitted under human rights law (📖 p.IV.418), but not in all circumstances
- Psychiatric evidence of a high risk of suicide if a person were deported has led to courts ruling against deportation, but only in 'very exceptional' cases. This does not necessarily include, for example, cases in which the deported person will receive no treatment and has no family to support them in the country of origin
- People subject to restrictions (📖 p.IV.412) under mental health law can be deported but only after specific consideration of their case; mentally disordered offenders are exempt from automatic deportation. In such cases it is lawful for the relevant minister to order discharge from hospital in order to facilitate deportation
- Detained patients can also be repatriated under mental health law: that is, they can be transferred as an inpatient to another country which has undertaken to continue their treatment.

Extradition

Extradition is not strictly part of immigration law, but is closely allied: it allows one country to surrender an individual to another country to face trial. The rules vary depending on the extradition treaties individual countries have signed with each other. Neither the UK nor RoI extradite those suspected of political offences, or where the country requesting extradition applies the death penalty to the alleged offence.

- If a person has a physical or mental condition that would make it unjust or oppressive to extradite them, and if the condition is likely to improve or resolve with treatment, the hearing should be adjourned.
- Extradition, like deportation, can be refused altogether if there is a serious mental disorder that is unlikely to improve, but the threshold for this is very high.

Common psychiatric issues in immigration and extradition

- The presence of any severe mental disorder
- PTSD (📖 p.II.70) and adjustment or other disorders relating to traumatic experiences
- Prognosis in relation to decisions on deportation or extradition
- The availability of treatment and support in the proposed destination, and the impact of not receiving necessary treatment.

A potential ethical dilemma of deportation

You are in charge of the care of a mentally disordered patient who has no permission to stay in your country. You know that as soon as you discharge her, she will be deported to a country where no adequate treatment or continuing rehabilitation will be available for her schizophrenia. Is there an ethical dilemma in treating her successfully, and/or in taking the decision to discharge her after recovery?

Inquests

Most deaths do not require any legal inquiry: the cause of death will be clear, uncontested, and involve no suspicious circumstances, and a doctor will be permitted to issue a death certificate. However, a death should be reported[*] to the coroner (or Procurator Fiscal in Scotland) if it occurred in any of the following circumstances:

- If the cause of death is unknown, or not clearly due to natural causes
- If a doctor did not see the deceased after death, or within the 14 days before death, or during their last illness
- Following accident or injury, however it occurred
- Following an industrial disease
- If the death was violent or there was a history of violence
- If there was a history of neglect, self-neglect, self-harm, or overdose
- During or shortly after a surgical operation (including any medically-induced termination of pregnancy) or recovery from an anaesthetic;
- During or shortly after detention in police custody, in prison or under mental health law
- If there were any other suspicious circumstances.

Postmortems and inquests

The coroner will frequently order a postmortem examination to clarify or confirm the cause of death. That will often be the end of the matter, but the coroner must usually hold an inquest if any of the circumstances in Box 19.4 apply. In addition, the coroner has discretion to hold an inquest in other circumstances if they think it necessary.

---

[*] Usually by GPs, hospitals and the police, but any person may report a death.

> **Box 19.4 Main grounds for an inquest or Fatal Accident Inquiry**
>
> - If the death was in prison, police custody or mental health detention
> - If it was violent or unnatural (in Scotland, or sudden or suspicious)
> - If the cause of death is still uncertain after a postmortem
> - In Scotland, after an accident at work
> - Certain deaths overseas, if the body is returned.[*]

Inquests are fact-finding inquiries, to establish who the deceased person was and when, where and how they died. They usually occur 3–9 months after death, but some may take years to conclude, particularly if they are adjourned while separate criminal trials and/or a public inquiry take place. Approximately 25,000 inquests are held every year in E&W.

The equivalent in Scotland in the Fatal Accident Inquiry, presided over by the Procurator Fiscal. Approximately 50–60 are held each year.

Relevant legislation

- *E&W* Coroners and Justice Act 2009; Coroners Act 1988[†]
- *Scotland* Fatal Accidents and Sudden Deaths Inquiry (Scotland) Act 1976
- *NI* Coroners Act (NI) 1959; *RoI* Coroners Act 1962.

Who is involved?

- The coroner, a doctor or lawyer responsible for the investigation (the vast majority are lawyers); or in Scotland, the Sheriff
- A coroner's officer, often a former police officer, who investigates and assists the coroner (in Scotland, staff at the Sheriff's office)
- In E&W, NI, and RoI, a jury of between 6 and 12 people (e.g. 7–11 in E&W) must be involved in the inquest if
  - The deceased died in custody or detention, and either the death was a violent or unnatural one, or the cause of death is unknown
  - The death resulted from an act or omission of a police officer, or a member of a service police force, or
  - The death was caused by a notifiable accident, poisoning or disease
- The coroner and jury are responsible for deciding the facts but may not directly find criminal or civil liability (this may follow later)
- Parents, children, spouses, and civil partners may attend, ask questions and be legally represented, as may be anyone whose acts or omissions may have caused or contributed to the death
- Witnesses may be called by the coroner or Sheriff, including psychiatrists and other mental health professionals.

---

[*] Except in Scotland—although, following a review of Fatal Accident Inquiries in 2009, the deaths of service personnel overseas can be the subject of an Inquiry in Scotland.
[†] At the time of writing, the 1988 Act is still in force; the 2009 Act is not due for full implementation until 2013, though some provisions may be brought in earlier. One notable change in the new Act is the requirement that all death certificates must be scrutinised by official Medical Examiners.

Inquest verdicts and Sheriff's determinations

At the end of the inquest or Fatal Accident Inquiry, the coroner or jury will issue a verdict, or the Sheriff will make a determination. Sheriff's determinations are always 'narrative': they set out the facts of the death in detail and explain the apparent causes. Coroners frequently give narrative verdicts, but may also give one of the following summary verdicts:

- Natural causes
- Accident (or misadventure, though this term is no longer approved)
- Suicide ('took their own life')
- Unlawful (or lawful) killing
- Industrial disease
- Open verdict (insufficient evidence for any other verdict).

Psychiatric involvement

Psychiatrists may be involved because the deceased was under their care, or as an expert advising the Coroner or Sherriff (or the family of the deceased) on issues such as the deceased's diagnosis or the quality of psychiatric care they received before death.

Chapter 20

The psychiatrist in court*

* This chapter describes the law and practice at the time of writing. However, the
Law Commission for E&W has recently published a proposal for sweeping reform
of this area of law, aimed at ensuring expert evidence (specifically including expert
psychiatric evidence) is not admitted without greater certainty about its reliability.
If accepted and enacted by the government, restrictive new rules on admissibility
(📖 p.IV.318) of expert evidence will apply in E&W within the next few years.

Principles & law of expert evidence

An expert's opinion is admissible to furnish the court with information that is likely to be *outside the experience and knowledge* of a judge or jury. If the judge or jury can form their own conclusions without help, then the opinion of an expert is unnecessary (*R v Turner*, 📖 p.App. 3.647).

Who is an expert, and what amounts to expert evidence?

There is no list of people who can be experts; in law, expertise is not defined solely by qualification, but more broadly in the following terms:

- Whether a person without instruction or experience in the area of knowledge or human experience would be able to form a sound judgement on the matter without the assistance of a witness possessing special knowledge or experience
- Whether the subject matter of the opinion forms part of a body of knowledge or experience which is sufficiently organized or recognized to be accepted as a reliable body of knowledge or experience, a special acquaintance with which by the witness would render his opinion of assistance to the court
- Whether the witness has acquired by study or experience sufficient knowledge of the subject to render his opinion of value in resolving the issues before the court

If detailed testing of the admissibility of expert evidence is not practical then the court may consider:

- Whether the expert's methodology accords with established practices in the profession or field, and
- The extent to which the basis of the expert's opinion can be properly explained and shown to be sound.

Fact and opinion

In criminal trials ordinary witnesses (📖 p.V.534) give evidence of fact. Only expert witnesses can also give their opinion. The judge determines what amounts to fact or opinion. Fact can include 'medical fact' which is attested to only by doctors, but distinguished from medical expert opinion:

> *Fact and opinion*
>
> A junior casualty doctor called to give evidence of what he found when he examined a victim of a knife attack might give factual medical information such as 'He had a single clean wound extending 6cm across the left side of the face, which had penetrated the muscle'.
>
> If, however, the doctor was then to answer the question 'Is it likely that the wound was made by a knife such as the one I am now holding up?' then this would amount to an expert medical opinion.

In some circumstances fact and inference from fact (i.e. opinion) can be clearly distinguished, for example:

- 'He was walking down the street and was unsteady on his feet' is clearly fact, albeit with some element of judgement contained within it, 'He was, at the time, suffering from multiple sclerosis' and 'his gait as observed was consistent with that diagnosis' is expert opinion

- 'He was suffering grief at the loss of his wife' might be a reasonable inference drawn by an ordinary witness (albeit subject to challenge in cross-examination), whereas 'he was suffering from an arrested grief reaction' would appear to require expert knowledge.

Expert evidence and hearsay

Evidence by a medical or psychological expert within a criminal trial will often include things said to the expert by the defendant and others. If presented to court by the expert, such evidence is essentially hearsay (📖 p.IV.319) in character. However, it is admissible, because it forms part of the information (📖 p.IV.297) upon which the expert properly formed their opinion, and is not given as evidence per se that is necessarily true. This distinction is a fine one and can be problematic, since the court (or a jury) is required to accept that the information is relevant to the view the expert formed, but to ignore it as regards proof of other matters.

Disagreement

In the UK, in both civil and (increasingly) criminal proceedings, where there is conflicting expert evidence experts are commonly asked to attend an experts' meeting and to issue a joint statement summarizing the areas of agreement and disagreement, making clear the basis for any disagreement (e.g. because experts accept different data, or draw different inferences from the same data).

Joint statements are encouraged over multiple supplementary reports by each expert, each responding to the last 'rebuttal' of their opinion by the other expert. They should be brief and focused on describing disagreements and the reasons for them. In some civil cases, the court may instead appoint a single joint expert (📖 p.V.535).

Other principles

Experts should:
- Provide impartial, unbiased evidence
- Be clear what legal questions they are answering
- Give reasons for their opinion and reasons for rejecting alternatives
- Cite evidence both for and against their opinion
- Give 'conditional' opinions where their opinion would vary depending on what findings of fact the court makes
- Be prepared to change their opinion in response to new information
- Acknowledge the limits of their expertise (and point out where the opinion of an expert from another profession would be useful)
- Refrain from being an advocate

Beyond various legal duties (📖 p.V.536), and duties laid down in codes of practice (📖 p.V.538), the expert has an ethical duty (📖 p.App. 3.651), to the court and to the profession, to be impartial. Expert work is subject to scrutiny by professional bodies just like clinical work, and poor or unethical performance may lead to professional liability proceedings (📖 p.V.522).

Witnesses, experts, & expert evidence

Types of witness in the UK and Ireland
There are three main types of witness to the court:
- An ordinary witness (i.e. witness to fact)
- A professional witness
- An expert witness.

Ordinary and professional witnesses may only describe factual matters and not give opinion evidence; ultimately, the court makes the distinction between fact and opinion (📖 p.V.532).[*]

Professional and expert witnesses in the UK
Factual and professional witnesses most commonly write, often with assistance from the police or a solicitor, *statements* that will become part of the case papers. Experts write *reports* to the court (although a report can also sometimes be transformed into a statement). All types of witness may then be required to give oral evidence, including being cross examined.

Professional and expert witnesses in RoI
In RoI, no distinction is made between expert and professional witness, at least where consultants giving evidence in their speciality are concerned. If a patient is under the care of a psychiatrist then that treating doctor becomes the expert witness in any relevant proceedings. They are ethically bound to do so[†] by the Medical Council of Ireland. The 'other side' will appoint its own expert.

Who can be an expert?
Expert witnesses may be from a range of disciplines and the types of evidence given may vary. Psychiatric evidence is more often categorical (the patient did or did not have this disorder), as opposed to dimensional psychological evidence (they scored this on that test, 📖 p.II.96).

The roles of the expert
There are various potential roles of an expert witness in the legal system which may be pursued either singly or sometimes together, including:
- *Clinical* This role requires direct contact with a defendant/witness and involves making an assessment (📖 p.II.89) of mental condition, perhaps including the use of psychometric tests (📖 p.II.96) of mental functioning.
- *Experimental* This is an impersonal role and does not necessarily require direct contact with the patient/defendant/witness. It is useful for obtaining facts and extracting them in situations relevant for a jury. For example, the reliability of eyewitness testimony.

---

[*] Some civil legal situations blur the distinction between factual evidence and expert opinion, such as when a treating psychiatrist (in theory a professional witness) is asked by a Tribunal whether the legal criteria for detention are met in respect of their patient (a matter of opinion).
[†] According to section 9 of the Medical Council of Ireland's Ethical Guide (Medical Council, 1998). Failure to comply with a request to provide an expert report could result in professional conduct proceedings (📖 p.V.521).

- *Advisory* In this capacity the expert may be asked to examine the evidence of another expert and provide a critique of it, within an adversarial context (see 📖 p.V.545). This role has had greater prominence in recent times and reports by an expert are increasingly being subjected to peer review by experts appointed by the other side. This role can feel uncomfortable but is necessary if a lawyer is to gain a real understanding of the strengths and weaknesses of an opinion expressed within a science of which they have little or no knowledge.
- *Actuarial* This is when the expert presents evidence of the probability of some event or of the prevalence of some condition in the population. It can be achieved through literature searches or by fieldwork: e.g. average earnings related to intelligence. It is based on probabilistic reasoning and the use of statistics and is increasingly applied in judicial proceedings.

Where an expert is required to be advisory after having been clinical in role, this necessitates good boundary-keeping. For example, it is common practice in a criminal trial for an expert to give unbiased evidence (clinical role) and then to sit behind counsel for the side that called them and to suggest questions to be put to the other opposing expert (advisory role).

Relevance and admissibility of expert evidence

For expert evidence to be allowed into legal proceedings it has to be both relevant and admissible (📖 p.IV.319). Relevance is determined by the 'probative value' of the evidence in a given case, i.e. how much it tends to prove or disprove a relevant fact, or state of mind. There are a number of specific legal rules (📖 p.V.536) governing what psychiatric evidence is relevant or admissible in certain types of cases.

It is the judge's prerogative to determine the competency of a witness to give expert evidence and whether what the expert intends to assert is relevant and admissible. In some circumstances, the judge may accept the expert's qualifications, but exclude part or all of their evidence.

The single joint expert

In civil proceedings, there may be a request for a psychiatrist to act as a joint expert, where both sides agree on one expert to provide an opinion. One solicitor will be appointed as the lead solicitor to instruct them. In cases where a party then wants to instruct another expert, this will need to be agreed separately by the judge with a clear rationale given. At the time of writing, criminal proceedings do not use joint experts.

Specific legal rules of expert evidence

The rules specific to mental health experts in the UK and Ireland need to be considered alongside the general rules of evidence (📖 p.V.532), both expert and non-expert (📖 p.V.534). The evidence of psychiatrists and other mental health experts has frequently been considered in the higher courts, but the rulings have not always been consistent, making it difficult to describe a clear set of rules that can be generalized to all settings. This page lists specific legal rules issued by higher courts.

Most of the rules on this page come from courts in E&W, many of which also directly apply in NI and a few in Scotland. Similar principles are followed in all jurisdictions, but courts in Scotland and RoI tend to allow much more discretion in the admissibility of evidence (📖 p.IV.319).

Compulsory evidence

In certain circumstances, psychiatric evidence may be deemed compulsory before a court can make certain decisions. For example:
- All jurisdictions require psychiatric evidence from two registered medical practitioners to support a finding of insanity (📖 p.IV.489)
- Psychiatric evidence is compulsory before an order for compulsory treatment (📖 p.IV.405), such as a hospital order, can be made
- A psychiatric report is recommended under sentencing guidelines in E&W after a conviction for arson (📖 p.IV.350) and certain sexual offences
- Psychiatric evidence may be practically essential in other areas but not required by statute, such as when considering a risk assessment order (📖 p.IV.408) in Scotland, before imposing an indeterminate sentence of imprisonment (📖 p.IV.364) in some cases, or before making a community order (📖 p.IV.368) with a mental health treatment requirement.

How mentally disordered?

Courts refuse to hear expert evidence on issues they consider within the everyday experience of ordinary people (*R v Turner*, 📖 p.App. 3.647). Therefore:
- There cannot be evidence from a psychiatrist in regard to psychological functioning of someone who is not in some way mentally abnormal
- Evidence of psychiatric abnormality (e.g. relating to a propensity to violence) is not admissible for the purpose of determining whether a defendant committed an offence, or which of two defendants committed the offence (*R v Kemp*, 📖 p.App. 3.639)
- Diagnostic evidence is usually allowed as it is founded on scientific principles
- Evidence relating to intellectual disability has tended to be allowed if a formal assessment shows or suggests an IQ of less than 70
- Psychiatric evidence is inadmissible when the issue concerns how an ordinary person reacts to stress (*R v Weightman*, 📖 p.App. 3.647); however,
- Expert evidence on complex psychological phenomena such as learned helplessness as a basis for a defence of duress by threats (📖 p.V.502) may be admissible (*R v Emery*, 📖 p.App. 3.636), and
- Psychiatric evidence relating to complex reactions to trauma is often allowed.

Specific examples of issues

Reliability

- Psychiatric evidence must be relevant and reliable (*R v Mohan*, 📖 p.App. 3.642)
- An expert may comment on the reliability of a witness if there is a mental disorder that makes a witness incapable of giving, or less likely to give, reliable evidence (*R v O'Brien*, 📖 p.App. 3.642). This may include personality disorder
- Expert evidence concerning the reliability of confessions (📖 p.IV.479) when related to mental disorder or related personality features such as unusual suggestibility or compliance (📖 p.II.123) is allowed
- Where interviews have been conducted with a defendant who was mentally disordered expert evidence is allowed as to the likely reliability of the content of the interview, if relevant
- Evidence from psychiatrists or psychologists as to which of two defendants the more likely to be violent is not usually allowed.

Veracity

- An expert may not bolster a witness's credibility (*R v Robinson*, 📖 p.App. 3.645); however, evidence is admissible of 'disabilities' which the jury, or court, should know about in properly interpreting the witness's evidence
- Child psychiatrists have been allowed to give evidence on whether children's evidence that they have been abused is likely to be reliable (*In Re M & R*, 📖 p.App. 3.640).

Intent, mens rea, and recklessness

- There may be a need to distinguish between intent (📖 p.IV.334) and capacity to form intent (📖 p.IV.481)
- An expert may give evidence on the issue of mens rea or capacity to form intent if there is mental disorder
- An expert may not give evidence on the intent of an ordinary person, unless there is a medical condition that may affect it, such as hypoglycaemia (*R v Toner*, 📖 p.App. 3.647).

Capacity to consent

- In sexual offences (📖 p.IV.348) an expert may consider the defendant's capacity to assess another person's ability to consent.

Criminal convictions

- There is a general rule that no criminal conviction can be based on expert evidence alone.[*]

---

[*] This comes from a series of notorious miscarriages of justice between 1990 and 2005 in which parents were convicted of killing their children primarily on the basis of (unintentionally) false or misleading evidence from paediatrician Professor Sir Roy Meadow about the unlikelihood of such deaths occurring naturally. Meadow was struck off the medical register, but reinstated after an appeal to the High Court and the Court of Appeal.

Codes of practice and experts

Some jurisdictions have specific codes of practice for experts, which in some cases are general in nature, and in E&W are detailed and specific, and separated into civil and criminal work. Box 20.1 contains an abridged version of the E&W Criminal Procedure Rules for expert witnesses (CPR33); the sections of the Civil Procedure Rules and Family Procedure Rules referring to expert witnesses (CivPR35, FPR25), and other jurisdictions' codes, embody similar principles. The Rules are often supplemented by more detailed Practice Directions issued by the courts which explain how the Rules should be complied with.

Box 20.1 E&W Criminal Procedure Rules for expert witnesses (CPR33)

33.1 A reference to an 'expert' in this Part is a reference to a person who is required to give or prepare expert evidence for the purpose of criminal proceedings, including evidence required to determine fitness to plead or for the purpose of sentencing.

33.2 An expert must help the court by giving objective, unbiased opinion on matters within his expertise. This duty overrides any obligation to the person from whom he receives instructions or by whom he is paid. This duty includes an obligation to inform all parties and the court if the expert's opinion changes from that contained in a report served as evidence or given in a statement.

33.3 An expert's report must:
- give details of qualifications, relevant experience and accreditation;
- give details of any literature or other information relied on;
- contain a statement setting out the substance of all facts given to the expert which are material to the opinions expressed in the report, or upon which those opinions are based;
- make clear which of the facts stated in the report are within the expert's own knowledge;
- say who carried out any examination, measurement, test or experiment which the expert has used for the report and:
  - give their qualifications, relevant experience and accreditation;
  - say whether or not the expert supervised them, and
  - summarize the findings on which the expert relies;
- where there is a range of opinion on the matters dealt with:
  - summarize the range of opinion, and
  - give reasons for the expert's own opinion;
- if the opinion requires qualification, state the qualification;
- contain a summary of the conclusions reached;
- contain a statement that the expert understands his duty to the court, has complied and will continue to comply with that duty; and
- contain the same declaration of truth as a witness statement.

Box 20.1 (*Contd.*)

33.4 A party who wants to introduce expert evidence must serve it on the court officer, and each other party; serve it as soon as practicable; and if another party so requires, give that party a copy of, or a reasonable opportunity to inspect any relevant records etc.

33.5. A party who serves on another party or on the court a report by an expert must, at once, inform that expert of that fact.

33.6 Where more than one party wants to introduce expert evidence, the court may direct the experts to:
• discuss the expert issues in the proceedings; and
• prepare a statement for the court of the matters on which they agree and disagree, giving their reasons.

Except for that statement, the content of that discussion must not be referred to without the court's permission.

33.7 Where more than one defendant wants to introduce expert evidence on an issue at trial, the court may direct that the evidence on that issue is to be given by one expert only. Where the co-defendants cannot agree who should be the expert, the court may:
• select the expert from a list prepared or identified by them; or
• direct that the expert be selected in another way.

33.8 Where the court gives a direction under rule 33.7 for a single joint expert to be used, each of the co-defendants may give instructions to the expert. When a co-defendant gives instructions to the expert he must, at the same time, send a copy of the instructions to the other co-defendant(s). The court may give directions about:
• the payment of the expert's fees and expenses; and
• any examination, measurement, test or experiment which the expert wishes to carry out.

The court may, before an expert is instructed, limit the amount that can be paid by way of fees and expenses to the expert. Unless the court otherwise directs, the instructing co-defendants are jointly and severally liable for the payment of the expert's fees and expenses.

33.9 The court may:
• extend (even after it has expired) a time limit under this Part; or
• allow the introduction of expert evidence which omits a detail required by this Part.

A party who wants an extension of time must—
• apply when serving the expert evidence for which it is required; and
• explain the delay.

Consent & confidentiality in court

There are specific issues relating to consent and confidentiality in court proceedings; however, it is important also to refer to the general medical duty of confidentiality (📖 p.III.263).

Consent

When undertaking assessments for court proceedings, the expert should be mindful of particular pressures on individuals to engage, especially if they have been instructed by the courts to do so. This is particularly important in assessment for criminal proceedings where the defendant may receive an indeterminate sentence (📖 p.IV.364) and where consent to risk assessment (📖 p.III.284) is an issue. Thus proper concern to obtain consent can be paramount. It is important to obtain consent from the defendant, and also to speak to other informants, e.g. family or other professionals, before writing the report (📖 p.V.560).

Confidentiality and related issues

- When acting as an expert witness, the medical duty of confidentiality is overridden by duties to the court and the instructing solicitor, and an expert should not offer or guarantee confidentiality to a party
- The expert witness has a duty to disclose all the evidence that they have used to form their opinion. When citing references in a report or in court, it is vital to have read the original source and cite the reference correctly
- If you are a junior psychiatrist or other professional seeking supervision (📖 p.III.252) prior to going to court, or discussing the finer points of a case with colleagues, then it is essential that you are sure the content of these discussions will not be disclosed by your supervisor or colleagues, as the information given to them, if it became commonly known might prejudice the case
- You should also ensure that your instructing solicitors understand you will be making limited disclosures to colleagues for the purposes of supervision or advice. Likewise, prior to discussing the specifics of a case with other experts, permission should be obtained from the instructing parties*
- In court, when placed under oath as a witness, you must answer the questions posed despite any duty of confidentiality you may be under, unless the judge orders that you do not need to answer the question. If your report was based upon information that you would not wish disclosed in this way, such as specific questions and scoring criteria in certain psychometric tests (📖 p.II.101), you should discuss this advance with your instructing solicitor, and if necessary with the judge.
- When giving evidence in a Magistrate's Court it is important to remember that the magistrates will not have been provided with a copy of your report and will not be subject to information that could prejudice the outcome of a case e.g. prior convictions of a defendant. Therefore it is important that you do not give this information in oral evidence, even though it was written in your report. In higher courts, if there is a jury, the same applies to evidence given when the jury is present.

---

* This does not exclude the possibility of limited disclosure when there is a serious and immediate risk of harm, such as when the assessment has revealed significant suicidal ideation.

Applied ethics and testimony

Judicial ethics & jurisprudence

Law and ethics are discussed elsewhere (📖 p.II.237) as forms of social discourse about how people relate to each other; and about what happens when the interests of one individual clash with those of another, or with society. Ethics is the discourse of values in relationships; the law is the codification of a social consensus about what is socially valuable.

Judicial ethics is a specific area of ethics, concerning the values held important by judges, which differ from those of psychiatrists (📖 p.III.294). *Jurisprudence* is the theory and philosophy of law and legal decision-making.

Jurisprudence

The law clearly has one central moral value at its heart:, justice. However, what 'justice' means in practice, and how it relates to competing values such as 'fairness', 'duty', and 'right', is the core study of jurisprudence. Descriptive jurisprudence analyses how these values shape what the law is in a society; normative jurisprudence extrapolates from such values to state what the law should be. Important normative jurisprudential theorists include John Rawls and Ronald Dworkin. Within descriptive jurisprudence there are three main schools of thought:

Natural law theorists hold that there are natural, absolute foundations to law (which might be considered laws of nature), and that these can be deduced by the power of reason. Hobbes and John Finnis are two of the most significant natural law theorists.

Legal positivists argue that law is wholly distinct from morality, and that societies adopt laws to reflect their social and political structures and power relationships. Within this there is much disagreement about how the relationship between law and society should be analysed. Key authors in this field include HLA Hart (a 'soft' positivist) and Joseph Raz (a 'hard' positivist).

Legal realism is an alternative sociological view of law, arguing that it is defined by what legal actors (judges, lawyers, clients, juries, legislators) do, not what they or others say it is or ought to do. Legal *pragmatists* following this approach argue that the law should be determined by the desired social outcome, not other ideals such as coherence or fidelity to a statute. *Critical legal studies* is a more radical derivative of legal realism.

Judicial ethics and judges

Judges have an important role in society and are entrusted with exercising considerable power. Judicial ethics is made up of the norms and standards that impacts on judges, and includes such matters as maintaining independence and impartiality, and avoiding impropriety.

This are considerable debate about how laws should be enacted to reflect justice. One view sees this as arising in judicial decisions, and indeed in the ethical mindset of individual judges. Different judges favour different ethical theories (📖 p.III.233): some may be more communitarian, for example, whilst others favour liberal individualism. The importance of these schools of thought can be seen in judicial appointments, especially to each country's Supreme Court (📖 p.IV.308), as the decisions of these courts can determine how all other courts interpret and apply the law.

- The European Court of Human Rights (📖 p.IV.326) has set out principles by which judges need to abide
- The United Nations has adopted the six 'Bangalore Principles' of judicial ethics, which have been endorsed and elaborated in detail by the Scottish judiciary and others. The principles are shown in Box 21.1.

Box 21.1 The Bangalore Principles of judicial ethics

All judges must:
- Be independent of all outside influences
- Be impartial between the different parties, cases, and views
- Maintain personal and professional integrity at all times
- Behave properly, and be seen to behave with propriety
- Ensure all are treated equally by the courts
- Exercise their duties competently and diligently.

Political influence

- Jurisprudence, ethics and politics affect the ways that laws are made
- Left wing governments often favour utilitarian ethics, and pass laws accordingly
- Right wingers generally support rights based/individualist ethical theories, and their laws reflect those values
- This is how it is possible to have laws that some would consider morally bad, and why it is thought to be important to have an independent judiciary.

Ethics, the psychiatrist, and court

Psychiatrists operate under unusual ethical circumstances when assessing for courts and providing reports, in that their role is entirely non-medical (📖 p.III.261). This is so even though the effect may sometimes be to result in treatment of the individual. Identifying and observing appropriate professional boundaries (📖 p.III.246) is therefore crucial.

Individual psychiatrists may be challenged by having to operate within a legal process, or with legal concepts that express values incongruent with their own. However, practicing forensic psychiatry requires at least an overall acceptance of the legal system within which it is necessary to function. Where values clash, in the end the law holds sway.

Addressing the ultimate issue

The term *ultimate issue* refers to the final decision before a court. For example, in a trial for murder, the ultimate issue is whether the defendant committed the actus reus (📖 p.IV.332) with the requisite mens rea (📖 p.IV.334). Whether the defendant was mentally ill at the time of the killing is an intermediate issue, properly subject to expert evidence.

Experts must limit themselves to matters within their expertise that are beyond the experience of the jury or judge and not directly address the ultimate issue before the court. This is because deciding the ultimate issue requires choosing between disputed facts or interpretations, and might involve making assumptions. It is a fundamental principle in common-law jurisdictions (📖 p.IV.306) that such decisions are matters for ordinary people or those representing them, not for experts.

In the USA, addressing the ultimate issue is prohibited by federal rules of evidence;[*] in the UK and RoI there is no explicit rule, but such conduct is likely to be censured by the judge.

Experts and the ultimate issue

Forensic psychiatric experts are particularly likely to be drawn into discussing the ultimate issue in the following areas:

- The defence of insanity (📖 p.V.489)—the expert should state whether the defendant suffered from a *disease of the mind* and the effects of that disease, but not whether those effects rendered them unable to know the nature and quality of their actions, or whether they were wrong
- The partial defence of diminished responsibility (📖 p.V.491)—the expert should state whether the defendant suffered from, say, an abnormality of mental functioning but not whether that abnormality substantially impaired their mental responsibility for their actions[†]
- In child protection cases (📖 p.V.511)—where questions may be asked of the expert that assume that disputed facts have been proved (e.g. that a child has been harmed in a particular way); the expert should either not accept such instructions until the relevant facts have been adjudged by the court, or give a conditional opinion (if X is proved, then my opinion would be . . .).

Guidelines

The following guidelines will help you avoid unintentionally addressing the ultimate issue:

- Obtain detailed instructions in advance from the relevant solicitor or court; request clarification if they ask legal questions (e.g. 'did Mr P have diminished responsibility?') instead of psychiatric ones (e.g. 'was Mr P suffering from an abnormality of mind, and if so what were its effects?')
- Ensure that every statement you make is based firmly on the evidence cited earlier in your report
- Do not make assumptions or value judgements
- Use medical or psychological rather than legal terminology, particularly when addressing specific legal tests
- Distinguish in the opinion section of your report clearly between psychiatric opinion and the legal implications of that opinion
- Ensure that the report is expressed in a way that can best assist the court in translating (📖 p.IV.300) from the medical diagnosis or formulation into the legal tests, rather than expressing a view per se on whether those tests are met.

---

[*] Rule 704(b): 'No expert witness . . . may state an opinion or inference as to whether the defendant did or did not have . . . an element of the crime charged . . . Such ultimate issues are matters for the trier of fact alone.'
[†] Unless specifically invited to do so by the judge, as the Court of Appeal has ruled is permissible.

Giving expert advice to one side

Advice instead of giving a report to the court

A clear distinction must be drawn between submitting a report to the court (irrespective of the source of instructions) and giving advice to lawyers. The former requires independence and an acknowledgement that the ultimate duty of the expert is to the court. Giving expert advice, which is most likely to involve reading and critiquing of the report, and/or clinical notes and process, of another psychiatrist (and which should never involve direct clinical assessment of the individual), represents assistance to one side within an adversarial process (🕮 p.IV.314).

Often giving advice will be in written form. This should be carefully constructed so as to make plain:

- The nature of the instructions
- The nature of what you are providing
- The distinction between such advice and a report which might be used directly in the legal proceedings.

Advice after completing a report

Where a psychiatrist has already provided a report to the court, usually based upon his or her own clinical assessment, they have an established duty of impartiality to the court.

If they then also give advice to the lawyers that instructed them, knowing it will be used in an adversarial fashion, this creates an ethical tension, requiring extreme caution concerning what is being done when. The advice might be in conference with counsel or the instructing solicitor, or through, for example, passing notes to counsel when they are cross-examining another expert, advising them of particular lines of questioning, or of particular detailed questions to ask.

This ethical tension is unavoidable, in that lawyers may not be able to understand the strengths and weaknesses of an opposing expert report without advice. Assisting the lawyers on one side of a case by explaining your own report to them, as well as its strengths and weakness, is acceptable, as is explaining the strengths and weakness of other experts' reports. However, pursuing impartiality in writing the original report, and in giving oral evidence to the court, and yet also advising counsel for the side that has instructed you, requires constant vigilance, in order to ensure that you do not yourself become adversarial.

Record-keeping when giving advice

As in all medico-legal situations, you must make good clinical notes, and also deal with all legal communications, on the assumption that they may be used or tested legally, whatever your role. It is therefore good practice to keep contemporaneous notes of discussions, and of the participants. Documents need to be checked, signed, and dated. It is also worth keeping a careful record of the oral information received and advice given, any documentation one has seen, and also (if known) what one has not seen. If it is known that facts are in legal dispute, then it is essential to make clear that this is also known by you, and that you have not taken a position in advance of legal determination of the relevant facts.

Controversial clinical concepts in court

Clinical concepts may be new or controversial. They may pose specific challenges for the legal system and experts. In general terms a number of general principles apply for experts:

- Present scientific information in simple terms
- Identify clearly any value judgements inherent in a particular diagnosis
- Acknowledge any limitations associated with a specific opinion
- Observe rules relating to expert opinion including giving the whole range of possible opinion and state why yours is preferred
- Ensure, that where you are dealing with a controversial issue you clearly reference, and can describe, the relevant scientific evidence
- Be prepared to explain and educate, rather than argue a particular side of a debate.

Neuroscience

Knowledge about the relationship between violence and neurobiology (🕮 p.II.28) is rapidly expanding. The main issues are whether biological correlates of violence exist, and whether they can be used to assess culpability in legal processes. The answer to the first question is evolving into a more certain yes despite methodological complexity. An answer to the second is likely to remain elusive. There should be extreme caution in drawing conclusions about any mental disorder, risk, or prognosis directly from the results of biological investigations. The exceptions to this are where an investigation is established as diagnostically important, such as an EEG in sleep disorders or epilepsy.

Recovered or false memories

The main debate is whether such memories (usually of sexual abuse) are a product of suggestions that have been made to the individual in the course of therapy (*false memories*), or whether they reflect an uncovering of true childhood memories of repressed, stressful events (*recovered memories*). Whilst an opinion about the nature of recalled events may be necessary, any court should be informed of the controversial nature of the concepts, and that:

- Memory is rarely an exact replication of true events
- Memory is likely to incorporate some distortion of events
- Recall of events can be influenced by suggestion (🕮 p.II.123)
- Repression is a psychological theory with limited scientific evidence for its existence

Controversial diagnoses

Many of the most controversial diagnoses relate to responses to stress and trauma.

- *Complex PTSD* has a degree of clinical validity but is not yet present in diagnostic classifications. There is overlap with the features of BPD (🕮 p.II.61). There is potentially legal significance to making one or other of these diagnoses: for example, in mitigation (🕮 pV.506), the diagnosis of complex PTSD (🕮 p.II.70) might be less likely to be accepted by the court, but that of PD might be more stigmatizing
- *Adjustment disorders* are recognized conditions but can be subject to criticism with respect to the utility of expert evidence because of their

intuitive nature. There may also be a view that they simply represent normal reactions to stress

- Certain disorders and diagnoses can be controversial because they may be diagnosed by use of one diagnostic manual and not the other:
  - PTSD: there is limited cross-manual reliability (between DSM-IV and ICD10, 📖 p.II.109) for this diagnosis
  - Paranoid schizophrenia is subject to different requirements for duration of symptoms (6 months DSM-IV and 1 month ICD-10)
- *Dissociative identity disorder* (or multiple personality disorder, 📖 p.II.73) is subject to continuing controversy regarding its validity as a diagnosis
- *Sex addiction* Although this is not included in DSM, the APA is recommending the addition of a new condition, 'hypersexual disorder'
- *Episodic dyscontrol syndrome* There is some evidence for the existence of this syndrome (📖 p.84) of explosive and apparently uncontrollable violence related to abnormalities of the temporal lobes and/or other brain regions, and it has been recognised as contributing towards a defence to murder (📖 p.IV.345), but it is not generally accepted.

Crime-related amnesia

Although much less controversial per se, there are multiple possible psychological and biological reasons for amnesia (📖 p. V.504), which may have legal consequences if the amnesia is accepted as due to an underlying mental disorder. As with other controversial conditions, this should be assessed and described carefully.

Case example

When Jane was 32 she started to see a hypnotherapist to help her to address issues of low self-esteem and symptoms of an eating disorder. She was told at the beginning of treatment that she would 'remember things that you do not want to remember, but they will come flooding back'. After several sessions of hypnotherapy, Jane began to describe memories of being sexually abused by her stepfather when she was 9 years old. Although Jane felt that many of her current problems were due to difficulties that she experienced during her childhood, she also reported that she had no memory of any episodes of abuse prior to starting hypnotherapy. She later made a complaint to the police alleging sexual abuse by her stepfather.

Did the sexual abuse happen? Can evidence from the hypnotherapist assist in that determination? What aspects of the memory are important in assessing its veracity?

Opinions in sentencing

Traditionally, psychiatrists give evidence or advice on disposal to courts solely for the purpose of treatment. However, as sentencing (📖 p.IV.361) has become progressively more concerned with public protection (📖 p.IV.294) and with the ongoing risk of harm to others (📖 p.II.189) posed by offenders, including mentally disordered offenders, the courts have increasingly expected psychiatrists to make and interpret risk assessments

(📖 p.II.127) or to give opinions on dangerousness (📖 p.V.549)—as well as to consider treatment in the context of more punitive sentences.

Recommending inpatient treatment

A recommendation for court-ordered treatment (📖 p.IV.405) such as a hospital order should be based on a view that the defendant will benefit from treatment, as well as meeting the relevant legal criteria. Particularly in E&W, those criteria have been loosened legally—for example, by the removal of the former treatability test (📖 p.IV.383). However, simply because people exhibiting psychopathy (📖 p.II.66), paedophilia, or other sexual deviancy (📖 p.II.74) might fall within the legal criteria justifying detention does not imply they should be detained and offered treatment, unless there are clear reasons for believing they will benefit (📖 p.III.282).

Penal sentences

No expert should ever recommend a penal disposal or punishment (eg 'he may have schizophrenia, but he knew exactly what he was doing in committing the offence and, in my view, should go to prison'). Where no psychiatric disposal is indicated, you should make no recommendation. It is then for the court to decide how to sentence.

With the great increase in indeterminate sentences (📖 p.IV.364), mental health professionals are increasingly called upon to carry out assessments of risk or 'dangerousness' (📖 p.V.549) directed towards determining whether such a sentence should be imposed. Even if a psychiatrist normally refuses such requests, they may have given a report for trial and then be drawn into such issues at sentencing, when hospital disposal is not under consideration. This raises a major ethical issue (📖 p.III.265), since it amounts to clinical assessment directed at a solely punitive objective.

Moreover, the law on what can be taken into account by the court is complex, especially in E&W: a psychiatrist who does decide to give an opinion on 'dangerousness' should seek guidance from their instructing solicitor on what issues should be addressed.

Hybrid orders and hospital directions

The hybrid order (📖 p.IV.408) in E&W and the hospital direction (📖 p.IV.408) in Scotland combine elements of treatment and punishment, and were created by the UK and Scottish governments because they believed that hospital orders did not always 'reflect an element of appropriate punishment', as well as because of concerns about 'dangerous' patients being released early when treatment had failed, or because the diagnosis made at sentence proved later to be wrong, and the basis for continued detention therefore lapsed.

The orders require the doctor to state that all the conditions are satisfied for the making of a hospital order or equivalent; the judge may then choose to impose a hybrid order or hospital direction instead. There are no guidelines to assist the judge in choosing between the alternative orders, and the judge may ask the psychiatrist for advice on this point.

If asked, it is important for you to remain within your professional role (📖 p.III.246). It is acceptable to state an honest opinion that treatment, though legally possible, has a low probability of achieving a significant risk reduction (📖 p.III.265); it is probably not acceptable to go beyond this and specifically recommend the hybrid order or hospital direction, which is tantamount to recommending a punishment.

Community orders with a condition of treatment

A community order (📖 p.IV.368) is essentially a punitive sentence but it may have a condition of mental health or drug treatment attached to it, such that if the offender fails to comply with the requirements of the treating psychiatric team, they may be 'breached' by their supervising probation officer and returned to court.

Your report should state what treatment you think necessary, if any, and where it may be offered (e.g. as an inpatient, or in the community). If you think that treatment is more likely to succeed if there is an element of supervision, it is acceptable to recommend a condition of treatment, as long as you are careful not to recommend the community order itself, as this is essentially a punitive sentence. A *conditional recommendation* is the easiest way of achieving this: e.g. 'Should the court be minded to impose a community order, I would recommend a mental health treatment requirement specifying . . . '.

However, before making any such recommendation you should obtain the agreement of the probation officer (or in Scotland, criminal justice social worker) who would supervise the order. It is also important to consider the functions of the treating psychiatrist and supervising officer; if either appears to have no obvious role, the order is inappropriate.

It is also wise to consider in advance the possibility that you, as the treating psychiatrist, will have evidence that your patient is in *breach* of the order, such as by refusing to comply with an aspect of treatment. What will the supervising officer expect you to disclose, and what will you agree to disclose? What is the threshold for breach?

Mitigating and aggravating factors

You should not explicitly give mitigating evidence (📖 p.V.507) on behalf of a defendant, even if they happen to be your patient. However, if instructed to do so, you may give medical information in response to specific questions (e.g. what impact would the mental disorder have had on the defendant's understanding of the seriousness of their actions?)

You should never raise the issue of aggravating factors (📖 p.V.506), or accept instructions to produce a report on them. You should likewise be aware of the possibility that a report you write for other purposes may later be used by the court as evidence of aggravating factors.

Courts' assessments of dangerousness

Sentencing (📖 p.IV.361) is becoming increasingly concerned with protecting society from dangerous offenders, rather than solely with punishing (📖 p.IV.297) the offender. In order to match sentences to 'dangerousness', courts need some way of determining offenders' dangerousness, and often turn to psychiatrists and psychologists to help. This is ethically controversial where any risk is reasonably perceived to be related to mental disorder, but even more so where the psychiatrist or psychologist is called upon to address risk in isolation from mental disorder, or even where there is no mental disorder. In the absence of mental disorder the psychiatrist has no expertise upon which to rely and should resist requests for assessment or an opinion.

Dangerousness and risk compared

'Dangerousness' is not a psychiatric concept, but rather a legal one referring to the perceived likelihood of harm to the public. As with many other legal concepts (📖 p.IV.296), it is superficially similar to the related psychiatric concept of risk of harm (📖 p.II.127), but differs in important ways: dangerousness is conceived as a simple, static, global characteristic of an individual, whereas risk of harm is specific to a given harm at a given time and in a given set of circumstances. Within a clinical paradigm, 'dangerousness' does not exist, only the risk of harm in given circumstances.

Should clinicians help courts consider dangerousness?

Clinicians may be called upon to assist a court with its assessment of dangerousness where:
- They have previously written a report on a defendant with mental disorder, and the court is now considering sentencing them, or
- They have not previously been involved in the case, but are specifically asked to assess dangerousness, such as under a risk assessment order (📖 p.IV.408) in Scotland.

Arguments against assisting
- Some psychiatrists refuse to offer such evidence, on the basis that it amounts to using medical techniques directed solely at a non-medical purpose, which is intended directly to influence punishment (see 📖 p.III.246); there is a risk of doing harm to the defendant/patient
- Risk assessment is inherently too unreliable reasonably to be offered to courts, especially when attempted by a single clinician who has not had the benefit of substantial data collection and investigation whilst the patient has been in hospital
- It may well be inherently invalid to use risk assessment techniques as a 'snapshot' of dangerousness for a court, as opposed to as part of a continuous process of risk management (📖 p.II.189) and re-assessment, within a therapeutic relationship
- Many risk assessment tools, or parts of them, utilize actuarial data based upon groups and do not refer to the individual patient, whereas justice in sentencing requires an individual approach.
- The courts seek an assessment of dangerousness, a non-medical concept, within their own legal paradigm (📖 p.IV.296), and medical concepts of risk are not valid in this context.

Arguments in favour of assisting
The chief argument is that the court will make an assessment of dangerousness regardless of whether a clinician assists, and if the defendant has mental disorder, better that the assessment is informed by expert psychiatric or psychological evidence than carried out solely by those without such training.

A further complexity concerns situations in which a psychiatrist compiles a report on issues other than 'dangerousness', but then finds that the information they have collected and which is in the report will be used by the court in an assessment of dangerousness. An expert who does not wish to assist such an assessment might decide simply to report their conclusions, without listing the data relied upon, thus preventing its use by the court in this way. However, this may breach rules on expert evidence (📖 p.V.536) and the expert might in any event be subpoenaed (📖 p.IV.314) to court to explain their conclusion.

Practical considerations

If an expert decides to assist (or not to frustrate) a court's assessment of dangerousness, the following should be considered.

- When seeking the patient's consent (📖 p.III.284) to assessment and to the completion of a report, you should explain the uses to which the report could be put by the court, beyond the requested purpose
- The risk assessment must be of the highest quality achievable, and should clearly set out its assumptions and limitations
- The report or evidence must be framed in medical terminology concerning risk, leaving the court to make inferences about dangerousness: you should not cross the divide (📖 p.IV.299) and attempt to address the legal concepts directly
- The report must absolutely not make recommendations about management of the risk by way of a particular sentence, unless you are recommending treatment (📖 p.IV.405).

Values influencing objective opinion

Effecting and affecting justice

There is a crucial distinction between applying expert knowledge so as to help to *effect* justice; and giving expert testimony with the intention to *affect* justice. Effecting justice (that is, doing what is required by the criminal justice process, 📖 p.IV.330) is the proper role of the expert: attempting to affect it—to alter what the outcome would otherwise have been—is not.

▶The expert should have no personal interest in the outcome of a case and should not be drawn therefore into the adversarial process by taking sides (📖 p.V.545).

This is a rule that is sometimes hard to adhere to. Psychiatrists may meet cases that involve their personal values and beliefs; and as doctors, they are trained to be both sympathetic and empathetic with people's stories. Psychiatrists' professional identities encourage them to do good for people; and establish a therapeutic alliance if they can. The ethical imperatives to 'first do no harm' and to favour beneficence (📖 p.III.233) may make it extremely difficult for a doctor to be objective about a person whom they are evaluating for litigation purposes. However, such factors should not influence how medical answers to legal questions are expressed.

Attempting objectivity

The risk of personal values intrusion makes it all the more important that the doctor should consciously attempt objectivity. Total objectivity is an impossible goal, but honesty in attempting to achieve objectivity is not. It is also the expert's ethical and legal duty to the court (📖 p.V.532) to maintain impartiality and avoid bias.

Some situations tend more than others to bring doctors' natural *inclination to care* into play, most obviously where they write reports on patients whom they are, or have been, caring for (eg in civil litigation for cases of PTSD (📖 p.II.70), or inpatients coincidentally involved in criminal proceedings), and especially where the therapeutic relationship is longstanding. For this reason it is recommended that treating doctors do not give expert testimony (as opposed to professional testimony, 📖 p.V.534) in cases involving their patients whenever possible.

By contrast, it may be easier to be objective when assessing a client who is a stranger, or whom one will never see again. However, there are then risks that one *fail to recognize a medical duty to them*: for example, in a criminal case when acting for the prosecution, one may unconsciously emphasize evidence that the defendant is mentally well; or in civil compensation (📖 p.V.514) cases, one may look for evidence that the client is malingering (📖 p.II.87) and dismiss signs of distress that go against this.

In addition, the doctor may have professional *'hobby horses'* that lend themselves to one side of a case or another. Such experts may make names for themselves, always seeking to put an particular point of view irrespective of the facts of the case, and appearing only for one side. Some doctors may have personal beliefs that influence how they give expert testimony: for example, some religious and other beliefs emphasize free will and reject the influence of mental illness on offending choices.

There is no obvious way to resolve the tension between doctors' duties to the court and those to patients: if doctors only give evidence that benefits patients (whether defendants or plaintiffs) then the court will not have access to relevant evidence that does not benefit those individuals; and the justice process will be unbalanced. However, it may be difficult for the subject of an evaluation to appreciate that the doctor assessing them, unlike other doctors they have known, is not acting in their interests.

Can objective opinion be value-free?

There are some reasons to think that it is difficult for doctors to be completely or even highly objective:.

- The argument from sociology that a speaker always speaks from their position, and tends to assume that their perspective is the most real and thus the most true
- The psychological argument that all individual personal memory and experience affects later cognitive appraisal and interpretation of facts
- The vexed question of the extent to which the expert is influenced by the legal team that instructs them; especially if that team is paying them, and if the expert makes their living chiefly from expert witness work (an expert who is perceived as tailoring their opinion to suit the side instructing them is often called a 'hired gun').

It is also important to be aware of one's own value systems and prejudices, and to reflect upon how they may influence opinion. Such beliefs need not preclude one from being an expert, but may indicate potential blind spots. Unconscious value systems may be harder to access! Colleagues, however, may be able to tell one about less consciously held beliefs and values, this being one of the benefits of attending professional development and reflective groups (📖 p.III.253).

Finally, it is good practice to ask oneself: 'What are the arguments against my position?' and to carefully consider the evidence against your arguments; even if they initially seem repugnant or foolish.

Providing reports

The aims and methods of report-writing

For expert evidence to be allowed into legal proceedings it has to be both relevant and admissible to the questions at issue. Relevance is determined by the probative value of the evidence in a given case.

Aims

The main aims of a medico-legal report are to provide the Court with an opinion concerning any mental disorder that may be, or may previously have been present, its potential legal implications, and any recommendations in terms of either further investigation that might be required or any disposal, interim or definitive, that might be recommended. The psychiatrist's role is to assist the Court and not the party instructing them. It is the expert's duty to provide the Court with not only their opinion but also sufficient details regarding the information they have relied upon in order for the Court to be able to evaluate the basis, plus likely reliability and validity, of the expert's opinion and conclusions. Data collected and/or used should therefore be clearly distinguished by source; and data, in turn, should be set out separate from the opinion and recommendations expressed. There should be a coherent architecture evident within the report, constructed so that the data, as well as the sources, and reasoning of the opinion are evident on its face.

Comprehensive psychiatric skills are required in order to assess defendants, appellants, or other litigants, and specific forensic psychiatric skills are necessary to present psychiatric evidence within legal proceedings in a fashion which can best assist the court, by maximizing its ability to understand the potential legal implications of such evidence.

What providing a report involves

Assessment prior to writing the report involves gaining and/or interpreting and presenting clinical information, plus any legal information potentially having clinical relevance, towards answering not medical questions but legal ones. The task for the psychiatrist is to present psychiatric findings in a way that can be understood by the Court, including assisting the court in their necessary translation into legal constructs (📖 p.IV.296) as best as can be achieved.

There is nothing intrinsically different between assessment for court proceedings and for clinical purposes; indeed it is important not to distort normal clinical practice because there is a legal purpose to the assessment. However, the content and format of the report is likely to vary from clinical reports. Also, whereas data that are considered irrelevant for clinical purposes may be excluded from clinical reports, court reports should be written so as not to be open the accusation of being 'selective' in the data used. Also, no presumptions should be made about the veracity of particular information; the report should usually include a section dealing with the likely validity of any diagnostic or formulatory conclusions. Finally, reports for court should be written so that the clinical findings can easily be read in terms of their potential legal implications, with a section included which deals with those implications (though not definitively, given the ultimate issue rule, 📖 p.V.543).

It is crucial to write any report in the knowledge that any aspect of it can be open to challenge under cross-examination. The foundation of well presented and defensible expert oral evidence is therefore a carefully constructed assessment, plus careful written presentation.

Most reports are based upon clinical assessment and investigation, plus consideration of medical records and legal papers, sometimes also other medical reports, either for the current or previous proceedings. Anything potentially of relevance either to your clinical opinion or its legal implications should be included in the report. Some reports offer clinical opinions based solely upon consideration of medical records, and/or legal papers (for example. in retrospective assessment of others' clinical practice within clinical negligence litigation, 📖 p.V.512).

Why there is expertise in being an expert

Most jurisdictions are moving towards recognition of the importance of the expertise of presenting medical evidence into legal proceedings, and the possible need for accreditation of experts. The reasoning is that there is a need to understand the relationship between medical and legal constructs (📖 p.IV.296) and their interface (📖 p.IV.299), *and* to develop expertise in handling and medically interpreting evidence that may not be solely medical, and then in integrating that evidence into the process of forming a medical opinion to present within a legal case.

For example, in a criminal trial it is necessary not only to assess the defendant with the usual medical techniques and tools available but also to consider ordinary evidence within the case (such as witness statements) that may bear upon whether, at the time of the alleged offence, the defendant was mentally disordered.

Consideration of the relevance of any disorder for strictly legal issues also requires an understanding of how courts will properly question medical evidence in that regard. Hence, merely being capable of making a diagnosis is inadequate. The doctor must have skills in presenting the diagnosis *in relation to* the legal questions to which it may be relevant.

Such skills also include the skills necessary robustly to validate the medical diagnosis in the first place, in the special circumstance of a legal case where there will inevitably (and properly) be a measure of scepticism about the veracity of the 'patient's' presentation when the evidence may be used to assist him as a defendant facing a serious criminal charge, or as a civil litigant in gaining compensation.

Expertise in being an expert does not infer being a 'court room hack', or 'hired gun'; in fact the reverse, since knowledge of the interface between legal and medical constructs and role makes policing the boundary for oneself much easier, so as to inhibit the influence of one's own values on the opinion expressed (📖 p.V.551).

Preparation and taking instructions

Preparation for a medico-legal report should be thorough and comprehensive, in terms of being confident of the legal questions to which the referrer considers psychiatric evidence relevant and of ensuring that you have investigated, with the referrer, all potential sources of information that could be relevant to your opinion on clinical matters and its legal implications. Often the referring solicitor will not themselves know what information may be relevant to your purposes.

The source of the request

'Receiving instructions' is the term usually used when there is a formal request for assistance in a case.

Requests for medico-legal reports may come from a variety of sources:

- For criminal reports this could be the defence solicitors, the prosecution, the court or the Criminal Cases Review Commission (📖 p.V.449).
- For civil proceedings, again instructions may come from either the claimant (pursuer) or defendant; sometimes both sides may agree to appoint the same expert, or the court may require that there should be a joint expert (📖 p.V.535). One solicitor will be appointed as lead solicitor. However, there should be an agreed letter of joint instruction, originating from all sides and representing the questions that all sides wish considered. Requests for reports for Mental Health Tribunals can arise from any party with an interest, plus the tribunal itself.

Taking and refusing legal instructions

- Before accepting instructions you should confirm that you are not only adequate as an expert for the case but also likely to be the best type of expert
- You should also make sure that you can do the report in the timeframe required
- It is usually necessary to provide the instructing body with an itemized estimate of the time and costs for your report. This should include: discussing the referral in detail, reading all background and other papers relevant to the case, the clinical assessment, analysis and scoring of tests (if relevant), writing the report, travel time and time necessary for discussion of any issues with the referring solicitor—falling short of attending a conference with counsel (a 'con'), which will usually be funded separately after there has been consideration of the relevance and 'use' of your report. The likely costs associated with appearing in court are often dealt with and funded separately, by the court itself
- You should also alert the referring body of any potential court days to avoid
- You should ensure that you receive clear instructions concerning the legal questions to which the assessment and report will be directed. Do not become drawn into dealing with something that emerges once you are into the case if you consider that you are being asked to deal with something outside your area of expertise (this is an easier error to make than avoiding taking on a case per se that is outside your expertise)

- There are often ethical considerations in a case, for example you may not wish to take on a request for an independent psychiatric assessment of a patient who is in your hospital or Trust, or of a current patient of your own, or in any other situation that would give rise to a conflict of interest (📖 p.III.244)
- Similarly, you may become aware of relevant legal questions towards which you have not been directed in your instructions and have to decide what to do about this
- Make sure you understand the legal issues in the case and that you are familiar with the relevant legal constructs and terminology
- Trainees should ensure that they will receive adequate supervision (📖 p.III.252)
- Once you have agreed to act as an expert witness, you must ensure you receive a letter of instruction and source documents as follows:

Letter of instruction

This is in effect an agreement between you and the solicitor, although it is advisable (and required in some cases) to accompany it with formal terms and conditions. It sets out the remit of your instructions and you should ensure that you address all the questions in the letter and, normally, do not deviate from these.

However, the letter may sometimes present an ethical problem if you become aware of an issue that the solicitors quite deliberately do not wish you to consider. If you identify issues that are relevant to the case but you have not been instructed to address, it certainly is necessary that you contact the instructing body. It is best to obtain any amended instructions in writing.

Sources of information

- Before seeing the patient, you should ensure you have obtained copies of all relevant documents, whether from the instructing agents or from other sources (with the client's consent). Consider whether you should receive each of the source documents shown on 📖 p.II.107
- You will need to check that you have been sent everything listed in the index of the bundle that has been sent to you, and that the bundle contains everything that you might need to see
- Read all the background information prior to seeing the client (or you may discover, after you have used up your allowed interview time and gone home, that you should have asked the defendant about a particular allegation in the witness statements, for example).

Before writing the report

The assessment

Your assessment of the patient should have been conducted with writing the report in mind—see the guidance on ☐ pp.II.90–II.125. If it was not, you might need to see the patient again to obtain specific consent (☐ pp.II.112, III.284) and to address issues not usually covered in a routine clinical assessment. The quality of your report will depend upon the care with which you performed this assessment (and read the relevant legal paperwork); any inadequacies are likely to be exposed during cross-examination (☐ p.V.588).

Assessing the defendant

Unless the diagnosis, or the lack of any disorder, is crudely obvious, forensic psychiatric assessment (☐ p.II.90) usually involves fairly lengthy interviewing. It is unusual to be able to complete an adequate assessment of someone facing a serious criminal charge in less than 3 or 4 hours (this excludes time considering past medical records and the papers in the case or time gaining data from informants).

The circumstances of the assessment are also of great importance, particularly in criminal proceedings. Psychiatric assessment often touches upon issues that are profoundly personal, and adequate assessment is therefore dependent upon the use of a quiet and emotionally safe environment. A defendant who, for example, was subjected to serious sexual abuse as a child is unlikely fully to divulge such information, or the effects upon his emotional or sexual functioning, unless he is approached with care in a quiet and confidential environment. It follows that it is wholly unacceptable to assess a defendant facing a serious charge, other than in relation to a simple issue, in the cells just before, or during, trial.

What makes assessment for a court report different

Although in essence the assessment is no different from those conducted in ordinary clinical contexts, there are several important matters to address which will bear upon the assessment:

- Consider the environment in which the assessment is to take place and the logistics associated with this (such as a prison setting, ☐ p.II.113)
- Explain very clearly to the defendant your role, including who you are, who has instructed you and the limits of confidentiality (☐ p.II.112)
- Explain that they can decide whether to comply with the assessment.— and what will happen if they do not
- At the end of your inquiries, ask the client whether there are any matters that you have not asked about that he considers important
- On completion of the assessment, it is usually not appropriate to give feedback about the results, since your conclusions will be placed into the context of all of the other information in the case in terms of determining its ultimate implications and potential for use (if it has been instructed by the defence); also the client is not your 'patient'
- Inform the defendant what will happen next, including repeating your description of who will receive the report
- At some stage ask staff, including medical staff if possible, about their observations of the prisoner.

After assessing the defendant

- If the defendant is in prison or hospital, make an entry in their inmate medical record (📖 p.II.115) or medical notes. However, you should be cautious of entering the conclusions of your report, as they may be 'owned' by the person who instructed you (see 📖 p.V.558)—although even if this is the case, you may have to breach confidentiality (📖 p.III.263) if the patient discloses evidence of, say, significant risk of death or serious harm to others
- Obtain consent from the defendant to speak to other informants, e.g. family, other professionals involved, etc; remember that if they refuse then you are still at liberty to approach them and to listen to what they tell you, since breaching confidence refers to giving away confidential information proffered to you by the defendant. However, if you are instructed by the defence in a criminal case, check that none of these is a prosecution witness (special permission will have be to sought by defence lawyers for you to have access to them)
- If it is necessary to collect other further information following your assessment ask the instructing body to do this, or do it yourself if it that is easier and appropriate.

The importance of good record-keeping

You need to treat every legal communication, and relevant clinical communication, on the basis that it may be used or tested legally (whatever your role). It is good practice therefore to keep contemporaneous notes of discussions, and with whom they were had. Documents need to be checked, signed and dated. It is also worth keeping a careful record of any verbal information given, any documentation one has seen, and also (if known) what one has *not* seen. If it is known that facts are in legal dispute, then it is essential to make clear that this is also known by you (and that you have not taken a position in advance of legal determination).

General aspects of report-writing

Psychiatric disorder

The psychiatric report to court arising from the assessment and tests, sometimes supplemented by a separate report from a clinical psychologist, will describe any disorder likely to have been present at the time of the alleged offence, or relevant to any legal issue of current importance.

Legal implications

It should also describe how the disorder may be (or not) relevant to particular legal issues. This may well be couched in conditional terms, in that the relevance may be dependent upon the particular narrative of the events relating to the alleged offence adopted, often in dispute. Nevertheless, however presented, you should not purport to address the legal issues directly, only to describe how they might be informed by the psychiatric diagnosis or formulation.

Causation, where relevant, in the strict scientific (not legal) sense is inherently usually impossible to argue (to a scientific standard). Rather, expert evidence can usually offer an 'understanding' of the relevance of a disorder in terms of how it can reasonably be seen as making a contribution to the narrative of the alleged offence (criminal), or litigated event (civil). Its contribution may, of course, be different depending upon what other aspects of narrative the court accepts as valid from non-medical evidence.

Rules

Reports intended to be used as evidence in court, and those preparing them, are subject to a variety of rules for expert witnesses (pp.V.532, V.536) because of the privileged status of experts (p.V.532), in being permitted to offer opinion evidence, unlike other witnesses. Before writing the report, you should be familiar with these rules and your duties to the court and your patient. The UK General Medical Council has in the past reviewed the fitness to practise (p.V.522) of psychiatrists and other doctors because of failings in the expert evidence they have given.

Context

The report should be written with the relevant legal context in mind. Reports for different legal purposes (such as criminal proceedings, p.V.569, mental health tribunals, p.V.567, and family proceedings, p.V.573) will demand different approaches, all of which are different from a standard clinical report such as a discharge summary or referral letter. Remember also that once released, the report might be reused in other settings—for example, a report in a criminal trial might be passed on to the prison service if the defendant is imprisoned.

Structure

The general structure of the report should separate out the following. A more detailed list of report sections, derived from one recommended by the Law Society, is shown on p.V.564.
- Instructions
- Sources of information
- The factual information relevant to your opinion, identified by source
- That opinion, distinguished into psychiatric opinion and potential legal implications (not directly addressing the legal issues)
- Recommendations in relation to disposal (if relevant and required).

Data by source

Ensure that your report indicates the source for all the data you describe, so that, to the extent that your opinion rests on a particular fact or set of facts, the court can weigh the evidence (p.IV.297) according to its perception of its reliability and validity. (For example, patients' self-report might be readily accepted in clinical settings, but might not be by the court if the patient is shown to have lied; unless, for example, there is other corroborating evidence.) Important factual evidence should also be linked to your opinion by a clear chain of reasoning. Evidence available to you which does not support your opinion, including arising from other experts' reports, should also be included or referred to, and the reason for, and interpretation of, the discrepancy should be explained.

Opinion

Responsible opinion

In giving an opinion, you should be confident that your opinion would be shared by a responsible body of practitioners,[*] especially where your opinion is based on novel or newly-developed areas of practice.

Using diagnostic systems

Adopting accepted systems of description such as the DSM-IV or ICD10 (📖 p.II.109) ensures rigour, improves communication and adds weight to your opinion. However, this can open the expert up to cross-examination which misunderstands the nature of diagnosis and the proper use of diagnostic classification systems. This is particularly the case with the DSMIV, which adopts an approach of 'n of m' required criteria in order to make the diagnosis. Such an approach can be open to inappropriate forensic dissection, in a 'cookbook' fashion, which the DSMIV itself warns against. The DSMIV is intended as a guide to diagnosis, and not as strict criteria the application of which can validly over-ride clinical judgement. Its function is to enhance the inter-rater reliability of clinicians diagnostically, and not to be a substitute for individual clinical judgement.

Diagnostic validation

Although the possibility of feigning or malingering (📖 p.II.87) is borne in mind by a psychiatrist in any context, clinical assessment for a legal purpose almost always carries an increased risk of it. That should not divert the clinician from ordinary and proper practice (eg it is impossible in medicine to avoid asking what lawyers call 'leading questions') but it does mean that particular attention should be paid to the possibility of feigning or exaggeration. It is important to recognize the possibility of feigning in the report and to list points for and against the possibility where relevant.

Keeping within the medical boundary

The expert should be aware of the importance of keeping within the medical boundary and role. Hence, for example, a doctor could reasonably give evidence relating to a plea of diminished responsibility (📖 p.V.491) suggestive of an abnormality of mental functioning at the time of an alleged murder, and could reasonably describe the detail of any abnormalities of perception, emotion, thinking, volition or consciousness at the time of the offence, but should fall short of addressing the ultimate issue of whether the abnormalities, taking into account of all the other evidence in the case, some in dispute, were sufficient to amount to the defence of diminished responsibility.

Dealing with potential legal implications

It is important to distinguish therefore between diagnosis (📖 p.II.108) and formulation (📖 p.II.110), or any other description of psychiatric or psychological status, and the legal implications. The former is clearly within the role of the expert; the latter should amount to offering the court an

---

[*] Although this standard originates from the *Bolam* test (📖 p.App. 3.631) within clinical negligence (📖 p.V.516) litigation, it is equally applicable to opinion expressed about clinical matters in terms of their potential relevance to legal questions.

understanding of the relevance of the expert's findings to the legal questions under consideration.

Stick to your area of expertise

Forensic psychiatrists, like all expert witnesses, should ensure that they only express opinions that are firmly based on the evidence available to them and that reflect the application of their specialist expertise—opinions that the court, without that expertise, could not otherwise reach. The consequences of giving evidence often go beyond medical benefit to the patient, and the psychiatrist giving evidence should be aware of the numerous ethical dilemmas that may result (📖 pp.III.239, III.255, III.271).

Style

A style of writing, format, and presentation should be adopted which acknowledges that the reader is not an expert. Technical language should be kept to the minimum necessary to allow another expert to assess the details of your assessment and opinion, and all technical terms should be explained.

A suggested report structure

- Cover page
- Basic details, such as name of client, date of birth, where seen, date of appointments, total amount of time seen
- Name and address of referral agent
- Purpose of assessment as per letter of instruction
- Sources of information
- Details of information obtained from interview with the defendant/litigant
- Mental state examination
- Details of information obtained from other sources which is relevant; including other interviews; medical records; other records (eg school, social services); legal papers (eg witness statements, police interviews, proofs of evidence)[*]
- Brief description of tests applied by author and others, both medical and psychometric (care may be needed in describing some psychometric tests in detail)
- Information from other reports (including for the 'other side')
- Psychiatric opinion, expressed in medical terms
- Legal Implications, explaining the relevance of the psychiatric opinion to the legal issues raised in the instructions, whilst avoiding addressing the ultimate issue (📖 p.V.543)

---

[*] It is sometimes important to include information from legal papers, since they can represent an important source of effectively clinical information (eg witness statements concerning whether a defendant appeared to have mental symptoms prior to an alleged offence). However, deciding which papers, and how much to extract may not be straightforward. Over-inclusion can make a report excessively long; omission of important information may represent a hostage to fortune ('doctor why did you not include that statement in your weighing of the case?'). The key rule is not to be selective, either between or within documents.

- Recommendations; this should address clinical issues within the particular legal context; for example, sentencing under mental health law (within criminal proceedings), or treatment aimed at improving prognosis (within civil litigation in personal injury, 📖 p.V.514)
- Summary (of clinical opinion and potential legal implications)
- Appendices—for example, raw data from psychometric tests
- A brief, relevant descriptive CV, giving name, professional status, professional address, qualifications, and affiliation of author; sometimes it may be appropriate to add details of experience, including particular clinical experience and medico-legal experience, to allow the court to weigh your evidence (📖 p.IV.297)appropriately
- Declaration—a statement of truth and a declaration of their independence, and the lack of influence upon their opinion arising from the legal source of instruction is mandatory (📖 p.V.538).

How long should a report be?

The necessary and proper length of the report[*] will depend upon the size, in terms of the quantity of data, and the clinical and legal complexity of the case. However, the following factors should be borne in mind:

- It must be of sufficient length to demonstrate its architecture and how the opinion follows from the data available and your reasoning upon the data
- Sufficient detail can save much court time by obviating the need for follow-up questions, and may allow a hearing to be avoided (especially in civil proceedings, but even in criminal proceedings)
- It can also avoid any appearance of not having been balanced in approach
- If there is a long time lapse between preparation of the report and giving oral evidence, or otherwise having to consider the report again, then sufficiency in terms of comprehensive data combined with evident architecture of your opinion, can quickly get you back into the case without having to read again all the source documents you considered previously
- But, excessive length, which includes extraneous data, merely wastes dictation, typing, reading and court time and may make it harder for the reader to understand what you are saying and why.

The inclusion of a summary at the end of the report, perhaps equivalent to the one page report of a bygone era,[*] can ensure that the reader can quickly become aware of the nub of your opinion, Some authors prefer to put the summary at the beginning of the report for this reason.

---

[*] The first Professor of Forensic Psychiatry at the Institute of Psychiatry and Maudsley Hospital, London, Professor Trevor Gibbens, famously wrote, 50 years ago, 'A court report should be no longer than a page'. This reflected an era when the courts wished only to know the expert's opinion; indeed, an era when experts in the witness box would commonly be somewhat affronted if their expert opinion was questioned ('that is my opinion, born of X years clinical experience, young man'). Modern day medico-legal practice enjoys no such luxury (if, indeed, it was such, or served justice). An expert report written now is no better than the extent to which it evidently reflects comprehensive addressing of relevant data and to which it displays balanced, coherent and cogent reasoning.

After writing the report

Failing to submit a report on time can be grounds for a formal complaint. If you are unable to comply with the required timetable then you have a responsibility to inform those instructing you at the earliest opportunity. A late report can result in proceedings being delayed at great expense and inconvenience to the legal system.

Disclosure

- When you have completed the report, do not forget its origin. If it was requested by a third party such as a solicitor, it is likely to be the property of that third party, and you will not be at liberty to disclose it without their permission, or where confidentiality can lawfully be breached (📖 p.III.263)
- The only exceptions to the rule are where there is a significant risk of death or serious harm to others arising from non-disclosure (*W v Egdell*, 📖 p.App. 3.635) or where it is in the public interest that it be disclosed for the proper administration of justice. This includes disclosing it to the court itself, for example, if the defence has decided to withhold it because it is not seen as helpful to their case.

Changing and adding to reports

- Experts must not be asked to, and must not, amend, expand or alter any part of a report in a manner that distorts the expert's true opinion or withholds information that it is not acceptable to withhold from the court (see 📖 p.III.250)
- However, it may be appropriate sometimes to agree to exclude information that is covered by legal privilege and which is not relevant to the medical opinion expressed. Also, the opinion may be altered by newly acquired information or newly submitted evidence
- Sometimes experts are asked to provide addendum reports addressing additional issues, and/or new information. Care should be taken to link the two reports, for ease of reading them together. Commonly this arises where the 'other side' have filed a report and it is helpful to the court that your position is clarified or explained on particular points as they have emerged through the other expert's report
- What is not helpful is a long sequence of argument by addendum reports. Increasingly even in criminal proceedings it is common for the court, once it has seen the reports of all experts, to request an experts' meeting and joint statement or joint report (it is almost universal practice in civil proceedings where experts disagree).

Subsequent meetings

Any meeting and statement/report should be based wholly upon an agreed agenda between the lawyers for all parties and not made up by the experts (unless the lawyers specifically ask the experts to draft an agenda for their consideration). Also, the purpose of the meeting and statement/report is to clarify the areas of agreement and disagreement, and the key underlying issues. It is not an appropriate forum for experts to argue their case by rehearsing the reasons for their opinion beyond the minimum necessary to establish the areas of disagreement. The latter should be evident from each expert's own detailed report, and the reports of all the experts 'sit behind' the joint statement/report.

Reports for mental health tribunals

Reports for Mental Health Tribunals present particular challenges as well as ethical dilemmas for the psychiatrist, especially in terms of having to justify diagnosis, current treatment, or future management of a patient, usually in front of the patient.[*]

The report should contain a comprehensive (but not over-long) summary of the patient's history and current condition, and should outline the specific details of their mental disorder and explain the risk assessment (📖 p.II.127). The general advice on legal report-writing (📖 p.V.561) should also be referred to. Avoid copying and pasting from computerized clinical notes. This results in long and tedious reports that are unhelpful to the Tribunal.

Essential elements of a report for a mental health tribunal

- Patient's name, address, date of birth, and reference number
- Legal powers under which they are detained or treated
- Date compulsory detention and/or treatment started
- Name of the RC/RMO (📖 p.IV.379) and, if different, author's name[†]
- Names of care coordinator and any other key staff members
- Date of the report
- Duration of illness and other important details of history
- Why admission or outpatient treatment was needed
- Why informal treatment was not possible
- The grounds for compulsory detention and/or treatment (e.g. the health or safety of the patient, protection of others etc.)
- Progress during the use of compulsory powers
- Current mental state, insight and attitude to treatment
- Diagnosis, using standard (ICD or DSM, 📖 p.App. 1.601) terminology, and codes
- Risk assessment (📖 p.II.127)
- Current treatment (📖 p.II.145) and risk management (📖 p.II.189) plan
- Aftercare (📖 p.IV.398) plan in the event of discharge
- Opinion (psychiatric) and recommendations (psychiatric and legal).

Summary, diagnostic formulation, plan, and opinion

These are the key sections of the report, in which the information in the body of the report is summarized and synthesized into a final recommendation to the Tribunal on the use of compulsory powers.

An opinion can be expressed with regard to the issues that the Tribunal will have to address, such as absolute or conditional (or deferred) discharge, recommendation for transfer, or continued detention in current location. Whatever the recommendation, it is vital to explain the reasons clearly, citing the legal criteria (📖 p.IV.373) for detention that you believe are fulfilled. Especially where a recommendation is made for continued

---

[*] And potentially also in public: although the vast majority of Tribunals are held in private, it is possible for the parties to agree to make the hearing, or part of it, public.
[†] If the RC/RMO is not the author of the report, they should countersign it. This is good practice in all cases, and a specific requirement for reports on restricted patients.

detention to allow safe arrangements for discharge to be made (and by extension, where the recommendation is for delayed discharge, 📖 p.IV.416, or in the case of restricted patients, 📖 p.IV.412, for deferred conditional discharge, 📖 p.IV.417), the report must explain what further arrangements need to be made (such as obtaining funding for a hostel place, or identifying a community care co-ordinator) and how long this is likely to take.

Even where the clinical team is strongly opposed to discharge now or in the near future, the report must contain an aftercare (📖 p.IV.398) plan at least in outline form, to indicate what would be done if the Tribunal made a decision to discharge the patient.

Dilemmas

There are four main dilemmas that you may face when making recommendations to a Tribunal:

- *The incompletely treated patient* (including non-medical treatment)—it may then not be possible to make recommendations for discharge, but it will be necessary to explain what further treatment is required
- *The patient recently in remission*—without overt symptoms of mental illness it may be difficult to justify why the patient should not be discharged. However, it may not have been possible to test out the improvements through degrees of individual responsibility and freedom[*]
- *Restricted patients for whom the RC/RMO recommends discharge contrary to the recommendations of the relevant minister*[†]—in these cases it is necessary to highlight the risk of relapse of mental disorder, or harm to self or others, and of subsequent offending
- *Patients suffering from primary personality disorder*—the dilemma here is when a patient is suffering from personality disorder that does not appear to be amendable to treatment because of either a lack of ability or motivation to cooperate with therapy. The psychiatrist will need to explain what intervention has been offered, the reasons why it was not successful and hence why discharge is appropriate.

It is also important to be mindful of the issue of power in the therapeutic relationship and the potential impact and effects of the outcome of the Tribunal on the individual patient.

---

[*] In E&W, for example, this might involve arguing that although the *degree* of the patient's mental disorder no longer warrants detention, the *nature* of their condition is such that without careful testing and discharge planning, relapse (and possibly consequent violence) is likely.
[†] The Secretary of State for Justice in E&W, the Secretary of State for Health, Social Security and Public Safety in NI, the Scottish Ministers, or the Minister of Justice in RoI.

Reports for criminal cases

Reports for criminal proceedings, for example, addressing trial issues such as criminal responsibility (📖 p.IV.338) or admissibility of police interviews (📖 p.IV.318) because of a defendant's suggestibility (📖 p.II.123), present an acutely focused form of the general problem of translation (📖 p.IV.299) between psychiatry and law. The general advice on legal report-writing (📖 p.V.561), is therefore especially pertinent.

Evidence, both written and then oral, addressing sentencing rather than guilt or innocence, is less exposed to these problems but by no means free from them, for example because of distinct legal and medical conceptions of dangerousness (📖 p.V.549) and risk of harm (📖 p.II.127) respectively.

This core disparity should be constantly in mind in assessing for, and writing reports for criminal courts, and in giving oral evidence.

Pitfalls

There are a number of pitfalls that you should be particularly aware of when writing a report to be used in a criminal context:

- The law uses different concepts of mental disorder in different criminal contexts and they are always distinct from medical concepts—for example, abnormality of mind or abnormality of mental functioning in diminished responsibility (📖 p.V.491) or defect of reason in relation to insanity (📖 p.V.489)
- Legal concepts of mental disorder used within trials are often different from those applied at sentencing
- Increasingly psychiatrists are asked to assess a defendant's risk of violence to others when the court is considering extended or indeterminate periods of imprisonment, such as a life sentence or sentence of imprisonment for public protection (📖 p.IV.364). This poses particular ethical dilemmas (see 📖 p.III.265)
- Advice on risk for punitive sentencing may include requests where there is no diagnosable mental disorder but where the court considers that there are mental factors which would benefit from expert comment. This raises ethical dilemmas at a further level (📖 p.V.547), and many forensic psychiatrists would not provide an opinion in this situation
- It is important not to give recommendations, explicitly or implicitly, on punishment or other non-medical matters, other than in the context of response to a request concerning risk (assuming you take the position of responding to such requests)
- There will often be a temptation to be helpful by giving recommendations that go beyond your instructions—for example, to give advice on psychiatric sentencing options in a report on diminished responsibility. This should not be indulged without prior discussion with your instructing solicitor
- There can be circumstances where the doctor considers they have a ethical duty, within their role as a doctor, voluntarily to disclose information to the court; this may occur in the context of having been asked for a report, or through deciding to provide a voluntary report to the court on a patient the doctor is treating without being asked for such.

Keeping your eye on a next stage

From the moment that you start work on a case, even before assessing the case clinically, have in mind that everything you do or advise is potentially subject to subsequent scrutiny, including in open court through cross exam-ination. Throughout the process of assessment, build the foundations of your report with care and the building will not later topple when exposed to hostile winds. When writing the report, have in mind that the particular words you use will be the words that you may have to defend in oral evidence. Words matter.

> #### Case example
>
> You are asked to see a 67–year-old man who has been charged with theft. His solicitors are concerned about his cognitive functioning and his memory as he does not seem to retain information from meetings with them. He also reports no memory of the theft with which he has been charged. His pre-trial hearing is coming up. What clinical issues does this raise? How do these relate to the legal issues?

Reports for the Parole Boards

Situations when reports are needed

There are different situations in which a psychiatrist may have to write a report for the Parole Board:[*]

- A prison psychiatrist may write a report for a hearing in relation to a prisoner who has not had psychiatric treatment outside of the prison system
- A supervising psychiatrist in hospital may write a report for a hearing where a prisoner has been transferred to hospital and has received a recommendation for discharge by a mental health tribunal (📖 p.IV.417)
- An independent psychiatrist may write a report following instruction by a solicitor, either for the prisoner of for the Ministry of Justice.

Some psychiatrists sit on the Board, either as a regular assessor or as a Board member, but their role is quite distinct from that of a psychiatrist providing a report to the Board.

Instructions

The Parole Board or prisoner's solicitor may issue specific instructions prior to a hearing and if they do not it is reasonable to ask for these. If instructions posed as questions are unanswerable then they should be resisted. Where the report is prepared for a prisoner, sometimes with no history of psychiatric treatment in the health service, great caution needs to be taken to avoid straying beyond one's areas of expertise as a psychiatrist (📖 p.III.244).

---

[*] There is a separate Parole Board for each of the three UK jurisdictions and for RoI. In NI, the reference is usually to the 'Parole Commissioners' rather than to a Board.

Most parole reports by psychiatrists are likely to relate to prisoners under some form of indeterminate imprisonment, where the tariff (📖 p.IV.365) has passed and where the focus is on risk of harm to others and management of that risk if released.

Where the doctor is the supervising psychiatrist for a transferred patient it will be automatic that they will provide a report to the Board, triggered by the previous Tribunal recommendation.

Assessment

Clinical assessment is similar to that for a tribunal report if the prisoner is currently transferred to hospital; however, notice will have to be taken of the additional model of risk assessment adopted by the Board, which is criminological and not psychiatric.

In preparing the Parole Board report the author will need to read the parole file and to be fully acquainted with the prisoner's prison history, beyond knowing their health records. They will also need to have read psychology reports, usually prepared by prison-based forensic psychologists (whose training and role is very different from clinical psychologists: see 📖 p.I.10.). There will need to be collaboration with the relevant probation officer, who will also be preparing a report. Particular attention should be paid to the nature and extent of post-release liaison between health and probation, including monitoring and arrangements for considering recall.

Report content

General aspects of report writing apply when considering reports for the Parole Board (see also reports for tribunals, 📖 p.V.567). The role of the psychiatrist is limited to those hearings where there is a psychiatric issue. The psychiatric or psychology member of the board (if there is one) will have a role in interpreting these reports. The report should always cover:

- Prisoner's psychiatric history
- Psychiatric factors associated with offending
- History of psychiatric treatment
- Mental health during imprisonment (and any hospital admission)
- Impact of changes in mental health on risk on future offending.

There may be specific questions asked by the Parole Board:

- Is the inmate's condition treatable?
- Can the mental disorder be treated post-release?
- Can advice be given about appropriate services?
- Are there specific hospitals or psychiatrists that can be recommended?
- Is the prisoner likely to cooperate with any treatment?
- Should there be any required mental healthcare input should he be released?
- Conditions of release relevant to mental healthcare.

There may also be reference to a system for recall if necessary, including for deterioration of mental health associated with increased risk of harm to others (since the prisoner may not be subject to mental health law once discharged and released, recall might only be possible via the prison and probation system, and this can cause difficulties if the person needs hospital care; this possibility requires careful planning of liaison between probation and health services).

Rules for the Lifer Panel in E&W

- Reports for the review can be withheld from the prisoner on the grounds that its disclosure would adversely affect:
  - National security, or
  - The prevention of disorder or crime, or
  - The health or welfare of the prisoner or others
- A report from a forensic psychologist will only be required in tariff-expired cases where there has been substantive psychological input to the case or where the Parole Board have particularly requested that such a report is made available for the review.
- Psychiatric reports are only required if there are mental health issues.

Reports for the family courts

What's different about the family court?

The family court[*] hears family law (📖 p.V.510) cases: where there are disputes within or about families, and matters such as adoption, child protection, and divorce. The over-riding duty of the family court is to the welfare of the child or children involved in proceedings.

In theory, the family court is not adversarial (📖 p.IV.307), and the rules of evidence (📖 p.IV.317) are looser than in other civil courts, and much looser than in criminal courts. However, different parties often have very different views of what is in a child's best interest, and disputes are frequently acrimonious and highly adversarial. To avoid this acrimony leading to every party instructing their own experts, judges in E&W often appoint a Single Joint Expert (📖 p.V.535) under the Family Procedure Rules (📖 p.V.538).

The family court specifically seeks to avoid overseeing gladiatorial clashes between experts; and where more than one expert has been instructed the court expects those experts to meet, confer, and set out for the court areas of agreement and disagreement in a joint statement.

Who are the parties?

In the family court there are usually at least three parties to child welfare proceedings, and often more. In such cases the parties may include:

- The mother
- The father
- The children, represented by (for example) a Guardian ad Litem
- Other relatives who seek to be involved in the children's care
- The State, most often the local council responsible for child protection.

Which experts?

Most family court work is properly conducted by experts in *child and family psychiatry* and psychology, and involves assessment not just of the individual parents and children but of interactions between the parents, and between the parents and the children. Often social work evidence may sit alongside expert psychiatric and psychological evidence.

Where one or more of the adults involved in the case appears to suffer from a mental disorder, it may be appropriate for a *general adult psychiatrist* to be appointed to assess them, or a *forensic psychiatrist* if they are thought to pose a significant risk of violence or sexual offending. The role of the adult or forensic psychiatrist is limited to describing the parent's disorder and its general implications for parenting or risks to the child. Most adult and forensic psychiatrists do not have the expertise to advise on parenting ability, which requires training, experience and systematic observation. Psychiatrists who give evidence beyond their expertise may be the subject of professional disciplinary procedures (📖 p.V.521).

---

[*] In E&W, NI and RoI the High Court, County Court, District Court, and Magistrates' Court are known as the 'Family Court', 'Family Care Centre' or 'Family Proceedings Court' when dealing with family matters. In Scotland, the Sheriff Court and Court of Session deal with family matters. The term 'family court' is used here to cover all these courts.

Case example

You are asked to see a single mother who has a severe somatizing disorder, and is known to local mental health services. She also has a criminal record for ABH (📖 p.IV.346). She has recently had her first baby, which she wishes to keep. The Local Authority are seeking to take the baby into care with a view to adoption. You are instructed as a single joint expert to address questions concerning the mother's mental disorder, potential for treatment, and risk of harming the baby.

In such a case, working alongside a child and family psychiatrist, you will need to see all the medical records, including GP records, You will also need the criminal, social services, and other records. You will need to interview the mother, and possibly relatives and professionals. The court will want you to address the following issues, supporting your opinion by reference to publications where appropriate:

• The nature and consequences of her mental disorder, and its prognosis
• The risk of harming or neglecting others, particularly her child, she may pose as a result of her mental disorder
• The possibilities for treatment of her disorder, the probability of success and the timescale, and the effect successful treatment might have on the risks she poses

Addressing factual issues

It is common for facts to be in dispute in family proceedings. The expert should not take a view as to which of completing narratives is the correct one. Therefore usually it will be appropriate to give alternative 'conditional' opinions in terms 'if X is accepted then . . . , if Y then . . . '.

On occasions, parties attempt to use expert psychiatric opinion to prove one particular version of events. For example, consider a case where a child has died without any clear explanation how, and the parents were not prosecuted because the lack of explanation meant there was no realistic prospect of conviction (📖 p.IV.330). A second child is born and the local authority seeks to take the child into care. They may wish to argue that the presence of a mental disorder proves that a parent is a risk, e.g. 'Given that the mother has borderline personality disorder, is it not likely that she killed her previous child?'. Psychiatric experts cannot and should not answer these questions, and must say so.

Reports for civil compensation cases

Reports for cases involving psychiatric injury should follow the general advice on report-writing (📖 p.V.561). Experts are also bound by civil procedure rules (📖 p.V.538).

Who are the parties?

The claimant will bring a claim against the defendant. The psychiatric expert may be instructed by either party and should request clear instructions (📖 p.V.558), as in any legal case. The claimant will be seeking damages and so the expert's report is likely to be used not only to establish the presence of a recognized psychiatric injury (📖 p.V.515) but also to assist in assessing the quantum of damages (📖 p.V.513), for example by way of assessing current disability and prognosis.

Which experts?

The expert in a compensation after injury case should only accept instructions relating to mental disorders in relation to which they have expertise. For example, the sequelae of brain injury may be an area in which psychiatrists with general experience have little expertise.

Main issues

- *The presence of a recognized mental illness* will be addressed by reference to whether any psychiatric diagnosis exists. Courts will often expect clinical judgement to be supported by widely-used, validated diagnostic procedures or measures
- *The relationship with the act or omission* alleged to have caused the psychiatric disorder, relevant to establishing causation
- *Prognosis with or without treatment* in psychiatric and functional terms., relevant to quantum This may include giving a view as to the likely capacity to work (📖 p.V.523), now and in the future
- *Opinions regarding treatment* including the likelihood of benefit.

Dilemmas

The issue of *causation* of mental disorders is rarely straightforward (and ultimately a legal issue), but can be addressed medically by considering:

- A very clear and detailed history is the best approach to establishing the apparent relationship between the event and the mental disorder, although on its own it is prone to malingering
- The report should contain details of any pre-existing symptoms, the timing and relationship of new symptoms, and explanations for the relationship between any event and the development of mental disorder, with a clear formulation of any additional factors that may be relevant
- The presence of symptoms relating directly to the event, such as in PTSD, re-experiencing symptoms; evident changes in mental state on discussion of the litigated event; evidence of avoidance of treatment or legal appointments

- Any particular psychological significance of the event should be recorded; this may include there having been *priming* events similar to and prior to the index (litigated) event
- The presence of predisposing factors such as personality structure
- If there are alternative explanations for the mental disorder these should be recorded, including other life events and the natural history of a pre-existing mental disorder.

Distinguishing an ordinary response from mental disorder can be complex. A clear approach using a specified diagnostic system should be used. There may be controversial diagnostic categories (📖 p.V.546), particularly adjustment disorders or acute stress reactions. The law does not recognize every classifiable disorder as amounting to psychiatric injury.

Malingering (📖 p.II.87) or *feigning* of symptoms is more likely to arise in cases involving compensation.

- Any symptoms that can be assessed by objective testing (📖 p.II.96) should be, using recognized instruments, and if necessary involving clinical psychology colleagues
- Specifically, administer (or ask a psychologist to administer) recognized tests of malingering such as the TOMM or SIRS (📖 p.II.104)
- A detailed history, with use of all available sources of information may be the most helpful way to assess this issue with consideration of discrepancies, exaggerations, and false claims
- Lack of cooperation with any assessment should be considered relevant (although in PTSD it may represent trauma-related avoidance)
- Presence of highly unusual symptoms should be considered suspicious
- Description of a 'full house' of symptoms is suspicious
- Answering 'no' to symptoms that are consistent with the putative diagnosis is less consistent with feigning
- Observation of inconsistency in physical symptoms (eg back pain) said to be causal of mental symptoms (eg walking differently when thought to be unobserved)
- Evidence in medical records of somatization in the past
- Video surveillance evidence, usually presented as suggestive of feigning.

If there is a dispute amongst experts that cannot be resolved then ultimately the court will decide the issue, unless both sides agree settlement to avoid the financial risk of proceeding to a court hearing.

Case example

You are asked to assess a nurse who was assaulted by a patient when she was working in A&E 7 months previously. She has not returned to work since. She reports flashbacks of the assault, nightmares, and feeling extremely anxious. She does not want to return to work as she is fearful that she will be attacked again. She reports that prior to the incident she was having some marital problems that were causing her stress.

Is she suffering from a recognized mental disorder? If so, is this causally related to the assault?

Reports in clinical negligence cases

Situations where reports are needed

There are various situations in which a psychiatrist may be asked to write a report in relation to alleged clinical negligence, either by one party or as a single joint expert (📖 p.V.535):

- Since the test of negligence in medicine is 'peer review' (in terms of the *Bolam* and *Bolitho* tests, 📖 p.V.516), the court may receive expert testimony from (usually senior) doctors in the field about reasonable practice and standards of care that would be expected, at the time of the event. Establishing an agreed professional standard of care assists the court in determining whether a breach of duty (📖 p.V.513) occurred
- The court will also expect to receive testimony addressing whether the failure to meet the standard of care was the cause of any harm to the patient
- Psychiatrists may be asked to provide expert testimony in cases of alleged failures of psychiatric care.

Assessment and reporting

Assessment for clinical negligence cases is time-consuming, detailed, and often complex. Where the claimant is alive it will usually include a clinical interview; but many cases are assessed 'on the papers', by way of thorough reading and analysis of the medical records, inquiry documents, and inquest statements and transcripts, and other relevant legal papers. It is important to be certain that you have the expertise to do this.

Expert testimony can be distinguished between:

- Testimony in relation to whether there is psychiatric disorder caused by alleged medical/psychiatric negligence, and
- Testimony as to whether there was psychiatric negligence.

Usually the two are not addressed together, but may be where, for example, alleged negligence in treating a psychiatric condition allegedly led to worsening of psychiatric disorder.

Always ground any opinion, wherever possible, in published textbooks, guidance and respected mainstream papers, and cite them; this includes citing and commenting upon sources which go against the opinion you have reached.

Subsequent work

After providing a report, if it is helpful to the side instructing you then you are likely to be asked later to read through draft documents within the legal 'pleadings'. This is entirely acceptable and ensures that the barrister acting for the claimant or defendant understands fully the nature and effect of your opinion. At a later stage you may be asked to review a medical report for the other side, as well as 'pleadings' from that side.

Pitfalls

There are several pitfalls that you should be aware of when writing a report to be used in a clinical negligence context.

- Generally it is unwise for junior professionals to take on medical negligence cases

- It is very unwise for a specialists to offer an opinion on a different a specialty (e.g. a psychiatrist commenting on psychotherapeutic care)
- Keeping an unbiased approach is difficult: a common pitfall is thinking 'What would I have done?'. The question rather should be 'Do I know responsible doctors who would have done as the doctor did?'
- There is also a crucial legal distinction between a breach of duty of care and an 'error of judgement'
- You should not provide expert testimony in a negligence action in relation to peers or colleagues one knows well or with whom one has had a professional relationship. This can be difficult to hold to in complex cases and small medical subspecialties (such as types of paediatric surgery or specialists in rare conditions)
- Expert evidence should address 'what was the process?' (e.g. what steps were taken in deciding not to detain a patient under mental health law who went on to kill themselves), not 'what does the outcome infer about the process?'
- Absence of good record keeping is relevant to addressing process, but it is not definitive evidence of bad process; there may be other evidence (eg within statements or transcripts within inquiries or inquests that can offer valid description of process, although they are more suspect than good contemporaneous notes.

Hindsight bias, especially where the outcome has been tragic, must be guarded against; it is easy for an expert to be outraged on behalf of either the grieving relatives or the hapless defendant doctor who is being criticized.

Safety in balance

It is advisable to avoid always being instructed for either defendants or claimants—though this can be difficult to achieve, given that solicitors tend to act for one class of litigant or the other, and to build natural relationships with experts.

Reports for employment tribunals

The scope for the use of psychiatric evidence in employment tribunals is limited, but as with any request for a psychiatric report clear instructions (📖 p.V.558) should be sought from the instructing solicitor. The general advice on report writing (📖 p.V.561) should also be followed.

An area that is likely to be relevant to the psychiatrist is whether the claimant is suffering from a disability, which is defined as a protected characteristic under equality law (📖 p.V.523). Other actions may relate to work-related stress; harassment, sexual or other; or bullying.

Which expert?

Occupational physicians may be involved in preparing reports for employment tribunals and there is a subgroup of psychiatrists who have special expertise in mental health at work. Forensic psychiatrists may be involved in preparing reports for employment tribunals because of their particular experience in legal settings where the condition at issue is a common psychiatric disorder. General or forensic psychiatrists may also be asked for reports on their own patients who face employment proceedings, though care must be taken to avoid bias in this situation.

Common issues

- Presence and diagnosis of mental disorder
- Distinguishing ordinary stress from mental disorder
- Does it amount to a relevant 'mental impairment' or disability?
- Assessment of risk of harm to self or others (📖 p.II.137)
- Duration of impairment; is it long term (longer than 12 months)?
- Prognosis
- Formulation (📖 p.II.110) of mental disorder specifically in relation to work experience as a precipitant or cause, or as a perpetuating factor
- The impact of mental disorder on a person's capacity to work in relation to their job or particular aspects of it
- The relationship of specific aspects of mental disorder to work and other day-to-day activities
- Recommendations to employers on minimizing the impact of work on an employee's mental health problems (e.g. proposing measures to make the job less stressful or better matched to the patient's abilities).

Issues when assessing fitness to work

- Worker's health and safety risk
- Third-party health and safety risk
- Psychological capacity for work
- Predicted performance and absenteeism
- Are there any factors that will enable work?

Assessment

This involves clinical interview, plus reading all NHS and occupational medical records, plus the employment record, plus any legal papers relating to the action.

Pitfalls

- Confusing psychiatric constructs (📖 p.IV.296) with legal ones, e.g. 'disability'
- Stating an opinion on the ultimate issue (📖 p.V.543), e.g. discrimination.

Case example

You are asked to assess a 55-year-old man who has not been going into work. He is employed as a driver for a small minicab company. He reports difficulties sleeping, low mood, poor appetite, and an increase in drinking since his wife left him for another man several months previously.

Does he have a mental disorder? If so, does it impact on his ability to work as a driver?

Reports in immigration cases

Some clinicians feel uncomfortable writing reports in such cases, where there may be major consequences for the subject of the report—though serious criminal cases also involve major potential consequences.

Situations when reports are needed

Reports may be requested by lawyers acting for people facing deportation or by the department attempting to deport them (e.g. the UK Border Agency) or directly by the body considering the issue—an immigration tribunal. Reports are likely to be requested where there is mental disorder, suspected mental disorder (often because of a history of past trauma) or risk of suicide. Often, reports will be requested after a failed asylum claim.

Instructions

There are likely to be instructions relating to the following. As with any report, you should ensure you receive clear instructions (📖 p.V.558) specifying what psychiatric issues you are to consider; and you should not comment directly on the ultimate issue (📖 p.V.543), such as whether deportation would amount to a breach of human rights, for example.
- Diagnosis (PTSD, 📖 p.II.70, is commonly relevant)
- Prognosis with or without treatment
- Treatment needs
- Suicide risk and the likely impact of deportation, including the impact of any possible lack of psychiatric treatment at the destination
- Impact of detention on mental health
- Impact of travel on mental health
- The nature and quality of care received while detained pending appeal
- The adequacy of the treatment likely to be received in the destination country (based upon information from your instructing solicitor about what that likely treatment would be)
- Direct questions relating to human rights law (📖 p.IV.418).

Assessment

- Ordinary methods of assessment apply, taking care to consider any transcultural issues (📖 p.II.26)
- There may be other medical reports regarding physical injuries relating to alleged torture, which you should read beforehand
- It is more likely that an interpreter will be required; if so, extra time may need to be allowed for the assessment
- The assessment should be carefully conducted, particularly when assessing the history of trauma
- As with other types of medico-legal work, there may be a need to consider (and possibly rule out) malingering (📖 p.II.87) or feigning of symptoms, as there may be strong motivation not to return to a country where mistreatment, discrimination or torture may be feared.

Report content

The general recommendations for report writing (📖 p.V.561) should be followed. You should be extremely cautious about offering any view as to the veracity of a person's claims to have been tortured; if this or other similar evidence is crucial to your opinion, consider giving a conditional opinion ('If this is the case, then my opinion would be X; if it is not, then Y'). There may be situations, for example, in which a person has no physical signs of torture but has significant post-traumatic symptoms. A report may describe these symptoms but should not go further.

Avoiding pressure

As with other medico-legal work an expert can be subjected to emotional pressure. However, this is especially so in immigration cases, and it could be easy to become drawn into the issue, and one's own notion of natural justice, and away from the pursuit of honest objectivity (📖 p.V.551). Immigration law can appear harsh, but it is not the role of doctors to bend assessments to counter its effects.

Case example

You are asked to see a 42-year-old woman who is currently facing deportation back to the Congo. She has been in the UK for almost 2 years. She has not worked since entering the country and has been living with relatives, together with her 2-year-old son. She reports that her husband was a politician and was killed in front of her during the civil unrest. She says that she was raped by several militia men before escaping the Congo, and that her son is a product of these rapes. She reports frequent flashbacks about the rapes and the death of her husband. She also describes difficulties in coping without him and states that life is not worth living.

You have been instructed to determine whether she suffers from any mental disorder, what risks there are to her mental health and safety, and what the impact of deportation would be on her. What issues does this raise?

Reports for inquests

It is likely that psychiatric evidence to an inquest will be requested if you have had clinical involvement with a patient immediately preceding their death. Otherwise psychiatrists can be instructed as an independent expert on a death by a Coroner or Sheriff, or by a lawyer representing the deceased's family (📖 p.V.527).[*]

---

[*] Relatives of a deceased person who may be considering legal action relating to the death commonly instruct counsel to represent them at the inquest. Your report may be in the form of an independent report for the inquest, or advice to counsel (📖 p.V.545) to assist in cross-examination. Depending on the outcome of the inquest, your report (or a subsequently commissioned report) may lay a foundation for subsequent litigation.

The information that follows applies to inquests in E&W, NI, and RoI, and Fatal Accident Inquiry reports in Scotland. The general advice on report writing (📖 p.V.561) should also be followed.

Special considerations

- If you were involved in treating the deceased there is a legal obligation to prepare a report if this is requested, and later to attend court
- Be clear about the nature of your involvement and whether you are writing a report as a professional or an expert witness (📖 p.V.534). In the latter case, you may give opinions if relevant and within your area of expertise; in the former, you should not give opinions unless you are describing a relevant opinion that you held at a material time before the death, which in this context is a fact, not an opinion
- If you are preparing a report on any patient you have had clinical involvement with then there is a possibility of criticism of your clinical practice; be prepared for this, and consult your defence union and/or your employer if necessary
- The Coroner or Sheriff may ask your report to focus only on very specific issues and areas, but a comprehensive psychiatric history and diagnosis. should still be included
- If preparing an expert report you may be required to provide an opinion on a colleague's practice. This should be borne in mind before accepting any instruction of this nature, whether from the coroner or lawyers for the family.

Preparation of a report

Your report should be based upon reading all relevant clinical records, both proximate to the death and also relevant earlier records (e.g. that indicate issues or risks that should have been considered close to the time of the death). It should explain what was known about the patient at the time, what should have been known (by way of obtaining records, or other enquiry) and how should that have been interpreted. Where there are witness statements prepared for the inquest these should also be considered, as well as any statements collected by the police. It may be necessary to read policy documents of the hospital or prison concerned, or relevant national policy guidelines. You may also need to gain an understanding of relevant local protocols and procedures, such as the ACCT (📖 p.II.115) system in prisons.

As with any report for legal purposes, expect to be told what questions you are to answer, and do not address other questions you might yourself consider relevant, or re-word questions as you would expect them to be. Notably, the standard of care expected is for the Coroner or Sheriff to determine (if the report is to the coroner) or for the lawyer instructing you to decide upon; do not assume that the standard is identical to that in negligence proceedings (📖 p.V.512). Although the results of the inquest may be relevant to any subsequent litigation, the legal concepts and definitions are distinct.

Where the death was of a patient in custody, either prison or secure hospital, it may be necessary to consider whether the patient was in the right facility, and this may involve consideration of national guidelines on transfer to hospital, as well as consideration of pressure on secure hospital beds.

What to avoid

- Improperly justifying your or your colleagues' clinical practice (let alone misrepresenting facts or distorting your opinion in order to avoid criticism)—you have a duty to be honest
- Inappropriate speculation, even if based on recognized techniques such as psychological autopsy (see Box 22.1)
- Directly commenting on the ultimate issue (📖 p.V.543), in this case the legal cause of death. It is not for the psychiatrist to say whether the death was by way of suicide, or aggravated by lack of care, or otherwise to give an opinion on the correct verdict.

> **Box 22.1 Psychological autopsy**
>
> Psychological autopsy is a method employed by psychologists and psychiatrists to provide an opinion on the mental state of a person at the time of death. It is not used in inquests in the UK and RoI. Psychological autopsy also refers to a research methodology often used to study the relevant antecedents of suicide.

Submitting reports without giving oral evidence

Giving oral evidence is not an inherent or necessary feature of every medico-legal endeavour. It is therefore essential that reports address all the areas set out in the legal instructions and are written in a way that can be understood by the court without the need for further explanation (see 📖 p.V.556). A well-written report can be so cogent as to avoid the need for oral evidence, and in the majority of civil cases settlement occurs out of court. A report should be distinguished from advice to counsel (📖 p.V.545), where the expert is offering assistance to a lawyer within the adversarial process per se.

Reasons for requiring oral evidence

Courts prefer to receive written evidence because it keeps down costs, and the court will only need to hear oral evidence if, for example:

- Statute requires it (e.g. the imposition of a restriction order, 📖 p.IV.412, under mental health law)
- Parties in the legal proceedings request it (e.g. in care proceedings, the Local Authority may ask for oral evidence to be heard even though all the other parties are content with written evidence). This is usually because counsel for the interested party considers they may be able to make a point from your evidence; or an opposing barrister may wish

to cross examine on particular aspects of written evidence. It is worth trying to find out what this point is; although, of course the decision as to whether to call oral evidence is not for you

- The expert evidence is disputed; either by the parties represented in terms of its legal implications or where there is conflicting expert testimony per se
- The report is poorly written and needs further explanation, even though it addresses all the relevant evidence and questions.

Avoiding the need for a hearing

Sometimes, to save court time, judges will ask conflicting experts to meet and provide a joint statement (📖 p.V.566) setting out areas of agreement and disagreement, which can then be submitted into evidence, without the need for any of the experts to be present.

There may also be occasions where solicitors, counsel, or even judges may ask for an opinion on a technical medical matter, not an opinion on a particular individual. This may be expressed solely as a written opinion. It is important to establish at the outset:

- Exactly what question is being asked
- How the answer is going to be used
- Who will have access to it
- Whether it could possibly be used in evidence, and by whom.

As with all forensic activity, it is important to be cautious, circumspect, and not to address questions beyond one's expertise. Lawyers and courts, however, may need assistance to know what questions psychiatry can and cannot address, and there is an ethical duty (if only as a citizen) to assist legal processes if possible.

Giving evidence

Giving evidence in court

This topic offers advice on giving evidence to courts, and in particular criminal courts (with further detail for criminal courts on 📖 p.V.590). However, much of the advice is applicable to other types of hearing.

Giving evidence in a court or tribunal can be an anxiety provoking, demanding, and intimidating experience for the expert witness. Poor performance can reduce the credibility of the written report, and undermine the cogency of the evidence as it should properly be understood and influence consideration of the case. High-quality provision of oral evidence depends not on learning tricks, but on a real understanding of the interface (📖 p.IV.299) between psychiatry and law, the disparities between psychiatric and legal constructs and process (📖 p.IV.296), and the difficulties of translating medical information into legal evidence. Beyond that, of course, quality depends crucially upon knowing the case, including relevant legal papers, inside out. If all that is achieved then oral evidence, including cross-examination, should hold no fears, since a good forensic psychiatrist who knows their case should be more than a match for a barrister who probably has only a very superficial understanding of psychiatry.

In order to maximize quality, it is therefore crucial to be well prepared and also to know the court's expectations of the expert witness. However, ultimately the quality of the oral evidence you are able to give will be constrained by the quality of the report you provided earlier. Good oral evidence is founded upon a comprehensive, balanced, and well-argued report.

Preparation

Preparation is vital. So:
- Obtain any court dates well in advance and block these out in your diary—request leave and arrange potential cover at your usual job
- Contact the instructing body to check whether there has been any new information which you have not been sent
- Ensure you understand fully the psychiatric and psychological issues you addressed, and why and how you did so
- Understand the legal questions to which psychiatric evidence is relevant and how your psychiatric opinion abuts onto those questions
- Read any reports prepared by other experts and consider the implications of differing opinions. Consider what points (if any) you should concede, and what not, and why
- Be very familiar with the case—re-read your report, as well as any notes you wrote on the background information with which you were provided
- Think of the arguments or data that go against your opinion, and know how to deal with them, including simply conceding them
- If the case is complex, consider whether making evidential notes, for example in the form of a 'mind map', will assist you in communicating your opinion, and its justification, to the court (thereby avoiding fumbling through pages of a long report searching for elements of opinion or data, when you should be looking at the jury, or judge)

- Alternatively, mark up your report with a highlighter pen, so as effectively to create a form of evidential notes, for ease of reference
- Ensure you have also marked up all directly relevant papers, including others' reports, past medical records, and legal papers. Know the papers inside out, and the implications of extracts, so that you are not caught on the hop under cross-examination
- Think what lines of questioning are likely, in terms of attack both on the validity of your psychiatric opinion and of its legal implications
- Remember that giving evidence is akin to education, and requires similar skills of communication, simplification, and précis. Prepare with this in mind
- Psychiatry is abstract and difficult for lay people to comprehend, especially for juries. Think of concrete analogies that may be helpful in getting over difficult concepts
- Bring all your handwritten notes with you, including original psychometric tests, as you may be asked to refer to them when giving evidence, or the other side may wish to scrutinize them
- Since it is essential to have a discussion with the barrister before giving your evidence, ensure this occurs (even if they don't think of it). In a complex case a conference prior to giving evidence will be necessary. Resist having a conference at the courtroom door if you consider this will be inadequate (remember, you understand your evidence and its problems better than the barrister does and it is you that will be on the spot in the witness stand)
- If you are inexperienced, practice with colleagues what you want to say in court during your evidence-in-chief and how you will respond to what might be asked in cross-examination. Ideally, obtain supervision from an experienced senior or colleague.

Arriving on the day
- Dress smartly but make sure you feel comfortable
- Ensure you know which court you are attending and how to get there (you may want to check whether there is parking nearby if you drive)
- On arrival, you may need to pass through a security scanner
- Ensure that your mobile phone is switched off at all times
- Once in court find the court listings sheet
- Ensure you meet the instructing lawyer in good time before you are due to give evidence
- Ask for the usher, clerks, or other court staff, if you cannot speak to a relevant lawyer, as they will be able to aid you with any questions that you may have about the proceedings
- Accept that you may be required to hang around for long periods of time, so bring reading material (or read through materials in the case if you need further time to do this)
- Clarify with the instructing lawyer whether you will be sitting in court whilst other evidence is being given (eg by the defendant, or another expert witness)
- Make notes of relevant parts of oral evidence to which you listen, and note its relevance to your psychiatric opinion or legal implications.

The courtroom process

- *Examination in chief* This is the start of the process of giving evidence, called by the side instructing the expert. The aim of it is to elicit your psychiatric opinion and its factual and scientific justification, as well as to explore its potential legal implications (though you will never opine on the ultimate issue (📖 p.V.543).
- *Cross-examination* by the barrister for the other side will then follow. This is likely to be challenging and will usually amount to testing the strength of, and attempting to undermine some or all of, the expert's evidence
- *Re-examination* will follow cross-examination. The counsel that called the expert will use this to repair any damage they perceives to have occurred to their client's case during cross examination.

For more information, see 'Court procedures' (📖 p.IV.314).

Giving evidence: practicalities

- Be familiar with court etiquette, including standing and bowing to the judge when he or she enters or leaves the room, and how to address the judge (see Box 23.1).
- You will hear how the judge is addressed before you start to give your evidence, or you can ask the lawyer or court clerk
- The Clerk of the Court will ask you whether you wish to swear or affirm: to swear an oath, or merely to make a solemn promise, that your evidence will be the truth, the whole truth, and nothing but the truth. In Scotland the choice is either to swear on the Bible or to affirm; in other jurisdictions you will be asked on which holy book you wish to swear, unless you are affirming
- Use the opportunity for swearing the oath or affirming to notice how it feels to be speaking in the court, and to get used to the sound of your own voice. Speak slowly and deliberately, and look at the jury (or the judge in civil proceedings), so as to set the tone of how you will give your evidence
- You will then be asked to state your name, professional address, qualifications, and experience
- If you are nervous try to minimize obvious indicators—shuffling feet, rushed or quiet speech; for example, clasp your hands behind your back if you wish to avoid wringing your hands anxiously; or have a glass of water with you at the witness box to allow you to pause for sips
- Always stand so that you are looking at the jury (in a criminal trial, though appropriately at the judge when he addresses you) or the judge in a civil trial
- Do not look at counsel, even your own. Counsel ask questions on behalf of the court (even hostile questions) and your answers should be to the court. Being examined is not a conversation with counsel. Moreover, looking at counsel allows them to use their body language to intimidate you if they are cross-examining you. Doctors find this a particularly difficult rule to stick to, but it is not rude in this context not to look at the person who is speaking to you
- Focus on a point just above a juror's head (or the judge's as appropriate) as a means of blocking out extraneous perceptions and of focusing on your own thoughts
- Make eye contact with the judge and watch their body language if he or she asks questions, but always watch the judge's pen (out of the corner

of your eye as you look towards the jury) to ensure you are not too far ahead of his or her note-taking; be ready to slow down and pause at times to allow him or her to keep up.

> ### Box 23.1 Titles for addressing the judge
>
> - Magistrate: Sir or Madam
> - County Court Judges: Your Honour
> - Circuit Judges (E&W): Your Honour
> - Senior Judges: Your Lordship/Ladyship, or My Lord/Lady.

Giving evidence: answering and educating

- Speak slowly, clearly, and with as few words as will get over the point you are making; the more words you use the more the risk of contradicting yourself inadvertently, or of creating hostages to fortune in cross examination
- In a spirit of educating the court, simplify, so long as you are still being honest and giving the 'essence' of the truth (excessive detail may be 'the whole truth' but is counterproductive to the court's needs if detail confuses). Remember that the judge and jurors are (hopefully) intelligent laypeople, not fellow psychiatrists
- However, avoid lecturing or patronizing the court
- During evidence in chief and re-examination be led by the barrister asking you questions, although do not be constrained if the questions do not infer the evidence you wish to put over: give a more wide-ranging answer than the question demands, or ask the judge whether you can expand on what you have said in answering the question
- Use resonant words and phrases, and vivid examples where appropriate, to assist the court in remembering the points you are making
- Do not use more than one word or phrase for one point, apart from giving a sentence or more to explain what it means
- So far as you properly can, and so far as the judge allows, make use of answers beginning 'Yes, but . . .'. Barristers often try to disaggregate evidence in cross-examination, like picking away at one or two bricks of a building in the hope that the entire edifice will collapse. Keep the whole building in view for the jury and judge
- If the form of a question in cross-examination will itself distort the evidence you are giving, turn to the judge and say so (for example, when asked to answer 'yes' or 'no' to a question, your response might be 'My Lord, if I answer the question as put my reply will be misleading to the court'). It is then for the judge to umpire the interchange
- Try to see where a line of cross examination is going, not so as to thwart a proper line, or to distort your evidence, but so as to see how best to frame your answers in order, overall, to get over the essence of what you are saying
- Be careful not to introduce evidence which may be inadmissible in front of the jury (eg past convictions); if in doubt, don't say it, or look towards counsel or the judge with an appropriate facial query and he will get the point and intervene to assist you. If necessary, turn to the judge and state explicitly that you cannot answer the question without introducing evidence that you believe to be inadmissible

- Finally, do not let emotion enter your evidence; above all do not see cross examination as 'personal'; it is merely the means of 'testing your evidence', however hostile may be the technique used. If you allow yourself to become angry, you will appear to have lost the argument and your evidence, however valid, may be given less weight.

Giving evidence: keeping and showing balance

- Be balanced in your answers and do not become defensive or adversarial
- Concede points validly made against your position
- Do not be afraid to say you don't know
- If it becomes apparent that you have made an error or exclusion, either of fact or interpretation, acknowledge the error and apologize to the court at the first opportunity
- If new evidence is presented to you, consider it, and its impact on your opinion; if it is admissible you must take it into account even if only recently made available.

After giving evidence

- Do not be upset if your evidence is not accepted—it does not mean that your opinion was necessarily wrong psychiatrically; the court may have translated the evidence into a legal outcome different from that sought by the side that instructed you.
- Ask for a transcript, or oral account, of relevant parts of judge's summing-up, in order to know how your evidence was received, including by comparison with that of the other side, and to learn for the future
- Keep all of your papers, at least until you know there will not be a re-trial, or appeal possibly followed by a re-trial (and at least for the period required by the data protection legislation, 📖 p.App. 2.622.)

Giving evidence in criminal courts

For general advice see also 'Giving evidence in court' (📖 p.V.586), much of which is relevant to criminal courts. However, the following additional advice may assist.

Preparation

- Understand in detail both the psychiatric and the legal questions or issues, and how they relate (e.g. how does the issue of low IQ relate to the defendant's fitness to plead, 📖 p.V.474? How does the defendant's hearing voices relate to diminished responsibility, 📖 p.V.491?)
- Be aware of potential distortions of your evidence that may arise from its presentation within a very restrictive evidential process, and in relation to legal constructs, both of which are highly autopoetic (📖 p.IV.297)
- Think of ways of minimizing any likely distortion through the way you frame your evidence
- Be particularly aware of the distinction between your medical opinion and your understanding of the legal implications of your opinion
- Be clear in your mind where your expertise stops, so as to avoid addressing issues beyond your expertise

- If the evidence is to be given in front of a jury, or even lay magistrates, plan (with the solicitor or barrister if possible) how you will communicate your evidence effectively
- It is normal practice for a expert witnesses to sit in court whilst other witnesses are giving evidence, often in order to know whether the evidence given varies from the statements that are in the case (the oral evidence is all that matters ultimately) or to know of new evidence
- Sitting in court can also be invaluable in getting to know how it is that each side is putting their case and to assist in preparing for the types of questions you are likely to be asked particularly in cross examination.

Giving evidence before a jury

- Ensure that you address all your responses to the jury, or where appropriate the judge. It may help to turn your body towards the judge when answering a question from them
- Treat the exercise as one of 'education' (📖 p.V.589), bearing in mind that there will be a wide range of intellectual abilities and experiences represented within the jury. Use simple, non-technical language, and concrete analogies where likely to be helpful
- Criminal courts are highly adversarial and barristers play to the jury; some use emotional techniques rather than calm reason. This can be used against an expert, with attempts to belittle evidence by simplistic approaches, or concentration on emotive words rather than on rational argument. Do not get drawn into the adversarial process. Stay rational in the face or tactics pursued with an eye to jury impression
- Offer the jury not only technical diagnosis and formulation but, where appropriate, also offer a narrative, expressed in terms of the mental disorder in relation to the narrative of the offence
- The judge will be writing down your responses in a good deal of detail, so that they are able to rehearse it in their summing up to the jury; keep an eye on the judge's pen and wait until the judge has stopped writing before you continue speaking
- If your evidence goes into a period of adjournment, you are not permitted to talk to anyone about the case; and this rule applies until you have completed your evidence
- Rarely the judge may give permission for you to discuss the case with counsel for your side, where an issue has arisen which has to be dealt with outside of your evidence per se, but which cannot be put off until your evidence is finished
- Often the jury will be asked to leave whilst there is legal argument. Usually you will not be asked to leave
- Above all, remain calm and good humoured, and do not become irritated (if cross-examining counsel becomes irritated you are almost certainly being effective in your evidence)
- After giving evidence the expert may be asked to stay and to sit behind counsel so as to advise on the evidence of another expert (📖 p.V.545).

Giving evidence in a voir dire

Before a jury is empanelled, on occasions there will be a 'trial within a trial', heard before the judge alone, to determine whether, for example, a piece of evidence should be placed before the jury. A voir dire can also arise during a trial, during which the jury are asked to leave. Sometimes a voir dire will address issues to which psychiatric evidence is relevant, for example, the admissibility of confession evidence (📖 p.V.479) where there is concern raised over the reliability of the police interviews, in relation to alleged suggestibility or compliance (📖 p.II.123). This will be a different and somewhat calmer experience for the expert, since counsel are unlikely to apply the types of emotional techniques often used in front of juries. The approach may be no less challenging for that, however.

The summing up

Following presentation of all the evidence and closing speeches by counsel for each side, the judge will sum up the case and the jury will then retire to consider their verdict. On their return to the courtroom the chairman of the jury will announce the verdict when asked by the judge. If they cannot reach a unanimous verdict, in some jurisdictions the judge will ask them to determine whether they can reach a verdict on a majority of 10:2. If the verdict is ultimately guilty then pleas in mitigation (📖 p.V.506) will be heard and the judge will determine the sentence (📖 p.IV.361), or there may be an adjournment for reports, including potentially psychiatric reports (your report for the trial may well not have dealt with sentencing matters).

Giving evidence to mental health tribunals

Who will be there?

- The President of the tribunal panel will be an experienced lawyer or (for restricted patients, 📖 p.IV.412) a High Court judge or equivalent
- The panel will also have a medical member and a lay member
- The patient and their legal representative
- The responsible clinician (or RMO) or their deputy
- The social worker or other author of the social circumstances report
- For inpatients, a nurse from the ward where the patient is detained
- Other professionals where relevant, including independent witnesses
- Family or friends invited by the patient, if the panel consents
- Occasionally there will be a legal representative for the responsible authority (the hospital's managers), if there are contentious legal issues.

Tribunal procedure

- The hearing will be at the hospital where the patient is or was detained
- All parties will be seated at the hearing, with the panel members on one side of a long table, and the parties and witnesses on the other
- The President will introduce the panel and explain the purpose of the hearing and the procedure it will follow
- The witnesses will then be questioned as shown in Box 23.2, beginning with the RC/RMO, and continuing in the order listed under 'Who will be there?', 📖 p.V.592
- Witnesses may request to leave after giving evidence, although the tribunal prefers them to remain for the entire hearing

- At the end there will be submissions from the legal representatives for the patient and (potentially) the responsible authority
- All parties will be asked to leave the room whilst the panel deliberate
- The decision is then delivered orally (and subsequently in writing)

Box 23.2 Procedure for giving evidence at a tribunal

1. The President will invite the witness to confirm that their opinion remains the same as that stated in their report, and to describe any changes or give any updates as needed.
2. The panel members will question the witness in turn (beginning with the medical member for the RC/RMO, and the lay member for the social worker)
3. The patient's legal representative will then question the witness
4. If the responsible authority is represented at the tribunal (either by the RC, or by a lawyer), that representative may then question the witness.

Psychiatrists as witnesses

Forensic or other psychiatrists may attend in different capacities:
- As the patient's responsible clinician (RC) or RMO
- As an independent expert witness instructed by the patient's solicitor
- As a representative of the hospital (the responsible authority).

Representing the responsible authority

In E&W, where the RC wishes to represent the responsible authority (and then be entitled to cross examine other witnesses and sum up the case) they must state this intention at the outset of the tribunal. Generally, it is advisable to refrain from adopting this role, and to suggest instead that the hospital obtain its own legal representative.

Preparation

General advice on giving evidence (📖 p.V.586) should be followed. If you have prepared a report then reread the report, other reports and relevant parts of the clinical notes before the tribunal.

Prepare your answers to obvious questions relating to the *legal criteria* for detention (or for the community order, 📖 p.IV.394):
- What is the diagnosis, and the important symptoms, etc.?
- What is your assessment of risk (📖 p.II.127) to the patient and others?
- What is your treatment plan, and the prognosis?
- Under which of the relevant statutory criteria (📖 p.IV.373) do you seek to justify the compulsory detention or treatment? How does your evidence show that those criteria are met?

Prepare your answers to *likely questions*, such as:
- Has the situation changed since your report? If so, how?
- What progress has been made? What treatment is still needed?
- Could this treatment be provided in the community? If not, why not?

- Why are compulsory powers needed to give this treatment?
- If the patient is ready for discharge but you are waiting for arrangements to be made (e.g. funding for a hostel), how do you legally justify continued detention? Could the patient safely be cared for elsewhere for a short time (e.g. at a family home) while arrangements are made?
- What is your contingency plan in the event of discharge? (There may be a legal requirement to have such a plan.)
- What do you believe would happen (and how would you respond) if after discharge the patient stopped treatment, relapsed, or reoffended?

For *restricted patients*, you might also be asked:
- If, as is often the case, the relevant minister (🕮 p.V.464) has opposed your recommendation for conditional or absolute discharge (🕮 p.IV.416), why do you disagree with their opinion?
- If the tribunal is considering conditional discharge, what conditions do you recommend and why?

Giving evidence to the Parole Board

Who will be there?
- The chair will be a senior legally qualified person
- If the prisoner under discussion has mental health problems, one of the members will be a psychiatrist or psychologist
- The third member of the panel will be a criminologist, a Probation Officer, or an independent member
- The prisoner and their legal representative (though this is now uncommon)
- A representative for the victim (e.g. probation Victim Liaison Officer and/or members of their family)
- Other witnesses including probation officers, prison psychologists, or other mental health professionals.

What is it like?
- The hearing will be in a prison (or hospital if the person is a transferred prisoner who has been recommended for discharge by a Tribunal, 🕮 p.IV.414)
- There may be a victim statement read at the outset of the hearing, often by a member of the victim's family, if present
- Each witness will be questioned by the panel
- Representatives of the prisoner and other parties may question the witness
- The main focus will be risk. Any issues relating to mental disorder will be geared towards mental disorder as a risk factor.

Psychiatrists as witnesses
A psychiatrist (forensic or otherwise) may be attending the Parole Board in different capacities
- As a professional witness where the patient has been under their care or they have had some clinical involvement
- As an expert witness where they are asked to give an opinion on specific issues.

Preparation

The general advice on giving evidence (📖 p.V.556) should be followed. If you have prepared a report then reread the report. If not, then it is reasonable to prepare notes relating to your involvement with the person concerned.

- As a professional witness you are likely to be asked about your risk assessment as this is the main focus of the parole board
- You are likely to be asked to comment on prognosis and the requirement for treatment
- Anticipate questions and consider your own involvement critically prior to any hearing, to assist in this process
- Consider the questions described in preparing reports for the Parole Board
- Remember that it is not necessary for the psychiatrist to justify detention in a parole hearing in the same way that they may be required to do in a mental health tribunal.

Giving evidence in civil courts and tribunals

For general advice see also 'Giving evidence in court' (📖 p.V.586). The civil courts operate separately from the criminal courts and have different rules and procedures, including the civil procedures rules (📖 p.V.538).

- Civil courts (📖 p.IV.308) are usually presided over by a Judge sitting alone without a jury
- A tribunal consists of a panel which is led by a chairman (judge) and two lay members. In employment tribunals one lay member may be from a HR background and the other may be from a trade union background.

Preparation

You should make sure you attend a pre-trial conference which will provide you with an opportunity to liaise with other experts and to understand the role of your evidence and the legal questions at hand. In relation to other experts you may well have already produced a joint statement (📖 p.V.566) concerning areas of agreement and disagreement.

Procedures in civil courts

In the case of a civil trial there is no prosecutor. The case is brought by a claimant ('plaintiff' in NI or 'pursuer' in Scotland) and defended by a defendant ('defender' in Scotland). The claimant may bring a litigation representative (eg, a solicitor) with them. Similar procedures (📖 p.IV.314) to those in criminal trials are broadly followed; however, there are some differences which are outlined next.

General advice

- You will initially be asked to swear or affirm (that is, to promise that you will give evidence truthfully and fully)
- After being asked your name, professional address, qualifications, and experience you will then be taken to a copy of your sworn statement

or report. You will be provided a copy in the witness box and will be asked to confirm the contents of your report as your evidence
- If you have any corrections to your report, this is the time to state what they are
- Unlike criminal proceedings, in E&W your report will usually stand as your examination in chief (💷 p.V.588): that is, you will not be questioned by the solicitor or barrister that instructed you; but you may be cross-examined by the other side
- On occasion an expert may be required to give oral evidence without being able to make reference to their report, so ensure that you are familiar with its contents in detail before beginning your testimony
- You will then be subject to cross examination, and may be asked questions by a number of different lawyers representing the different parties involved.

At the end of the trial or hearing

At the end of the trial or hearing, the Sheriff, judge or tribunal President will usually retire to consider their judgement and will deliver this in writing later.

Giving evidence at inquests

You should also read the general advice on giving evidence (💷 p.V.586).

Who will be there?
- The coroner, usually a specially-trained doctor or senior lawyer
- The coroner's officer (typically a former police officer), who acts as clerk and usher
- A jury of 6–12 members in many cases (except in Scotland; see 💷 p.V.528)
- Witnesses, including police, pathologists, GPs, and prison staff may be present
- Interested parties, who may have their own legal representatives
- The hearing will be public and so reporters may be present.

What is it like?
- It need not be held within a court but may be in local municipal offices, or in a hospital or police station. In most cases, however it will be held in a Coroner's court (or Sheriff Court in Scotland)
- The initial hearing will usually be adjourned after basic details of the death have been recorded
- Witnesses are called and examined by the coroner (fiscal in Scotland)
- A coroner is usually addressed as Sir or Madam
- The coroner may indicate whether you should sit or stand to give evidence
- Other interested parties and their representatives may examine the witness
- The jury (if present) may ask the witness questions
- Interested parties may make submissions on points of law
- The coroner will sum up the evidence and either reach a verdict themselves, or tell the jury which verdicts are legally open to them.

Psychiatrists as witnesses

A psychiatrist (forensic or otherwise) may attend an inquest in different capacities:

- As an ordinary witness to a death
- As a professional witness (📖 p.V.534) where the person who died was a patient who had been under your care or with whom you had had some clinical involvement
- As an expert witness where you are asked to give an opinion on specific issues relevant to the death.

Preparation

It is particularly important to familiarize yourself with the material you are likely to be examined on as there may have been a significant length of time between your assessment or involvement and the hearing. Also, if you are a professional witness who is giving evidence because you were clinically involved, think about how the fact of the death puts a new perspective on what you thought at the time: be ready to explain your reasoning, based upon the information available to you then.

The court is also likely to have access to other inquiries relating to the death, and if possible you should obtain and review these.

- As a professional witness you are likely to be asked about your risk assessment and the notion of risk assessment and prediction (📖 p.II.128)
- If you have been critical of other professionals you may face more rigorous or even hostile questions
- There may be questions concerning the relationship of different factors with suicide risk (📖 p.II.137). Prepare for any that may arise: for example, if the person had recently been started on a new medication then prepare to answer questions relating to any possible link between this and their death
- Anticipate questions and consider your own involvement critically prior to the hearing
- Ensure you have had a thorough discussion with your employer prior to the hearing if appearing as a professional witness; consider seeking advice from your defence union
- Bear in mind that the deceased's family are likely to be present; be sensitive in the way you express yourself.

Appendices

Diagnostic classifications: DSM & ICD

The following table lists the diagnoses and diagnostic codes from the International Classification of Diseases, 10th edition (ICD10) and the APA Diagnostic and Statistical Manual, 4th edition, text revision (DSM-IV-TR). The DSM codes are in fact those of the previous edition of the ICD (ICD9.CM).

There are many more specific diagnoses in ICD10 than in DSM-IV-TR; the diagnostic terms listed are therefore those of the ICD10.

The new version of DSM in preparation at the time of writing, due in 2013, introduces several major changes, some of which are summarized at the end of this appendix.

ICD10 code	DSM code	Diagnosis
F00–09		*Organic mental disorders*
F00.0	290.10	Dementia in Alzheimer's disease with early onset
F00.1	290.0	Dementia in Alzheimer's disease with late onset
F00.2	294.1	Dementia in Alzheimer's disease, atypical or mixed type
F00.9	294.1	Dementia in Alzheimer's disease, unspecified
F01.0	290.40	Vascular dementia of acute onset
F01.1	290.40	Multi-infarct dementia
F01.2	290.40	Subcortical vascular dementia
F01.3	290.40	Mixed cortical and subcortical vascular dementia
F01.8	290.40	Other vascular dementia
F01.9	290.40	Vascular dementia, unspecified
F02.0	290.10	Dementia in Pick's disease
F02.1	290.10	Dementia in Creutzfeldt-Jakob disease
F02.2	294.1	Dementia in Huntington's disease
F02.3	294.1	Dementia in Parkinson's disease
F02.4	294.1	Dementia in human immunodeficiency virus [HIV] disease
F02.8	294.1	Dementia in other specified diseases classified elsewhere

F03	294.8	Unspecified dementia
		A fifth character may be added to F00-F03, as follows:
	.x0	Without additional symptoms
	.x1	Other symptoms, predominantly delusional
	.x2	Other symptoms, predominantly hallucinatory
	.x3	Other symptoms, predominantly depressive
	.x4	Other mixed symptoms
F04	294.0	Organic amnesic syndrome, not substance-induced
F05.0	293.0	Delirium, not superimposed on dementia, so described
F05.1	293.0	Delirium, superimposed on dementia
F05.8	293.0	Other delirium
F05.9	780.09	Delirium, unspecified
F06.0	293.82	Organic hallucinosis
F06.1	293.89	Organic catatonic disorder
F06.2	293.81	Organic delusional [schizophrenia-like] disorder
F06.3	293.83	Organic mood [affective] disorders
F06.30	293.83	Organic manic disorder
F06.31	293.83	Organic bipolar affective disorder
F06.32	293.83	Organic depressive disorder
F06.33	293.83	Organic mixed affective disorder
F06.4	293.84	Organic anxiety disorder
F06.5	293.9	Organic dissociative disorder
F06.6	293.9	Organic emotionally labile [asthenic] disorder
F06.7	294.9	Mild cognitive disorder
F06.8	293.9	Other specified mental disorders due to brain damage etc.
F06.9	293.9	Unspecified mental disorder due to brain damage etc.
F07.0	310.1	Organic personality disorder
F07.1	310.1	Postencephalitic syndrome
F07.2	310.1	Postconcussional syndrome
F07.8	310.1	Other organic personality and behavioural disorder
F09	293.9	Unspecified organic or symptomatic mental disorder

F10-19		*Mental and behavioural disorders due to substance use*
F10.00	303.00	Acute alcohol intoxication—uncomplicated
F10.01	303.00	Acute alcohol intoxication—with bodily trauma or injury
F10.02	303.00	Acute alcohol intoxication—with other medical complications
F10.03	291.0	Acute alcohol intoxication—with delirium
F10.04	303.00	Acute alcohol intoxication—with perceptual distortions
F10.05	303.00	Acute alcohol intoxication—with coma
F10.06	303.00	Acute alcohol intoxication—with convulsions
F10.07	303.00	Acute alcohol intoxication—pathological intoxication
F10.1	305.00	Harmful alcohol use
F10.20	303.90	Alcohol dependence—currently abstinent
F10.21	303.90	Alcohol dependence—abstinent in a protected environment
F10.22	303.90	Alcohol dependence—on a maintenance/replacement regime
F10.23	303.90	Alcohol dependence—abstinent, receiving drug treatment
F10.24	303.90	Alcohol dependence—currently using alcohol
F10.25	303.90	Alcohol dependence—continuous use
F10.26	303.90	Alcohol dependence—episodic use (dipsomania)
F10.30	291.81	Alcohol withdrawal—uncomplicated
F10.31	291.81	Alcohol withdrawal—with convulsions
F10.40	291.0	Alcohol withdrawal—with delirium but without convulsions
F10.41	291.0	Alcohol withdrawal—with delirium and convulsions
F10.50	291.9	Alcohol-induced psychosis, schizophrenia-like
F10.51	291.9	Alcohol-induced psychosis, predominantly delusional
F10.52	291.9	Alcohol-induced psychosis, predominantly hallucinatory
F10.53	291.9	Alcohol-induced psychosis, predominantly polymorphic
F10.54	291.9	Alcohol-induced psychosis, predominantly depressive
F10.55	291.9	Alcohol-induced psychosis, predominantly manic
F10.56	291.9	Alcohol-induced psychosis, mixed

F10.60	291.1	Alcohol-induced amnesic syndrome
F10.70	291.9	Alcohol-induced residual disorder—with flashbacks
F10.71	291.9	—with personality or behaviour disorder
F10.72	291.9	—with residual affective disorder
F10.73	291.2	—with dementia
F10.74	291.9	—with other persisting cognitive impairment
F10.75	291.9	—with late-onset psychotic disorder
F10.80	291.9	Other mental/behavioural disorder related to alcohol use
F10.90	291.9	Unspecified mental/behavioural disorder related to alcohol use

Conditions related to use of substances other than alcohol follow the same general pattern. Each has a different DSM code for harmful use (abuse) and for dependence (all subtypes). The digit shown as 'x' in the ICD codes indicates the substance concerned, as follows:

	Abuse	Dependence	Substance
x=1	305.50	304.00	Opioids
x=2	305.20	304.30	Cannabinoids
x=3	305.40	304.10	Sedatives or hypnotics
x=4	305.60	304.20	Cocaine
x=5	305.90	304.90	Other stimulants, including caffeine
x=6	305.30	304.50	Hallucinogens
x=7	305.90	305.10	Tobacco
x=8	305.90	304.60	Volatile solvents
x=9	305.90	304.90	Multiple drugs or other substances
F1x.00	292.89		Acute intoxication—uncomplicated
F1x.01	292.89		Acute intoxication—with trauma or other bodily injury
F1x.02	292.89		Acute intoxication—with other medical complications
F1x.03	292.89		Acute intoxication—with delirium
F1x.04	292.89		Acute intoxication—with perceptual distortions
F1x.05	292.89		Acute intoxication—with coma
F1x.06	292.89		Acute intoxication—with convulsions

F1x.07	292.89	Acute intoxication—pathological intoxication
F1x.1	above	Harmful use
F1x.20	above	Dependence—currently abstinent
F1x.21	above	Dependence—abstinent in a protected environment
F1x.22	above	Dependence—on a maintenance/replacement regime
F1x.23	above	Dependence—abstinent, receiving drug treatment
F1x.24	above	Dependence—currently using the substance
F1x.25	above	Dependence—continuous use
F1x.26	above	Dependence—episodic use
F1x.30	292.0	Withdrawal state—uncomplicated
F1x.31	292.0	Withdrawal state—with convulsions
F1x.40	292.0	Withdrawal state—with delirium but without convulsions
F1x.41	292.0	Withdrawal state—with delirium and convulsions
F1x.50	292.9	Substance-induced psychosis, schizophrenia-like
F1x.51	292.9	Substance-induced psychosis, predominantly delusional
F1x.52	292.9	Substance-induced psychosis, predominantly hallucinatory
F1x.53	292.9	Substance-induced psychosis, predominantly polymorphic
F1x.54	292.9	Substance-induced psychosis, predominantly depressive
F1x.55	292.9	Substance-induced psychosis, predominantly manic
F1x.56	292.9	Substance-induced psychosis, mixed
F1x.6	292.83	Substance-induced amnesic syndrome
F1x.70	292.9	Substance-induced residual disorder—with flashbacks
F1x.71	292.9	—with personality or behaviour disorder
F1x.72	292.9	—with residual affective disorder
F1x.73	292.82	—with dementia
F1x.74	292.9	—with other persisting cognitive impairment
F1x.75	292.9	—with late-onset psychotic disorder
F1x.8	292.9	Other substance-related mental/behavioural disorders
F1x.9	292.9	Unspecified substance-related mental/behavioural disorder

F20–29		*Schizophrenia, schizotypal and delusional disorders*
F20.0	295.30	Paranoid schizophrenia
F20.1	295.10	Hebephrenic schizophrenia
F20.2	295.20	Catatonic schizophrenia
F20.3	295.90	Undifferentiated schizophrenia
F20.4	311	Post-schizophrenic depression
F20.5	295.60	Residual schizophrenia
F20.6	295.90	Simple schizophrenia
F20.8	295.90	Other schizophrenia
F20.9	295.90	Schizophrenia, unspecified
		A fifth character may be used to classify course:
	.x0	Continuous
	.x1	Episodic with progressive deficit
	.x2	Episodic with stable deficit
	.x3	Episodic remittent
	.x4	Incomplete remission
	.x5	Complete remission
	.x6	Other
	.x9	Course uncertain, period of observation too short
F21	301.22	Schizotypal disorder
F22.0	297.1	Delusional disorder
F22.8	297.1	Other persistent delusional disorders
F22.9	297.1	Persistent delusional disorder, unspecified
F23.0	298.9	Acute non-schizophreniform polymorphic psychotic disorder
F23.1	295.40	Acute schizophreniform polymorphic psychotic disorder
F23.2	295.40	Acute schizophrenia-like psychotic disorder
F23.3	297.1	Other acute predominantly delusional psychotic disorders
F23.8	298.8	Other acute and transient psychotic disorders
F23.90	298.8	Acute/transient psychotic disorder with acute stress

F23.91	298.8	Acute/transient psychotic disorder without acute stress
F24	297.3	Induced delusional disorder
F25.0	295.70	Schizoaffective disorder, manic type
F25.1	295.70	Schizoaffective disorder, depressive type
F25.2	295.70	Schizoaffective disorder, mixed type
F25.8	295.70	Other schizoaffective disorders
F25.9	295.70	Schizoaffective disorder, unspecified
F28	298.9	Other nonorganic psychotic disorders
F29	298.9	Unspecified nonorganic psychosis
F30-39		*Mood [affective] disorders*
F30.0	296.00	Hypomania
F30.1	296.03	Mania without psychotic symptoms
F30.2	296.04	Mania with psychotic symptoms
F30.8	296.00	Other manic episodes
F30.9	296.00	Manic episode, unspecified
F31.0	296.40	Bipolar disorder, current episode hypomanic
F31.1	296.43	Bipolar disorder, manic without psychotic symptoms
F31.2	296.44	Bipolar disorder, manic with psychotic symptoms
F31.30	296.52	Bipolar disorder, mild or moderate non-somatic depression
F31.31	296.52	Bipolar disorder, mild or moderate somatic depression
F31.4	296.53	Bipolar disorder, severe non-psychotic depression
F31.5	296.54	Bipolar disorder, severe psychotic depression
F31.6	296.60	Bipolar disorder, current episode mixed
F31.7	296.66	Bipolar disorder, currently in remission
F31.8	296.7	Other bipolar affective disorders
F31.9	296.7	Bipolar affective disorder, unspecified
F32.00	296.21	Mild depressive episode without somatic syndrome
F32.01	296.21	Mild depressive episode with somatic syndrome
F32.10	296.22	Moderate depressive episode without somatic syndrome
F32.11	296.22	Moderate depressive episode with somatic syndrome

F32.2	296.23	Severe depressive episode without psychotic symptoms
F32.3	296.24	Severe depressive episode with psychotic symptoms
F32.8	311	Other depressive episodes
F32.9	311	Depressive episode, unspecified
F33.00	296.31	Recurrent depression, mild without somatic syndrome
F33.01	296.31	Recurrent depression, mild with somatic syndrome
F33.10	296.32	Recurrent depression, moderate without somatic syndrome
F33.11	296.32	Recurrent depression, moderate with somatic syndrome
F33.2	296.33	Recurrent depression, current episode severe non-psychotic
F33.3	296.34	Recurrent depression, current episode severe psychotic
F33.4	296.36	Recurrent depression, currently in remission
F33.8	296.30	Other recurrent depressive disorders
F33.9	296.30	Recurrent depressive disorder, unspecified
F34.0	301.13	Cyclothymia
F34.1	300.4	Dysthymia
F34.8	296.90	Other persistent mood [affective] disorders
F34.9	296.90	Persistent mood [affective] disorder, unspecified
F38.0	296.90	Mixed affective episode
F38.1	296.90	Recurrent brief depressive disorder
F38.8	296.90	Other specified mood [affective] disorders
F39	296.90	Unspecified mood [affective] disorder
F40-49		*Neurotic, stress-related and somatoform disorders*
F40.00	300.22	Agoraphobia without panic disorder
F40.01	300.21	Agoraphobia with panic disorder
F40.1	300.23	Social phobias
F40.2	300.29	Specific (isolated) phobias
F40.8	300.29	Other phobic anxiety disorders
F40.9	300.29	Phobic anxiety disorder, unspecified
F41.0	300.01	Panic disorder [episodic paroxysmal anxiety]

F41.1	300.02	Generalized anxiety disorder
F41.2	300.00	Mixed anxiety and depressive disorder
F41.3	300.00	Other mixed anxiety disorders
F41.8	300.00	Other specified anxiety disorders
F41.9	300.00	Anxiety disorder, unspecified
F42.0	300.3	Predominantly obsessional thoughts or ruminations
F42.1	300.3	Predominantly compulsive acts [obsessional rituals]
F42.2	300.3	Mixed obsessional thoughts and acts
F42.8	300.3	Other obsessive–compulsive disorders
F42.9	300.3	Obsessive–compulsive disorder, unspecified
F43.0	308.3	Acute stress reaction
F43.1	309.81	Post-traumatic stress disorder
F43.20	309.9	Brief depressive reaction
F43.21	309.9	Prolonged depressive reaction
F43.22	309.9	Mixed anxiety and depressive reaction
F43.23	309.9	With predominant disturbance of other emotions
F43.24	309.9	With predominant disturbance of conduct
F43.25	309.9	With mixed disturbance of emotions and conduct
F43.28	309.9	With other specified predominant symptoms
F43.8	308.3	Other reactions to severe stress
F43.9	308.3	Reaction to severe stress, unspecified
F44.0	300.12	Dissociative amnesia
F44.1	300.13	Dissociative fugue
F44.2	300.15	Dissociative stupor
F44.3	300.15	Trance and possession disorders
F44.4	300.15	Dissociative motor disorders
F44.5	300.15	Dissociative convulsions
F44.6	300.15	Dissociative anaesthesia and sensory loss
F44.7	300.15	Mixed dissociative [conversion] disorders
F44.80	300.11	Ganser's syndrome

F44.81	300.14	Multiple personality disorder
F44.82	300.11	Transient childhood & adolescent dissociative disorders
F44.88	300.11	Other specified dissociative [conversion] disorders
F44.9	300.15	Dissociative [conversion] disorder, unspecified
F45.0	300.81	Somatization disorder
F45.1	300.82	Undifferentiated somatoform disorder
F45.2	300.7	Hypochondriacal disorder
F45.30	300.82	Somatoform autonomic dysfunction—cardiovascular system
F45.31	300.82	Somatoform autonomic dysfunction—upper GI tract
F45.32	300.82	Somatoform autonomic dysfunction—lower GI tract
F45.33	300.82	Somatoform autonomic dysfunction—respiratory system
F45.34	300.82	Somatoform autonomic dysfunction—genitourinary system
F45.38	300.82	Somatoform autonomic dysfunction—other organ or system
F45.4	307.80	Persistent somatoform pain disorder
F45.8	300.82	Other somatoform disorders
F45.9	300.82	Somatoform disorder, unspecified
F48.0	300.82	Neurasthenia
F48.1	300.6	Depersonalization—derealization syndrome
F48.8	300.9	Other specified neurotic disorders
F48.9	300.9	Neurotic disorder, unspecified
F50-59		*Behavioural syndromes associated with physical factors*
F50.0	307.1	Anorexia nervosa
F50.1	307.1	Atypical anorexia nervosa
F50.2	307.51	Bulimia nervosa
F50.3	307.51	Atypical bulimia nervosa
F50.4	307.50	Overeating associated with other psychological disturbances
F50.5	307.50	Vomiting associated with other psychological disturbances
F50.8	307.50	Other eating disorders

F50.9	307.50	Eating disorder, unspecified
F51.0	307.42	Nonorganic insomnia
F51.1	307.44	Nonorganic hypersomnia
F51.2	307.45	Nonorganic disorder of the sleep-wake schedule
F51.3	307.46	Sleepwalking [somnambulism]
F51.4	307.46	Sleep terrors [night terrors]
F51.5	307.47	Nightmares
F51.8	307.47	Other nonorganic sleep disorders
F51.9	307.47	Nonorganic sleep disorder, unspecified
F52.0	302.71	Lack or loss of sexual desire
F52.10	302.79	Sexual aversion
F52.11	302.79	Lack of sexual enjoyment
F52.2	302.72	Failure of genital response
F52.3	302.70	Orgasmic dysfunction
F52.4	302.75	Premature ejaculation
F52.5	306.51	Nonorganic vaginismus
F52.6	302.76	Nonorganic dyspareunia
F52.7	302.9	Excessive sexual drive
F52.8	302.70	Other sexual dysfunction, not caused by organic disorders
F52.9	302.70	Unspecified non-organic sexual dysfunction
F53.0	293.9	Mild puerperal mental and behavioural disorders
F53.1	293.9	Severe puerperal mental and behavioural disorders
F53.8	293.9	Other puerperal mental and behavioural disorders
F53.9	293.9	Puerperal mental disorder, unspecified
F54	316	Psychological/behavioural factors of other disorders
F55.0	305.90	Abuse of non-dependence-producing antidepressants
F55.1	305.90	Abuse of non-dependence-producing laxatives
F55.2	305.90	Abuse of non-dependence-producing analgesics
F55.3	305.90	Abuse of non-dependence-producing antacids
F55.4	305.90	Abuse of non-dependence-producing vitamins

F55.5	305.90	Abuse of non-dependence-producing steroids or hormones
F55.6	305.90	Abuse of non-dependence-producing herbal or folk remedies
F55.8	305.90	Abuse of other non-dependence-producing substances
F55.9	305.90	Abuse of unspecified non-dependence-producing substances
F59	300.9	Unspecified behaviour syndromes with physiological disturbances
F60-69		*Disorders of adult personality and behaviour*
F60.0	301.0	Paranoid personality disorder
F60.1	301.20	Schizoid personality disorder
F60.2	301.7	Dissocial personality disorder
F60.30	301.9	Emotionally unstable personality disorder, impulsive type
F60.31	301.83	Emotionally unstable personality disorder, borderline type
F60.4	301.50	Histrionic personality disorder
F60.5	301.4	Anankastic (obsessive-compulsive) personality disorder
F60.6	301.82	Anxious [avoidant] personality disorder
F60.7	301.6	Dependent personality disorder
F60.8	301.81	Narcissistic personality disorder
F60.8	301.9	Other specific personality disorders
F60.9	301.9	Personality disorder, unspecified
F61.0	301.9	Mixed personality disorders
F61.1	301.9	Troublesome personality changes
F62.0	301.9	Enduring personality change after catastrophic experience
F62.1	301.9	Enduring personality change after psychiatric illness
F62.8	301.9	Other enduring personality changes
F62.9	301.9	Enduring personality change, unspecified
F63.0	312.31	Pathological gambling
F63.1	312.33	Pathological fire-setting [pyromania]
F63.2	312.32	Pathological stealing [kleptomania]
F63.3	312.39	Trichotillomania

F63.8	312.30	Other habit and impulse disorders
F63.9	312.30	Habit and impulse disorder, unspecified
F64.0	302.85	Transsexualism
F64.1	302.85	Dual-role transvestism
F64.2	302.6	Gender identity disorder of childhood
F64.8	302.6	Other gender identity disorders
F64.9	302.6	Gender identity disorder, unspecified
F65.0	302.81	Fetishism
F65.1	302.3	Fetishistic transvestism
F65.2	302.4	Exhibitionism
F65.3	302.82	Voyeurism
F65.4	302.2	Paedophilia
F65.5	302.9	Sadomasochism
F65.6	302.9	Multiple disorders of sexual preference
F65.8	302.9	Other disorders of sexual preference
F65.9	302.9	Disorder of sexual preference, unspecified
F66.0	302.6	Sexual maturation disorder
F66.1	302.6	Egodystonic sexual orientation
F66.2	302.6	Sexual relationship disorder
F66.8	302.6	Other psychosexual development disorders
F66.9	302.6	Psychosexual development disorder, unspecified
F66.90	302.6	Psychosexual development disorder, heterosexual
F66.91	302.6	Psychosexual development disorder, homosexual
F66.92	302.6	Psychosexual development disorder, bisexual
F66.98	302.6	Psychosexual development disorder, other including prepubertal
F68.0	300.9	Elaboration of physical symptoms for psychological reasons
F68.1	300.19	Factitious disorder
F68.8	301.9	Other specified disorders of adult personality and behaviour
F69	301.9	Unspecified disorder of adult personality and behaviour

F70-79		*Mental retardation [learning disability]*
F70	317	Mild mental retardation
F71	318.0	Moderate mental retardation
F72	318.1	Severe mental retardation
F73	318.2	Profound mental retardation
F78	319	Other mental retardation
F79	319	Unspecified mental retardation
		A fourth character may be used for behavioural impairment
	F7x.0	No, or minimal, impairment of behaviour
	F7x.1	Significant behavioural impairment requiring treatment
	F7x.8	Other impairments of behaviour
	F7x.9	Without mention of impairment of behaviour
F80-89		*Disorders of psychological development*
F80.0	315.39	Specific speech articulation disorder
F80.1	315.31	Expressive language disorder
F80.2	315.32	Receptive language disorder
F80.3	307.9	Acquired aphasia with epilepsy [Landau-Kleffner syndrome]
F80.8	307.9	Other developmental disorders of speech and language
F80.9	307.9	Developmental disorder of speech and language, unspecified
F81.0	315.00	Specific reading disorder
F81.1	315.2	Specific spelling disorder
F81.2	315.1	Specific disorder of arithmetical skills
F81.3	315.9	Mixed disorder of scholastic skills
F81.8	315.9	Other developmental disorders of scholastic skills
F81.9	315.9	Developmental disorder of scholastic skills, unspecified
F82	315.4	Specific developmental disorder of motor function
F83	315.4	Mixed specific developmental disorders
F84.0	299.00	Childhood autism
F84.1	299.80	Atypical autism

F84.2	299.80	Rett's syndrome
F84.3	299.10	Other childhood disintegrative disorder
F84.4	299.80	Overactive disorder of mental retardation [LD], with stereotyped movements
F84.5	299.80	Asperger's syndrome
F84.8	299.80	Other pervasive developmental disorders
F84.9	299.80	Pervasive developmental disorder, unspecified
F88	299.80	Other disorders of psychological development
F89	299.80	Unspecified disorder of psychological development
F90-98		*Childhood & adolescent behavioural and emotional disorders*
F90.0	314.9	Disturbance of activity and attention
F90.1	312.81	Hyperkinetic conduct disorder
F90.8	314.9	Other hyperkinetic disorders
F90.9	314.9	Hyperkinetic disorder, unspecified
F91.0	312.89	Conduct disorder confined to the family context
F91.1	312.89	Unsocialized conduct disorder
F91.2	312.89	Socialized conduct disorder
F91.3	313.81	Oppositional defiant disorder
F91.8	312.89	Other conduct disorders
F91.9	312.89	Conduct disorder, unspecified
F92.0	312.89	Depressive conduct disorder
F92.8	312.89	Other mixed disorders of conduct and emotions
F92.9	312.89	Mixed disorder of conduct and emotions, unspecified
F93.0	309.21	Separation anxiety disorder of childhood
F93.1	300.29	Phobic anxiety disorder of childhood
F93.2	300.23	Social anxiety disorder of childhood
F93.3	V61.8	Sibling rivalry disorder
F93.8	313.9	Other childhood emotional disorders
F93.9	313.9	Childhood emotional disorder, unspecified
F94.0	313.23	Elective mutism
F94.1	313.89	Reactive attachment disorder of childhood

F94.2	313.89	Disinhibited attachment disorder of childhood
F94.8	313.9	Other childhood disorders of social functioning
F94.9	313.9	Childhood disorder of social functioning, unspecified
F95.0	307.21	Transient tic disorder
F95.1	307.22	Chronic motor or vocal tic disorder
F95.2	307.23	de la Tourette's syndrome
F95.8	307.20	Other tic disorders
F95.9	307.20	Tic disorder, unspecified
F98.0	307.6	Nonorganic enuresis
F98.1	307.7	Nonorganic encopresis
F98.2	307.59	Feeding disorder of infancy and childhood
F98.3	307.52	Pica of infancy and childhood
F98.4	307.3	Stereotyped movement disorders
F98.5	307.0	Stuttering [stammering]
F98.6	307.9	Cluttering
F98.8	313.9	Other specified childhood/adolescent disorders
F98.9	313.9	Unspecified childhood/adolescent disorders
F99		*Unspecified mental disorder*
F99	293.9	Mental disorder, not otherwise specified

DSM-5 revisions

Both DSM and ICD* are, at the time of writing, undergoing major revisions. DSM-5†, which will be published in April 2013, makes significant changes to the classification of diagnoses—for example, conceptualizing and organizing them developmentally and in terms of disease clusters and spectra rather than in the existing groups. At the same time, dimensional assessments applicable to all disorders are being introduced (e.g. of depressed mood, or anxiety level, or substance use), and the criteria for many disorders are being changed. Notable alterations include:

- New forms of eating disorder within a general category alongside anorexia and bulimia
- Removal of the subtypes of schizophrenia (paranoid, hebephrenic, catatonic, simple)

---

*ICD11 is due to be published in 2015, and there is currently too much uncertainty about its eventual form to make any useful comments in this handbook.
† The DSM is switching from Roman to Arabic numerals, to allow successive smaller revisions in future (DSM5.1, 5.2 etc.).

- A new attenuated psychosis syndrome, designed to facilitate early recognition and treatment of young people at risk of developing full-blown psychotic disorders
- New hoarding disorder, olfactory reference syndrome (a preoccupying belief that one has a foul odour), and premenstrual dysphoric disorder
- Simplification and reduction of the somatic symptom (previously somatoform) disorders, and
- A reformulation of personality disorder.

The changes to personality disorder are particularly relevant to forensic psychiatrists. The details are not yet fixed, but it seems likely that a mixed dimensional and categorical system will be adopted: to make a diagnosis, an impairment of general personality functioning will need to be demonstrated, as well as matching the patient to a PD trait or domain; both impairment and type/domain will have to be stable over time.

Statutes

Most of the statutes listed on these pages made several changes to the law; some are highly complex, with many different effects. The brief summaries provided here focus on the most important elements of each statute, from the perspective of the handbook. Elements of each Act not relevant to forensic psychiatry are not mentioned.

Statutes

Adults with Incapacity (Scotland) Act 2000 This provides ways to help safeguard the welfare and finances of individuals who lack mental capacity (📖 p.IV.424).

Adult Support and Protection (Scotland) Act 2007 This Act enables people who are unable to care for themselves (📖 p.IV.440) to be removed to a hospital or other place of safety. It also provides a range of measures for safeguarding vulnerable adults (📖 p.II.202).

Age of Legal Capacity (Scotland) Act 1991 This sets out that a person under the age of 16 years has no legal capacity to enter into any transaction, where as a person over age 16 years has full capacity to enter into any form of agreement. See 📖 p.IV.428.

Age of Majority (NI) Act 1969 This Act relates to capacity in children and adolescents, that is those under age 18 years. See 📖 p.IV.428.

Children Act 1989, 2004 *E&W* **1995** *Scotland* **2001** *RoI* These Acts changed the law in regard to children and introduced the notion of parental responsibility. They simplified child protection legislation and increased the powers of (and also the scrutiny of) child welfare and education departments. See 📖 pp.IV.510, IV.429.

Civic Government (Scotland) Act 1982 This Act modified and simplified the Scottish law relating to acquisitive offences (📖 p.IV.354).

Constitutional Reform Act 2005 UK This removed the judicial functions of the House of Lords and created a Supreme Court (📖 p.IV.308).

Coroners & Justice Act 2009 E&W, NI This Act substantially revised the legal test for diminished responsibility (📖 p.V.491), and replaced provocation with a new defence of loss of control (📖 p.V.498).

Courts (Establishment and Constitution) Act 1961 RoI
Courts Service Act 1998 RoI These Acts established the modern court system in RoI, and provided rules for their management, appeals, and the appointment of judges etc. See 📖 p.IV.324.

Crime and Disorder Act 1998 E&W This introduced ASBOs (📖 p.IV.372) and a variety of other community sentences (📖 p.IV.368) and related orders. It also abolished the rule that children between 10 and 14 could only be convicted of an offence if they knew what they were doing was wrong (*doli incapax*, 📖 p.IV.338), and established new rules for sentencing children (📖 p.IV.363).

Criminal Evidence (Witness Anonymity) Act 2008 E&W, NI This Act allows the courts to grant protection, most notably anonymity, to vulnerable or intimidated witness where this does not prevent a fair trial. See 📖 p.II.119.

Criminal Justice Act 2003 UK This amends large areas of the law relating to police powers, bail, disclosure, allocation of criminal offences, prosecution appeals, hearsay, bad character evidence, sentencing and release on licence, affecting E&W more than Scotland or NI. The Act replaced automatic life sentences for certain serious offences with IPPs (📖 p.IV.364). It allows offences to be tried by a judge without a jury in cases where there may be threats of interference with jury. It also allows a defendant to be tried twice for the same offence (double jeopardy) if new and compelling evidence has been found. This Act also revised and simplified community sentences (📖 p.IV.368).

Criminal Justice Act (NI) 1966 This created the statutory defence of diminished responsibility (📖 p.V.491) for NI in terms similar to those in the E&W Homicide Act 1957 (see later in list). It also decriminalized suicide, clarified the special verdict of not guilty by reason of insanity (📖 p.V.489), and refined the rules for inferring mens rea (📖 p.IV.334) from behaviour and for criminal liability when intoxicated (📖 p.V.489).

Criminal Justice and Licensing (Scotland) Act 2010 This Act created the Scottish Sentencing Council (📖 p.IV.363), abolished short periods of imprisonment (📖 p.IV.366), created new offences including one of stalking (📖 p.IV.358), revised criminal procedure and rules of evidence (📖 p.IV.317), and replaced common law rules on insanity (📖 p.V.490) and fitness to plead (insanity in bar of trial, 📖 p.V.474) with new statutory rules.

Criminal Justice and Public Order Act 1994 *E&W* This increased the police power (📖 p.V.450) to stop and search suspects, and restricted the right to silence (📖 p.V.451) by allowing courts to draw inferences from it. It also criminalized previous civil torts (📖 p.V.512), including disruptive trespass, squatting, and unauthorized camping.

Criminal Justice (Public Order) Act 1994 *RoI* This Act modified the available public order offences (📖 p.IV.352) and changed the law on acquisitive offences (📖 p.IV.354).

Criminal Justice (Theft and Fraud Offences) Act 2001 *RoI* This is the main statement of the law relating to fraud and other acquisitive offences (📖 p.IV.354).

Criminal Law Act 1967 *E&W* **1967** *NI* **1997** *RoI* These Acts clarified powers of citizen's arrest (📖 p.V.450) or in RoI police arrest, and what amounts to reasonable force (📖 p.IV.341) in certain situations.

Criminal Law (Insanity) Act 1997, 2006 *RoI* These Acts provide a statutory definition and restatement of the test for criminal insanity (📖 p.V.490), changed the plea to not guilty by reason of insanity, introduced a new plea of diminished responsibility (📖 p.V.492) in cases of murder, and brought in new provisions in relation to a person's fitness to plead (📖 p.V.476). It amended the law on infanticide (📖 p.IV.345), provided new rules on transferring prisoners to hospital (📖 p.IV.410), and established a new independent Review Board to supervise them.

Criminal Law (Rape) Act 1981 *RoI* This legislation, and the subsequent Criminal Law (Rape) (Amendment) Act 1990, defined new offences of rape (📖 p.IV.348) and certain other sexual offences.

Criminal Lunatics Act 1800 *UK* This Act established, for the first time, the principle that mentally disordered offenders found not guilty by reason of insanity (📖 p.V.489) who pose a risk of harm to the public should be treated compulsorily rather than automatically released. It provided for their indefinite detention in an asylum (or prison). See 📖 p.II.216.

Criminal Procedure (Insanity) Act 1964 E&W This revised the special verdict of not guilty by reason of insanity (📖 p.V.490), and established procedures for a trial of the facts (📖 p.V.476) after a finding of unfitness to plead. It also sets out the court orders (📖 p.IV.409) available after a finding of insanity or unfitness to plead. The current version of the Act is the result of amendments by the Criminal Procedure (Insanity and Unfitness to Plead) Act 1991 and Domestic Violence, Crime and Victims Act 2004.

Criminal Procedure (Scotland) Act 1995 This consolidating Act is now the primary source of Scottish criminal procedure. It raised the age of criminal responsibility (📖 p.IV.338), introduced new mental health disposals including the compulsion order (📖 p.IV.405), created the risk assessment order (📖 p.IV.408), and created or revised a number of community sentences (📖 p.IV.368).

Data Protection Acts 1984, 1998 UK **1988, 2003** RoI These Acts implemented EU law (📖 p.IV.326) on the protection of personal data, and set down many detailed rules on the processing and retention of personally-identifiable and confidential (📖 p.III.263) information.

Domestic Violence Crime and Victims Act 2004 E&W This Act focuses on the legal protection and assistance to victims of crime (📖 p.IV.442), particularly domestic violence. It amended the Criminal Procedure (Insanity) Act 1964 (also listed here) to change the disposals available after a finding of unfitness to plead (📖 p.IV.477), and established new rules for informing victims when restricted patients (📖 p.IV.412) and other patients sentenced to treatment (📖 p.IV.405) are discharged (see also 📖 p.IV.442).

Enduring Powers of Attorney (NI) Order 1987 This Act relates to decisions over property and affairs after the donor loses capacity. See powers of attorney (📖 p.IV.432).

Equality Act 2004 RoI **2010** UK These Acts implemented EU law (📖 p.IV.326) updating rules against discrimination (📖 p.V.524) on the basis of sex, race and disability, amongst other characteristics. The UK also merged a number of previous bodies into a single Equality Commission.

European Convention on Human Rights Act 2003 RoI This legislation made the European Convention on Human Rights (📖 p.IV.420) directly applicable in Irish courts.

Extradition Acts 2003 *UK* **1965, 2001** *RoI* These cover the extradition of people from the UK or RoI to face criminal trial in other countries. See 📖 p.V.526.

Family Law Reform Act 1969 *E&W* This Act presumes children aged 16 or 17 to have capacity to consent (📖 p.IV.428) to medical or surgical treatment.

Fraud Act 2006 *E&W* This Act replaced various previous specific acquisitive offences such as obtaining property by deception with a set of new general offences of fraud (📖 p.IV.354).

Health & Safety at Work etc. Act 1974 *UK;* **Health & Welfare at Work Act 2005** *RoI* These Acts place duties on employers (📖 p.V.523) to their employees, including people with mental disorder, to ensure a safe workplace and safe working practices. There is also a duty to ensure the mental health of employees.

Homicide Act 1957 *E&W* This was introduced as a partial reform of the common law offence of murder in English law by abolishing the doctrine of constructive malice and reforming the partial defence of provocation (📖 p.V.499). It introduced the partial defences of diminished responsibility (📖 p.V.491) and suicide pact (📖 p.IV.343).

Human Rights Act 1998 *UK* This Act made the European Convention on Human Rights (📖 p.IV.420) directly applicable in British courts, saving the need to appeal to the European Court of Human Rights in Strasbourg. It also requires all public bodies to carry out their duties in ways that conform with the Convention.

Immigration Acts 1971–2006 *UK* **1999–2010** *RoI* These complex sets of Acts set out the rules on who can claim British or Irish citizenship, who may enter and remain in either country, who may be granted asylum, and whom the government may legally deport. See 📖 p.V.525.

Life Sentences (NI) Order 2001 This Order provides for the release and recall of offenders serving a life sentence (📖 p.IV.364) in NI. It also makes changes to the way such sentences and sentences of detention at the Secretary of State's pleasure are made in court.

Lunacy Acts 1845-1891 *UK* These Acts, and the associated County Asylums Act 1888 and Trial of Lunatics Act 1883, established a network of asylums across E&W, Scotland and Ireland; defined rules for admission, transfer, leave and discharge; and instituted a system of inspection by Commissioners who could order minimum standards of treatment and the release of patients. See 📖 p.IV.374.

Lunacy Regulation (Ireland) Act 1871 This Act remains the primary legislation in RoI for managing the affairs of people who lack mental capacity (📖 p.IV.424), although at the time of writing it is under review and may be replaced.

Mental Capacity Act 2005 *E&W* This provides a framework to empower and protect adults who lack capacity (📖 p.IV.424) to make decisions for themselves on medical treatment and other matters. It also enables people to plan ahead for when they may lack capacity, such as by making advance statements (📖 p.IV.430).

Mental Capacity (Health, Welfare and Finance) Bill *NI* This is due to be introduced in summer 2011, and would unify mental health and mental capacity law in a single, comprehensive capacity-based framework. Its guiding principles, set out at the start of the Bill, are respect for autonomy, justice, beneficence and non-maleficence (see 📖 p.III.233)—compare the existing principles of mental health laws (📖 p.IV.373) and principles of mental capacity law (📖 p.IV.424). If the Bill becomes law, it will be a major international innovation. At the time of writing, however, the details of the proposed legislation are unclear and subject to considerable change, and are therefore not referred to in detail in this handbook.

Mental Deficiency and Lunacy (Scotland) Act 1913 Mental Deficiency Act 1913 *E&W* These Acts set up specific institutions for the care and control of people with learning disability, with a Board of Control to inspect them. See 📖 p. IV.375.

Mental Health Act 1983 *E&W* This Act, which was heavily modified by the Mental Health Act 2007 in particular, is the primary mental health law (📖 p.IV.373) in E&W. It deals with the detention in hospital of people with mental disorders, as well as other compulsory measures including guardianship and supervised community treatment (📖 p.IV.394). It sets out the criteria (📖 p.IV.381) that must be met before compulsory measures can be taken, as well as protections and safeguards for patients. It also introduced the deprivation of liberty safeguards (DoLS, 📖 p.V.436) for patients lacking capacity.

Mental Health Act 2001 *RoI* This is the primary Irish mental health law (📖 p.IV.373), and covers the circumstances in which a patient may be admitted to hospital for mental health treatment against their will. The Mental Health Commission is the statutory independent body which oversees the Act's implementation and use.

Mental Health (Care & Treatment) (Scotland) Act 2003 This Act enables medical professionals to detain and treat people against their will; it is Scotland's primary mental health law. Unlike the equivalents elsewhere, the main ground for detention of people with mental disorder is their lack of capacity (📖 p.IV.377).

Mental Health (NI) Order 1986 This Order is the primary mental health legislation (📖 p.IV.373) for NI, and also contains provisions on unfitness to plead (📖 p.V.474) and insanity (📖 p.V.489).

Mental Treatment Acts 1930 *E&W* **1932** *NI* **1945** *RoI* These Acts permitted voluntary admission to, and outpatient treatment within, psychiatric hospitals. The RoI Act went much further and abolished the need for judicial orders for admission. See 📖 p.IV.375.

National Assistance Act 1948 *E&W* This Act formally abolished the Poor Laws (📖 p.IV.374), and provided basic social welfare for people who were not eligible to receive services because they did not pay National Insurance contributions (e.g. the homeless, unmarried mothers and the severely disabled). It includes powers to move unwilling people unable to care for themselves (📖 p.IV.440) to a hospital or nursing home.

Non-Fatal Offences Against the Person Act 1997 *RoI* This is the principal Act that defines the offences of assault (📖 p.IV.346) that does not amount to homicide.

Offences against the Person Act 1861 *E&W, NI* This is one of a group of Acts sometimes referred to as the criminal law consolidation Acts of 1861. It is the foundation for prosecuting assault (📖 p.IV.346), short of murder, in the courts of E&W and NI. In Ireland (both NI and RoI) this Act continues to be the basis of the ban on abortion.

Police and Criminal Evidence Act 1984 *E&W* This and the associated codes of practice provide the core framework of police powers (📖 p.V.450) and safeguards around stop and search, arrest, detention, investigation, identification and interviewing suspects. Its aim is to achieve a proper balance between the powers of the police and the rights and freedoms of the public.

Powers of Attorney Act 1996 *RoI* This Act relates to decisions over property, money and personal care after the donor loses capacity. See powers of attorney (📖 p.IV.432).

Prisoners and Criminal Proceedings (Scotland) Act 1993 This is the legislation that relates to detention, transfer (except to hospital) and release of imprisoned offenders (📖 p.V.456) in Scotland.

Probation of Offenders Act 1907 *E&W, NI and RoI* This Act gave judges the discretion to dismiss a charge against a defendant after a summary trial (📖 p.IV.330) even when the court is of the opinion that it is proved, or to conditionally discharge a defendant (whether charged on an indictment or summarily). The judge could also dismiss a case under the Act on condition that the defendant pay a contribution to charity, or repay costs arising from his actions, or if the case was seen as trivial. The Act established a system of probation of offenders (📖 p.V.462) that continues today in modified form.

Public Order Act 1986 *E&W* **Order 1987** *NI* This Act and Order respectively created a new set of public order offences (📖 p.IV.352), replacing the common law offences of riot, unlawful assembly and affray that had by then become confused.

Sexual Offences Act 2003 *E&W* **2009** *Scotland* **Order 2008** *NI* These Acts and this Order each consolidated and replaced the older common law and statutory sexual offences (📖 p.IV.348), redefining the offences more clearly and explicitly. Several new offences were created in some cases, such as non-consensual voyeurism, assault by penetration, penetration of any part of a corpse and causing a child to watch a sexual act. Rape was redefined to include male rape in Scotland. The law was also amended to make it clear that only a reasonable and genuine mistaken belief that the other party consented could be a defence to rape.

Theft Acts 1968, 1978 *E&W* **1969** *NI* These Acts replaced the over-complicated and confusing common law offences of larceny with a new set of theft offences (📖 p.IV.354).

Vagrancy Acts 1774–1898 *UK* These laws were introduced to deal with the large numbers of soldiers and others returning after the Napoleonic Wars, who were often homeless and out of work. It became an offence to sleep on the streets or beg. See 📖 p.IV.374.

Legal cases

The cases referred to in the handbook are listed here and summarized briefly on the following pages. In these summaries, we have focused on the elements most relevant to the topic in the handbook that refers to the case. With a few cases, this means that the summary we have given might not reflect other significant points made in the judgment.

Cases

A-G's ref In this case, the defendant had killed two people by driving his lorry into parked cars on the side of the motorway. He claimed to be in an automatic state caused by 'repetitive visual stimulus experienced on long journeys on straight flat roads'. The trial court accepted the defence of automatism; the Attorney-General appealed, and the Court of Appeal ruled that, on the medical evidence, the defendant had partial control over his actions and the defence of automatism therefore did not apply, stating 'the defence of automatism requires that there was a total destruction of voluntary control on the defendant's part'. See ⬚ p.V.483. *Attorney-General's Reference (No. 2 of 1992)* [1993] 3 WLR 982.

A-G v Whelan Mr Whelan knowingly received stolen goods (⬚ p.IV.354), and was convicted despite the jury accepting he had acted under duress (⬚ p.V.502) from Farnon, who was known to carry a revolver. The Court of Criminal Appeal overturned the conviction, and set down the test for duress in RoI. See ⬚ p.V.503. *Attorney General v Whelan* [1934] IR 518.

R v Ahluwalia The defendant was a woman in an arranged marriage who had suffered years of abuse and violence from her husband. One evening, after an argument in which he threatened to beat her in the morning, she set him alight in his sleep, killing him. She pleaded provocation (⬚ p.V.498) but was convicted of murder on the ground that the time that elapsed between the argument and the killing meant that her loss of self-control, if any, had not been 'sudden and temporary'. This was upheld by the House of Lords, but a retrial was ordered to allow her to claim diminished responsibility (⬚ p.V.492) on the grounds that she suffered from 'battered woman syndrome', a form of PTSD (⬚ p.II.70); her conviction was later reduced to manslaughter on these grounds. The law was later changed by statute: see ⬚ p.V.500. *R v Ahluwalia* [1992] 4 AllER 889.

R (Ashworth Hospital) v MHRT H had been detained at Ashworth, a high security hospital, under section 3 (⬚ p.IV.388) since 1994; he had been transferred after seriously assaulting a junior doctor at a medium secure unit. A Tribunal discharged him on the ground that he had recovered from schizophrenia, despite opposition from the hospital and the local services, and despite the lack of any aftercare arrangements; it considered adjourning but said that it did not believe Ashworth Hospital would make the necessary arrangements. The RMO re-detained him under section 5(2), then section 3, and the hospital applied for judicial review of the Tribunal's decision. The decision was ruled unlawful, because it was *Wednesbury* unreasonable not to adjourn, and because the

Tribunal had not given adequate reasons for its decision. The new section was also held to be unlawful: the hospital should instead have applied to the High Court for a stay of the Tribunal's decision. See 📖 p.IV.311. *R (on the application of Ashworth Hospital) v Mental Health Review Tribunal for West Midlands and Northwest Region; R (on the application of H) v Ashworth Hospital Authority and others* [2002] EWCA Civ 923.

Miss B was tetraplegic and could only live on a mechanical ventilator. She regarded her quality of life as unacceptably low, and requested that the ventilator be disconnected. Her doctors would not agree; but she applied to the High Court (📖 p.IV.320), which ruled that she had the right to refuse ventilation, even though she would die as a result. See 📖 p.III.279. *Re B (Adult: Refusal of treatment)* [2002] 2 FCR 1.

R v Bell While driving, Mr Bell collided with a number of objects and cars, but avoided pedestrians. He was charged with driving recklessly. He described giving no thought of the consequences of his actions by virtue of his mental illness. The judgment stated that the only alternative verdict if insanity was rejected was conviction. See 📖 p.V.489. *R v Bell* 1984 Crim. LR 685

R v Bentley Derek Bentley was a 19-year-old who had twice suffered serious head injuries and had low IQ. He and a 16-year-old, Christopher Craig, were caught by the police after breaking into a warehouse. Bentley allegedly shouted 'Let him have it, Chris', after which Craig shot a police officer, wounding him. Bentley was arrested, and shortly afterwards another officer was shot and killed (by Craig, it was alleged). Craig was convicted of murder (📖 p.IV.345) but, as a child, received an indeterminate sentence (📖 p.IV.364) and was released ten years later. Bentley was also convicted on the basis of joint enterprise (📖 p.IV.340), the key evidence being his alleged shout, which implied that he knew Craig had a gun. As an adult, he was sentenced to death. The case generated great public unease, and Bentley received a posthumous pardon in 1993, with his conviction formally being quashed several years later. See 📖 p.IV.340. *R v Bentley* (1952, unreported); *R v Bentley (Deceased)* [2001] 1 CrAppR 307.

Black v Forsey Dr Forsey was a Scottish SHO who detained Mr Black using a second assessment section (📖 p.IV.383) on the instructions of her consultant, despite this being illegal under Scottish mental health law at the time. The hospital claimed that, although the purported section was unlawful, it had a common law power to detain Mr Black nevertheless. The court confirmed the existence of a common law power to detain 'a person of unsound mind who is a danger to himself or others', 'in a situation of necessity', but held that it could only apply to a private individual, not to a hospital or other authority that can detain patients under mental health law. See 📖 p.IV.440. *Black v Forsey* [1988] SC (HL) 28.

Bolam Mr Bolam was a patient at a mental hospital. He agreed to undergo ECT (📖 p.II.158), at a time when the risk of mortality with muscle relaxants was widely believed to outweigh the benefits, and the use of restraints was thought to increase the risk of injury. He suffered a fractured acetabulum and sued, claiming negligence. The claim was dismissed, on the grounds that the doctors at the hospital had followed a practice accepted as proper by a responsible body of medical opinion. This remains the key test in clinical negligence (📖 p.V.516). *Bolam v Friern Hospital Management Committee* [1957] 1 WLR 583.

Bolitho A 2-year-old child suffered three bouts of respiratory difficulty, during the third of which he had a cardiac arrest and sustained brain damage. The parents claimed negligence, because no doctor had attended and the child had not been prophylactically intubated after the earlier respiratory difficulty. The claim was dismissed and this was upheld on appeal by the House of Lords, as a body of paediatric opinion held that such intubation would have been inappropriate. However, the House of Lords also ruled that if the body of opinion 'was incapable of withstanding logical analysis', it would not be a defence to negligence. See 📖 p.V.516. *Bolitho v Hackney Health Authority* [1998] AC 232.

Bournewood In this case, a 48-year-old man with severe autism who frequently harmed himself was admitted informally to hospital after becoming very agitated at a day centre. He lacked capacity, but did not express a refusal of treatment. The RMO (📖 p.IV.379) indicated that she would detain him under section 5(2) (📖 p.IV.386) if he tried to leave, for his own safety. His carers sued on his behalf, claiming false imprisonment (📖 p.IV.358). The House of Lords found (reversing the Court of Appeal's earlier decision) that he was lawfully detained, but suggested that Parliament review the situation. The case was then taken to the European Court of Human Rights, where it was known as *HL v UK* (see later in list). See 📖 p.III.278. *R v Bournewood Community & Mental Health NHS Trust, ex parte L* [1999] 1 AC 458.

R v Bowen Mr Bowen was convicted of fraud offences, despite claiming that he had acted under threats that his family would be petrol-bombed if he did not commit the offences. He appealed on the grounds that, although a reasonable person would not have experienced duress (📖 p.V.502), his low IQ and suggestibility should have been taken into account. The appeal was dismissed. See 📖 p.V.503. *R v Bowen* [1996] 2 CrAppR 157.

R v Bonython. Mr Bonython was convicted of forgery and uttering a request for money. He was alleged to have forged the signature of Miss Bell;

a police handwriting expert gave evidence that the handwriting was not that of Miss Bell. This was the subject of appeal. The Supreme Court of South Africa laid down rules stating that expert evidence was admissible if it falls within the class of subjects on which expert testimony is permissible, which requires considering whether the witness's expertise is necessary, and whether the opinion forms part of a recognized body of knowledge or experience. *R v Boynthon* (1984) 38 SASR 45.

R v Brady Mr Brady was a patient at Ashworth Hospital with a severe personality disorder. He sought to have part of his Tribunal heard in public, apparently in order to publicize his case against detention (while keeping medical evidence confidential). The hospital applied for judicial review of the Tribunal's preliminary decision to allow a partially public hearing. In a judgment that overturned this decision, the High Court accepted in principle the argument that Mr Brady might lack capacity (📖 p.IV.424) to request a public hearing on the ground that his desire to manipulate others distorted his process of weighing information in the balance. See 📖 p.IV.424. *R (on the application of Mersey Care NHS Trust) v Mental Health Review Tribunal (Brady and another, interested parties)* [2005] 2 AllER 820.

Bratty v A-G NI Mr Bratty was convicted of strangling an 18-year-old girl. He had psychomotor epilepsy, and had claimed (amongst other defences) that he had suffered from an automatism. The House of Lords held that there were two types of automatism, insane and non-insane, that an insane automatism could only be caused by disease of the mind, and that 'any mental disorder which has manifested itself in violence and is prone to recur is a disease of the mind'. See 📖 p.V.483. *Bratty v Attorney-General for Northern Ireland* [1963] 1 AC 386.

R v Burgess The defendant in this case caused GBH while sleep-walking. The High Court ruled on appeal that the sleep-walking, while transient, was still a disease of the mind (and therefore an insane automatism) because it was 'due to an internal factor . . . had manifested itself in violence and might recur' See 📖 p.V.484. *R v Burgess* [1991] 2 QB 93.

R v Byrne. In this case Mr Byrne strangled a young woman and mutilated her corpse. There was evidence that from an early age Mr Byrne was subject to perverse violent desires and that the impulse or urge associated with these desires was stronger than normal. The High Court ruled that the term 'abnormality of mind' in relation to diminished responsibility should be taken to mean the mind's activities in all its aspects, not only the perception of physical acts and matters; and the ability to form a rational judgement whether an act is right or wrong but also the ability to exercise will-power to control physical acts in accordance with that rational judgement. See 📖 p.V.492. *R v Byrne* [1960] 2 QB 396.

Re C concerned a patient with schizophrenia detained in long stay residential psychiatric care. He had gangrene in his leg and was advised to have an amputation, but refused. The Court ruled that he had capacity to refuse surgical treatment even though his delusions included the belief that he was an expert in surgery and therefore knew that he would survive without amputation. (In the event, he turned out to be right: he recovered without surgery.) The ruling set down the common law rules on mental capacity, which still apply in NI. See pp.III.279, V.426. *Re C (Adult: Refusal of treatment)* [1994] 2 FCR 151.

Caldwell set fire to a hotel where he had been employed, because of a grudge against the proprietor; he was so drunk that he did not consider the risk that anyone's life might be endangered. The House of Lords upheld his conviction on the grounds that a reasonable person would have considered the risk, undermining the subjective nature of recklessness (📖 p.IV.336). It was overturned 22 years later by R v G, see later in list. See 📖 p.IV.337. *Metropolitan Police Commissioner v Caldwell* [1982] AC 341.

Camplin The defendant, at the age of 15, killed a man by hitting him on the head with a heavy pan. He claimed that the victim had forcibly raped him and then taunted him, i.e. that he had been provoked. The jury was instructed to decide whether the reasonable person (i.e. an adult) would have done so, not a 'reasonably boy', and convicted him. The House of Lords ruled that the trial judge had misdirected the jury, and that they should have been allowed to take his age into account (i.e. the reasonable person test was made more subjective). See 📖 p.V.500. *DPP v Camplin* [1978] UKHL 2.

Caparo v Dickman Caparo bought a struggling company, Fidelity, intending to make a profit. However, when it gained control, it realised Fidelity was in a far poorer condition that its accounts had revealed, meaning Caparo would make a loss. Caparo sued for negligence in the production of the accounts. The House of Lords ruled that Caparo was not owed a duty of care by the accountant Dickman, who prepared Fidelity's accounts. It laid down the 'threefold test' of a duty of care in negligence cases. See 📖 p.V.513. *Caparo Industries PLC v Dickman* [1990] 2 AC 605.

Clunis Christopher Clunis had schizophrenia, and was often violent when psychotic; his condition responded well to antipsychotics when detained in hospital, but after discharge he invariably defaulted from treatment, and avoided contact with community mental health staff. Eventually he killed a man, Jonathan Zito, on a tube station platform because of his persecutory delusion that Mr Zito was about to attack him. He was convicted of manslaughter on the grounds of diminished responsibility (📖 p.V.491). Following the Ritchie report (📖 p.App. 5.656), he sued one of the responsible health authorities over the standard of care received, but his case was dismissed by the Court of Appeal and the European Court of Human Rights on the ground that he bore primary responsibility for his own criminal acts. See 📖 p.V.502. *R v Clunis* (unreported); *Clunis v UK* [1998] ECHR 116.

R v Crozier Mr Crozier attacked his sister with an axe; he pleaded guilty to attempted murder. A psychiatrist found that he suffered from psychopathic disorder (📖 p.II.66) and recommended detention in high security (📖 p.II.209). The report was not submitted, and the court passed a sentence of 9 years' imprisonment; the psychiatrist (who had arrived to give evidence) gave the report to the prosecution counsel, who successfully applied to vary the sentence to a hospital order with restrictions (📖 p.IV.412). Mr Crozier appealed, claiming a breach of confidentiality (📖 p.III.263); this was dismissed, on the ground that the public interest in the disclosure of the report outweighed the patient's right to confidentiality. See 📖 p.III.264. *R v Crozier* [1991] CrimLR 138.

R v Dietschmann Mr Dietschmann killed a man whilst under the influence of alcohol. He believed the victim had insulted his dead aunt. At trial psychiatrists agreed that he was suffering from an abnormality of mind for the purposes of diminished responsibility: a delayed grief reaction or adjustment disorder. The trial judge directed the jury to consider whether if he had not consumed alcohol he would still have killed. At appeal this was challenged. The underlying condition was the relevant issue, not whether he would have still killed had he not consumed alcohol. See 📖 p.V.488. *R v Dietschmann* [2003] UKHL 10.

R v Dix Mr Dix shot a friend of his 'to put her out of her misery'. He later claimed diminished responsibility on the basis of his odd behaviour and claims after the killing. The trial judge ruled that the defence required medical evidence, and could not be proved on the basis of ordinary evidence, no matter how odd. This was upheld at appeal. See 📖 p.V.492. *R v Dix* [1982] CrimLR 302.

Donoghue v Stevenson Donoghue drank some ginger beer bought for her by her friend. They later realized the bottle contained the decomposing remains of a snail. Donoghue suffered gastroenteritis. She claimed £500 damages from Stevenson, the manufacturer. The House of Lords ruled in a preliminary hearing that Stevenson owed her a duty of care even though she had not purchased the drink: the manufacturer ought to have had the ultimate consumer, not merely the purchaser, in mind. The case laid the foundations of the modern law of negligence (📖 p.V.512). *Donoghue v Stevenson* [1932] UKHL 100.

Dooley v Cammell Laird The plaintiff was a crane driver whose employer had fitted his crane with a defective rope; the rope snapped, dropping the load into the hold of a ship where the driver's fellow employees were working. Mr Dooley received compensation for the psychiatric illness he suffered because of his fears for their safety, even though in fact they were not injured; the court held he was an 'involuntary participant' in the creation of the dangerous situation. See 📖 p.V.514. *Dooley v Cammell Laird* [1951] 1 Lloyd's Rep 271.

DPP v Morgan The defendant invited three younger men to his house for sex with his wife, telling them that she was 'kinky' and would only pretend to resist. In fact she did not consent, and was raped by all four men. They were convicted on the ground that they had no sufficient reason to believe that she consented. The Court of Appeal ruled that the test was subjective, and that a genuine mistaken belief prevented conviction for rape (but also upheld the conviction on the ground that the defendants did not have such genuine beliefs). The law was later changed to reverse this ruling. See 📖 pp.IV.344, IV.337. *DPP v Morgan* [1976] AC 182.

Drury v HM Advocate This controversial case concerned a man who killed his wife with a hammer after discovering her affair. The Court of Criminal Appeal redefined murder as requiring 'wicked intent' or wicked recklessness, such that provocation (if the violence was in proportion to it) made the intent no longer wicked. Conversely, a provoked defendant who used excessive violence could still be convicted of murder. This conflicts with other principles of the provocation defence. See 📖 p.V.499. *Drury v HM Advocate* [2001] SCCR 583.

R v Duffy Mrs Duffy was the victim of repeated domestic violence by her husband, who had refused to allow her to leave with their child. Seeing no alternative, she later killed him with a hatchet while he slept. The Court of Criminal Appeal upheld the trial judge's direction that provocation (📖 p.V.498) required a sudden and temporary loss of self-control. This rule was later changed in E&W, but it remains the law in RoI. See 📖 p.V.500. *R v Duffy* [1949] 1 AllER 932.

W v Egdell W was a patient detained in a special hospital after shooting and killing or wounding seven people. He applied to a Tribunal, seeking transfer to an RSU (📖 p.II.210). His solicitor commissioned an independent psychiatric report, which strongly opposed transfer and commented on his continued interest in firearms and explosives. W then withdrew his application. The independent psychiatrist, Dr Egdell, was concerned that the treating hospital lacked key information and disclosed his report to the hospital, breaching W's confidentiality. The Court held that Dr Egdell did owe W a duty of confidentiality, but that the breach of it was justified by the public interest in preventing further very serious offending by W. See 📖 p.III.263. *W v Egdell* [1990] 1 AllER 835.

R v Emery The defendant, a teenage mother, was acquitted of assaulting her 11-month-old daughter (but convicted of failing to protect her from multiple, ultimately fatal, assaults by the father). The acquittal was partly based on evidence from psychologists that Miss Emery suffered from 'battered woman syndrome' and behaved as she did because of learned helplessness. The Court of Appeal upheld the trial judge's admission of this evidence, even though it was not evidence of a recognized mental disorder, because it was 'complex and not known by the public at large'. See 📖 p.V.536. *R v Emery* [1993] 14 CrAppR(S) 394.

R v Erskine Mr Erskine had been convicted of a series of murders of elderly people in 1988, many of whom he had also sexually assaulted. His behaviour after arrest was bizarre, and it was later accepted that there would have been grounds for a plea of diminished responsibility (📖 p.V.491). However, at the time he did not allow this plea to be put forward, because of his beliefs arising from his mental disorder. The Court of Appeal rejected the contention that Mr Erskine would have been unfit to plead at the original trial, ruling that a defendant is not unfit 'merely because he will not accept . . . eminently sensible advice from his legal advisors'. However, it went on to substitute a verdict of manslaughter on the grounds of diminished responsibility 'in the interests of justice'. See 📖 p.V.475. *R v Erskine* [2009] EWCA Crim 1425.

Fitzpatrick This was the first case in which an Irish court set down the common law definition of mental capacity (📖 p.IV.424) in that jurisdiction, founding it on the principles in Re C (📖 p.App. 3.633). It concerned a Jehovah's Witness who wished to refuse a life-saving blood transfusion. See 📖 p.IV.426. *Fitzpatrick & Another v K & Another* [2008] IEHC 104.

Freeman v Home Office Mr Freeman was a life sentence prisoner with personality disorder and intermittent depression, who was administered antipsychotic drugs in Wakefield Prison. He later sued, claiming that his apparent consent was not valid because, amongst other reasons, the Prison Medical Officer was acting as a disciplinary agent of the prison rather than as a doctor. The Court of Appeal ruled that prisoners were capable of giving or withholding consent, notwithstanding the disciplinary nature of staff. See 📖 p.II.148. *Freeman v Home Office* [1984] 1 AllER 1036.

R v G and another This case was similar on the facts to *Caldwell*, listed earlier. Two young boys, out camping, entered a disused building and set fire to some newspapers, thinking they would extinguish themselves. The fire spread and damaged nearby shops. The boys were initially convicted because a reasonable person would have recognized the risk of the fire spreading, but the conviction was overturned by the House of

Lords on appeal. Recklessness (📖 p.IV.336) was returned to its original, subjective, definition. See 📖 p.IV.337. *R v G and another* [2004] 1 AC 1034.

Galbraith v HM Advocate Ms Galbraith killed her husband and was convicted of murder. She appealed her conviction on the grounds that she was abused for many years by the deceased and was suffering from a form of PTSD. The court ruled that the test in HM Advocate v Savage should not be interpreted narrowly: diminished responsibility required some form of abnormality of mind sufficient to have a substantial effect on a person's mind and in relation to his act, but it was not necessary to prove that the accused's mental state bordered on insanity. See 📖 p.V.492. *Galbraith v HM Advocate* (2002) JC 1.

Gillick In this case, a mother sought a declaration that a Department of Health guideline allowing doctors to prescribe contraception to under-16-year-olds was unlawful. The House of Lords ruled that it was lawful, and that a child under 16 could consent to treatment in their own right if they have 'sufficient understanding and intelligence to understand fully what is proposed'. See 📖 p.IV.428. *Gillick v West Norfolk and Wisbech Area Health Authority* [1985] 3 All ER 402.

Gillon v HM Advocate The defendant did not dispute that he had killed the victim by repeatedly hitting him on the head with a spade, but claimed that the victim had provoked him by first attacking him with the spade. The Appeal Court reaffirmed the rule in *Robertson v HM Advocate* (see later in list) that the violence must be proportionate to the provocation, and rejected an alternative rule based on what an ordinary person might do. See 📖 p.V.499. *Gillon v HM Advocate* [2007] SC(JC) 24.

R v Gotts. Mr Gotts was charged with attempted murder. He claimed to have been ordered by his father to kill his mother. He claimed a defence of duress. The trial judge ruled that duress was not available as a defence to attempted murder. The trial judge's direction was upheld on appeal. See 📖 p.V.503. *R v Gotts* [1992] 2 WLR 878.

R v Hardie Mr Hardie lived with a woman at her flat. Their relationship broke down and she asked him to leave. As a result of his upset he took a quantity of diazepam, making him voluntarily intoxicated (📖 p.V.486), in which state he started a fire in the flat. The judge at his trial for arson directed that the self-administration of the drug was irrelevant, but this was overturned on appeal. The jury should have been directed to consider whether the taking of the drug did negate mens rea, and if it did, whether the taking of the drug was reckless (📖 p.IV.336). See 📖 p.V.486. *R v Hardie* [1985] 3 AllER 848.

R v Hasan Mr Hasan was convicted of an aggravated burglary. He had claimed that he had acted under duress (📖 p.V.502), having been threatened by another person (who had boasted of murdering others) that if he did not commit the burglary, he and his family would be harmed. The House of Lords upheld the conviction and set down the requirements of the defence of duress by threats. See 📖 p.V.502. *R v Hasan* [2005] UKHL 22.

R v Hennessy Mr Hennessy had diabetes, and not having taken insulin for several days, experienced a hyperglycaemic episode in which he took and drove off a car. He claimed this was an automatism; the trial judge ruled that as it was due to an intrinsic cause, the disease of diabetes, the only available defence was insanity. The Court of Appeal ruled that the trial judge was correct, and moreover that stress, anxiety and depression, while perhaps 'external', lacked the 'feature of novelty or accident' required of causes of non-insane automatism. See 📖 pp.V.483, V.489. *R v Hennessy* [1989] EWCA Crim 1.

HL v UK This was the continuation of the *Bournewood* case (listed earlier) at the European Court of Human Rights (📖 p.IV.326). The court found, contrary to the decision of the House of Lords in the UK, that the lack of procedural safeguards in detaining HL, and the lack of access to a Tribunal, made his detention unlawful. The government responded by using the Mental Health Act 2007 to add Deprivation of Liberty Safeguards (DoLS) to the Mental Capacity Act 2005. See 📖 p.IV.436. *HL v UK* [2004] 40 EHRR 761.

Holley Mr Holley, an alcoholic, killed his girlfriend with an axe while drunk. He claimed provocation, stating that she had taunted him about having an affair. There was disagreement at his various trials about whether he was voluntarily intoxicated (📖 p.V.486), and whether he suffered from personality disorder that made it hard for him to control his drinking. The Privy Council (📖 p.IV.327) reversed the decision of the House of Lords in *Morgan Smith* (see later in list), and stated that the Homicide Act 1957 required the reasonable person test to be a purely objective test, meaning that none of the special characteristics of the defendant could be taken into account. The government replaced this Act with the Coroners and Justice Act 2009, and returned the test to a mixed subjective and objective test, in order to overturn this ruling. See 📖 p.V.500. *HM Attorney-General for Jersey v Holley* [2005] UKPC 23.

Home Office v Dorset Yacht Co A group of detainees at a Borstal (a type of youth detention centre) were working in a harbour under the direction of prison officers. They absconded with a yacht which they crashed into another boat, damaging it. The owners of the second yacht sued for damages. The court upheld their claim, stating that the prison officers had failed to exercise proper control over the detainees and that their behaviour, and the consequent damage, was of a kind that was reasonably foreseeable if they were not properly controlled. See 📖 p.V.519. *Home Office v Dorset Yacht Co* [1974] 2 AllER 294.

R v Jason Cann The defendant had paranoid schizophrenia and was detained in hospital. He killed a nurse whom he believed, because of delusions, intended to rape him. Appealing against conviction for manslaughter on the grounds of diminished responsibility (📖 p.V.491), he claimed that he should have been allowed to plead self-defence (📖 p.IV.340). The Court of Appeal rejected this, ruling that the test of reasonable force was entirely objective, and his delusions were irrelevant. See 📖 p.IV.342. *R v Jason Cann* [2005] EWCA 2264.

K v Home Office The Home Office had issued a deportation order against Mr M, a Kenyan convicted of a sexual offence and burglary; however, it was not carried out, and he went on to rape Ms K. She sued the Home Office for the harm she had suffered from the rape, but her claim was dismissed on the ground that there was no proximity (📖 p.V.513) between her (at the time an unidentified member of the public) and the Home Office. See 📖 p.V.519. *K v Secretary of State for the Home Department* [2002] EWCA Civ 775.

R v Kemp Mr Kemp, who had assaulted his wife, suffered from arteriosclerosis. Transient cerebral ischaemia had caused a temporary 'lapse of consciousness' during which he attacked his wife. The High Court held that this amounted to an insane automatism, despite the temporary nature of the 'lapse', because arteriosclerosis was a disease affecting the mind. It does not matter whether the disease concerned has a physical or mental origin. See 📖 p.V.484. *R v Kemp* [1957] 1 QB 399.

R v Khan Mr Khan bludgeoned his roommate to death with a cricket bat. He claimed diminished responsibility, with psychiatric evidence in support, but was convicted of murder. He appealed, claiming that the judge should have directed the jury that they should accept the plea of diminished responsibility. The Court of Appeal upheld the conviction, ruling that the issue was for the jury to decide. See 📖 p.V.493. *R v Khan* [2009] EWCA 1569.

R v Kimber The defendant was charged with indecent assault on a female patient in a mental hospital. He claimed that she had known what he was doing and had consented. The trial judge told the jury that the sole issue was whether the victim had truly consented or not. The Court of Appeal held that the judge had erred, and that a mistaken belief that consent had been given would lead to acquittal. (However, it upheld the conviction on the grounds that the defendant lacked any such mistaken belief.) See 📖 p.IV.344. *R v Kimber* [1983] 1 WLR 1118.

R v Kingston Mr Kingston was charged with indecently assaulting (📖 p.IV.349) a 15-year-old boy. He contended that he had been drugged by a co-defendant (with triazolam, a benzodiazepine) and that he would not have acted as he had done if he had not been drugged. The jury were directed that if he was found to have intent (📖 p.IV.334) then the fact he was drugged was not relevant. In other words, the involuntary intoxication (📖 p.V.485) would have had to make him incapable of forming intent (📖 p.V.481). The jury found that the photographs and audiotapes of Kingston's behaviour in assaulting the boy demonstrated that he must have intended assault at the time, notwithstanding his intoxication. This was upheld at appeal. See 📖 p.V.486. *R v Kingston* [1994] 3 WLR 519.

Laporte This case concerned protesters demonstrating against the Iraq War, who were arrested for breach of the peace. The House of Lords made it clear that not only police officers but all citizens could arrest people to prevent a breach of the peace (i.e. the use or threat of violence). See 📖 p.IV.441. *R (on the application of Laporte) v Chief Constable of Gloucestershire* [2006] UKHL 55.

Lewisham v Malcolm Mr Malcolm had sub-let his council flat, in breach of his tenancy agreement. He had schizophrenia (although the council did not know this) and had not been taking his medication. Lewisham sought an order for possession (i.e. to evict him), and was granted one; Mr Malcolm appealed. The House of Lords eventually dismissed his appeal, stating that because the council had treated him in exactly the same way as it would have treated anyone else, there was no discrimination. This ruling was overturned by the Equality Act 2010, which provided for cases in which a consequence of a disability made it more difficult for someone to comply with a requirement. See 📖 p.V.524. *Lewisham London Borough Council v Malcolm* [2008] UKHL 43.

R v Lloyd Mr Lloyd strangled his wife to death. On trial for murder, there was psychiatric evidence that he suffered from an abnormality of mind due to depression, but none of the psychiatrists thought that this would have 'significantly' affected his mental responsibility for the killing. The trial judge ruled that 'significant' had to mean less than total, but more than trivial or minimal, and the jury convicted him of murder. The trial judge's direction was approved by the Court of Appeal. See 📖 p.V.495. *R v Lloyd* [1967] 1 QB 175.

In re M & R A local authority applied to take four children into care, alleging their mother had sexually abused them. The judge in the family court accepted that there was 'a real possibility' that the abuse had occurred, but that it had not been proved (📖 p.IV.317) to the requisite standard under the Children Act 1989 (that the judge was 'satisfied' the abuse had occurred), and refused a full care order (but made interim care orders on the grounds that there was 'reasonable cause to believe' the abuse had occurred). Although the Court of Appeal dismissed the local authority's appeal, it ruled that the judge could admit evidence from child psychiatrists as to the reliability of the child witnesses. See 📖 p.V.537. *In re M and R (Child abuse: evidence)* [1996] 2 FLR 195.

R v M The defendant had been convicted on several counts of sexually abusing his granddaughter, and appealed on the ground that the jury would have found him unfit to plead because of anterograde amnesia, if the trial judge had not 'set the bar too low' in the way he described the *Pritchard* test of fitness to plead. The Court of Appeal dismissed the appeal, and restated the test in clear language. See 📖 p.V.474. *R v M (John)* [2003] EWCA Crim 3452.

DPP v Majewski Mr Majewski had used large quantities of alcohol and drugs over 48 hours, and then assaulted several people, including police officers; his convictions for assault were upheld by the House of Lords, despite the lack of specific evidence of intent to assault or recklessness as to the risk of assaulting others. The House of Lords confirmed that voluntary intoxication (📖 p.V.486) is no defence for offences of basic intent (📖 p.IV.335), although it may be for offences of specific intent (📖 p. IV.335). The rule that a person may be deemed to intend or foresee the 'natural and probable consequences' of their acts enabled the trial jury to conclude that the defendant would have foreseen that he might commit assault while drunk, and was therefore reckless (📖 p.IV.336). See 📖 p.V.487. *DPP v Majewski* [1977] AC 443.

R v Martin Mr Martin was disqualified from driving. His wife's son was late for work; she threatened suicide if he did not drive him to work. He was caught and convicted of driving while disqualified. He appealed on the ground of necessity, supported by medical evidence that she was likely to have attempted suicide if he refused to drive. His conviction was quashed on the ground that the jury should have been allowed to consider whether the facts supported duress of circumstances (📖 p.V.503); in the judgment, the House of Lords set out the requirements of the defence. See 📖 p.V.503. *R v Martin* [1989] 1 AllER 652.

R v Martin (Anthony) The defendant had been convicted of murder for shooting a burglar who broke into his isolated farmhouse at night; his claim of self-defence had been rejected. He had paranoid personality disorder and depression, and appealed on the ground that his symptoms made him perceive more threat from the burglar than a reasonable person would, and that the force used was therefore reasonable. The court held that this was not relevant to the objective standard of whether a reasonable person would have used that degree of force in what he defendant believed to be the circumstances. Instead, he was convicted of manslaughter on the grounds of diminished responsibility (📖 p.V.491). See 📖 p.IV.342. *R v Martin (Anthony)* [2002] 1 CrAppR 27.

R v Mohan Dr Mohan, a paediatrician, was charged with sexually assaulting four teenage patients. In a voir dire (📖 p.IV.319), psychiatric 'profiling' (📖 p.V.454) evidence that the assaults were probably committed by someone with characteristics Dr Mohan lacked (e.g. psychopathy) was ruled inadmissible because it was not sufficiently relevant; addressed the ultimate issue (📖 p.V.543); and was unreliable, given the poor evidence base for such profiling. See 📖 p.V.537. *R v Mohan* [1994] 2 SCR 9.

Morgan Smith The defendant fatally stabbed a man whom he believed had stolen his carpentry tools. He claimed provocation (📖 p.V.498), based upon a diagnosis of depression. The trial judge, in directing the jury, limited the scope for them to take his depression into account in determining what the reasonable person would have done. The House of Lords allowed an appeal, ruling that the reasonable person should have been deemed to have depression, like the defendant. This case was the high-water mark of the subjective form of the reasonable person test. See 📖 p.V.499. *R v Smith (Morgan)* [2001] 1 AC 146.

Moss v Howdle Mr Moss was driving on the motorway when his passenger suddenly cried out and was clearly in severe pain. Mr Moss broke the speed limit in order to get to the nearest service station quickly, where he could assist his passenger. He appealed against conviction for breach of the speed limit, claiming that the circumstances amounted to necessity (📖 p.V.503). The High Court of Justiciary set down the rules for the defence, and concluded that it did not apply because Mr Moss could have stopped at the side of the motorway rather than breaking the speed limit to get to a service station. See 📖 p.V.503. *Moss v Howdle* [1997] SCCR 215.

Munjaz Mr Munjaz was a patient at Ashworth special hospital (📖 p.II.209) who had been repeatedly secluded for long periods. The hospital's original seclusion policy was found to be unlawful because it provided for substantially fewer reviews than the MHA Code of Practice; a revised policy with more reviews, but still fewer than in the Code, was upheld on appeal to the House of Lords. At an earlier stage of the case, the Court of Appeal had ruled that, separate to the MHA, there is a general common law power to take reasonable necessary and proportionate steps to prevent significant harm, even from people with full capacity (📖 p.IV.424), and that this included a power to seclude patients. See 📖 p.IV.440. *Munjaz, v. Ashworth* [2005] UKHL 58; *Munjaz v Mersey Care NHS Trust* [2003] EWCA Civ 1036.

R v O'Brien Mr O'Brien and his co-defendants robbed and seriously assaulted Mr Saunders, who died 5 days later. All three were convicted of murder, largely on the evidence of the co-defendant Hall, and sentenced to custody for life (📖 p.V.464), as they were under 21. Some years later, the Criminal Cases Review Commission (📖 p.V.449) referred the case to the Court of Appeal on the grounds that Hall had a high level of compliance (📖 p.II.124)—but no diagnosed mental disorder—that predisposed him to lie and fantasize, casting doubt on the convictions. The court ruled that the expert evidence could be admitted even in the absence of a diagnosis, because it showed 'a very significant deviation from the norm'. See 📖 p.V.537. *R v O'Brien, Hall & Sherwood* [2000] EWCA Crim 3.

Page v Smith Page was involved in a moderately severe car accident caused by Smith's negligent driving. Nobody was physically injured, but Page later suffered a recurrence of chronic fatigue syndrome (📖 p.II.74). The House of Lords held that Page was a primary victim and that Smith owed a duty of care to avoid causing injury, including psychiatric illness, since it was reasonably foreseeable that he might suffer some form of injury (in this case physical injury): there was no need for the specific harm caused to be foreseeable. See 📖 p.V.514. *Page v Smith* [1996] AC 155.

Palmer v Tees Mrs Palmer's 3-year-old daughter had been abducted, raped and murdered by Mr Armstrong. He had been in psychiatric hospitals on various occasions after suicide attempts, and had allegedly disclosed his fantasies about sexually abusing and killing young children. Mrs Palmer sued the health authority for the trauma she had suffered, but the claim was dismissed because there was insufficient proximity (📖 p.V.513) between her and the hospital. The judges noted that, even if Mr Armstrong's actions had been found to be reasonably foreseeable, there was no treatment the hospital could have given that would have protected Mrs Palmer's daughter, nor was Mrs Palmer identifiable in advance as someone who could have been warned. See 📖 p.V.519. *Palmer (administratrix of the estate of Palmer) v Tees Health Authority* [1999] AllER 722.

R v Podola Mr Podola was charged with murder. He claimed that he was suffering from hysterical amnesia rendering him unfit to plead and was insane at the material time. The court ruled that amnesia for the offence could not amount to unfitness to plead because a defendant might still be able to understand the trial process (and that Mr Podola was able to do so). It also emphasized that where the defence raise a defence of insanity and this is contested by the prosecution, the burden of proof is on the defence. See 📖 p.V.474. *R v Podola* [1960] 1 QB 325.

R v Pritchard Pritchard was a person of sound mind who was charged with bestiality. He could not easily communicate with others because he was both deaf and mute. The trial judge stated the rule for the jury to follow in deciding whether he was fit to plead (📖 p.V.474). *R v Pritchard* [1836] 7 CP 303.

R v Quick Mr Quick was a nurse at a mental hospital in Somerset. He and a co-defendant were charged with assaulting a patient. Quick had diabetes; that morning, he had taken insulin but then drunk spirits and eaten too little food, resulting in hypoglycaemia. The High Court allowed his appeal against conviction, holding that a 'transitory effect . . . of some external factor' could not be a disease of the mind (and therefore could not amount to insanity), but that it could be an automatism. See 📖 p.V.483. *R v Quick* [1973] 1 QB 910.

R v Rabey Mr Rabey was a student who had unreciprocated feelings for a fellow student. He found a note amongst her books in which she described him as one of a 'bunch of nothings'. He felt 'hurt and angry' and entered a dissociative state in which he hit her on the head with a rock and then strangled her. At trial, he was acquitted on the ground of non-insane automatism. The Supreme Court of Canada ruled that the dissociation was internal to the mind and could therefore only amount to an insane automatism; the 'ordinary stresses and disappointments of life' do not amount to a 'psychological blow' that would make the automatism non-insane. A retrial was ordered. See 📖 p.V.484. *R v Rabey* [1980] SCR 513.

R v Reynolds Miss Reynolds, aged 18, killed her mother, then arranged matters to make it appear there had been a burglary. This happened a few weeks after she gave birth to a child who was immediately given up for adoption; she had concealed the pregnancy and the identity of the father from her family. There was psychiatric evidence that she was suffering from post-natal depression and pre-menstrual tension. She was convicted of murder at trial, but the Court of Appeal accepted that the psychiatric evidence had not been properly dealt with and substituted a verdict of manslaughter on the grounds of diminished responsibility. See 📖 p.V.492. *R v Reynolds* [1988] CrimLR 679.

Robertson v HM Advocate Mr Robertson killed a man who made homosexual advances towards him and also threatened him with a knife. He claimed provocation (📖 p.V.498). The High Court of Justiciary refused his appeal against conviction for murder, holding that provocation required not only a loss of self-control, but also a reasonably proportionate relationship between the provocation and the reaction to it. See 📖 p.V.499. *Robertson v HM Advocate* [1994] SC(JC) 245.

R v Robertson The defendant in this case was charged with murder, but before the case began the prosecution raised the issue of his fitness to plead (📖 p.V.474), claiming that he was unable 'properly' to instruct counsel or defend himself. The medical evidence was that he could understand the relevant requirements, but because of his 'persecution mania' might make unwise decisions or fail to defend himself 'properly'.

In the Crown Court he was found unfit, but this finding was quashed by the Court of Appeal, which ruled that the fact that he might not act in his best interests was insufficient to render him unfit. The fact that the issue was raised by the prosecution and opposed by the defendant might have been a significant factor in this controversial ruling. See 📖 p.V.475. *R v Robertson* [1968] 3 AllER 557.

R v Robinson A 15-year-old girl with learning disability was allegedly raped by her stepfather. The trial judge allowed a psychologist to give evidence that nevertheless she was not particularly suggestible or likely to fantasize. On appeal, the conviction was quashed on the ground that there had been no claim that the victim was suggestible or liable to fantasise, and that therefore the psychologist's evidence amounted to an attempt by the prosecution to improve the reliability of witness evidence. See 📖 p.V.537. *R v Robinson* [1994] 3 AllER 346.

R v Sanderson Mr Sanderson was convicted of murdering his girlfriend after hitting her over a hundred times with a wooden stave. At trial Mr Sanderson was described as having a paranoid psychosis exacerbated by drug use by the defence expert, but having paranoia due to drug use by the prosecution psychiatrist. The judge directed that where the paranoia was caused by drugs this was not an abnormality of mind (for the purposes of diminished responsibility) unless it had caused disease or injury to the brain. This was successfully appealed, however. See 📖 p.V.492. *R v Sanderson* (1994) 98 Cr.App.R 325.

HM Advocate v Savage Mr Savage was charged with the murder of Jemima Grierson by cutting her throat. It was argued that because of his mental condition the verdict should be culpable homicide and not murder. The judgement led to the view that there must be aberration or weakness of mind; that there must be some form of mental unsoundness; that there must be a state of mind which is bordering on, though not amounting to, insanity; and that there must be a mind so affected that responsibility is diminished from full responsibility to partial responsibility. This test was later replaced by the test from *Galbraith v HM Advocate* (listed earlier). See 📖 p.V.492. *HM Advocate v Savage* (1923) JC 49.

R v Stephenson The defendant had schizophrenia. One night, he went to sleep in a haystack, having made a small fire in order to keep warm. The haystack erupted into fire. Medical evidence suggested that because of his disorder he was unable to foresee the fire as a possible consequence of his actions. He was acquitted by the Court of Appeal, which held that what was required for recklessness (📖 p.IV.336) was actual foresight. The fact that a reasonable person would have foreseen the risk of fire was not relevant. See 📖 p. IV.336. *R v Stephenson* [1979] QB 695.

R v Stewart Mr Stewart had an alcohol dependence syndrome. He was homeless and killed another man. One of the psychiatrists at trial gave evidence that drinking in the context of alcohol dependence syndrome could never be involuntary: there is always some degree of choice. Mr Stewart appealed but his conviction was upheld because the jury had had the option of rejecting the evidence of the psychiatrist. See 📖 p.V.485. *R v Stewart* [2010] EWCA Crim 2159.

R v Sullivan Mr Sullivan seriously assaulted a man while suffering an epileptic fit. The House of Lords upheld the trial judge's ruling that epilepsy was a disease of the mind, and also that in this case the fit had rendered Mr Sullivan insane at the time of the assault. (The defendant changed his plea to guilty to avoid the then-automatic hospital order with restrictions, 📖 p.IV.412, for a verdict of not guilty by reason of insanity, 📖 p.V.489.) See 📖 p.V.484. *R v Sullivan* [1984] 1 AC 156.

Surrey v McManus The council's social services department was in contact with Keith Waite, who went on to sexually abuse the three McManus children. They later sued the council. The claim for negligence was struck out on the grounds that the council could not reasonably have know the children were at risk and therefore did not owe them a duty of care (📖 p.V.512). See 📖 p.V.519. *Surrey County Council v McManus and others* [2001] EWCA 691.

R v T The defendant was raped and suffered PTSD. Three days after being raped, she stabbed a victim and reached into her car to take her bag, while in a dissociative state. The Crown Court ruled that the defence of non-insane automatism was available, because the rape was a severe external psychological blow. (However, the jury did not accept the defence, and convicted her.) See 📖 p.V.484. *R v T* [1990] CrimLR 256.

R v Tandy Ms Tandy, an alcoholic, strangled her daughter after drinking most of a bottle of vodka. The judge directed the jury to decide whether she suffered from an abnormality of mind or whether her abnormality was due to her drunkenness. She was convicted and appealed. Her conviction was upheld and three conditions were stated that needed to be demonstrated for diminished responsibility: that she had an abnormality of mind; that this was induced by the disease of alcoholism; and that the craving for drink (or drugs) was involuntary (an 'irresistiable impulse'). If brain damage had occurred then this could in itself be an abnormality of mind. See 📖 p.V.492. *R v Tandy* [1989] 1 WLR 350.

Tarasoff Mr Poddar, a student at the University of California, became friends with Tatiana Tarasoff. He misinterpreted her kiss on New Year's Eve, and became resentful when she rebuffed him subsequently. He began stalking her. He saw a psychologist, and revealed his intent to kill her. The psychologist arranged for the campus police to detain him for psychiatric assessment, but he was thought to be rational and was released.

He stopped seeing the psychologist and no further action was taken. He went on to kill Miss Tarasoff. Her family sued the university, and the court found in their favour, ruling that a mental health professional has a duty to protect third parties who may be harmed by their patient. See 📖 p.V.519. *Tarasoff v Regents of the University of California* 17 Cal 3d 425.

R v Toner Mr Toner had been fasting for a prolonged period, broke his fast, and went on to strangle his wife. He was charged with attempted murder. Medical evidence on the effect of the fast and of breaking it was excluded by the trial judge. A retrial was ordered by the Court of Appeal on the ground that the jury should have heard the evidence because Mr Toner was not simply an ordinary person; he was affected by a medical condition. See 📖 p.V.537. *R v Toner* [1991] 93 CrAppR 382.

R v Turner Mr Turner killed his girlfriend with a hammer after she taunted him about her having an affair. There was no evidence of mental disorder, but the defence attempted to introduce psychiatric evidence that he had felt a 'deep emotional relationship' with his girlfriend that had been shattered in what might amount to provocation (📖 p.V.498). The court ruled it inadmissible because it dealt with matters within the jury's 'common knowledge and experience'. See 📖 p.V.532. *R v Turner* [1975] QB 834.

Wednesbury A cinema chain challenged the local council's power to impose sweeping conditions on Sunday opening. It lost its case, because of the very wide powers granted to the council under the relevant legislation, but the case was notable because the Court of Appeal laid down the grounds for judicial review of administrative decisions: taking inappropriate matters into account, ignoring appropriate matters, or unreasonableness. The test of unreasonableness was stated vividly by Lord Diplock in *Council of Civil Service Unions v Minister for the Civil Service* [1983] UKHL 6 as a decision 'so outrageous in its defiance of logic or accepted moral standards that no sensible person who had applied his mind to the question to be decided could have arrived at it.' See 📖 p.IV.309. *Associated Provincial Picture Houses Ltd v Wednesbury Corporation* [1948] 1 KB 223.

R v Weightman In this complex case, a defendant suspected of having histrionic personality traits (but not necessarily a personality disorder) was charged with killing her 2-year-year-old daughter. She had confessed the murder (which had initially been thought by the coroner to be accidental asphyxiation) to her husband, probation officer and police. At her trial, she did not plead diminished responsibility or insanity. The judge refused an application to call evidence from a psychiatrist who had attended the police interviews. The Court of Appeal upheld her conviction, ruling that expert psychiatric evidence was inadmissible when its effective purpose was to tell the court how a person without mental disorder would 'react to the stresses and strains of life'. See 📖 p.V.536. *R v Weightman* [1990] 92 CrAppR 291.

R v Windle Mr Windle married an older woman who was believed to suffer from mental disorder, who repeatedly threatened suicide. He became obsessed with this and discussed it continually with his workmates, one of whom, exasperated, eventually suggested giving her 'a dozen aspirin'. He gave her a hundred, causing her death. He was diagnosed with folie à deux (📖 p.II.56), but not found insane because he knew he was 'doing an act which the law forbade'. The Court of Criminal Appeal held that the fact that he believed he was not doing anything morally wrong was irrelevant. See 📖 p.V.490. *R v Windle* [1952] 2 QB 826.

R v Wood Mr Wood was an excessive drinker who went to the flat of an acquaintance after consuming large amounts of alcohol. He claimed that he fell asleep and awoke to find the victim trying to perform oral sex on him. He killed him using a meat cleaver. At trial four psychiatrists concluded that he had alcohol dependency syndrome. The trial judge directed that a verdict of diminished responsibility was only open to Mr Wood if his drinking was truly involuntary and that a craving was not equivalent to this. This was overturned at appeal. See 📖 p.V.488. *R v Wood* [2008] EWCA Crim 1305.

X v UK A patient on a restriction order appealed to the European Court of Human Rights because a Tribunal had ruled that he should be discharged, but the Home Secretary had ignored its ruling, as the law then allowed. The Court held that this was a breach of article 5(4) of the ECHR (📖 p.IV.420) and the government was forced to amend the Mental Health Act to make Tribunals' decisions binding. *X v United Kingdom* [1981] 4 EHRR 188.

Ethical codes

The following pages reproduce extracts from ethical codes and professional guidelines (p.III.240) that are particularly relevant to forensic psychiatrists.

General Medical Council
Good Medical Practice (2006)
Writing reports and CVs, giving evidence and signing documents
- You must be honest and trustworthy when writing reports, and when completing or signing forms, reports and other documents
- You must always be honest about your experience, qualifications and position, particularly when applying for posts
- You must do your best to make sure that any documents you write or sign are not false or misleading. This means that you must take reasonable steps to verify the information in the documents, and that you must not deliberately leave out relevant information
- If you have agreed to prepare a report, complete or sign a document or provide evidence, you must do so without unreasonable delay
- If you are asked to give evidence or act as a witness in litigation or formal inquiries, you must be honest in all your spoken and written statements. You must make clear the limits of your knowledge or competence
- You must cooperate fully with any formal inquiry into the treatment of a patient and with any complaints procedure that applies to your work. You must disclose to anyone entitled to ask for it any information relevant to an investigation into your own or a colleague's conduct, performance or health. In doing so, you must follow the guidance in Confidentiality: Protecting and providing information
- You must assist the coroner or procurator fiscal in an inquest or inquiry into a patient's death by responding to their enquiries and by offering all relevant information. You are entitled to remain silent only when your evidence may lead to criminal proceedings being taken against you.

Royal College of Psychiatrists
Good Psychiatric Practice (Third Edition, 2009)
Patients, their carers, their families and the public need good psychiatrists. Good psychiatrists make the care of their patients their first concern: they are competent; keep their knowledge up to date; are able and willing to use new research evidence to inform practice; establish and maintain good relationships with patients, carers, families and colleagues; are honest and trustworthy, and act with integrity. Good psychiatrists have good communication skills, respect for others and are sensitive to the views of their patients, carers and families.

A good psychiatrist must be able to consider the ethical implications of treatment and clinical management regimes. The principles of fairness, respect, equality, dignity and autonomy are considered fundamental to good ethical psychiatric practice. A good psychiatrist will take these issues into account when making decisions, and will need to pay particular attention to issues concerning boundaries and the vulnerability of individual patients. A good psychiatrist will not enter into a relationship with a patient or with someone who has been a patient. . . .

Good Psychiatric Practice: Confidentiality and Information-Sharing

- Express consent should be sought where sharing of information outside the healthcare team is anticipated
- Competent refusals made before death should be respected after death unless there are overriding circumstances
- Information should not be shared within inter-agency teams without consent
- At CPA meetings, the psychiatrist's duty of confidentiality must be acknowledged and respected if information is to be shared
- If non-team members are to be involved in your patient's care (including attending team meetings), you should discuss it with the patient
- If you attend a meeting arranged by an outside agency, consider and record your decisions about disclosure to them. Remember, the agency to which you disclose information may apply standards of confidentiality different from your own
- In situations with dual obligations you must be clear in explaining your role to your patient, and in seeking consent
- For court proceedings, you do not have to disclose in the absence of a court order unless you have consent or there are grounds to override refusal
- It is sometimes justifiable for a psychiatrist to pass on patient information without consent or statutory authority. Such situations include:
  - Where death or serious harm may occur to a third party, whether or not a criminal offence (e.g. disclosure of threat of serious harm to a named person, on the expectation that this would prevent the harm)
  - When a disclosure may assist in the prevention, detection or prosecution of a serious crime, especially crimes against the person; or conversely in situations where it is necessary to the defence of a case to ensure that there is no miscarriage of justice
  - Where the patient is a health professional and the psychiatrist has concerns over that person's fitness to practise
  - Where a psychiatrist has concerns over a patient's fitness to drive
  - Where a psychiatrist has concerns over a patient's fitness to hold a firearms licence
- When deciding to disclose you must take a wide range of factors into account. You must communicate with your patient; it is advisable to discuss the proposed disclosure with appropriate colleagues or organizations
- You have a duty to cooperate with MAPPA. You do not have an obligation to disclose. Public interest will be an important factor for your consideration

- You should normally seek written consent before drafting a report. However, where there is a statutory obligation or there are overriding considerations, consent is not required. Remember to make your role clear to the patient when seeking consent, and disclose only the necessary information.

American Academy of Psychiatry and the Law

Ethical Guidelines for the Practice of Forensic Psychiatry

... Forensic psychiatrists practice at the interface of law and psychiatry, each of which has developed its own institutions, policies, procedures, values, and vocabulary. As a consequence, the practice of forensic psychiatry entails inherent potentials for complications, conflicts, misunderstandings and abuses.

Psychiatrists in a forensic role are called upon to practice in a manner that balances competing duties to the individual and to society. In doing so, they should be bound by underlying ethical principles of respect for persons, honesty, justice, and social responsibility. However, when a treatment relationship exists, such as in correctional settings, the usual physician-patient duties apply.

Confidentiality

... Psychiatrists should maintain confidentiality to the extent possible, given the legal context. Special attention should be paid to the evaluee's understanding of medical confidentiality. A forensic evaluation requires notice to the evaluee and to collateral sources of reasonably anticipated limitations on confidentiality. Information or reports derived from a forensic evaluation are subject to the rules of confidentiality that apply to the particular evaluation, and any disclosure should be restricted accordingly ... Psychiatrists should indicate for whom they are conducting the examination and what they will do with the information obtained. At the beginning of a forensic evaluation, care should be taken to explicitly inform the evaluee that the psychiatrist is not the evaluee's 'doctor.' Psychiatrists have a continuing obligation to be sensitive to the fact that although a warning has been given, the evaluee may develop the belief that there is a treatment relationship ...

Consent

At the outset of a face-to-face evaluation, notice should be given to the evaluee of the nature and purpose of the evaluation and the limits of its confidentiality. The informed consent of the person undergoing the forensic evaluation should be obtained when necessary and feasible. If the evaluee is not competent to give consent, the evaluator should follow the appropriate laws of the jurisdiction ...

It is important to appreciate that in particular situations, such as court-ordered evaluations for competency to stand trial or involuntary commitment, neither assent nor informed consent is required. In such cases, psychiatrists should inform the evaluee that if the evaluee refuses to participate in the evaluation, this fact may be included in any report or testimony. If the evaluee does not appear capable of understanding the information provided regarding the evaluation, this impression should also be included in any report and, when feasible, in testimony.

Absent a court order, psychiatrists should not perform forensic evaluations for the prosecution or the government on persons who have not consulted with legal counsel when such persons are: known to be charged [or] under investigation . . .

Consent to treatment in a jail or prison or in other criminal justice settings is different from consent for a forensic evaluation. Psychiatrists providing treatment in such settings should be familiar with the jurisdiction's regulations governing patients' rights regarding treatment.

Honesty and Striving for Objectivity

When psychiatrists function as experts within the legal process, they should adhere to the principle of honesty and should strive for objectivity [despite being] retained by one party to a civil or criminal matter . . .

Psychiatrists practicing in a forensic role enhance the honesty and objectivity of their work by basing their forensic opinions, forensic reports and forensic testimony on all available data. They communicate the honesty of their work, efforts to attain objectivity, and the soundness of their clinical opinion, by distinguishing, to the extent possible, between verified and unverified information as well as among clinical 'facts,' 'inferences,' and 'impressions.'

Psychiatrists should not distort their opinion in the service of the retaining party. Honesty, objectivity and the adequacy of the clinical evaluation may be called into question when an expert opinion is offered without a personal examination . . .

In custody cases, honesty and objectivity require that all parties be interviewed, if possible, before an opinion is rendered. When this is not possible, or is not done for any reason, this should be clearly indicated in the forensic psychiatrist's report and testimony. If one parent has not been interviewed, even after deliberate effort, it may be inappropriate to comment on that parent's fitness as a parent. Any comments on the fitness of a parent who has not been interviewed should be qualified and the data for the opinion clearly indicated.

Contingency fees undermine honesty and efforts to attain objectivity and should not be accepted. Retainer fees, however, do not create the same problems in regard to honesty and efforts to attain objectivity and, therefore, may be accepted.

Psychiatrists who take on a forensic role for patients they are treating may adversely affect the therapeutic relationship with them. Forensic evaluations usually require interviewing corroborative sources, exposing information to public scrutiny, or subjecting evaluees and the treatment itself to potentially damaging cross-examination. The forensic evaluation and the credibility of the practitioner may also be undermined by conflicts inherent in the differing clinical and forensic roles. Treating psychiatrists should therefore generally avoid acting as an expert witness for their patients or performing evaluations of their patients for legal purposes.

Treating psychiatrists appearing as 'fact' witnesses should be sensitive to the unnecessary disclosure of private information or the possible misinterpretation of testimony as 'expert' opinion. In situations when the dual role is required or unavoidable (such as Workers' Compensation, disability evaluations, civil commitment, or guardianship hearings), sensitivity to differences between clinical and legal obligations remains important. . . .

Qualifications

Expertise in the practice of forensic psychiatry should be claimed only in areas of actual knowledge, skills, training, and experience.

When providing expert opinion, reports, and testimony, psychiatrists should present their qualifications accurately and precisely . . .

World Psychiatric Association Declaration of Madrid

Psychiatry is a medical discipline concerned with the prevention of mental disorders in the population, the provision of the best possible treatment for mental disorders, the rehabilitation of individuals suffering from mental illness and the promotion of mental health. Psychiatrists serve patients by providing the best therapy available consistent with accepted scientific knowledge and ethical principles. Psychiatrists should devise therapeutic interventions that are *least restrictive* to the freedom of the patient and seek advice in areas of their work about which they do not have primary expertise. While doing so, psychiatrists should be aware of and concerned with the *equitable allocation* of health resources.

It is the duty of psychiatrists to keep abreast of *scientific developments* of the specialty and to convey updated knowledge to others. Psychiatrists trained in research should seek to advance the scientific frontiers of psychiatry.

The patient should be accepted as a partner by right in the therapeutic process. The psychiatrist-patient relationship must be based on mutual trust and respect to allow the patient to make free and informed decisions. It is the duty of psychiatrists to provide the patient with all *relevant information* so as to empower the patient to come to a rational decision according to personal values and preferences.

When the patient is gravely disabled, incapacitated and/or incompetent to exercise proper judgement because of a mental disorder, the psychiatrists should consult with the family and, if appropriate, seek legal counsel, to safeguard the human dignity and the legal rights of the patient. *No treatment should be provided against the patient's will*, unless withholding treatment would endanger the life of the patient and/or the life of others. Treatment must always be in the *best interest* of the patient.

When psychiatrists are requested to assess a person, it is their duty first to inform and advise the person being assessed about the purpose of the intervention, the use of the findings, and the possible repercussions of the assessment. This is particularly important when psychiatrists are involved in third party situations.

Information obtained in the therapeutic relationship is private to the patient and should be *kept in confidence* and used, only and exclusively, for the purpose of improving the mental health of the patient. Psychiatrists are prohibited from making use of such information for personal reasons, or personal benefit. Breach of confidentiality may only be appropriate when required by law (as in obligatory reporting of child abuse) or when serious physical or mental harm to the patient or to a third person would ensue if confidentiality were maintained; whenever possible, psychiatrists should first advise the patient about the action to be taken . . .

Appendix 5

Important inquiries and reports

Barrett inquiry Sometimes also known as the *Robinson inquiry* after its chair, this was an inquiry into the circumstances that led to a recently readmitted (but not recalled, 📖 p.V.467) forensic psychiatric patient, John Barrett, being allowed leave (📖 p.IV.392) from the secure unit, during which he stabbed a member of the public to death. The consultant forensic psychiatrist involved was heavily criticized in the inquiry report (but not in the subsequent court case) for prioritizing the working relationship with the patient over acting on the concerns raised by other members of the clinical team about an increased risk of harm to others.

Bennett inquiry An inquiry into the death of David 'Rocky' Bennett in a psychiatric unit, after a controversial incident during which he was restrained in the prone position, with staff pressing down on his back. The inquiry found that misunderstanding of, or discrimination against, Mr Bennett because of his Afro-Caribbean background was a contributory factor and recommended the employment of a greater proportion of staff from black and minority ethnic (BME) groups.

Blom-Cooper inquiry The first of the two inquiries into Ashworth Hospital, this 1992 inquiry examined conditions at the hospital and in particular the deaths of two patients (only one by suicide) and the abuse of two others. It concluded that there were serious deficiencies in standards of care. Seven staff members were disciplined and/or charged as a result.

Bradley Report This report was chaired by Lord Bradley and published in April 2009. The review focused on people with mental disorder and learning disability in the criminal justice system. The report recommended a wide range of measures to improve detection and treatment of mental disorder within the CJS and to facilitate transfer to hospital if needed. It required substantial additional resources and therefore, at the time of writing, has not been implemented.

Butler inquiry An influential 1974 report, of the Committee on Mentally Abnormal Offenders, which was set up after a patient released from Broadmoor, Graham Young, committed murder. It recommended (amongst other things) the creation of Regional Secure Units (📖 p.II.210).

The **Falling Shadow** This inquiry related to the killing of Georgina Robinson by Andrew Robinson in 1993. The inquiry was published as a book under the title The Falling Shadow by its chair, Louis Blom-Cooper. Andrew Robinson had a long history of mental illness and had been admitted to a high security hospital following a previous offence. The report is highly critical of a number of aspects of his clinical care. There was particular criticism of the failure to observe the legal requirements for leave relating to detained patients. There was a specific recommendation to extend powers for compulsory treatment to patients in the community, which resulted in the introduction of supervised discharge in 1995 (a precursor to the Community Treatment Order, 📖 p.IV.394).

Fallon inquiry A second inquiry into Ashworth Hospital (📖 p.II.209), in this case into the operation of the Personality Disorder Unit in 1996. It found that security policies were ignored, pornography was widely available, and a child visitor was groomed for paedophile abuse. It recommended that the hospital close, although this did not happen.

Glancy report The report in 1974 of the Working Party on Security in NHS Psychiatric Hospitals, it recommended that psychiatric hospitals establish secure wards for patients (whether offenders or not) whose behaviour could not be safely managed on open wards.

Lukewarm Luke inquiry This inquiry concerned the killing of Susan Milner by the then Michael Folkes in 1994 (he later changed his name to Lukewarm Luke). Mr Folkes was under the care of forensic psychiatric community services, following discharge by a tribunal against medical and Home Office advice. A condition of his discharge was to take antipsychotic medication. He subsequently stopped taking depot medication in favour of oral medication and at the time of the killing was not taking anything. He had presented to hospital the day before the killing. Criticism focused on communication between members of the clinical team and the decision to allow him to stop depot medication. There was also criticism of the decision not to discharge him to a staffed hostel.

Michael Stone inquiry Michael Stone had a severe personality disorder (📖 p.II.58) and misused substances; in 1996, he committed a very high-profile multiple murder, that of Lin Russell and her daughter Megan (her other daughter Josie was seriously injured, but survived). Despite the inquiry's finding that mental health and probation services had done everything that could reasonably be done to help Mr Stone (with some minor criticisms), the case was one used by the New Labour government of the time in support of its programme of detention of 'dangerous' people with severe personality disorder (DSPD, 📖 p.II.211).

National Confidential Inquiry The National Confidential Inquiry into Suicide and Homicide by People with Mental Illness (NCI/NCISH, 📖 p.V.471) is a research project funded by the Scottish Government and the English and Northern Irish Departments of Health. All incidents of suicide and homicide by people in contact with mental health services in the UK are examined. A variety of research studies have been published since the Inquiry was founded.

ONS studies A series of studies carried out by the Office of National Statistics and, before that, the Office of Population Censuses and Surveys, of the epidemiology of psychiatric condition. One key study in 1997 of over 3000 prisoners established the prevalence of psychosis in prison as 7–14%, and all mental disorders as 90%.

The **Reed Report** This report produced by the Department of Health in 1992 concerned mentally disordered offenders. The report contained multiple recommendations with a general theme that the care provided to mentally disordered offenders should be equivalent to that available to other patients. There were also significant recommendations relating to multi-agency working.

Ritchie report An inquiry into the killing of Jonathan Zito by Christopher Clunis (📖 p.App. 3.633), a man with paranoid schizophrenia who had repeatedly defaulted from treatment, in 1992. The report highlighted numerous failings of community care services in London, and recommended better quality risk assessment (📖 p.II.127), a change of professional culture including inter-agency working across boundaries, more resources, more hostels, a form of compulsory community treatment (📖 p.IV.394), and special services for patients who were difficult to follow up. (Also an alternative name for the Ledward inquiry, see following entry).

The **Shipman, Ayling, Ledward, Neale**, and **Kerr-Haslam** inquiries concerned a series of grave breaches of trust by doctors: GP Clifford Ayling indecently assaulted his patients; gynaecologists Rodney Ledward and Richard Neale carried out dangerous operations with poor post-operative care resulting in unnecessary deaths, and Neale moved from one hospital and country to another to avoid investigation; psychiatrists William Kerr and Michael Haslam indecently assaulted vulnerable patients; and most notoriously, GP Harold Shipman murdered over 200 elderly patients. They resulted in a series of reforms to government regulation of the medical profession in the UK, requiring amongst other things 'revalidation' of doctors' professional qualifications and subsequent appraisal and professional development every 5 years.

Tilt report This report into the level of security (📖 p.II.152) at the three English high security hospitals (📖 p.II.209) was commissioned to comply with a recommendation of the Fallon inquiry (listed earlier). It recommended that external physical and procedural security at the hospitals should be increased, to allow a reduction in internal procedural security measures (such as internal escorting within the site); and that long-term medium secure facilities should be developed for patients whose slow progress and risk to others prevented movement through the usual medium secure system to the community, but who no longer warranted high security.

Mental health law: quick reference

Table 24.1 shows the pages on which each important section of mental health law is covered. The pages on which other Acts are covered are listed in the appendix on statutes (📖 p.App. 2.618).

Mental health law statutes in each jurisdiction

E&W:	Mental Health Act 1983
Scotland:	Mental Healthcare and Treatment Act 2003 and
	Criminal Procedure (Scotland) Act 1995 (prefixed by C)
NI:	Mental Health (Northern Ireland) Order 1986
RoI:	Mental Health Act 2001 and
	Criminal Law (Insanity) Act 2006 (prefixed by C).

Table 24.1 Quick Reference Guide

E&W	Scotland	NI	RoI	Provision	Page
			C4,5	Committal for examination/treatment	403
2		4	9	Civil admission for assessment	383
		12		Removal by police officer	400
3			15	Civil admission for treatment	388
			C15	Transfer of prisoner	410
4				Emergency civil admission	386
5		7	23	Emergency detention of inpatient	386
7				Guardianship	394
		12		Civil detention for treatment	388
17		15	26	Leave from hospital	392
17A				Community treatment order	394
		18		Guardianship	394
	25–27			Aftercare	398
35		42		Remand to hospital for assessment	403

(continued)

Table 24.1 (Contd.)

E&W	Scotland	NI	Rol	Provision	Page
36		43		Remand to hospital for treatment	403
	36			Emergency detention order	386
	44			Short-term detention order	383
	41,53			Suspension of detention	392
	C52B-S			Assessment and treatment orders	403
37	C57A	44		Hospital order or compulsion order	405
38	C53	45		Interim hospital or compulsion order	405
	57			Compulsory treatment order	388
	C58			Court-ordered guardianship	434
41	C59	47		Restriction order (on hospital order)	412
45A	C59A			Hospital (and limitation) direction	408
47		53		Transfer of sentenced prisoner	410
48		54		Urgent transfer of other prisoner	410
49		55		Restriction direction (on transfer)	412
56–64		62–69	56–61	Consent to treatment	390
	C60B			Intervention order	434
	C60C			Urgent detention of acquitted persons	408
117		112–3		Aftercare	398
	127,179			Suspension of detention	392
	136			Transfer of prisoner for treatment	410
	C200			Remand for pre-sentence report	403
	C210B			Risk assessment order	408
135	293	129		Removal from private premises	400
136	297	130		Removal from public place	400
	221,224			Suspension of detention	392
	233–249			Consent to treatment	390
	299			Nurse's holding power	386

Index

W